The Metallome in Motion

The Metallome in Motion

Insights into Ecosystem and Food Chain Toxicodynamics

Edited by

Vandana Singh
Department of Microbiology, Sharda School of Allied Health Sciences, Sharda University, Greater Noida, Uttar Pradesh, India

Rouf Ahmad Bhat
Renowned Researcher and Instructor in Environmental Sciences, Department of School Education, Jammu and Kashmir, India

Gowhar Hamid Dar
Department of Environmental Science, Government Degree College Kulgam, Higher Education Department, Jammu and Kashmir, India

Karuna Singh
Sharda School of Allied Health Sciences, Sharda University, Greater Noida, Uttar Pradesh, India

ELSEVIER

ACADEMIC PRESS
An imprint of Elsevier

Academic Press is an imprint of Elsevier
125 London Wall, London EC2Y 5AS, United Kingdom
50 Hampshire Street, 5th Floor, Cambridge, MA 02139, United States

ISBN: 978-0-443-44299-5

For information on all Academic Press publications visit our website at https://www.elsevier.com/books-and-journals

Publisher: Mara Conner
Acquisitions Editor: Palak Gupta
Editorial Project Manager: Sweta Bharti
Production Project Manager: M. Balakrishnan
Cover Designer: Mark Rogers

Typeset by Integra Software Services

Dedicated to our parents, teachers, and friends …

Contents

4 Metal bioavailability: Speciation, complexation, and redox dynamics

Sania Gupta and Niharika Shanker

5 Metal–radical interactions: Synergistic effects on food chain toxicodynamics

Safeera Akbar, Sumira Tyub, Farheen Mushtaq, Aabroo Fatima, Uzma Ali, and Syed Nasir Ahmad

8 Hidden metal reservoirs in the food chain: Soil microaggregates as metal sinks

Ananta Shrivastava, Kritika Singh, Kaushlendra Kumar, Hema Kumari, and Bushra Shaida

18 Intensive cropping systems reduce heavy metals in cotton fields

Sherif Ibrahim Abdel-Wahab, Tamer Ibrahim Abdel-Wahab, Eman Ibrahim Abdel-Wahab, and Mohamed Mourad Lamlom

19 Molecular toxicology of metal exposure: Oxidative stress induction and cytotoxic mechanistic pathways

Maneesh Kumar, Bibekananda Bhoi, and Suman Kumar

20 Molecular mechanism of metal-induced oxidative stress and cytotoxicity

Auroshree Sadhu, Surajit Ghosh, Kishore Dhara, Nimai Chandra Saha, Surjyo Jyoti Biswas, and Shubhajit Saha

Contributors

Eman Ibrahim Abdel-Wahab Food Legumes Research Department, Field Crops Research Institute, Agricultural Research Center (ARC), Giza, Egypt

Sherif Ibrahim Abdel-Wahab Crop Intensification Research Department, Field Crops Research Institute, Agricultural Research Center (ARC), Giza, Egypt

Tamer Ibrahim Abdel-Wahab Crop Intensification Research Department, Field Crops Research Institute, Agricultural Research Center (ARC), Giza, Egypt

Syed Nasir Ahmad Centre of Research for Development (CORD), University of Kashmir, Srinagar, India

Akansha Department of Nutrition and Dietetics, SSAHS, Sharda University, Greater Noida, India

Safeera Akbar Centre of Research for Development (CORD), University of Kashmir, Srinagar, India

Sateesh Alavala Cell Biology Division, ICMR-National Institute of Nutrition, Hyderabad, Telangana, India

Uzma Ali Centre of Research for Development (CORD), University of Kashmir, Srinagar, India

Aneesha Department of Nutrition and Dietetics, Manav Rachna International Institute of Research and Studies, Faridabad, Haryana, India

Gayatri Barabde Department of Environmental Science, The Institute of Science, Dr. Homi Bhabha State University, Mumbai, India

Bibekananda Bhoi Institutional Ethics Committee; Tata Memorial Centre, Homi Bhabha Cancer Hospital and Research Centre, Muzaffarpur, Bihar, India

Surjyo Jyoti Biswas Genetics and Cell Biology Laboratory, Department of Zoology, Sidho-Kanho-Birsha University, Purulia, West Bengal, India

A. Bobbili Amity Institute of Food Technology, Amity University, Noida, Uttar Pradesh, India

Akshay Botle Department of Environmental Science, The Institute of Science, Dr. Homi Bhabha State University, Mumbai, India

Shirsha Chakrabarty Department of Clinical Research, Sharda School of Allied Health Sciences, Sharda University, Gautam Buddha Nagar, Uttar Pradesh, India

Suresh Challa Cell Biology Division, ICMR-National Institute of Nutrition, Hyderabad, Telangana, India

Amit Pratap Singh Chouhan Department of Radiology, School of Allied Health Sciences, Galgotias University, Greater Noida, Uttar Pradesh, India

Shrabani Das Cell Biology Division, ICMR-National Institute of Nutrition, Hyderabad, Telangana, India

Kishore Dhara Department of Fisheries, Government of West Bengal, Kolkata, West Bengal, India

Aabroo Fatima Department of Botany, University of Kashmir, Srinagar, India
Surajit Ghosh Ecotoxicology Research Laboratory, Department of Zoology, The University of Burdwan, Burdwan, West Bengal, India
Charu Gupta School of Studies in Microbiology, Jiwaji University, Gwalior, Madhya Pradesh, India
Harshita Gupta Institute of Hotal Management, Lucknow, Uttar Pradesh, India
Mahendra K. Gupta School of Studies in Botany, Jiwaji University, Gwalior, Madhya Pradesh, India
Sania Gupta Amity Institute of Food Technology, Amity University, Noida, Uttar Pradesh, India
Ravi Prakash Jamalpur Cell Biology Division, ICMR-National Institute of Nutrition, Hyderabad, Telangana, India
Gaurav Kaushik Sharda School of Allied Health Sciences, Sharda University, Gautam Buddha Nagar, Uttar Pradesh, India
Ravinder Kaushik School of Health Sciences and Technology, UPES, Dehradun, India
Nasiruddin Khan Department of Food Sciences, College of Applied and Health Sciences, A' Sharqiuah University, Ibra, Oman
Swati Kimothi Department of Nutrition and Dietetics, Noida International University, Greater Noida, Uttar Pradesh, India
Ajay Kumar MRIT, Santosh Medical College, Uttar Pradesh, India
Anmol Kumar Department of Radiology, Santosh Medical College, Ghaziabad, Uttar Pradesh, India
Kaushlendra Kumar Department of Biomedical Science, School of Biosciences and Technology, Galgotia University, Greater Noida, India
Maneesh Kumar State-Virus Research and Diagnostic Laboratory, Department of Microbiology, All India Institute of Medical Sciences, Deoghar, Jharkhand, India
Pradeep Kumar MRIT, Santosh Medical College, Uttar Pradesh, India
Rahul Kumar Faculty of Pharmacy, Vidya University, Meerut, India
Suman Kumar State-Virus Research and Diagnostic Laboratory; Department of Microbiology, All India Institute of Medical Sciences, Deoghar, Jharkhand, India
Hema Kumari Department of Biomedical Science, School of Biosciences and Technology, Galgotia University, Greater Noida, India
Jyoti Kumari Department of Pharmacology, Sharda School of Allied Health Sciences, Sharda University, Gautam Buddha Nagar, Uttar Pradesh, India
Kavita Kushwah School of Studies in Microbiology, Jiwaji University, Gwalior, Madhya Pradesh, India
Mohamed Mourad Lamlom Crop Intensification Research Department, Agricultural Research Center (ARC), Field Crops Research Institute, Giza, Egypt
Prem Shankar Mishra Faculty of Pharmacy, Vidya University, Meerut, India
Rakhi Mishra Noida Institute of Engineering & Technology (Pharmacy Institute), Greater Noida, India
Farheen Mushtaq Centre of Research for Development (CORD), University of Kashmir, Srinagar, India
Shabir Ahmad Padder Govt. Degree College Kilam, Kulgam, Jammu and Kashmir, India
Tenzin Palden Department of Clinical Research, Sharda School of Allied Health Sciences, Sharda University, Gautam Buddha Nagar, Uttar Pradesh, India

Zeba Parveen Department of Clinical Research, Sharda School of Allied Health Sciences, Sharda University, Gautam Buddha Nagar, Uttar Pradesh, India
Mayuri Rastogi Department of Nutrition and Dietetics, Sharda University, Greater Noida, Uttar Pradesh, India
Varsha Rawat Department of Pharmaceutical Science and Research, SGT University, Gurugram, Haryana, India
Aditi Rikhari Department of Nutrition and Dietetics, SSAHS, Sharda University, Greater Noida, India
Auroshree Sadhu Ecotoxicology Research Laboratory, Department of Zoology, The University of Burdwan, Burdwan, West Bengal, India
Ashok Kumar Sah Department of Medical Laboratory Sciences, College of Applied and Health Sciences, A' Sharqiyah University, Ibra, Oman
Nimai Chandra Saha Harichand Guruchand University, Thakurnagar, West Bengal, India
Shubhajit Saha Ecotoxicology Research Laboratory, Department of Zoology, The University of Burdwan, Burdwan, West Bengal, India
Sayli Salgaonkar Department of Environmental Science, The Institute of Science, Dr. Homi Bhabha State University, Mumbai, India
Shaon Santaki Cell Biology Division, ICMR-National Institute of Nutrition, Hyderabad, Telangana, India
Jyotiram A. Sawale Krishna Institute of Pharmacy, Krishna Vishwa Vidyapeeth (Deemed to be University), Karad, Maharashtra, India
Mohammad Shadab Department of Clinical Research, Sharda School of Allied Health Sciences, Sharda University, Gautam Buddha Nagar, Uttar Pradesh, India
Bushra Shaida Center for Nutrition and Dietetics, SIST, Jamia Hamdard, New Delhi, India
Niharika Shanker Amity Institute of Food Technology, Amity University, Noida, Uttar Pradesh, India
Anushka Sharma Faculty of Pharmacy, Vidya University, Meerut, India
Mansi Sharma Calpro Specialties Pvt. Ltd, Gurigram, Haryana, India
S. Sharma Amity Institute of Food Technology, Amity University, Noida, Uttar Pradesh, India
Ananta Shrivastava Department of Biomedical Science, School of Biosciences and Technology, Galgotia University, Greater Noida, India
Ratnakar Shukla Department of Clinical Research, Sharda School of Allied Health Sciences, Sharda University, Gautam Buddha Nagar, Uttar Pradesh, India
Akruti Singh School of Health Sciences and Technology, UPES, Dehradun, India
Kritika Singh Department of Biomedical Science, School of Biosciences and Technology, Galgotia University, Greater Noida, India
Pratibha Singh Department of Nutrition and Dietetics, Manav Rachna International Institute of Research and Studies, Faridabad, Haryana, India
Tej Bhan Singh Department of Agriculture, Invertis University, Bareilly, India
Vandana Singh Department of Microbiology, Sharda School of Allied Health Sciences, Sharda University, Greater Noida, Uttar Pradesh, India
Divyanka Thakur Department of Environmental Science, The Institute of Science, Dr. Homi Bhabha State University, Mumbai, India
Rahul Tiwari Department of Chemistry Institute of Basic Science, Dr. B. R. Ambedkar University, Agra, India

Rohit Kumar Tiwari Department of Clinical Research, Sharda School of Allied Health Sciences, Sharda University, Gautam Buddha Nagar, Uttar Pradesh, India
Sumira Tyub Centre of Research for Development (CORD), University of Kashmir, Srinagar, India
Ankur Vashishtha Department of Medical Laboratory Technology, Sharda School of Allied Health Sciences, Sharda University, Gautam Buddha Nagar, Uttar Pradesh, India
Ankush Verma Department of Radiology, School of Allied Health Sciences, Galgotias University, Greater Noida, Uttar Pradesh, India
Piyush Verma School of Health Sciences and Technology, UPES, Dehradun, India
Pooja Yadav Cell Biology Division, ICMR-National Institute of Nutrition, Hyderabad, Telangana, India

About the editors

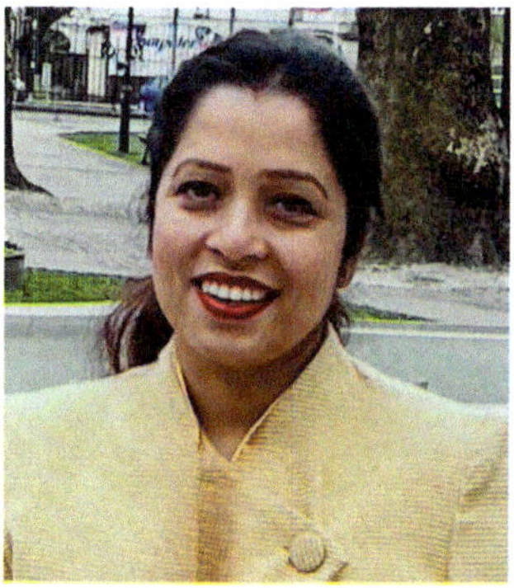

Dr. Vandana Singh is an associate professor in the Sharda School of Allied Health Sciences, Sharda University, India. She earned her M.Sc. in Microbiology from the University of Pune and completed her PhD in Microbiology at Noida International University. With more than 15 years of teaching and research experience, she has developed expertise across diverse domains of microbiology, including medical and environmental microbiology, food microbiology, microbial nanotechnology, nanomaterials, and microbial biotechnology. Her research is directed towards the application of microbiological and biotechnological approaches for sustainable environmental and health solutions, with a strong emphasis on microbial fuel cells, wastewater and biological treatment technologies, bioremediation of industrial and agricultural pollutants, biodegradation pathways, microbial food technology, and the molecular basis of biofilm and biosurfactant production. Her work integrates fundamental microbiology with applied nanotechnology and biotechnology, enabling the design of microbial and nano-based systems for environmental and biomedical applications. She has made significant scholarly contributions, reflected in her portfolio of numerous patents, research/review papers, edited books, and chapters with leading reputed publishers such as Elsevier, Springer, and CRC Press. She has also contributed extensively to curriculum design, academic training, and evidence-based microbiological education, while guiding numerous research projects at undergraduate, postgraduate, and PhD levels. Her long-term research vision focuses on advancing sustainable microbial and nanobiotechnological interventions for food technology, energy generation, pollutant remediation, and microbial resource management, thereby addressing critical challenges in health, food security, and environmental sustainability.

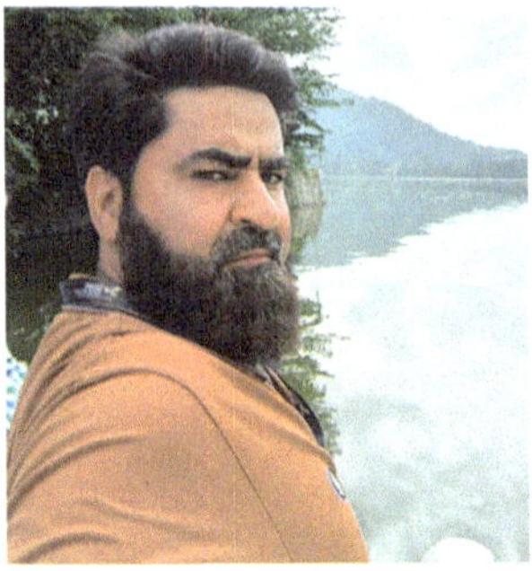

Dr. Rouf Ahmad Bhat pursued his doctorate at Sher-e-Kashmir University of Agricultural Sciences and Technology, Kashmir (Division of Environmental Sciences). He works in the Department of School Education, Government of Jammu and Kashmir. Dr. Bhat has been teaching for the past nine years and has authored over 55 research articles (h-index 36; i-index 64; total citation 5600) and 50 chapters, and has published more than 50 books with international publishers. Besides, he has worked as an associate environmental expert in World Bank-funded Flood Recovery Project and the environmental support staff in the Asian Development Bank funded development projects.

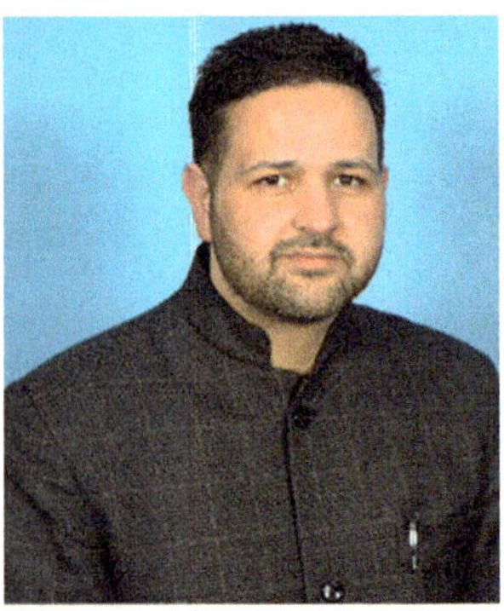

Dr. Gowhar Hamid Dar serves as a senior assistant professor and head of the department of Environmental Science at Government Degree College Kulgam, Higher Education Department, Government of Jammu & Kashmir, since 13 December 2023. Previously, he was posted at Government Sri Pratap College, Srinagar, from 21 February 2017 to 12 December 2023, where he played a key role in steering the institution's NAAC accreditation from Grade A to A+. During this tenure, he was actively involved in teaching postgraduate (M.Sc.) environmental science and undergraduate courses in environment and water management under Cluster University, Srinagar. Dr. Dar holds a PhD in Environmental Science from the University of Kashmir titled *"Profiling and Effect of Pathogenic Bacteria in Fishes of Jammu and Kashmir State and Correlation of Disease Incidence with the Trophic Status of Water Bodies."* He also earned an M.Phil. in environmental science from the same department, with research focused on *"Isolation, Identification and Characterization of Penicillium Isolates for Alpha-Amylase Activity."* His areas of specialization include environmental microbiology, fish microbiology and pathology, industrial microbiology, microbial taxonomy, pollution, and limnology. He has worked on a nationally funded research project sponsored by SERB-DST, Government of India, focusing on the assessment of bacterial and protozoan diseases in fish fauna of Jammu & Kashmir triggered by pollution and climate change. His research expertise includes the isolation, identification, and characterization of microbes, their pathogenic behavior, and the impact of pollution on fish health, with implications for industrial, economic, and environmental sustainability. Dr. Dar has an extensive publication record, with over 80 research publications (h-index: 19; i10-index: 27; total citations

>1400) in reputed national and international journals, including high-impact journals such as Science of the Total Environment and Chemosphere. He has also authored and edited several books and book chapters published by leading international publishers including Springer, Elsevier, CRC Press (Taylor & Francis), Apple Academic Press, John Wiley, and IGI Global. He supervises several PhD and Master's students in Environmental Science. In recognition of his contributions, he has received multiple awards and commendations for excellence in research, teaching, and scientific development. Dr. Dar has served as Principal Investigator and Coprincipal Investigator for research projects funded by JKST&IC, Government of J&K, and SERB-DST, Government of India. He is a member of the Board of Studies (BOS) and Board of Research Studies (BORS), Cluster University Srinagar, and has contributed to various academic and research committees.He also serves as Coordinator, Internal Quality Assurance Cell (IQAC) at Government Degree College Kulgam. Previously, he served as Nodal Officer, Interdisciplinary Research Centre/HUB for Biological Sciences at Sri Pratap College, Cluster University, Srinagar.

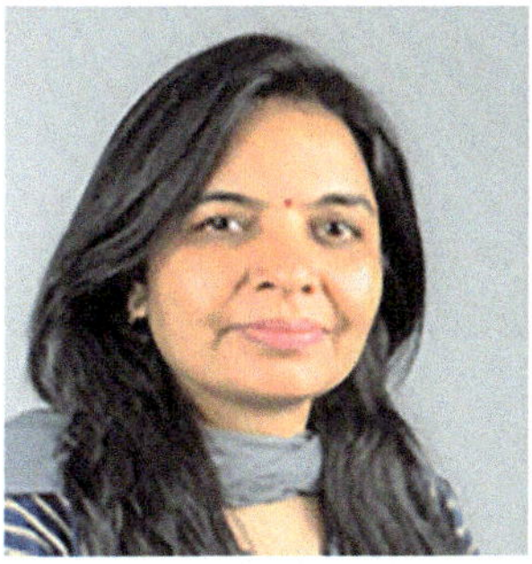

Dr. Karuna Singh servers as a professor and Dean at the Sharda School of Allied Health Sciences, Sharda University, India. She holds advanced academic qualifications in Foods and Nutrition from Vanasthali Vidyapeeth, Rajasthan, where she was a university rank holder and gold medalist, and completed her doctoral research in the area of food and nutrition sciences. With extensive experience in teaching, research, and academic leadership, she has developed strong expertise across diverse domains of public health nutrition, maternal and pediatric nutrition, functional foods, food safety, food therapeutics, nutrient bioavailability, food fortification, and sustainable food systems. Her research is primarily focused on translating nutritional science into practical health solutions, with particular emphasis on functional food development using natural ingredients, dietary interventions for health promotion, nutrition-based therapeutic strategies, and community nutrition approaches for vulnerable populations. Her work integrates fundamental nutritional science with applied food technology, enabling the development of innovative, health-oriented, and sustainable food solutions. In addition, she has also made significant scholarly contributions, reflected in her portfolio of numerous peer-reviewed research and review articles, edited and authored books, and several book chapters published with leading national and international academic publishers such as Springer Nature and AAP. She has been actively involved in externally funded research projects, industrial collaborations, and consultancies, and holds multiple published patents, including a granted patent for an innovative food-based technology. In addition to her academic responsibilities, she is actively engaged in community nutrition programs, awareness initiatives, and professional capacity-building activities. She also serves as a reviewer and editor for reputed scientific journals and is a life member of several professional bodies, contributing to the advancement of evidence-based nutrition science, food innovation, and public health outcomes.

Foreword

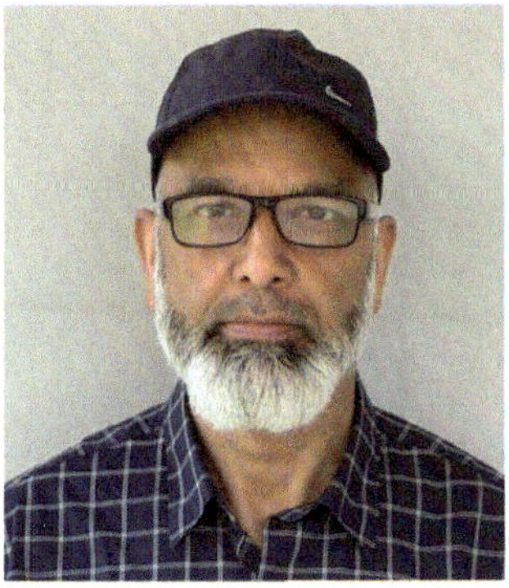

The movement of metals through ecosystems and food chains represents one of the most intricate challenges at the intersection of environmental science, toxicology, and public health. As a researcher and educator in this field, I find *The Metallome in Motion: Insights into Food Chain Toxicodynamics* to be an appropriate and rationally demanding contribution that captures the dynamic nature of metal–biological interactions with excellent precision.

This book advances our understanding of metal toxicodynamics by integrating metallomics, molecular toxicology, and ecological processes into a coherent framework. Of particular significance is its treatment of metal-induced epigenetic regulations, oxidative stress, and disruption of cellular homeostasis, which together explain how metals exert both immediate and long-term biological effects, including transgenerational impacts. The discussion of metalloproteins and metallochaperones further strengthens the mechanistic depth of the volume, providing valuable insight into metal transport, sequestration, and detoxification pathways.

A key strength of this book lies in its editorial leadership. The editors are highly experienced scholars with substantial academic and research expertise in *metallomics,* environmental toxicology, and related disciplines. In addition, the authors effectively connect geochemical and anthropogenic sources of metals with factors governing bioavailability, speciation, and trophic transfer. The examination of bioaccumulation and biomagnification across aquatic and terrestrial food webs clearly demonstrates how environmental contamination translates into agricultural and dietary exposure risks. The inclusion of advanced analytical and omics-based tools reflects current methodological advances and enhances the book's relevance for contemporary research and risk assessment.

Importantly, this volume extends beyond mechanistic science to address predictive modeling, regulatory perspectives, and sustainable management of metal contamination. Its interdisciplinary scope and scientific rigor align well with Elsevier's tradition of publishing authoritative academic resources.

I am confident that this book, "*The Metallome in Motion*", will serve as an essential reference for researchers, postgraduate/graduate students, and professionals seeking a comprehensive understanding of metal dynamics in ecosystems and food chains, and will stimulate further research aimed at mitigating metal-related risks to environmental and human health.

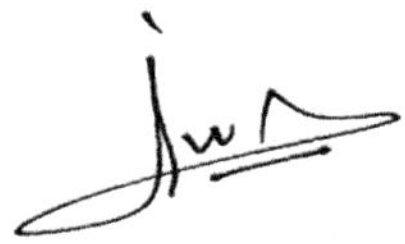

Javeed Iqbal Ahmad Bhat
Division of Basic Sciences & Humanities
SKUAST-Kashmir

Preface

Dear Reader,

The movement of metals through ecosystems and food chains corresponds to one of the most complex challenges at the intersection of environmental science, toxicology, and public health. As editors deeply immersed in metallomics and toxicodynamics, we conceived "*The Metallome in Motion: Insights into Food Chain Toxicodynamics*" to illuminate these complex interactions with clarity and rigor. This volume integrates metallomics, molecular toxicology, and ecological processes into a unified framework, revealing how metals drive epigenetic regulation, oxidative stress, and disruptions in cellular homeostasis—with profound implications for transgenerational health.

What follows is a comprehensive exploration of metal transport, bioaccumulation, and biomagnification across aquatic and terrestrial systems, from geochemical sources to human dietary risks. Guided by cutting-edge omics tools and predictive models, our contributing authors—leading experts in the field—bridge mechanistic insights with practical strategies for regulatory and sustainable management. We invite researchers, students, and professionals to engage with these pages, not only to deepen understanding but to inspire action against metal-related environmental threats.

With gratitude for your interest,

Vandana Singh
Rouf Ahmad Bhat
Gowhar Hamid Dar
Karuna Singh

Acknowledgments

The editors would like to acknowledge the efforts of the following contributors for rendering immense support while drafting this book and making this publication possible:

1. Rafia Rasool Gowhar
2. Hummara Sultan
3. Master Mohammad Zaeem Gowhar
4. All the authors of the various chapters
5. The supporting staff of Elsevier and Academic Press
6. The Editorial Project Manager

About the book

The Metallome in Motion: *Insights into Ecosystem and Food Chain Toxicodynamics* addresses the urgent need for a comprehensive understanding of metal contaminants within ecosystems and their cascading effects through food chains. This book fills a vital gap by integrating multidisciplinary research on how metals influence biological systems, food safety, and environmental health. As concerns over metal pollution grow, a resource that unites molecular, ecological, and regulatory perspectives is essential for researchers and practitioners. The book's contents span across a wide range of interrelated topics, beginning with metal-mediated epigenetic modifications and toxicodynamics at the molecular and cellular levels. It explores the geochemical and anthropogenic origins of contaminants, factors affecting metal bioavailability, and the synergistic effects of metal-radical interactions. Detailed chapters address the roles of metalloproteins, pathways of bioaccumulation and trophic transfer, transgenerational toxicity, and hidden reservoirs such as soil microaggregates. Advanced analytical methods, the emerging field of toxicometallomics, impacts of metals in agriculture, quantum effects of nanoparticles, and global regulatory frameworks are also thoroughly discussed. *The Metallome in Motion: Insights into Ecosystem and Food Chain Toxicodynamics* is an essential reference for postgraduate students in food science, as well as for academics and researchers in agriculture, plant science, environmental science, and biotechnology. It supports undergraduates, research scholars, and professionals in food processing, government, and regulatory sectors, providing critical knowledge for managing metal toxicity in food chains and protecting the ecosystem and human health.

Chapter 1

Metal-mediated epigenetic modifications: Implications for food chain toxicodynamics

Bibekananda Bhoi[a] and Maneesh Kumar[b]
[a]*Institutional Ethics Committee, Homi Bhabha Cancer Hospital and Research Centre, Muzaffarpur, Bihar, India*
[b]*State-Virus Research and Diagnostic Laboratory, Department of Microbiology, All India Institute of Medical Sciences, Deoghar, Jharkhand, India*

1.1 Introduction

Heavy metal contamination of the environment has emerged as a serious global issue, as its presence in natural systems is known to cause various detrimental effects. Rapid development of industry (particularly the agricultural and metallurgical industries), a lack of environmentally safe waste processing, and the intensive use of fertilizers and pesticides continue to lead to inorganic pollutants entering water, soil, and air (Mishra et al., 2018; Munir et al., 2021). This chapter discusses the pathways by which these metals enter various environmental compartments and how exposure and fate are controlled. Most metals affect vital organ functions and normal development; some of them accumulate in specific organs and cause fatal diseases such as cancer. It aids in understanding the pharmacokinetics and toxicological routes of each of the metals, which cause effects on the human body.

Over the last few years, there has been a shift from traditional toxicology to examining how metals affect the expression of genes, particularly without changing the DNA sequence. Metals and metalloids, including Cd, As, Pb, Hg, chromium (Cr), and nickel (Ni), are now considered strong modifiers of DNA methylation, histone conformation, and noncoding RNA function (Singh and Prasad, 2015; Zhao et al., 2022). As opposed to the relatively rare variants that drive evolution according to current models, these epigenetic modifications can reprogram cellular signaling pathways, metabolism, and stress responses through several trophic levels of an entire food web (Vogt, 2021). One issue of critical importance is that these epigenetic marks are not only dynamic but also

The Metallome in Motion. https://doi.org/10.1016/B978-0-443-44299-5.00001-8

inheritable, with effects that can be sustained after metal exposure has ceased. Metal-triggered methylation changes in plants, as well as the growth patterns, nutrient uptake, and defense responses of plants, affect herbivores and their predators (Key et al., 2024; Zhang et al., 2024). In aquatic systems, metals translocate within plankton, invertebrates, and fish, leading to the occurrence of epigenetic modifications that alter detoxification ability, immune defense and reproductive performance. Early disruption of these molecular pathways can alter population dynamics and ecosystem stability long before the onset of toxic effects (Samuel et al., 2023; Madesh et al., 2024).

The interplay between epigenetic responses to metals at various trophic levels, bioaccumulation, biomagnification, and species-specific differences in their metabolic capabilities results in a multilayered toxicodynamic process for metal exposure (Oros, 2025). Higher trophic-level predators, meanwhile, tend to experience increased levels of metals and greater accompanying epigenetic alterations that can affect their capacity for developmental plasticity and long-term health (Ghosh et al., 2022). In humans, toxic metal exposure via grain/produce consumption or animal/fish-based diets can lead to epigenetic markers that possibly cause prolonged traces on the genome profile, leading to chronic diseases, metabolic disorders, behavioral deficits, and immunological science deficits (Ryu et al., 2015). Such risks are further complicated by cooccurrence with pesticides, microplastics, and other environmental stressors that synergize with metals in the generation of more complex epigenetic marks. The food chain thus serves not only as a route of chemical transfer but also as a channel for molecule-level changes that affect organismal fitness, generation after generation (Sharma et al., 2025; Piergiacomo et al., 2022). Knowledge of metal-mediated epigenetic changes enhances our understanding of food chain toxicodynamics, connecting environmental pollution with subtle yet global consequences in gene regulation (Adegbola and Adetutu, 2024). From this perspective, more detailed studies on sentinel species, early-warning biomarkers, and intervention measures at ecological and agricultural interfaces should be encouraged. Ultimately, incorporating epigenetics into food chain toxicology will increase our ability to predict risks, develop less risky growing practices, and protect public health in areas where metal pollution remains a problem.

1.2 Sources and bioavailability of toxic metals in the food chain

The toxic metals from various environmental and anthropogenic sources are entering the food chain, and their transfer between different trophic levels is predominantly influenced by their chemical form and bioavailability. Natural sources also exist, such as the weathering of metal-rich rocks, volcanic outgassing, and geothermal processes, whereby metallic elements find their way into soil and water and are absorbed by plants (Saidon et al., 2024). However, human activities remain the main cause. Industrial processes, such as those employed in mining, smelting, metal plating, and battery production, release high levels of Pb, Cd, and Cr into the environment. Agriculture is also a major contributor, with Cd-contaminated phosphate fertilizers and pesticides containing As and Pb compounds. Heavy metal pollution refers to the accumulation of toxic heavy metals in the cycles of life. Metal ions enter plants from the soil mainly through roots (Zhao et al., 2022; Liang et al., 2024). Roots can often immobilize or sequester such metals in the soil matrix, thereby decreasing their overall bioavailability. Heavy metals are generally transported into plants through three major routes: (1) phytoextraction, in which plants absorb and store toxic metals from the contaminated soil; (2) phytostabilization, where heavy metal pollutants are either immobilized or their mobility is reduced in the environment to prevent further migration and spread; and (3) rhizofiltration, the direct absorption of pollutants by plant roots from water or soil. These accumulated metals can damage plant tissues and may even be transmitted to humans through the food chain, causing much more serious health issues (Jayakumar et al., 2021; Sharma et al., 2023) (Fig. 1.1).

Unprecedented industrial and technological development has led to increased exposure of both ecosystems and human populations to numerous toxic substances, including pesticides such as insecticides, fungicides, and herbicides.

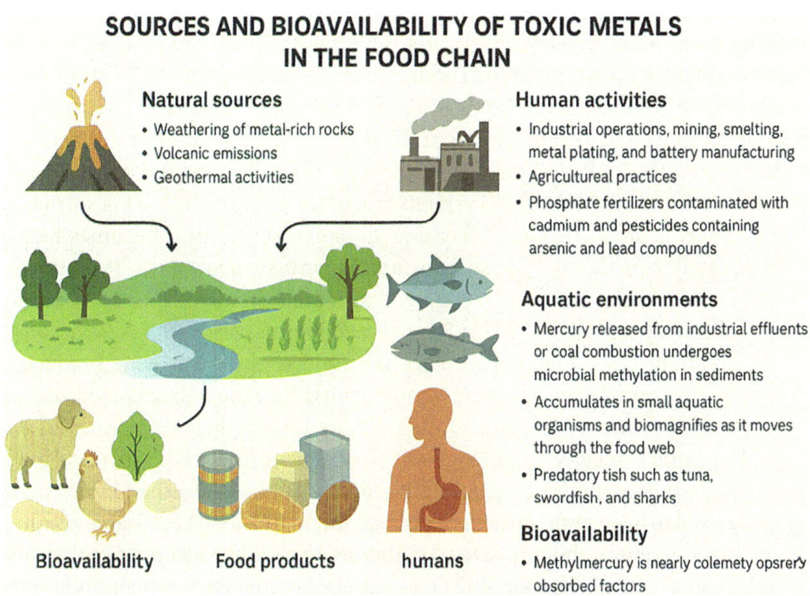

FIG. 1.1 Toxic metals enter ecosystems and accumulate through the food chain: The figure illustrates how toxic metals from the natural environment and human activities build up in soil, water, and crops before entering animals and ultimately moving up to humans. It also identifies the most significant sources of toxic metals, such as mining, fertilizers, and wastewater, and explains how these contaminants are absorbed by plants, animals, and fish. The figure highlights that bioavailability is an important factor for estimating human exposure.

Pesticides are man-made chemicals used in agriculture and other industries to kill pests, with insecticides being the most commonly used due to their efficiency and low cost. Nonetheless, overuse and uncontrolled application are resulting in the biomagnification of these substances within food webs, with potential implications for mammals and nontarget species (Maurya and Malik, 2016; Adegbola and Adetutu, 2024). Such factors directly or indirectly affect ecological equilibrium, while residues of pesticides are widely known to exist in plant tissues and parts, soil, air, and water. These residues are now recognized as major environmental pollutants and can persist in ecosystems for many years, with the potential to cause cancer in exposed populations (Derakhshan Nejad et al., 2018). In addition, metals are introduced into croplands via wastewater irrigation, sewage sludge application, and unregulated landfilling of municipal solid waste. For instance, the metal content in rice grains increases abnormally when irrigation is sourced from arsenic (As)-containing groundwater in the paddy fields of Bangladesh and West Bengal, leading to high levels of dietary As-related hazards. Likewise, vegetables grown around industrial areas may have high levels of Cd and Pb due to their accumulation from atmospheric emissions (Sarkar et al., 2012; Chowdhury et al., 2018). Bioavailability, which refers to how readily these metals are absorbed by plants, animals, and humans, depends on factors such as soil pH, organic matter, redox state, and the chemical form of the metal. Metals like Cd, Zn, and Pb are more soluble in acidic soils, making them more available to plants. This may explain the observation that leafy vegetables grown in low-pH soils generally have higher Cd levels (Kumar et al., 2017). Another major point of entry is through the aquatic environment. Metals in industrial discharges or from the combustion of coal are released as mercury (Hg), which transforms through microbial methylation in sediments into bioavailable and toxic methylmercury (methyl Hg). This substance accumulates in small fish and other aquatic organisms until it becomes highly concentrated in predatory fish, such as tuna, swordfish, and sharks. Human consumption of these fish is now recognized as a major global exposure route for methyl Hg (Ray and Shaju, 2023; Regnell and Watras, 2018).

In addition, toxic metals can enter the food chain via livestock animals. Animals that graze in pollution-contaminated pastures or are fed metal-contaminated feedstock accumulate Pb, Cd, and As in their tissues, milk, and eggs. For cattle subjected to mining belts, for instance, there is an increase in Cd levels in their liver and kidney tissue. In poultry, As-based feed additives traditionally used to accelerate growth have been found to leave measurable residues in meat and manure, though several countries have moved to restrict their use (Miclean et al., 2019; Kumar, 2021). Cross-contamination can occur while the food is being processed, compounded by storage. The Pb solder used in old canned food containers and surfaces that have been plated with Cd or even brass and copper products can contaminate food by allowing it to leach into the products themselves, especially when acidic substances are added (Rana et al., 2023). The bioavailability of metals to humans is not only dependent on their concentration but also on dietary constituents. Methyl Hg is almost 100% absorbed through the human gut, and because inorganic lead is increasingly absorbed from this exposure when calcium or iron is deficient (pregnant women and minerals are protein-bound), the two mechanisms together make children very susceptible. Food Cd is more easily absorbed by people with low Zn content. These observations illuminate the role of nutritional status in the impact of heavy-metal toxicity (Malik et al., 2023; Wu et al., 2024).

1.3 Epigenetic mechanisms altered by toxic metals

Environmental pollutants, especially toxic metals, are now recognized as important contributors to epigenome distortion. They can change the pattern of DNA methylation, which affects how genes are turned on, the tags placed onto histone proteins, and the expression of noncoding RNAs. These metals control transcription not just through mis-regulation of the epigenetic apparatus but also by directly binding to metal-responsive elements in gene promoters (Jurkowska, 2024). Epigenetic regulation is a key process in the maintenance of cellular homeostasis, and metal-related epigenetic modifications have received considerable attention due to their impact on long-term health effects and risk evaluation frameworks (Ozarde et al., 2025). Epigenetics involves the transmissible change in gene expression without modifying the DNA sequence. Together, these processes integrate transcriptional and posttranscriptional control of growth, lineage commitment, and environmental signaling (Faiz et al., 2025; Mititelu et al., 2025). The major epigenetic mechanisms are DNA methylation, posttranslational modification of histones, and the roles of noncoding RNAs. However, because these systems are sensitive to environmental tumors and insults, the loss of their normal function has been linked to the cause of many diseases. Among these mechanisms, DNA methylation is the best characterized (Desaulniers et al., 2021). It is also involved in other cellular processes such as genomic imprinting and X chromosome inactivation. Methylation is the process of adding a methyl group to cytosine at CpG sites, resulting in 5-methylcytosine. These marks are written and read by DNA methyltransferases, predominantly DNMT1, DNMT3A and DNMT3B (Edwards et al., 2017; Lyko, 2018) (Table 1.1).

The histone modification provides a second level of regulation that may be susceptible to toxic metals. Histones pack DNA into nucleosomes, and their tails undergo acetylation, methylation, phosphorylation, ubiquitination, and sumoylation (Zhang et al., 2023). More than a dozen histone marks have been identified so far that correlate with either transcriptional activation or repression, depending on the modified residue. For instance, H3K4me3 is employed to mark active promoter regions, and H3K27me3 and/or H3K9me3 characterize silent chromatin (Igolkina et al., 2019; Morgan and Shilatifard, 2020). Metals such as Ni, Cr, and Hg can be so blinding to those enzymes that mark addition or subtraction is impaired. These changes in chromatin structure modulate genes

TABLE 1.1 Toxic metals and their major epigenetic alterations.

Metal	Primary epigenetic changes	Biological impacts	Key examples
As	Global DNA hypomethylation, promoter hypermethylation, and altered microRNA expression	Genomic instability, oxidative stress, and cancer risk	Hypermethylation of p16, altered miR-21, and miR-200
Cd	DNMT activation; histone acetylation and methylation changes	Impaired DNA repair, inflammation, carcinogenesis	Increased H3K9me2 and disrupted methylation in tumor suppressor genes
Pb	Hypomethylation of CpG sites; altered microRNA patterns	Neurodevelopmental deficits, immune dysregulation	Reduced global 5-mC; altered miR-146a, miR-155
Ni	Histone demethylase inhibition: increased repressive histone marks	Transcriptional silencing, chromatin condensation	Enrichment of H3K9me2 and H3K27me3
Cr VI	DNA damage–associated methylation shifts; histone phosphorylation changes	Oxidative stress, impaired cell cycle regulation	Altered H3 phosphorylation, hypermethylation of repair genes
Hg	DNA methylation disruption; microRNA dysregulation	Neurotoxicity, metabolic dysfunction	Changes in miR-92, miR-370, and global methylation changes

involved in the cell cycle, DNA repair, and stress response. These dysregulations have been linked to cancer, neurological conditions, and developmental abnormalities (Alcántara-Mejía et al., 2024).

In addition to the above-mentioned coding proteins, noncoding RNAs (ncRNAs), such as miRNA and lncRNA, also add complexities to regulating the epigenome. MicroRNAs are gene expression regulators mediating translational repression or mRNA degradation (Bure et al., 2022). Thousands of mature microRNAs have been discovered so far, and their aberrant expression is associated with cancer, cardiovascular disease, or hereditary diseases. Poisonous metals may downregulate or upregulate the concentration of specific microRNAs involved in important inflammation, apoptosis, or cell cycle pathways (Kumar et al., 2020; De Rosa et al., 2014). Their stability in body fluids also makes them potential biomarkers of exposure and effect. Recent findings indicate that metals in the environment change the epigenetic structure on a large scale and for a lasting duration, not simply through direct interaction with the DNA. These modifications underpin how exposure to metals contributes to the risk of chronic diseases, transgenerational impact, and prolonged molecular dysfunction (Aguilera et al., 2010; Fasani et al., 2023).

While adaptive epigenetic responses to environmental cues do occur, inappropriate and overabundant changes increase disease susceptibility. All stages of life can be susceptible to exposure-induced epigenetic toxicity; however, early development is particularly vulnerable as it experiences a high degree of epigenetic reprogramming. The susceptibility of stem cells serves as a clear example of this (Abdolmaleky et al., 2025; Derakhshan Nejad et al., 2018). Pluripotent embryonic stem cells, which are isolated from the inner cell mass of blastocyst-stage embryos, can differentiate into endodermal, mesodermal, and ectodermal lineage cells. Multidifferentiated stem cells are of tissue origin and have the capacity for regeneration throughout life. This self-renewal potential and their differentiation potential make them essential for repair, but at the same time, this plasticity can be detrimental to normal function when environmental stress interferes with programs that regulate their behavior during repair processes, as heavy metals do. Increased utilization of metals in industry and poor disposal practices result in a continuous increase in the amounts people come into contact with at both the occupational and community levels, leading to constant environmental pollution as well as public health challenges (Abdolmaleky et al., 2025; Guo et al., 2025).

1.4 Environmental and agricultural sources of metal contamination

Environmental and agricultural systems have been increasingly contaminated with persistent metals, which bioaccumulate and translocate throughout the soil-water-plant continuum to enter the human food chain. Heavy metals are nondegradable toxicants and, if present in the environment and agricultural matrices, pose a potential health risk to humans by accumulating from soil and water into crops through the food chain (Ghori et al., 2016; Kumar et al., 2025). At present, the supply chain for crop production is highly dependent on land, fertilizer, and pesticide application intensity, which results in soil erosion, nutrient loss, and the accumulation of chemical residues. The accumulation of these metals in agricultural soils is further aggravated by poor solid waste management and deteriorating water quality, leading to distortions in plant metabolism, yield, and nutritional composition. However, with good agronomy, the "richness of soil" can be restored using microbial diversity and structure (Kumar and Akhtar, 2019). Amid all of this, climate change compounds the pressure, leaving agriculture at risk from extreme heat, salinity, and water scarcity. Veering away from pesticides, implementing precision agriculture, and using hardier crop species are some of the ways to make food production safer and better. Nevertheless, it is still largely contaminated by external sources. Cd, Pb Cr, Ni, and As are released into the environment through industrial processes such as the burning of fossil fuels and metallurgical industries (e.g., ore smelting and metal processing). These metals are also deposited on farmlands in the vicinity or carried into irrigation canals, thereby contaminating soils and increasing soil metal content over time (Kumar et al., 2023). Consequently, these contaminants modify soil chemistry and biology, playing a dual role in crop quality output. Severe health problems, including Cd-induced itai-itai disease and Minamata disease from Hg poisoning, emphasize the risks of metal exposure. Traditional remediation techniques, such as those used to remove or reduce pollutant regeneration, can be expensive, time-consuming, and environmentally devastating (Kumar et al., 2024, Kumar et al., 2025a). Phytoremediation has been developed as an acceptable alternative and environmentally friendly solution. This system leverages plants' natural ability to uptake, stabilize and detoxify pollutants. Phytoextraction is the process of using plants to absorb heavy metals (e.g., Cd, Pb, Ni, or Hg) into their tissues. Phytostabilization is a method to prevent the migration of metals in soil and reduce their dispersibility. Phytodegradation uses plants to degrade pollutants, while rhizofiltration involves the absorption of metals by plant roots. As a cost-effective, nondisruptive, and farmer-oriented tool, phytoremediation can provide a sustainable platform for field reclamation and food security (Shackira and Puthur, 2019; Ranjan et al., 2024).

Even agricultural inputs are a significant source of pollution. Cd is a contaminant and impurity present in phosphate fertilizers and enters the soil through repeated application, gradually raising Cd concentrations. Pesticides, especially older ones, may contain traces of arsenic (As), Pb, or Hg. Mixed sewage and livestock manure, applied as low-cost organic amendments, can introduce copper, zinc, Pb, and Cr, along with contaminants from feed composition, industrial waste in such feed, oil baths mixed in sewage, and additives used in animal husbandry. While these substances can increase soil fertility, they simultaneously serve as direct channels for metal accumulation. Irrigation water is also a significant source of pollution (Naja and Volesky, 2017; Younas et al., 2025). Areas that rely on groundwater often contend with heightened levels of As, fluoride, and other metals resulting from natural geochemical processes. In industrial belts, rivers and canals are often fed with raw effluents containing various metals, which are then reused for crop irrigation. This practice allows some toxic metals to be adsorbed onto soil colloids or taken up by plant roots, particularly in crops such as rice, leafy greens, and root vegetables (Brindha and Schneider, 2019) (Fig. 1.2).

Atmospheric deposition from heavy diesel emissions, coal, and waste burning also adds to the metal burden. Residues from old fuels and particles emitted through open waste burning on farmland are deposited directly onto the soil at the soil surface. Floodwaters in mining areas can transport polluted sediment to neighboring agriculturally utilized plains and spread metals over large areas (Kumar

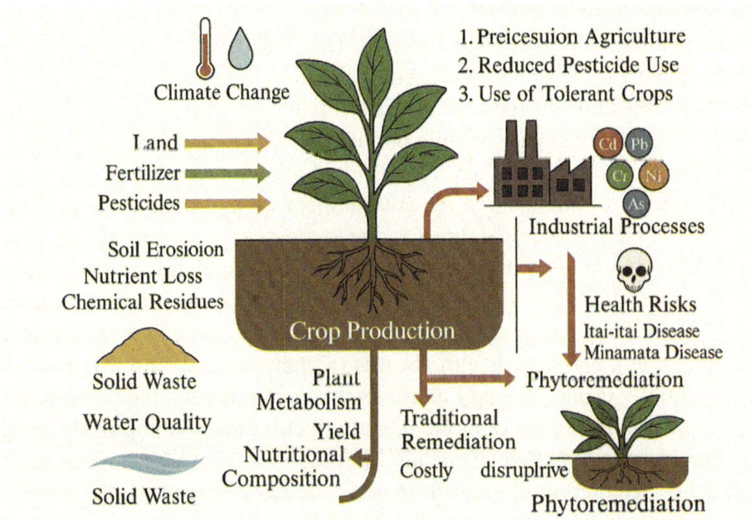

FIG. 1.2 The figure depicts key environmental and agricultural sources of metal exposure, illustrating how heavy metals make their way into the human food supply through soil, water, and crops.

et al., 2024). These intersecting inputs pose ongoing hazards to the environment and public health. Meanwhile, the floodwater itself provides significant contributions to water management, infrastructure, and resource use, along with supporting a range of social and environmental requirements. Water is a prerequisite for life and commerce, yet its extremes—droughts and floods—can also be catastrophic. In recent years, whether due to the dangers of climate change or human activities such as intensive farming, construction, charcoal burning, mining, and hunting, the world has witnessed an increase in both the magnitude and frequency of flooding and droughts. Such occurrences compromise water access and sustainable development in many countries. Soil with elevated metal concentrations can slow plant growth, decrease crop yields, and disturb populations of microbes that keep soil healthy (Rana et al., 2017). People can be exposed to metals through contaminated food, drinking water, or the air they breathe. Such pathways need to be understood for the development of soil remediation strategies, better utilization of fertilizers, improvement in wastewater treatment, and standard environmental monitoring. Enhancing regulatory systems and promoting sustainable agricultural techniques will continue to be key actions in minimizing metal pollution at its source (Kumar et al., 2025b).

1.5 Bioaccumulation and trophic transfer of epigenetically active metals

Epigenetically reactive metals are a class of environmental toxicants that can perturb gene regulation in the absence of direct DNA sequence changes. They exert their biological impact via alterations in DNA methylation, histone modification, and microRNA activity, thereby causing longstanding or even permanent alterations in cellular function. These metals, once released into ecosystems, persist for long periods, accumulate in living biota, and pass along the food chain, resulting in increased impacts at higher trophic levels over time. Heavy metals, unlike many organic pollutants, cannot be destroyed and tend to persist in the environment. They are adsorbed by sediments, soils, or biological tissues, and are introduced into the environment even in remote sites (Ganguly et al., 2024). Their ecological threat is due to their chemical persistence, formation of highly toxic derivatives, and efficient bioaccumulation followed by trophic chain transfer. Thus, heavy metals are currently priority pollutants in most parts of the world because they can change ecosystem structures, harm agricultural production, and pose health hazards (Kumar et al., 2017). Their build-up may potentially change the soil microorganism community, block plant physiological functions, reduce crop yield, and affect the functioning of the ecosystem. The biomagnification of metals like Cd and methyl Hg in humans and wildlife has been reported to result in neurological dysfunction, organ toxicity, and carcinogenesis (Lawal et al., 2021). This conclusion underscores the need to evaluate their long-term environmental behavior. Heavy metal contamination can be of natural or anthropogenic origin. Volcanic activity, rock weathering, and forest fires produce trace amounts of metals, which are normal components of geochemical cycles. However, anthropogenic activities have dramatically enhanced metal input into the environment. Contamination arises from industrial activities such as mining, smelting, burning fossil fuels, and electroplating, as well as the widespread use of agrochemicals (Kar, 2022). The situation is further compounded in many developing areas where a lack of regulation allows the movement of such metals across boundaries, presenting a regional or global exposure paradigm. In addition to metal concentration, intrinsic toxicity and biological availability play important roles in causing environmental impacts (Kumar et al., 2025b).

Bioaccumulation refers to the progressive increase of metals in organisms compared with those in their environment. Metals such as Cd, As, Hg, Pb, and Ni are poorly metabolized and have an affinity for tissue deposition (Nnaji et al., 2023). Aquatic organisms accumulate Cd by incorporating it into metallothioneins, where it elicits epigenetic regulation of the genes responsible for oxidative stress and apoptotic cell death. In agropastoral systems, Cd uptake by crops, particularly rice, has been found to silence growth-regulatory genes epigenetically, leading to poor development and reduced yield quantity of the plant (Greco et al., 2025). Bioaccumulated metals are transferred trophically from prey to predators, often leading to biomagnification. The most obvious example of this phenomenon is methyl Hg, which arises as a result of microbial transformations in sediment but gradually accumulates from plankton into fish, seabirds, and humans (Harding et al., 2018). Increased exposure at higher trophic levels is linked to global DNA hypomethylation and the downregulation of neurodevelopmentally related genes. Prenatal exposure in fish-eating populations has been associated with lasting epigenetic changes, resulting in cognitive and behavioral deficits (Perera and Herbstman, 2011; Zhao et al., 2022).

The As poisoning provides another example of how bioaccumulation can lead to trophic transfer across both aqueous and terrestrial food chains. In areas like Bangladesh and parts of India, arsenic can make its way into food chains through water plants and invertebrates that carry it onward to fish and humans (Kumar et al., 2017). Arsenic disrupts one-carbon metabolism, leading to the atypical methylation of essential tumor suppression genes, which may persist even after reducing exposure. Likewise, Pb accumulating in the invertebrates of soils moves to consumers higher up, where early life exposure results in long-term epigenetic alterations of neural plasticity. Together, the examples here demonstrate how the retention of metals and their transfer through food webs mediate environmental pollution to long-lasting biological and human health effects (Saidon et al., 2024; Nnaji et al., 2023).

1.6 Transgenerational and health impacts of epigenetic metal toxicity

Transgenerational effects emerge following disruption of the epigenome in germ cells (or during early embryogenesis). Exposure to As in utero is one of the most thoroughly investigated examples. Prenatal As exposure has been found to be associated with long-term DNA methylation changes in genes linked to immune function, metabolic regulation, and carcinogenesis in the next generation (Van Cauwenbergh et al., 2020). Experimental animal models have documented the heritability of such epigenetic modifications, which are known to predispose future generations to disease even in the absence of chronic exposure. Cd exposure exhibits similar effects, as it interferes with imprinting control regions and histone methylation, leading to altered developmental programming and impaired fertility in offspring. All these metals act through a range of epigenetic mechanisms, including abnormal methylation, dysregulation of microRNAs, and altered chromatin structure, to favor carcinogenesis as well as chronic disease (Cowley et al., 2018).

Millions of people are chronically exposed to As, mainly in low- and middle-income geographies. Increasingly, early-life exposure is also of interest; epidemiological and experimental evidence indicates that maternal or even preconceptional exposures may imprint the risk of disease in subsequent generations (Fall, 2013). This developmental programming can be seen in F1 offspring and subsequent effects on multigenerational (transgenerational) generations, many beyond the F3 generation. These findings underscore epigenetic inheritance as a mechanism through which environmental exposure early in life may be connected to disease in adulthood. In animal models, gestational arsenic exposure increased tumor formation in descendants, and human studies associated in utero exposure with greater risks for cancer, respiratory disease, and cardiovascular disease (Skinner, 2008; Darby et al., 2019).

Such epigenetic metal toxicity has far-reaching health effects and often presents subtle early symptoms that make it challenging to diagnose. Among these neurodevelopmental effects, the impact of exposure to Pb and methyl Hg during critical windows of development has been observed. These metals interfere with the epigenetic regulation of genes associated with synaptic plasticity, neurogenesis, and neurotransmitter signaling which helps explain cognitive impairments, behavioral disorders, and susceptibility to other dementing diseases (Ijomone et al., 2020). These risks may be difficult to detect at birth, and reliable follow-up of exposed populations over a sufficiently long period is crucial. Apart from the aforementioned neurological disorders, epigenetically active metals are also strongly associated with metabolic, cardiovascular, and oncological diseases (Gorini and Tonacci, 2023). Metal-driven methylation changes of tumor suppressor and DNA repair genes increase the likelihood of cancer, whereas Cd-induced inhibition of antioxidants and stress responses exacerbates chronic inflammation and tissue-injurious responses (Muthukumaran et al., 2023). Additionally, accumulating research has shown that metal exposure can disrupt the epigenetic control of insulin signaling and lipid homeostasis, thereby increasing the risk of metabolic syndrome and cardiovascular disease later in life. From a public health perspective, the trans-generational nature of epigenetic metal toxicity is a significant concern (Martins et al., 2023). The key issue here is that conventional risk assessment models, which emphasize acute or short-term toxicity, are inadequate for representing the long-lasting and trans-generational burden of epigenetic changes. Preventive actions and more stringent environmental protection measures should be implemented, along with long-term monitoring of exposed cohorts, to mitigate such risks for this and future generations (Gavito-Covarrubias et al., 2024).

1.7 Risk assessment and epigenetic biomarkers in food safety

Despite current procedures, the manifestation of food safety has predominantly been based on identifying chemical substances and estimating overexposure, as well as hazard endpoints (i.e., acute toxicity and carcinogenicity). However, growing evidence shows that different foodborne contaminants, such as heavy metals and persistent organic pollutants, can impact biological systems at the epigenetic level (Kumar et al., 2024). This work has expanded the horizon of risk evaluation to include concerns about subtle endpoints, such as cumulative, sustained biological responses that conventional systems might fail to detect. Scientists have developed applications of epigenetic biomarkers for improved measures of food safety (Fasani et al., 2023; Wisman et al., 2024). These biomarkers are associated with changes in DNA methylation, histone modifications, and noncoding RNA expression levels that result from exposure to toxicants such as As, Cd, Hg, or Pb via diet. Given that epigenetic marks may change at relatively low doses and can be sustained for extended periods, they provide early warning signs of biological perturbation preceding the development of symptomatic illness. For example, modified methylation of tumor suppressor genes and oxidative stress-related genes has been observed in subjects exposed to metal-contaminated food or drinking water, enabling precocious risk assessment (Dai et al., 2024; Nnaji et al., 2023) (Fig. 1.3).

These studies will support the breadth of chronic and cumulative exposure by integrating epigenetic biomarkers into food safety assessment. In contrast to conventional biomarkers, which may only convey recent exposures and offer limited insight into cumulative health risks, conditions such as cancer risk, metabolic disorders, and neurodevelopmental outcomes may benefit from a perspective that considers past exposure (Darby et al., 2019). Its importance is particularly apparent in vulnerable populations, such as pregnant women, infants, and children, who might be more sensitive during the early stages of their lives. Regulatorily, the use of epigenetic endpoints can help reduce exposure limits and assist in the identification of hazards by bridging molecular changes to apical health outcomes (Van Cauwenbergh et al., 2020; Harding et al., 2018). High-throughput epigenomic technologies are improving, which further supports the argument for their use in population-level surveillance. Community-level integration of epigenetic biomarkers for food safety risk assessment is essential. To sum up, the incorporation of epigenetic biomarkers in food safety risk assessment enables us to better identify, predict, and manage health risks due to food contamination and contributes to the development of more protective and forward-looking policies for food safety (Crépet et al., 2025).

1.8 Future perspectives and research gaps

Although there is increased awareness of the potential of epigenetic biomarkers for the evaluation of food safety risks, there are several important gaps that need to be addressed in order to fully realize the regulatory and public health potential of these biomarkers. A major issue to overcome is the lack of standardized epigenetic biomarkers that have been validated across populations, exposure levels, and food matrices. However, studies conducted so far have generally been small or population-based and are not directly applicable to routine food safety surveillance. Equally important knowledge deficiencies exist regarding dose–response relationships in dietary exposure and consequent epigenetic changes. Although the toxic effects of chemical exposure occur at relatively low levels, threshold responses that differentiate adaptive changes from deleterious effects are still poorly defined. Prospective studies are required to determine if these epigenetic signatures are reversible and/or whether they persist over time, promoting disease escalation. Future studies should also untangle the joint effects of several foodborne contaminants. In the natural environment, people are exposed to mixtures of metals, pesticides, and additives that have thousands

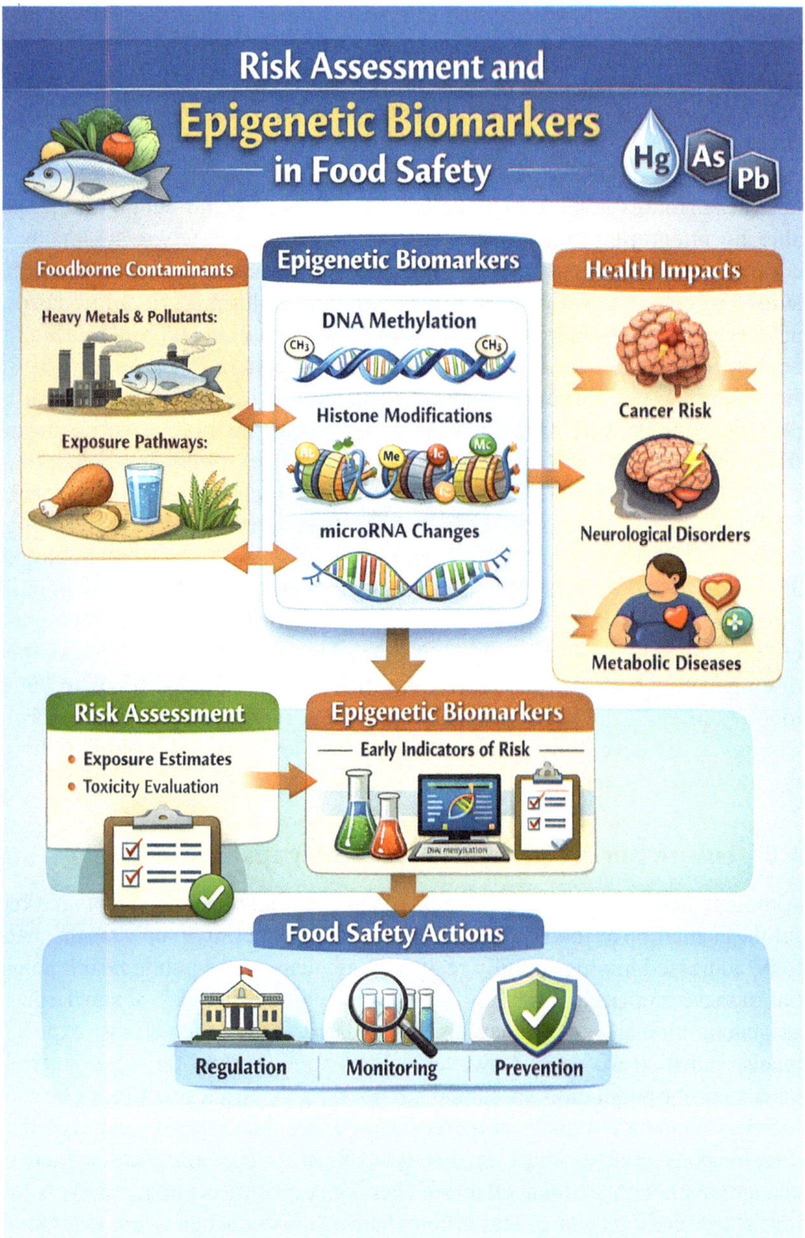

FIG. 1.3 Foodborne metal contaminants induce epigenetic changes, leading to early biomarkers indicative of dietary exposure-related health hazards—implications for food safety risk assessment and prevention strategies.

of years of history, while most epigenetic studies focus on single compounds. Knowledge of the interplay of interactive and cumulative epigenetic responses will be crucial for meaningful risk evaluation. The transgenerational relevance of foodborne epigenetic alterations is still poorly understood. Human data are scarce, but it has been proposed that dietary exposure in early life can affect disease susceptibility in subsequent generations. Well-powered, multigenerational cohort studies need to be conducted to define causality and patterns of inheritance. From a technical standpoint, the connections of these epigenomic data to standard toxicological or epidemiological endpoints have proven difficult. Future work should focus on building new and cost-effective platforms for high-throughput screening and generating bioinformatic procedures that are compatible with regulatory use. Closing these knowledge gaps will provide stronger value to food safety policymakers from an evidentiary standpoint regarding the inclusion of epigenetic biomarkers and additional predictive, prevention-focused risk assessment approaches.

1.9 Conclusion

These findings highlight the importance of epigenetic mechanisms in assessing long-term health effects from foodborne metal exposure. Unlike traditional toxicity end points, which typically focus on early or "high-dose" effects, epigenetic mechanisms explain chronic and subtle perturbations in biology that occur after extended exposure to environmental toxicants such as As, Cd, Hg, and Pb. These metal exposures disrupt DNA methylation, histone modification, and noncoding RNA regulation in experimental models and human epidemiological studies, which lead to neurological, developmental, metabolic, cardiovascular, and carcinogenic effects. Epigenetic biomarkers could potentially be considered in the risk assessment of food to more effectively represent early biological responses in susceptible subpopulations during periods of vulnerability. However, there are still challenges regarding the integration of biomarkers, the definition of exposure limits, and translating epigenetic findings into regulations. These gaps will require conclusions drawn from longitudinal, multiexposure, and population-based studies. In conclusion, the incorporation of epigenetic endpoints in food safety assessment is a critical advance in risk assessments toward complete risk evaluation, protecting public health, and ensuring the sustainable handling of risks from food contamination across generations.

References

Abdolmaleky, H.M., Nohesara, S., Zhou, J.R., Thiagalingam, S., 2025. Epigenetics in evolution and adaptation to environmental challenges: pathways for disease prevention and treatment. Epigenomics. 1750-192X. 17 (5), 317–333. Available from: https://www.tandfonline.com/journals/iepi20. doi:10.1080/17501911.2025.2464529.

Adegbola, P.I., Adetutu, A., 2024. Genetic and epigenetic modulations in toxicity: the two-sided roles of heavy metals and polycyclic aromatic hydrocarbons from the environment. Toxicol. Rep. 2214-7500. 12, 502–519. Available from: https://www.sciencedirect.com/science/journal/22147500. doi:10.1016/j.toxrep.2024.04.010.

Aguilera, O., Fernández, A.F., Muñoz, A., Fraga, M.F., 2010. Epigenetics and environment: a complex relationship. J. Appl. Physiol. 1522-1601. 109 (1), 243–251. Available from: http://jap.physiology.org/cgi/reprint/109/1/243. doi:10.1152/japplphysiol.00068.2010Spain.

Alcántara-Mejía, V.A., Álvarez-Barrera, L., Mateos-Nava, R.A., Rodríguez-Mercado, J.J., 2024. Metal-induced DNA damage, its impact on health, and activation of repair mechanisms: an overview. Toxicology 20, 1–18.

Brindha, K., Schneider, M., 2019. Impact of urbanization on groundwater quality. In: Venkatramanan, S., Prasanna, M.V., Chung, S.Y. (Eds.), GIS and Geostatistical Techniques for Groundwater Science. Elsevier, Germany, pp. 179–196. Available from: http://www.sciencedirect.com/science/book/9780128154137. doi:10.1016/B978-0-12-815413-7.00013-4.

Bure, I.V., Nemtsova, M.V., Kuznetsova, E.B., 2022. Histone modifications and non-coding RNAs: mutual epigenetic regulation and role in pathogenesis. Int. J. Mol. Sci. 1422-0067. 23 (10). Available from: https://www.mdpi.com/1422-0067/23/10/5801/pdf?version=1653205287. doi:10.3390/ijms23105801.

Chowdhury, N.R., Ghosh, S., Joardar, M., Kar, D., Roychowdhury, T., 2018. Impact of arsenic contaminated groundwater used during domestic scale post harvesting of paddy crop in West Bengal: arsenic partitioning in raw and parboiled whole grain. Chemosphere. 211, 173–184.

Cowley, M., Skaar, D.A., Jima, D.D., Maguire, R.L., Hudson, K.M., Park, S.S., Sorrow, P., Hoyo, C., 2018. Effects of cadmium exposure on DNA methylation at imprinting control regions and genome-wide in mothers and newborn children. Environ. Health Perspect. 1552-9924. 126 (3). Available from: https://ehp.niehs.nih.gov/wp-content/uploads/2018/03/EHP2085.alt_.pdf. doi:10.1289/EHP2085.

Crépet, A., Quénel, P., Garric, J., Kaufmann, A., Bonmatin, J.-M., Duché, P., Mathieu, A., Carsique, M., Jean, J., Sanders, P., Cravedi, J.-P., Schuler, M., Barouki, R., 2025. Integration of the exposome concept into health risk assessments: a challenge for health safety agencies. Environ. Res. 0013-9351. 286 (Pt 3), 123036. doi:10.1016/j.envres.2025.123036.

Dai, W., Qiao, X., Fang, Y., Guo, R., Bai, P., Liu, S., Li, T., Jiang, Y., Wei, S., Na, Z., Xiao, X., Li, D., 2024. Epigenetics-targeted drugs: current paradigms and future challenges. Signal Transduct. Target. Ther. 2059-3635. 9 (1). Available from: https://www.nature.com/sigtrans. doi:10.1038/s41392-024-02039-0.

Darby, J.R.T., Dollah, M.H.B.M., Regnault, T.R.H., Williams, M.T., Morrison, J.L., 2019. Systematic review: impact of resveratrol exposure during pregnancy on maternal and fetal outcomes in animal models of human pregnancy complications—are we ready for the clinic? Pharmacol. Res. 1096-1186. 144, 264–278. Available from: http://www.elsevier.com/inca/publications/store/6/2/2/9/3/1/index.htt. doi:10.1016/j.phrs.2019.04.020.

De Rosa, S., Curcio, A., Indolfi, C., 2014. Emerging role of microRNAs in cardiovascular diseases. Circ. J. 78 (3), 567–575.

Derakhshan Nejad, Z., Jung, M.C., Kim, K.H., 2018. Remediation of soils contaminated with heavy metals with an emphasis on immobilization technology. Environ. Geochem. Health 40 (3), 927–953.

Desaulniers, D., Vasseur, P., Jacobs, A., Aguila, M.C., Ertych, N., Jacobs, M.N., 2021. Integration of epigenetic mechanisms into non-genotoxic carcinogenicity hazard assessment: focus on DNA methylation and histone modifications. Int. J. Mol. Sci. 1422-0067. 22 (20), 10969. doi:10.3390/ijms222010969.

Edwards, J.R., Yarychkivska, O., Boulard, M., Bestor, T.H., 2017. DNA methylation and DNA methyltransferases. Epigenetics Chromatin. 1756-8935. 10 (1). doi:10.1186/s13072-017-0130-8.

Faiz, S., Lnu, N., Bibi, M., Joshi, N., Khan, I., Ukasha, M.H., Saud, S., Fahad, S., Adhikari, B., Asmatullah, Sarmad, M., 2025. Epigenetic regulation of abiotic stress responses. In: Tiwari, S., Gonzalez-Hernandez, J.L., Lata, C. (Eds.), Decoding Non-Coding RNA: Enhancing Plant Abiotic Stress Tolerance. Springer Nature Singapore, Singapore, pp. 79–124.

Fall, C.H.D., 2013. Fetal programming and the risk of noncommunicable disease. Indian J. Pediatr. 0019-5456. 80 (S1), 13–20. doi:10.1007/s12098-012-0834-5.

Fasani, E., Giannelli, G., Varotto, S., Visioli, G., Bellin, D., Furini, A., DalCorso, G., 2023. Epigenetic control of plant response to heavy metals. Plants. 2223-7747. 12 (18), 3195. doi:10.3390/plants12183195.

Ganguly, D., Kumar, P., Kumari, A., Kumar, M., 2024. Importance of microbial consortia and green chemistry in the removal of xenobiotics from the environment. In: Srivastav, A.L., Grewal, A.S., Tiwari, M., Pham, T.D. (Eds.), Role of Green Chemistry in Ecosystem Restoration to Achieve Environmental Sustainability. Elsevier, pp. 11–21.

Gavito-Covarrubias, D., Ramírez-Díaz, I., Guzmán-Linares, J., Limón, I.D., Manuel-Sánchez, D.M., Molina-Herrera, A., Coral-García, M.Á., Anastasio, E., Anaya-Hernández, A., López-Salazar, P., Juárez-Díaz, G., Martínez-Juárez, J., Torres-Jácome, J., Albarado-Ibáñez, A., Martínez-Laguna, Y., Morán, C., Rubio, K., 2024. Epigenetic mechanisms of particulate matter exposure: air pollution and hazards on human health. Front. Genet. 1664-8021. 14. doi:10.3389/fgene.2023.1306600.

Ghori, Z., Iftikhar, H., Bhatti, M.F., Sharma, I., Kazi, A.G., Ahmad, P., 2016. Phytoextraction: the use of plants to remove heavy metals from soil. In: Ahmad, P. (Ed.), Plant Metal Interaction. Elsevier, pp. 385–409.

Ghosh, D., Ghosh, A., Bhadury, P., 2022. Arsenic through aquatic trophic levels: effects, transformations and biomagnification—a concise review. Geosci. Lett. 9 (1), 20.

Gorini, F., Tonacci, A., 2023. Toxic metals in pregnancy and congenital heart defects. Insights and new perspectives for a technology-driven reduction in food sources. Explor. Cardiol. 1 (3), 114–140. doi:10.37349/ec.2023.00012.

Greco, E., Talarico, E., Guarasci, F., Camoli, M., Palermo, A.M., Zambelli, A., Chiappetta, A., Araniti, F., Bruno, L., 2025. Epigenetic mechanisms of plant adaptation to cadmium and heavy metal stress. Epigenomes. 2075-4655. 9 (4). Available from: https://www.mdpi.com/journal/epigenomes. doi:10.3390/epigenomes9040043.

Guo, Y.W., Liu, Y., Huang, P.C., Rong, M., Wei, W., Xu, Y.H., Wei, J.H., 2025. Adaptive changes and genetic mechanisms in organisms under controlled conditions: a review. Int. J. Mol. Sci. 1422-0067. 26 (5). Available from: http://www.mdpi.com/journal/ijms. doi:10.3390/ijms26052130.

Harding, G., Dalziel, J., Vass, P., 2018. Bioaccumulation of methylmercury within the marine food web of the outer bay of fundy, gulf of maine. PloS One. 13 (7), e0197220.

Igolkina, A.A., Zinkevich, A., Karandasheva, K.O., Popov, A.A., Selifanova, M.V., Nikolaeva, D., Tkachev, V., Penzar, D., Nikitin, D.M., Buzdin, A., 2019. H3K4me3, H3K9ac, H3K27ac, H3K27me3 and H3K9me3 Histone tags suggest distinct regulatory evolution of open and condensed chromatin landmarks. Cells. 2073-4409. 8 (9). Available from: https://www.mdpi.com/2073-4409/8/9/1034/pdf. doi:10.3390/cells8091034.

Ijomone, O.M., Ijomone, O.K., Iroegbu, J.D., Ifenatuoha, C.W., Olung, N.F., Aschner, M., 2020. Epigenetic influence of environmentally neurotoxic metals. Neurotoxicology. 81, 51–65.

Jayakumar, M., Surendran, U., Raja, P., Kumar, A., Senapathi, V., 2021. A review of heavy metals accumulation pathways, sources and management in soils. Arab. J. Geosci. 1866-7538. 14 (20). Available from: http://www.springer.com/geosciences/journal/12517?cm_mmc=AD-_-enews-_-PSE1892-_-0. doi:10.1007/s12517-021-08543-9.

Jurkowska, R.Z., 2024. Role of epigenetic mechanisms in the pathogenesis of chronic respiratory diseases and response to inhaled exposures: from basic concepts to clinical applications. Pharmacol. Ther. 0163-7258. 264, 108732. doi:10.1016/j.pharmthera.2024.108732.

Kar, S., 2022. Geochemical characteristics of mineral elements: arsenic, fluorine, lead, nitrogen, and carbon. In: Giri, B., Kapoor, R., Wu, Q.-S., Varma, A. (Eds.), Structure and Functions of Pedosphere. Springer Nature, India, pp. 209–254. doi:10.1007/978-981-16-8770-9_10.

Key, J., Gispert, S., Kandi, A.R., Heinz, D., Hamann, A., Osiewacz, H.D., Meierhofer, D., Auburger, G., 2024. CLPP-null eukaryotes with excess heme biosynthesis show reduced L-arginine levels, probably via CLPX-mediated OAT activation. Biomolecules. 2218-273X. 14 (2). Available from: http://www.mdpi.com/journal/biomolecules. doi:10.3390/biom14020241.

Kumar, M., 2021. In silico efficacy of [S]-8-gingerol (a derivative) with 6-gingerol against PT-domain of Polyketide synthase A (PksA). IP Int. J. Med. Microbiol. Trop. Dis. 2581-4753. 7 (1), 62–64. doi:10.18231/j.ijmmtd.2021.014.

Kumar, M., Akhtar, M.S., 2019. Application of microbial biotechnology in improving salt stress and crop productivity. In: Akhtar, M.S. (Ed.), Salt Stress, Microbes, and Plant Interactions: Mechanisms and Molecular Approaches, vol. 2. Springer Singapore, India, pp. 133–159. doi:10.1007/978-981-13-8805-7_7.

Kumar, M., Akhtar, M.S., Bhardwaj, H., Bhoi, B., Kumar, P., 2025a. Futuristic and prospective role of agricultural biotechnology in sustainable environment. In: Akhtar, M.S., Hakeem, K.R. (Eds.), Agricultural Biotechnology. Apple Academic Press, pp. 1–23.

Kumar, M., Akhtar, M.S., Ganguly, D., Kumari, L., Kumari, K., Agrawal, M., 2025b. Agroecosystem diversity and maintenance of soil and environment health. In: Akhtar, M.S., Hakeem, K.R. (Eds.), Agricultural Biotechnology. Apple Academic Press, pp. 155–176.

Kumar, M., Bharadwaj, H., Kumari, K., 2023. Plant adaptation to salinity stress: significance of major metabolites. In: Anjum, N.A. (Ed.), Making Plant Life Easier and Productive under Salinity-Updates and Prospects. IntechOpen, pp. 1–24.

Kumar, M., Bhoi, B., Kumar, H., Bhardwaj, H., 2024. Fungi's involvement in metal NPS synthesis and environmentally sustainable practices. In: Bhardwaj, A.K., Srivastav, A.L., Rai, S. (Eds.), Biogenic Wastes-Enabled Nanomaterial Synthesis: Applications in Environmental Sustainability. Springer Nature, India, pp. 149–170. Available from: https://link.springer.com/book/10.1007/978-3-031-59083-2. doi:10.1007/978-3-031-59083-2_6.

Kumar, M., Kumari, P., Kumari, A., 2025. Determinants of soil health and its role in environmental sustainability. In: Joshi, N.C., Leustek, T., Singh, P.K. (Eds.), Soil Health and Nutrition Management. CABI, GB, pp. 238–250.

Kumar, S., Gonzalez, E.A., Rameshwar, P., Etchegaray, J.-P., 2020. Non-coding RNAs as mediators of epigenetic changes in malignancies. Cancers. 2072-6694. 12 (12), 3657. doi:10.3390/cancers12123657.

Kumar, S.S., Kadier, A., Malyan, S.K., Ahmad, A., Bishnoi, N.R., 2017. Phytoremediation and rhizoremediation: uptake, mobilization and sequestration of heavy metals by plants. Plant-Microbe Interact. Agro-Ecol. Perspect. 2, 367–394. Available from: http://www.springer.com/in/book/9789811065927. doi:10.1007/978-981-10-6593-4_15.

Lawal, K.K., Ekeleme, I.K., Onuigbo, C.M., Ikpeazu, V.O., Obiekezie, S.O., 2021. A review on the public health implications of heavy metals. World J. Adv. Res. Rev. 2581-9615. 10 (3), 255–265. doi:10.30574/wjarr.2021.10.3.0249.

Liang, H., Tan, Y., Yin, J., Peng, Y., Wei, M., Chen, H., Chen, Q., 2024. Phosphate fertilizers' dual role in cadmium-polluted acidic agricultural soils: dosage dependency and passivation potential. Agronomy. 2073-4395. 14 (10), 2201. doi:10.3390/agronomy14102201.

Lyko, F., 2018. The DNA methyltransferase family: a versatile toolkit for epigenetic regulation. Nat. Rev. Genet. 1471-0056. 19 (2), 81–92. doi:10.1038/nrg.2017.80.

Madesh, S., Gopi, S., Sau, A., Rajagopal, R., Namasivayam, S.K.R., Arockiaraj, J., 2024. Chemical contaminants and environmental stressors induced teratogenic effect in aquatic ecosystem—a comprehensive review. Toxicol. Rep. 2214-7500. 13, 101819. doi:10.1016/j.toxrep.2024.101819.

Malik, D., Narayanasamy, N., Pratyusha, V.A., Thakur, J., Sinha, N., 2023. Microminerals and toxic heavy metals. In: Malik, D., Narayanasamy, N., Pratyusha, V.A., Thakur, J., Sinha, N., (Eds.), Textbook of Nutritional Biochemistry. Springer Nature Singapore, Singapore, pp. 447–504.

Martins, A.C., Ferrer, B., Tinkov, A.A., Caito, S., Deza-Ponzio, R., Skalny, A.V., Bowman, A.B., Aschner, M., 2023. Association between heavy metals, metalloids and metabolic syndrome: new insights and approaches. Toxics. 2305-6304. 11 (8). Available from: http://www.mdpi.com/journal/toxics. doi:10.3390/toxics11080670.

Maurya, P.K., Malik, D.S., 2016. Bioaccumulation of xenobiotics compound of pesticides in riverine system and its control technique: a critical review. J. Ind. Pollut. Control 0970-2083. 32 (2), 580–594. Available from: http://www.indiaenvironmentportal.org.in/taxonomy/term/8906.

Miclean, M., Cadar, O., Levei, E.A., Roman, R., Ozunu, A., Levei, L., 2019. Metal (Pb, Cu, Cd, and Zn) transfer along food chain and health risk assessment through raw milk consumption from free-range cows. Int. J. Environ. Res. Public Health. 1660-4601. 16 (21), 4064. doi:10.3390/ijerph16214064.

Mishra, S., Bharagava, R.N., More, N., Yadav, A., Zainith, S., Mani, S., Chowdhary, P., 2018. Heavy metal contamination: an alarming threat to environment and human health. In: Sobti, R.C., Arora, N.K., Kothari, R. (Eds.), Environmental Biotechnology: For Sustainable Future. Springer Singapore, Singapore, pp. 103–125.

Mititelu, M., Neacşu, S.M., Busnatu, Ş.S., Scafa-Udrişte, A., Andronic, O., Lăcraru, A.E., Ioniță-Mîndrican, C.B., Lupuliasa, D., Negrei, C., Olteanu, G., 2025. Assessing heavy metal contamination in food: implications for human health and environmental safety. Toxics. 2305-6304. 13 (5). Available from: http://www.mdpi.com/journal/toxics. doi:10.3390/toxics13050333.

Morgan, M.A.J., Shilatifard, A., 2020. Reevaluating the roles of histone-modifying enzymes and their associated chromatin modifications in transcriptional regulation. Nat. Genet. 1061-4036. 52 (12), 1271–1281. doi:10.1038/s41588-020-00736-4.

Munir, N., Jahangeer, M., Bouyahya, A., El Omari, N., Ghchime, R., Balahbib, A., Aboulaghras, S., Mahmood, Z., Akram, M., Ali Shah, S.M., Mikolaychik, I.N., 2021. Heavy metal contamination of natural foods is a serious health issue: a review. Sustainability. 14 (1), 161.

Muthukumaran, R.B., Bhattacharjee, P., Bhowmick, P., Zote, L., Malsawmtluangi, Kumar, N.S., Jahau, L., Cooke, M.S., Hu, C.W., Chao, M.R., 2023. Genetic and epigenetic instability induced by betel quid associated chemicals. Toxicol. Rep. 2214-7500. 10, 223–234. Available from: http://www.journals.elsevier.com/toxicology-reports/. doi:10.1016/j.toxrep.2023.02.001.

Naja, G.M., Volesky, B., 2017. Toxicity and sources of Pb, Cd, Hg, Cr, As, and radionuclides in the environment. In: Handbook of Advanced Industrial and Hazardous Wastes Management. CRC Press, Canada, pp. 855–903. Available from: http://www.tandfebooks.com/doi/book/10.1201/9781315117423. doi:10.1201/9781315117423.

Nnaji, N.D., Onyeaka, H., Miri, T., Ugwa, C., 2023. Bioaccumulation for heavy metal removal: a review. SN Appl. Sci. 5 (5), 125.

Oros, A., 2025. Bioaccumulation and trophic transfer of heavy metals in marine fish: ecological and ecosystem-level impacts. J. Xenobiotics. 2039-4713. 15 (2), 59. doi:10.3390/jox15020059.

Ozarde, Y., Purandare, D., Deshmukh, S., Gadhave, R., 2025. Heavy metals and cardiovascular health: uncovering links and health challenges. J. Trace Elem. Med. Biol. 0946-672X. 89, 127648. doi:10.1016/j.jtemb.2025.127648.

Perera, F., Herbstman, J., 2011. Prenatal environmental exposures, epigenetics, and disease. Reprod. Toxicol. 0890-6238. 31 (3), 363–373. doi:10.1016/j.reprotox.2010.12.055.

Piergiacomo, F., Brusetti, L., Pagani, L., 2022. Understanding the interplay between antimicrobial resistance, microplastics and xenobiotic contaminants: a leap towards one health? Int. J. Environ. Res. Public Health 20 (1), 42.

Rana, M., Asdari, R., Chowdhury, A.J.K., Munir, M.B., 2023. Heavy metal contamination during processing of canned fish: a review on food health and food safety. Desalin. Water Treat. 1944-3986. 315, 492–499. Available from: https://www.sciencedirect.com/journal/desalination-and-water-treatment. doi:10.5004/dwt.2023.30015.

Rana, S., Mahato, J.P., Kumar, M., Sarsaiya, S., 2017. Modeling and docking of cysteine protease-A (CPA) of Leishmania donovani. J. Appl. Pharm. Sci. 2231-3354. 7 (9), 179–184. Available from: http://www.japsonline.com/admin/php/uploads/2422_pdf.pdf. doi:10.7324/JAPS.2017.70924.

Ranjan, P., Kumar, M., Bhardwaj, H., Kumari, P., Kumari, A., 2024. Application of enzymes in biomass waste management. In: Srivastav, A.L., Bhardwaj, A.K., Kumar, M. (Eds.), Valorization of Biomass Wastes for Environmental Sustainability: Green Practices for the Rural Circular Economy. Springer, India, pp. 189–205. Available from: https://link.springer.com/book/10.1007/978-3-031-52485-1. doi:10.1007/978-3-031-52485-1_10.

Ray, S., Shaju, S.T., 2023. Bioaccumulation of pesticides in fish resulting toxicities in humans through food chain and forensic aspects. Environ. Anal. Health Toxicol. 2671-9525. 38 (3), e2023017. doi:10.5620/eaht.2023017.

Regnell, O., Watras, C.J., 2018. Microbial mercury methylation in aquatic environments: a critical review of published field and laboratory studies. Environ. Sci. Technol. 53 (1), 4–19.

Ryu, H.W., Lee, D.H., Won, H.R., Kim, K.H., Seong, Y.J., Kwon, S.H., 2015. Influence of toxicologically relevant metals on human epigenetic regulation. Toxicol. Res. 2234-2753. 31 (1), 1–9. Available from: http://ocean.kisti.re.kr/downfile/volume/ksot/DSHHBQ/2015/v31n1/DSHHBQ_2015_v31n1_1.pdf. doi:10.5487/TR.2015.31.1.001.

Saidon, N.B., Szabó, R., Budai, P., Lehel, J., 2024. Trophic transfer and biomagnification potential of environmental contaminants (heavy metals) in aquatic ecosystems. Environ. Pollut. 0269-7491. 340 (Pt 1), 122815. doi:10.1016/j.envpol.2023.122815.

Samuel, P.O., Edo, G.I., Oloni, G.O., Ugbune, U., Ezekiel, G.O., Essaghah, A.E.A., Agbo, J.J., 2023. Effects of chemical contaminants on the ecology and evolution of organisms a review. Chem. Ecol. 1029-0370. 39 (10), 1071–1107. Available from: www.tandf.co.uk/journals/titles/02757540.asp. doi:10.1080/02757540.2023.2284158.

Sarkar, S., Basu, B., Kundu, C.K., Patra, P.K., 2012. Deficit irrigation: an option to mitigate arsenic load of rice grain in West Bengal, India. Agric. Ecosyst. Environ. 0167-8809. 146 (1), 147–152. doi:10.1016/j.agee.2011.10.008.

Shackira, A.M., Puthur, J.T., 2019. Phytostabilization of heavy metals: understanding of principles and practices. In: Srivastava, S., Srivastava, A.K., Suprasanna, P. (Eds.), Plant-Metal Interactions. Springer International Publishing, Cham, pp. 263–282.

Sharma, J.K., Kumar, N., Singh, N.P., Santal, A.R., 2023. Phytoremediation technologies and their mechanism for removal of heavy metal from contaminated soil: an approach for a sustainable environment. Front. Plant Sci. 1664-462X. 14. Available from: https://www.frontiersin.org/journals/plant-science. doi:10.3389/fpls.2023.1076876.

Sharma, P., Dagariya, S., Sharma, S., Singh, M., 2025. Uncovering the nexus of human health hazards of nanoplastics, gut-dysbiosis and antibiotic-resistance. J. Environ. Sci. Health C. 2689-6583. 44, 1–60. doi:10.1080/26896583.2025.2578871.

Singh, A., Prasad, S.M., 2015. Remediation of heavy metal contaminated ecosystem: an overview on technology advancement. Int. J. Environ. Sci. Technol. 1735-1472. 12 (1), 353–366. doi:10.1007/s13762-014-0542-y.

Skinner, M.K., 2008. What is an epigenetic transgenerational phenotype? F3 or F2. Reprod. Toxicol. 0890-6238. 25 (1), 2–6. doi:10.1016/j.reprotox.2007.09.001.

Van Cauwenbergh, O., Di Serafino, A., Tytgat, J., Soubry, A., 2020. Transgenerational epigenetic effects from male exposure to endocrine-disrupting compounds: a systematic review on research in mammals. Clin. Epigenetics. 1868-7075. 12 (1). doi:10.1186/s13148-020-00845-1.

Vogt, G., 2021. Epigenetic variation in animal populations: sources, extent, phenotypic implications, and ecological and evolutionary relevance. J. Biosci. 0250-5991. 46 (1). doi:10.1007/s12038-021-00138-6.

Wisman, G.B.A., Wojdacz, T.K., Altucci, L., Rots, M.G., DeMeo, D.L., Snieder, H., 2024. Clinical promise and applications of epigenetic biomarkers. Clin. Epigenetics. 1868-7083. 16 (1). Available from: https://clinicalepigeneticsjournal.biomedcentral.com/. doi:10.1186/s13148-024-01806-8.

Wu, Y.S., Osman, A.I., Hosny, M., Elgarahy, A.M., Eltaweil, A.S., Rooney, D.W., Chen, Z., Rahim, N.S., Sekar, M., Gopinath, S.C.B., Rani, N.N.I.M., Batumalaie, K., Yap, P.S., 2024. The toxicity of mercury and its chemical compounds: molecular mechanisms and environmental and human health implications: a comprehensive review. ACS Omega. 2470-1343. 9 (5), 5100–5126. Available from: http://pubs.acs.org/journal/acsodf. doi:10.1021/acsomega.3c07047.

Younas, H., Nazir, A., Bareen, F.E., 2025. From sources to solutions: integrated approaches for Cd, Hg, and Pb remediation- a comprehensive review. Plant Soil. 1573-5036. 510 (1), 1–47. Available from: https://www.springer.com/journal/11104. doi:10.1007/s11104-024-06944-9.

Zhang, L., Liu, Z., Song, Y., Sui, J., Hua, X., 2024. Advances in the involvement of metals and metalloids in plant defense response to external stress. Plants. 2223-7747. 13 (2), 313. doi:10.3390/plants13020313.

Zhang, Y., Zhang, Q., Zhang, Y., Han, J., 2023. The role of histone modification in DNA replication-coupled nucleosome assembly and cancer. Int. J. Mol. Sci. 1422-0067. 24 (5), 4939. doi:10.3390/ijms24054939.

Zhao, L., Islam, R., Wang, Y., Zhang, X., Liu, L.-Z., 2022. Epigenetic regulation in chromium-, nickel- and cadmium-induced carcinogenesis. Cancers. 2072-6694. 14 (23), 5768. doi:10.3390/cancers14235768.

Chapter 2

Toxicodynamics of metals: Molecular and cellular mechanisms

Varsha Rawat[a] and Jyotiram A. Sawale[b]
[a]*Department of Pharmaceutical Science and Research, SGT University, Gurugram, Haryana, India*
[b]*Krishna Institute of Pharmacy, Krishna Vishwa Vidyapeeth (Deemed to be University), Karad, Maharashtra, India*

2.1 Introduction

Toxicodynamics is the investigation of the biochemical, molecular, and physiological actions of toxic compounds on living organisms, including the processes by which the effects are generated. In metals, toxicodynamics deals with the intricate pathways of interactions between metal species and biological systems, from their very first molecular identification up to the expression of cellular malfunction, tissue damage, and systemic toxicity (Wu et al., 2016). In contrast to the absorption, distribution, metabolism, and excretion of toxicants addressed in toxicokinetics, toxicodynamics is concerned with the "what the toxin does to the body" phenomenon, including receptor binding, enzyme inhibition, oxidative stress generation, and disruption of essential cellular signaling pathways (Lu et al., 2025). This mechanistic understanding is central not only to explaining the hazards of metals but also to designing targeted prevention, diagnostic, and therapeutic strategies. Heavy metals and metalloids like lead (Pb), mercury (Hg), cadmium (Cd), arsenic (As), chromium (Cr), and nickel (Ni) are known to be key environmental and occupational toxicants (Gao, 2024; Gong et al., 2022; Davidova et al., 2024). Their toxicodynamic profiles are significantly diverse based on their chemical speciation, oxidation state, and biological targets. Certain metals are trace micronutrients required in specific biological processes zinc (Zn), copper (Cu), and manganese (Mn)—but are toxic at larger doses, while others, like lead or cadmium, do not have any known useful biological function and are harmful even at very low dosages (Skalnaya and Skalny, 2018). The duality of such metals betrays the intricacy of their biological interactions and requires a multifaceted perspective

The Metallome in Motion. https://doi.org/10.1016/B978-0-443-44299-5.00022-5

when considering risk and therapeutic intervention. Ecologically, harmful metals are nonbiodegradable, persistent pollutants that can biomagnify and bioaccumulate via food webs. Both anthropogenic activities (mining, smelting, industrial processes, agricultural runoff, fossil fuel burning, disposal of electronic waste) and natural processes (volcanic eruptions, weathering of rocks, geothermal emanations) release them into the environment (Asamoah et al., 2020; Padoan et al., 2024). After release, these metals may adsorb to soil particles, dissolve in water bodies, or be taken up by plants and microbes, subsequently entering the food chain of humans and wildlife. The capacity of metals to pass through biological membranes and build up in target tissues, mainly the brain, liver, kidneys, and bones, is the basis of their chronic toxicodynamic effects (Ro et al., 2022). Toxic metals, at the molecular level, usually cause their effects by binding to functional groups of biomolecules, more specifically sulfhydryl (-SH), carboxyl (-COOH), and phosphate (-PO_4) moieties. Binding changes protein conformation and activity, inhibits essential enzymes, and upsets cellular homeostasis (López-Armada et al., 2022; Srivastava, 2016). For instance, mercury's strong binding to thiol groups in enzymes and structural proteins disrupts mitochondrial respiration, whereas arsenic can replace phosphate in adenosine triphosphate (ATP) formation, producing unstable adenosine analogs that compromise cellular energy metabolism (Seyfried and Chinopoulos, 2021). Furthermore, a broad range of toxic metals catalyze the formation of reactive oxygen species (ROS), causing oxidative damage to DNA, proteins, and lipids, triggering cascades of cellular damage that may end in apoptosis, necrosis, or unchecked proliferation. The cellular reactions to metal exposure are complex and entail stress response mechanisms like the mitogen-activated protein kinase (MAPK) cascade, activation of nuclear factor kappa B (NF-κB), and regulation of p53-mediated apoptosis (Goutam Mukherjee et al., 2022; Schrenk et al., 2020). Cells can try to offset metal toxicity by inducing metallothioneins, glutathione (GSH) production, and antioxidant enzymes, but such adaptive responses can be overcome under high-level or long-term exposure. The damage that ensues can cause organ-specific pathologies—neurotoxicity in the instance of lead and mercury, hepatotoxicity with arsenic and copper excess, nephrotoxicity due to cadmium, and cardiovascular complications resulting from chronic exposure to multiple metals (More et al., 2023). From a public health perspective, knowledge about the toxicodynamics of metals is important since diseases caused by metals have long latent periods, nonspecific early manifestations, and irreparable injury when clinically evident. Effect biomarkers—including DNA adducts, markers of oxidative stress, and changed gene expression patterns—provide promising approaches to earlier detection and intervention (Donaher and Van den Hurk, 2023). New omics technologies (genomics, proteomics, metabolomics) are widening the capacity to chart the complex web of metal-induced molecular changes, opening the door to predictive toxicology models that can inform regulatory policy and clinical practice. In addition, understanding toxicodynamic processes is critical to the identification of effective therapeutic strategies. Chelation therapy is currently still the gold standard in acute metal poisoning, but its drawbacks—such as failure to remove all metal, redistribution, and possible side effects—mandate the use of alternative or additive measures (Ali et al., 2019). Antioxidant nutraceuticals, nanotechnology-based detoxification systems, and targeted delivery of protective agents to involved organs are new frontiers that show promise. These strategies need to be based on a good knowledge of the particular molecular and cellular processes by which each metal is toxic.

2.2 Sources and environmental fate of toxic metals

Toxic metals are found naturally in the Earth's crust, but their distribution, chemical speciation, and ecotoxicological effects depend significantly on geological processes as well as anthropogenic processes. Knowledge of the source and environmental pathway of these metals is essential to understanding their toxicodynamics, as source properties tend to condition the concentration, chemical form, and bioavailability of metals in biota. The environmental destiny of metals—where they travel, change, and accumulate—ultimately determines their capacity for introduction into the food web and their long-term ecological and health impacts (Khan et al., 2017; Martínez-Alcalá and Bernal, 2020).

2.2.1 Natural sources

Natural geochemical cycling is a reference point source for metal occurrence in the biosphere. Such processes tend to release metals at low to moderate levels, frequently bound within minerals or geochemically stabilized. Key natural sources include:

- **Geological weathering**

  Weathering of metal-containing rocks and soils is the predominant natural route for the release of metals into the environment. Mechanical disruption and chemical degradation of minerals release metals like iron (Fe), manganese (Mn), copper (Cu), zinc (Zn), and small traces of toxic metals like arsenic (As), cadmium (Cd), and lead (Pb). Rates of weathering vary with rock type, climate, pH, and biological activity. Acidic conditions, for instance, promote metal sulfide dissolution, which augments metal mobility in groundwater and soil (Angon et al., 2024; Nieder et al., 2018).

- **Volcanic activity**

  Volcanoes release high amounts of metals and metalloids—especially mercury (Hg), arsenic, lead, and selenium—into the atmosphere via ash particles and volcanic gases. These may be transported long distances before depositing and forming a global background level of metals. Volcanic hot springs and fumaroles may also add metals directly to aquatic environments in soluble, frequently bioavailable forms (Chowdhury and Rahman, 2024; Kar, 2022).

- **Geothermal and hydrothermal systems**

  Land geothermal vents and ocean hydrothermal vents discharge metals such as copper, zinc, cobalt, and iron, usually accompanied by sulfur, to produce metal sulfides. Although some of these emissions sustain unique microbial communities, they are also known to cause local metal enrichment in sediments and biota (Ranaweera et al., 2023).

- **Wildfires and biomass burning**

While usually referred to as anthropogenically triggered, wildfires also occur naturally and release metals that are sequestered in plant tissue and organic soil matter. Metals such as manganese, copper, and chromium can volatilize or be adsorbed onto particulates in the air, affecting atmospheric transport (Awan et al., 2021).

2.2.2 Anthropogenic sources

Natural metal cycling has been greatly affected by human activities, both in terms of the magnitude and type of metal released. Anthropogenic sources tend to yield more soluble, reactive, and bioavailable metal species, heightening toxicodynamic potential (Zhang et al., 2023).

- **Mining and smelting**

Extraction of metal ores (e.g., gold, copper, lead, zinc) and smelting them afterward are some of the largest sources of environmental metal pollution. Waste rock, tailings, and smelter emissions release metals in dissolved and particulate forms. Acid mine drainage—formed when sulfide minerals are exposed to water and air—results in acidic solutions containing dissolved, metal-rich concentrations of Fe, Cu, Zn, Pb, and Cd, which can last for decades to centuries (Muchowska et al., 2017).

- **Industrial manufacturing**

Metals are extensively applied in manufacturing industries such as electronics (lead, cadmium, rare earths), plating and galvanizing (chromium, nickel, zinc), battery manufacturing (lead, cadmium, lithium), and pigment and dye making (cadmium, mercury, chromium). Uncontrolled disposal of industrial effluents, solid wastes, and by-products leads to enormous environmental loading (Fomina and Skorochod, 2020).

- **Agriculture**

Agricultural practices add metals to water and soil through the application of phosphate fertilizers (commonly cadmium-containing), pesticides (formerly arsenic-, mercury-, and copper-containing), and livestock feed additives (copper and zinc). Metal contamination of water used for irrigation can also increase soil metal concentrations, affecting crop uptake and entry into the human diet via the food chain (Li et al., 2021).

- **Combustion of fossil fuels**

Coal-fired power plants, oil refineries, and motor vehicle emissions release metals like mercury, lead, vanadium, and nickel into the air. These metals are usually associated with fine particulates ($PM_{2.5}$, PM_{10}), which are inhaled or deposited onto soil and water, eventually finding their way into terrestrial and aquatic food webs (Zitoun et al., 2024).

- **Urban waste and E-waste recycling**

  Municipal solid waste incineration emits metals such as lead, cadmium, and mercury. Backyard or inadequately controlled e-waste recycling is a rapidly growing source of toxins, particularly in the developing world. Acid leaching and open burning in e-waste recycling facilities pollute soil, water, and air, leading to localized toxic hotspots (Liu et al., 2024).

- **Military and defense activities**

  The use of lead-containing ammunition, cadmium-based components in military electronics, and heavy metals in propellants or armor plating contributes to localized contamination in training grounds, testing sites, and active combat zones. These activities release metals into surrounding soils, groundwater, and surface water, creating long-lasting environmental "hotspots" of contamination. Over time, these metals may leach into nearby ecosystems, accumulate in vegetation or wildlife, and pose chronic exposure risks to both military personnel and civilian populations (Sonke et al., 2023; Jin et al., 2025).

2.2.3 Bioavailability and food chain transfer

Environmental fate of toxic metals is controlled by their speciation—the chemical state in which the metal occurs. This determines solubility, mobility, and the ability for biological uptake. Metals in soluble or ionic complex forms are more bioavailable than those in mineral-bound or adsorbed states.

- **Soil and sediment interactions**

  Metals can be bound to soil particles, organic materials, or clay minerals, limiting mobility while producing long-term reservoirs. Acidification, salinity, and changes in redox potential mobilize bound metals, making them bioavailable. Sediments act as sinks and secondary sources of metals in aquatic environments (Feng et al., 2022).

- **Aquatic transport and uptake**

  In aquatic environments, metals may occur as free ions, inorganic compounds (e.g., chlorides, carbonates), or organic complexes (e.g., with humic substances). Aquatic organisms take up metals through gills, skin, or food. Mercury, especially, is transformed by microbial action into methyl mercury, a very toxic, fat-loving compound that biomagnifies through the aquatic food chain (Mahimairaja et al., 2005).

- **Biomagnification in terrestrial and aquatic systems**

  Bioaccumulation is defined as the accumulation of metals by an organism at a rate greater than removal, whereas biomagnification is the gradual increase in metal concentrations with increasing trophic levels. Apex predators—predatory fish, birds of prey, and humans—tend to be most threatened through ingestion of toxic prey. Some examples include higher levels of mercury in tuna and cadmium in rice crops cultivated on polluted soils (Shaheen and Tsadilas, 2018).

- **Influence of environmental and biological factors**

  Metal bioavailability and transfer efficiency are influenced by environmental parameters (pH, temperature, dissolved organic matter) and biological traits (species-specific uptake mechanisms, feeding habits, metabolic rates). For instance, filter-feeding bivalves efficiently accumulate metals from water and sediment, serving as bioindicators of contamination (Saidon et al., 2024).

- **Environmental persistence and long-term risks**

  Unlike most organic pollutants, metals are not biodegradable. Once released, they exist in the environment forever, cycling continually among air, water, soil, and biota. Exposure risks may be minimized by environmental remediation, but eradication is seldom possible. Consequently, even temporary contamination incidents can have long-lasting toxicodynamic effects.Climate change also makes the environmental destiny of metals more complex. Thawing permafrost can release formerly sequestered metals into the ecosystems of the Arctic, while ocean acidification can shift metal speciation, and thus potentially enhance bioavailability to marine organisms. Such environmental alteration may reconfigure the distribution and toxicity profiles of metals and influence both human and ecological well-being (Cao et al., 2023; Ghosh et al., 2022).

2.3 Molecular mechanisms of metal toxicity

The toxicodynamic action of metals stems from their ability to engage with basic molecular targets in cells, causing disruption of structural integrity, interference with biochemical processes, and induction of pathological cascades of signals. The degree of interaction is mostly determined by the physicochemical characteristics of metals, such as ionic radius, redox potential, electro negativity, and specificity for certain functional groups. While some mechanisms are metal-specific, many converge on common pathways such as protein dysfunction, membrane damage, metabolic inhibition, and oxidative stress. Understanding these mechanisms is crucial for linking exposure to observed toxic outcomes and for identifying potential therapeutic interventions (Wu et al., 2016).

2.3.1 Interaction with proteins and enzymes

Proteins are the main targets for metal binding because of the availability of reactive side groups in amino acids like cysteine, histidine, aspartate, and glutamate. Thiol (-SH) groups of cysteine residues are especially vulnerable to covalent or coordinate bond formation with metals like mercury (Hg), cadmium (Cd), and arsenic (As) (Kumar et al., 2018).

2.3.2 Binding to enzyme active sites

Metals can displace essential metal cofactors (e.g., Zn^{2+}, Mg^{2+}, Fe^{2+}) from binding sites on metalloenzymes, causing a loss of enzymatic activity. For instance, lead (Pb^{2+}) displaces calcium or zinc in proteins like δ-aminolevulinic acid dehydratase (ALAD), which inhibits heme biosynthesis and causes anemia (Davidova et al., 2024).

2.3.3 Allosteric modulation and structural alteration

Metal binding to noncatalytic sites can provoke conformational changes that lower catalytic performance or destabilize protein structure. The binding of mercury to sulfhydryl groups in tubulin suppresses microtubule assembly, disabling neuronal transport systems (Huang et al., 2017).

2.3.4 Cross-linking and aggregation

Certain metals encourage aberrant protein cross-linking, producing insoluble cross-linked aggregates that are proteolytically resistant. Chromium (Cr^{6+}), following intracellular reduction, can bind stably to proteins, potentially initiating immune responses and chronic inflammation (Norris and Hobbs, 2020).

2.3.5 Metal–protein complexes and signaling disruption

Metals may disrupt receptor–ligand interactions or signaling cascades by modifying the conformation of membrane-bound receptors. Cadmium, for example, can activate estrogen receptors in a ligand-independent manner, which is a form of endocrine disruption (Moubarak et al., 2024).

2.3.6 Disruption of membrane integrity

Biological membranes are essential for cellular compartmentalization and electrochemical gradients. Metals can disrupt membrane function both directly by interacting with lipid bilayers and indirectly by causing oxidative damage (Duché and Sanderson, 2024).

2.3.7 Lipid–metal interactions

Cationic metals are able to bind with negatively charged phospholipid headgroups, changing membrane packing as well as fluidity. Aluminum (Al^{3+}) and lead (Pb^{2+}) can disrupt lipid bilayer structure, impacting ion permeability and membrane potential (Sun et al., 2022).

2.3.8 Oxidative damage to lipids

Redox-active metals (e.g., Fe^{2+}, Cu^{2+}, Cr^{6+}) catalyze lipid peroxidation through Fenton or Haber–Weiss reactions, producing reactive radicals that degrade polyunsaturated fatty acids in membranes. This results in membrane damage, leakage of cellular contents, and inhibition of membrane-bound enzymes (Cheng et al., 2021).

2.3.9 Disruption of membrane proteins

Membrane transporters, ion channels, and receptors can be modified by direct metal binding or by alterations in membrane fluidity. For instance, cadmium and mercury interfere with Na^+/K^+-ATPase activity, disrupting ionic homeostasis and contributing to neurotoxicity (Cheng et al., 2021).

2.3.10 Mitochondrial membrane damage

Mitochondria are especially sensitive to metal-induced membrane damage. Mitochondrial membrane potential loss resulting from lipid peroxidation or protein damage hinders ATP synthesis and may initiate apoptotic pathways through cytochrome *c* release (Gashkina, 2024).

2.3.11 Inhibition of metabolic pathways

Metals inhibit critical metabolic processes by acting against enzymes, cofactors, and electron transport systems, resulting in energy loss and cellular malfunction (Gashkina, 2024).

2.3.12 Energy metabolism

Several metals interfere with glycolysis, the tricarboxylic acid cycle, and oxidative phosphorylation:

- Arsenic (As^{3+}) substitutes for phosphate in ATP-generating reactions, producing unstable ADP-arsenate, which rapidly hydrolyzes, depleting energy reserves.
- Mercury (Hg^{2+}) and cadmium (Cd^{2+}) impair mitochondrial electron transport chain (ETC) complexes, reducing ATP output and increasing ROS production (Soladogun and Zhang, 2024).

2.3.13 Heme biosynthesis

Lead binds to ALAD and ferrochelatase, inhibiting the conversion of protoporphyrin IX to heme. Oxygen transport, ETC function are compromised (Soladogun and Zhang, 2024).

2.3.14 Neurotransmitter synthesis and degradation

Excess manganese (Mn^{2+}) inhibits enzymes such as tyrosine hydroxylase, impairing dopamine metabolism and leading to Parkinsonian symptoms (Soladogun and Zhang, 2024).

2.3.15 Hormonal and endocrine disruption

Certain metals replace or inhibit the actions of hormones. Cadmium's capacity to bind to estrogen receptors changes patterns of gene expression in hormone-sensitive tissues, whereas mercury interferes with thyroid hormone metabolism and transport (Chen et al., 2025).

2.3.16 Formation of reactive oxygen species and oxidative stress

Oxidative stress is a common mechanism in the toxicity of most metals. It is caused by an imbalance between ROS generation and antioxidant defense capacity, which leads to damage to DNA, proteins, and lipids (Chen et al., 2025).

2.3.17 Redox-active metals and ROs generation

Metals such as iron (Fe^{2+}/Fe^{3+}), copper (Cu^{+}/Cu^{2+}), and chromium (Cr^{3+}/Cr^{6+}) undergo redox cycling, catalyzing the conversion of hydrogen peroxide into highly reactive hydroxyl radicals via the Fenton reaction:

$$Fe^{2+} + H_2O_2 \rightarrow Fe^{3+} + OH^{-} + \cdot OH$$

These radicals initiate chain reactions of lipid peroxidation and oxidative DNA damage (Zhou et al., 2023).

2.3.18 Redox-inactive metals and antioxidant depletion

Redox-inactive metals like cadmium, mercury, and lead indirectly cause oxidative stress by depleting GSH and inhibiting antioxidant enzymes such as superoxide dismutase (SOD) and catalase (CAT), tilting the cellular redox balance in a pro-oxidant direction (Zhou et al., 2023).

2.3.19 DNA damage and genotoxicity

ROS damage DNA bases and the sugar-phosphate backbone, generating lesions like 8-oxo-2'-deoxyguanosine (8-oxo-dG) and single- or double-strand breaks. Chromium(VI) metabolites can also induce DNA–protein crosslinks, disrupting replication and repair (Wise and Wise, 2019).

2.3.20 Activation of pro-inflammatory pathways

Oxidative stress has been shown to activate transcription factors such as NF-κB and AP-1, which increase the expression of inflammatory cytokines, tumor necrosis factor-alpha (TNF-α), interleukin (IL-6), and adhesion molecules. This pro-inflammatory condition worsens tissue damage and contributes to the development of chronic diseases (Wise and Wise, 2019).

2.3.21 Mitochondrial ROS amplification

Damaged mitochondrial ETC components leak electrons to oxygen, generating superoxide radicals. This creates a vicious cycle in which mitochondrial dysfunction increases R–OS production, which, in turn, further damages mitochondrial proteins, lipids, and DNA (Wise and Wise, 2019).

2.3.22 Integrated mechanistic perspective

Although these molecular pathways are commonly characterized individually, they are very interconnected. For instance, metal binding by proteins can inhibit antioxidant enzymes, increasing oxidative stress, which in turn destroys membranes and blocks metabolic pathways. In the same way, membrane disintegration can damage ion gradients, further disrupting mitochondrial function and speeding up ROS production. The combined actions of these pathways lead to the development of sub cellular injury, frank cellular dysfunction, and eventually tissue and organ disease (Fig. 2.1) (Boniolo and Campaner, 2018).

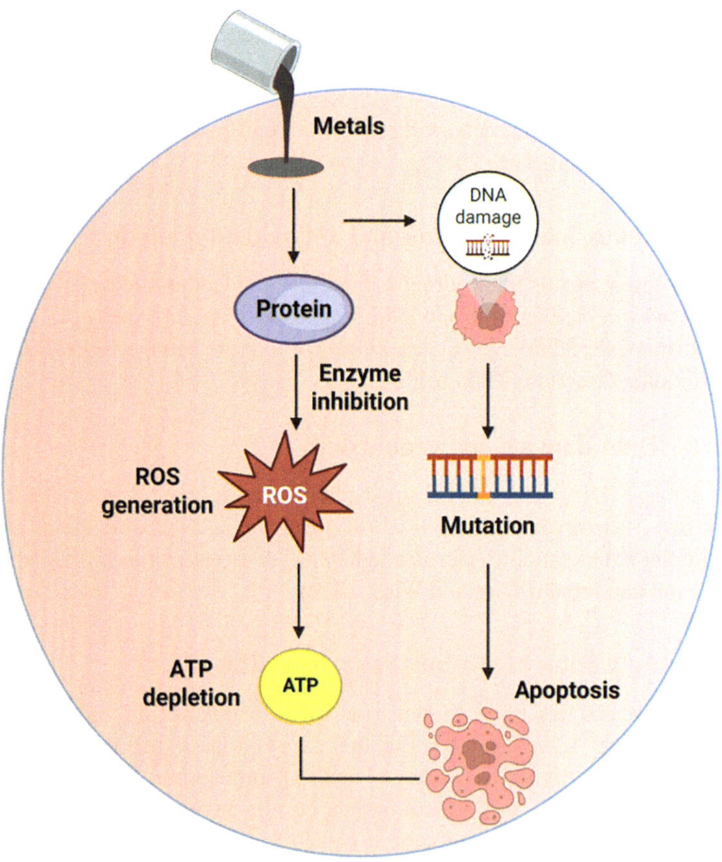

FIG. 2.1 Molecular mechanisms of metal toxicity.

2.4 Cellular responses to metal exposure

Although the molecular basis of metal toxicity determines the primary biochemical aberrations, the secondary cellular responses regulate the persistence, exaggeration, or alleviation of injury. After toxic metals bind to proteins, membranes, nucleic acids, and metabolic pathways, cells activate a variety of defensive and adaptive responses. When exposure exceeds these defense mechanisms, pathological effects such as organelle impairment, DNA damage, dysregulated signaling, and programmed cell death occur. These cell-level phenomena bridge the gap between submolecular interactions and tissue-level toxic effects (Sanders et al., 2023).

2.4.1 Bioaccumulation in cellular organelles

The distribution of metals in subcellular locations is important in determining the toxicity profiles of metals. Preferential accumulation of many metals in particular organelles results from electrochemical gradients, the specificity of transporters, or ligand interactions (Mititelu et al., 2025).

2.4.2 Mitochondria

Mitochondria are frequent targets because their negative membrane potential attracts cationic metal species. For example:

- Manganese (Mn^{2+}) accumulates in the mitochondrial matrix, impairing oxidative phosphorylation.
- Cadmium (Cd^{2+}) damages the mitochondrial permeability transition pore, triggering the loss of membrane potential and ATP collapse (Chowdhury and Rahman, 2024).

2.4.3 Lysosomes

Metals such as cobalt and nickel are sequestered in lysosomes via endocytosis or autophagic uptake. Lysosomal accumulation can lead to:

- Membrane permeabilization
- Release of cathepsins into the cytosol
- Initiation of apoptosis or necrosis (Chowdhury and Rahman, 2024)

2.4.4 Nucleus

A number of metals, such as chromium (Cr^{6+}) and arsenic (As^{3+}), easily interact with nuclear DNA or histone proteins, influencing gene expression and chromatin structure (Umapathi et al., 2022).

2.4.5 Endoplasmic reticulum

Lead (Pb^{2+}) and mercury (Hg^{2+}) interfere with endoplasmic reticulum (ER) calcium homeostasis, leading to ER stress and unfolded protein responses that can result in apoptosis (Umapathi et al., 2022).

2.4.6 DNA damage and genotoxicity

Genotoxicity is a crucial issue for metals since DNA damage can result in mutagenesis, carcinogenesis, or heritable effects (Umapathi et al., 2022).

2.4.7 Direct DNA binding

Platinum and chromium metals can directly bind to DNA bases through covalent adduct formation, blocking replication and transcription (Krawic and Zhitkovich, 2023).

2.4.8 Interference with DNA repair

Metals such as nickel and arsenic are known to inhibit DNA repair proteins like poly(ADP-ribose) polymerase and ligases. This results in the persistence of lesions, leading to an enhanced mutational burden (Krawic and Zhitkovich, 2023).

2.4.9 Epigenetic modifications

Exposure to metals results in global DNA hypomethylation or hypermethylation of specific promoter sequences, as observed in arsenic-induced suppression of tumor suppressor genes (Islam et al., 2022).

2.4.10 Disturbance of signaling pathways

Cellular signaling pathways are acutely sensitive to metal disturbances. Such disturbances can cause aberrant growth, inflammation, or apoptosis (Islam et al., 2022).

2.4.11 MAPK pathway activation

The MAPK cascades extracellular signal-regulated kinase (ERK), c-Jun N-terminal kinase (JNK) , and p38—are commonly activated by metal-induced oxidative stress. For example:

- Cadmium triggers JNK activation, promoting pro-apoptotic gene expression.
- Arsenic activates p38 MAPK, enhancing inflammatory cytokine production (Qu and Zheng, 2024).

2.4.12 NF-κB pathway

Metals such as lead and chromium activate NF-κB via IκB kinase signaling, leading to the transcription of pro-inflammatory mediators like IL-1β, TNF-α, and adhesion molecules (Qu and Zheng, 2024).

2.4.13 PI3K/Akt signaling

Certain metals, including nickel, abnormally activate the PI3K/Akt pathway and induce resistance to apoptosis in transformed cells and carcinogenesis (Qu and Zheng, 2024).

2.4.14 Calcium signaling disruption

Lead can substitute for calcium in neuronal cells, binding to calmodulin and altering neurotransmitter release and synaptic plasticity (Sukumaran et al., 2021).

2.4.15 Alterations in apoptosis and autophagy

Programmed cell death and autophagy machinery are strongly regulated to achieve homeostasis. Exposure to metals can tip this balance toward either unwanted cell death or the survival of injured cells (Sukumaran et al., 2021).

2.4.16 Apoptosis induction

Intrinsic (mitochondrial) pathway: Mercury and cadmium metals induce mitochondrial outer membrane permeabilization, leading to cytochrome *c* release and activation of caspase-9. Extrinsic pathway: Certain metals have the ability to sensitize cells to death receptor signaling through Fas/FasL or TNF receptor activation (Korotkov, 2023).

2.4.17 Apoptosis inhibition

Long-term low-dose exposure to some metals (e.g., arsenic) has been reported to inhibit apoptosis, permitting the survival of genomically unstable cells—a putative carcinogenic process (Korotkov, 2023).

2.4.18 Autophagy modulation

Metals are able to induce and inhibit autophagy:

- Induction: Cadmium induces autophagic vesicle formation as an adaptation to stress
- Blockade: Overload of copper can impair lysosomal degradative ability, leading to the accumulation of defective organelles (Korotkov, 2023)

2.5 Systemic and organ-specific toxicity

While molecular and cellular processes specify the inciting insult of metal exposure, the additive injury becomes apparent at the tissue and organ level, constituting clinically recognizable disease states. Organ tropism, characterized by a "preference" for accumulation and toxicity in specific organs, is a common feature of toxic metals and is influenced by variations in blood supply, transporter expression, metabolic rate, and detoxification capability. Table 2.1 outlines the primary organ systems involved, the principal toxic metals, mechanisms of injury, and representative clinical effects (Rieder et al., 2025) (Table 2.1).

The peripheral and central nervous systems are particularly sensitive to metal poisoning due to their high-oxygen-consumption rates, the lipid content of myelin sheaths, and their low intrinsic regenerative capacity. Metals impair neuronal integrity in a number of ways. Lead (Pb 2 +) is structurally similar to calcium ions and binds to proteins that affect neurotransmission

TABLE 2.1 Classification and examples of biomarkers (Santonen et al., 2022; Maćkiewicz et al., 2018; Molina-Villalba et al., 2015; Balali-Mood et al., 2021; Huang et al., 2025; Rerknimitr et al., 2019).

Organ/system	Key toxic metals	Primary mechanisms	Representative clinical outcomes
Nervous system	Lead, mercury, manganese, aluminum, arsenic	Disruption of Ca^{2+} signaling, mitochondrial dysfunction, myelin damage	Cognitive decline, learning deficits, tremors, and Parkinsonism-like symptoms
Liver	Arsenic, cadmium, copper, lead, mercury	Oxidative stress; mitochondrial injury; disruption of bile acid metabolism	Elevated liver enzymes, jaundice, fibrosis, and cirrhosis
Kidney	Cadmium, lead, mercury	Proximal tubule injury, glomerular damage, oxidative stress	Proteinuria, reduced GFR, and chronic kidney disease
Cardiovascular	Arsenic, cadmium, mercury, lead	Endothelial damage, myocardial oxidative stress, electrophysiological disturbances	Hypertension, atherosclerosis, arrhythmias
Immune System	Lead, mercury, arsenic, gold	T-cell suppression, autoimmunity induction, macrophage dysregulation	Increased infection risk, autoimmune exacerbation, and chronic inflammation

and calcium signaling. Manganese ($Mn2+$) and mercury ($Hg 2+$) disrupt the mitochondrial oxidative phosphorylation pathway, leading to lowered energy production in neurons, whereas aluminum and lead injure oligodendrocytes, causing them to demyelinate (Lin and Chen, 2023). These neurotoxic effects clinically manifest as symptoms of cognitive impairment, memory/learning deficits, Parkinsonism, motor impairment, and sensory disturbances, including tremors. The developing brain is especially vulnerable due to the absence of a complete blood-brain barrier and active synaptogenesis, making prenatal exposure particularly harmful. The liver is an important target of toxic metals as a key detoxifying organ with a high perfusion rate. Lipid peroxidation within hepatocyte membranes caused by arsenic and cadmium impairs structural stability, and in Wilson disease, caused by copper overload, ATP production by the mitochondria is impaired (**Reinhold and Rittner, 2017**). Lead and mercury affect the hepatic elimination of bile, which causes hepatic failure. The effects at the histopathological level include steatosis, fibrosis, cirrhosis, and hepatocellular necrosis. At the clinical level, these changes present as raised liver enzyme levels [alanine aminotransferase (ALT), aspartate aminotransferase (AST), alkaline phosphatase (ALP)], jaundice, and, with prolonged exposure, the development of chronic liver disease. The kidneys are among the most vulnerable organs, as they are involved in filtration and are constantly exposed to circulating metals. Cadmium binds strongly to metallothionein and accumulates in proximal tubular cells, where it induces lysosomal lysis, whereas lead contributes to the formation of immune-complex deposits in glomeruli, and mercury-mediated oxidative stress occurs in podocytes as well as tubular epithelial cells (**Forcella et al., 2022**). These disruptions contribute to proteinuria, the loss of β_2-microglobulin, and a decreased glomerular filtration rate (GFR), and subsequent progression to chronic kidney disease with continued exposure. The effects on the cardiovascular system include both direct (myocardial injury) and indirect (systemic alterations in vascular homeostasis) impacts. Arsenic and cadmium decrease nitric oxide availability, impairing vasodilation; mercury stimulates excessive production of ROS in the mitochondria of cardiomyocytes; and lead distorts cardiac ion channels, increasing the QT interval. These disturbances are associated with hypertension, atherosclerosis, arrhythmia, and a higher probability of heart attack. Metal-induced immune dysregulation is highly significant (**Bridle et al., 2021**). Lead and mercury inhibit T-cell proliferation and cytokine release, interfering with immune defense, while mercury and gold can break immunological tolerance and initiate autoimmune responses. Arsenic causes polarization of the macrophage balance in favor of a pro-inflammatory M1 phenotype, a factor that promotes low-grade chronic inflammation. Clinically, these immunotoxic effects are characterized by increased infection rates, enhanced autoimmune disease progression, and chronic inflammatory pathologies (Fig. 2.2) (**Li et al., 2023**).

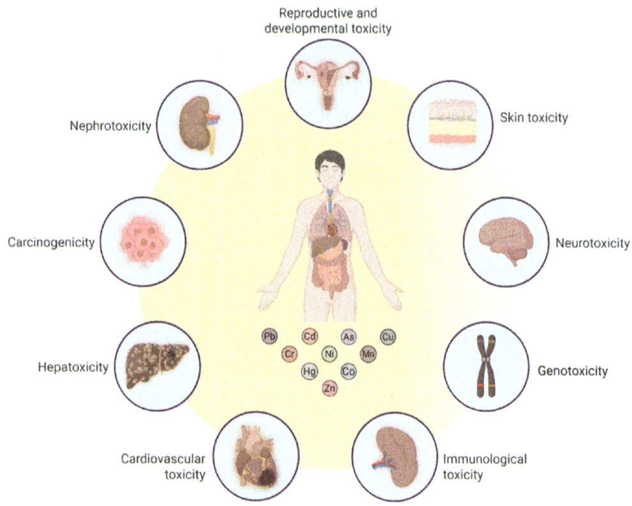

FIG. 2.2 An organ-specific toxicity map showing target organs for different metals.

2.5.1 Biomarkers of metal-induced toxicity

Biomarkers are quantifiable indicators of exposure, biological effects, or susceptibility to toxicants. For metal toxicodynamics, they establish an important link between mechanistic understanding and applications to clinical diagnosis, occupational risk, and environmental monitoring (Table 2.1). A good biomarker should be sensitive and specific, with a noninvasive methodology that detects early alterations before irreversible damage. Outside these general classes, cellular and 2′,7′-dichlorofluorescin diacetate (DCFH-DA) molecular biomarkers offer more mechanistic details (Table 2.2). Indicators of oxidative stress [e.g., ROS, malondialdehyde (MDA), 4-hydroxynonenal (4-HNE)], levels of antioxidant enzymes [(SOD, CAT, glutathione peroxidase (GPx)], and markers of DNA damage [comet assay, 8-hydroxy-2'-deoxyguanosine (8-OHdG)] represent quantifiable surrogates for subcellular metal-induced damage (Santonen et al., 2022; Vijiyakumar and Prince, 2024). Clinical biomarkers differ by organ system, like β_2-microglobulin and N-acetyl-beta-d-glucosaminidase (NAG) for renal damage, ALT/AST for hepatic damage, and alterations in nerve conduction velocity (NCV) for neurotoxicity. Ecotoxicological biomarkers, like metallothionein content in bivalves and induction of oxidative enzymes in fish gills, apply these uses to environmental monitoring (Andrade et al., 2017) (Table 2.2).

2.5.2 Molecular and cellular biomarkers

Markers of oxidative stress are sensitive indicators of early metal-induced injury. Excessive amounts of metals such as arsenic, cadmium, and mercury trigger an overreaction of ROS, overpowering cellular redox status. Indicators of ROS are

to trap mercury or arsenic and be removed from biological fluids with a magnet, or mesoporous silica nanoparticles could serve as vehicles to release chelators in a controlled-release manner. Nanozymes, such as cerium oxide nanoparticles with regenerative catalytic properties, mimic natural antioxidant enzymes to minimize ROS elicited by metals. Such solutions, however, have significant limitations, including potential nanotoxicity, the possibility of bioaccumulation, and regulatory obstacles before clinical translation (Muhammad et al., 2017; Rai et al., 2022).

2.6.5 Phytoremediation and environmental detoxification

Source-focused activities to prevent metal toxicity include ecosystem-level interventions. Currently, phytoremediation processes like phytoextraction, where plants like *Brassica juncea* and *Helianthus annuus* are used to accumulate metals in their biomass, and phytostabilization, where metals are immobilized so that they cannot enter water and cause contamination, can go a long way in helping to clean the soil and water of such contamination. Microbial bioremediation, through the use of metal-resistant bacteria (e.g., *Pseudomonas putida*) or fungi (e.g., *Aspergillus niger*), provides other means of bioaccumulation or biotransformation of metals into a less toxic form (Zhou et al., 2024).

2.6.6 Prevention policy-based prevention

At the population level, integrated regulation and surveillance will be necessary to restrict exposure. Screening of high-risk populations (miners and smelter workers) on a routine basis, as well as screening of water and food by the community and other sources, allows for early detection of contamination. Regulatory activities are important measures of prevention, including the enactment of permissible exposure limits, maximum contaminant levels, and the phasing out of toxic products like leaded fuels, mercury thermometers, and cadmium-based pigments. Risk communication, in the form of educating people about healthy fish consumption, occupational safety issues, and proper waste management procedures, goes a long way in reducing accidental exposure (Carter et al., 2024).

2.6.7 Integrative and future-oriented strategies

The next generation of metal detoxification emphasizes accuracy and individualization. Susceptibility screening genetic methods, such as metallothionein polymorphisms, can inform individualized therapy, including personalized antioxidant and/or chelation regimens. Combination treatments—such as the pairing of chelators and antioxidants or the sequencing of detoxification and rehabilitation treatments—will interlock advantages to combat both metal burden as well as oxidative stress. Future therapies, such as engineered metal-binding peptides, highly specific enzymes, and engineered gene therapy strategies to overcome downregulated endogenous detoxification pathways, have the potential to radically change the management of metal toxicity in the years to come (Aronica et al., 2022; Raza et al., 2022).

2.6.8 Future directions

Even with great progress in the conceptualization of metal toxicodynamics, important gaps continue to hamper the formulation of integrated risk assessments and effective interventions. One potential direction is to integrate multiomics technologies-genomics, transcriptomics, proteomics, and metabolomics-to create an integrated picture of metal–cell interactions and reveal molecular signatures of susceptibility (Gong et al., 2022). These datasets, if standardized and validated, may be the foundation for precision toxicology to allow focused preventive and therapeutic interventions. Computational modeling and predictive toxicology also have immense promise; in silico simulations and machine learning algorithms can predict metal behavior in biological systems, detect new exposure–disease associations, and inform regulatory choices. Nonetheless, the precision of such models is presently hampered by a lack of mechanistic information and the absence of rigorous validation against in vivo and human epidemiological data. Research in the future also needs to seek out sensitive and specific biomarkers that can identify metal exposure before the development of overt pathology (Ahmad et al., 2022). Specifically, epigenetic changes-DNA methylation and histone acetylation-constitute a novel category of biomarkers that could reflect the long-term biological signature of metal exposure. These must be validated in prospective studies to prove their predictive capacity. On the therapeutic side, there is an urgent need to develop chelating agents that are more selective for toxic metals relative to the essential micronutrients, as well as the development of innovations such as nanocarrier-based targeted drug delivery systems to damaged tissues. Gene-editing technologies, such as CRISPR, could ultimately provide a means to cure genetic vulnerabilities in at-risk populations of metal poisoning. Regulatory and public health-wise, conversion of mechanistic discoveries into actionable policy is still a challenge. Existing safety standards tend to understate the health hazards of chronic, low-dose exposures, and gaps remain in tracking metal contamination of the food chain, especially in low- and middle-income nations. Closing these gaps will demand greater integration of scientists, policymakers, and public health agencies, ensuring laboratory findings are implemented swiftly and effectively in real-world settings. In total, the following decade in metal toxicodynamics science ought to serve to bridge the gap between mechanistic knowledge and effective use, applying new technologies to inform prevention and protect both human and ecosystem health (Usmani et al., 2024).

2.7 Conclusion

Heavy metals are a long-standing global environmental and health hazard as a result of their nonbiodegradable nature, bioaccumulation, and multilevel toxicodynamic effects. This chapter has considered the molecular interaction of metals with cellular constituents, their systemic effects on human health, and the biomarkers and intervention strategies that can inform action. Metal toxicodynamics is a multiscale process—starting from molecular disturbance (protein binding, oxidative stress), moving through cellular reactions (DNA damage, disturbed signaling), and ending in organ-specific pathology. Knowledge of these pathways is not only crucial for successful treatment but also for the development of preventive policies that protect ecosystems and human populations. In the future, the convergence of multiomics technologies, computational prediction models, and precision medicine holds the promise to transform our capacity to detect, prevent, and treat metal toxicity. These advances, however, need to be complemented by strong regulatory systems and community-level interventions to provide equitable health protection. Ultimately, addressing the toxicodynamics of metals calls for a comprehensive approach—one that brings together scientific innovation, environmental stewardship, and public health dedication.

References

Abdallah, S.M., Muhammed, R.E., Mohamed, R.E., El Daous, H., Saleh, D.M., Ghorab, M.A., El-Sayyad, G.S., 2024. Assessment of biochemical biomarkers and environmental stress indicators in some freshwater fish. Environ. Geochem. Health 46 (11), 464.

Ahmad, A., Imran, M., Sharma, N., 2022. Precision nanotoxicology in drug development: current trends and challenges in safety and toxicity implications of customized multifunctional nanocarriers for drug-delivery applications. Pharmaceutics. 14 (11), 2463.

Ali, H., Khan, E., Ilahi, I., 2019. Environmental chemistry and ecotoxicology of hazardous heavy metals: environmental persistence, toxicity, and bioaccumulation. J. Chem. 2019 (1), 6730305.

Andrade, V.M., Aschner, M., Marreilha Dos Santos, A.P., 2017. Neurotoxicity of metal mixtures. Neurotox. Met. 10, 227–265.

Angon, P.B., Islam, M.S., Das, A., Anjum, N., Poudel, A., Suchi, S.A., 2024. Sources, effects and present perspectives of heavy metals contamination: soil, plants and human food chain. Heliyon. 10 (7), e28357.

Aronica, L., Ordovas, J.M., Volkov, A., Lamb, J.J., Stone, P.M., Minich, D., Bland, J.S., 2022. Genetic biomarkers of metabolic detoxification for personalized lifestyle medicine. Nutrients. 14 (4), 768.

Asamoah, R.B., Yaya, A., Nbelayim, P., Annan, E., Onwona-Agyeman, B., 2020. Development and characterization of clay–nanocomposites for water purification. Materials. 13 (17), 3793.

Awan, R.S., Liu, C., Yang, S., Wu, Y., Zang, Q., Khan, A., Li, G., 2021. The occurrence of vanadium in nature: its biogeochemical cycling and relationship with organic matter—a case study of the Early Cambrian black rocks of the Niutitang Formation, western Hunan, China. Acta Geochim. 40 (6), 973–997.

Balali-Mood, M., Naseri, K., Tahergorabi, Z., Khazdair, M.R., Sadeghi, M., 2021. Toxic mechanisms of five heavy metals: mercury, lead, chromium, cadmium, and arsenic. Front. Pharmacol. 12, 643972.

Ben, Y., Cheng, M., Liu, Y., Wang, X., Wang, L., Yang, Q., Zhou, Q., 2023. Biomarker changes and oxidative damage in living plant cells as new biomonitoring indicators for combined heavy metal stress assessment. Ecol. Indic. 154, 110784.

Boniolo, G., Campaner, R., 2018. Molecular pathways and the contextual explanation of molecular functions. Biol. Philos. 33 (3), 24.

Bridle, T.G., Kumarathasan, P., Gailer, J., 2021. Toxic metal species and 'endogenous' metalloproteins at the blood–organ interface: analytical and bioinorganic aspects. Molecules. 26 (11), 3408.

Cao, X., Lu, R., Xu, Q., Zheng, X., Zeng, Y., Mai, B., 2023. Distinct biomagnification of chlorinated persistent organic pollutants in adjacent aquatic and terrestrial food webs. Environ. Pollut. 317, 120841.

Carter, E.D., Stewart, D.E., Rees, E.E., Bezuidenhoudt, J.E., Ng, V., Lynes, S., Lee, A.C.K., 2024. Surveillance system integration: reporting the results of a global multicountry survey. Public Health. 231, 31–38.

Chen, L., Shen, Q., Liu, Y., Zhang, Y., Sun, L., Ma, X., Xie, J., 2025. Homeostasis and metabolism of iron and other metal ions in neurodegenerative diseases. Signal Transduct. Target. Ther. 10 (1), 31.

Cheng, H., Yang, B., Ke, T., Li, S., Yang, X., Aschner, M., Chen, P., 2021. Mechanisms of metal-induced mitochondrial dysfunction in neurological disorders. Toxics. 9 (6), 142.

Chowdhury, F.N., Rahman, M.M., 2024. Source and distribution of heavy metal and their effects on human health. In: Heavy Metal Toxicity: Human Health Impact and Mitigation Strategies. Springer Nature Switzerland, Cham, pp. 45–98.

Davidova, S., Milushev, V., Satchanska, G., 2024. The mechanisms of cadmium toxicity in living organisms. Toxics. 12 (12), 875.

Depledge, M.H., 2020. The rational basis for the use of biomarkers as ecotoxicological tools. In: Nondestructive Biomarkers in Vertebrates. CRC Press. pp. 271–295.

Donaher, S.E., Van den Hurk, P., 2023. Ecotoxicology of the herbicide paraquat: effects on wildlife and knowledge gaps. Ecotoxicology. 32 (9), 1187–1199.

Duché, G., Sanderson, J.M., 2024. The chemical reactivity of membrane lipids. Chem. Rev. 124 (6), 3284–3330.

Feng, X., Li, P., Fu, X., Wang, X., Zhang, H., Lin, C.J., 2022. Mercury pollution in China: implications on the implementation of the Minamata Convention. Environ. Sci. Process. Impacts 24 (5), 634–648.

Fomina, M., Skorochod, I., 2020. Microbial interaction with clay minerals and its environmental and biotechnological implications. Minerals. 10 (10), 861.

Forcella, M., Lau, P., Fabbri, M., Fusi, P., Oldani, M., Melchioretto, P., Urani, C., 2022. Is cadmium toxicity tissue-specific? Toxicogenomics studies reveal common and specific pathways in pulmonary, hepatic, and neuronal cell models. Int. J. Mol. Sci. 23 (3), 1768.

Gao, Y., 2024. Application of toxicokinetic–toxicodynamic models in the aquatic ecological risk assessment of metals: a review. Environ. Toxicol. Pharmacol. 110, 104511.

Gashkina, N.A., 2024. Metal toxicity: effects on energy metabolism in fish. Int. J. Mol. Sci. 25 (9), 5015.

Ghosh, D., Ghosh, A., Bhadury, P., 2022. Arsenic through aquatic trophic levels: effects, transformations and biomagnification—a concise review. Geosci. Lett. 9 (1), 20.

Gong, B., Qiu, H., Romero-Freire, A., Van Gestel, C.A., He, E., 2022. Incorporation of chemical and toxicological availability into metal mixture toxicity modeling: state of the art and future perspectives. Crit. Rev. Environ. Sci. Technol. 52 (10), 1730–1772.

Goutam Mukherjee, A., Ramesh Wanjari, U., Eladl, M.A., El-Sherbiny, M., Elsherbini, D.M.A., Sukumar, A., Valsala Gopalakrishnan, A., 2022. Mixed contaminants: occurrence, interactions, toxicity, detection, and remediation. Molecules. 27 (8), 2577.

Gulcin, İ., Alwasel, S.H., 2022. Metal ions, metal chelators and metal chelating assay as antioxidant method. Processes. 10 (1), 132.

Hernández-Jerez, A., Hougaard Bennekou, S., Hoogenboom, L., Mcardle, H., Pieper, C., Farcal, L., European Food Safety Authority (EFSA), 2024. Conceptual basis for the development of guidance for the use of biomarkers of effect in regulatory risk assessment of chemicals. EFSA J. 22 (12), e9153.

Huang, M., Li, H., Chen, J., Li, L., Zhan, Y., Du, Y., Lai, D., 2025. Blood lead levels and bladder cancer among US participants: NHANES 1999–2018. BMC Public Health. 25 (1), 416.

Huang, Y.W., Cambre, M., Lee, H.J., 2017. The toxicity of nanoparticles depends on multiple molecular and physicochemical mechanisms. Int. J. Mol. Sci. 18 (12), 2702.

Islam, R., Zhao, L., Wang, Y., Lu-Yao, G., Liu, L.Z., 2022. Epigenetic dysregulations in arsenic-induced carcinogenesis. Cancers. 14 (18), 4502.

Jin, X., Wu, Q., Peñuelas, J., Sardan, J., Peng, Y., Li, Z., Yue, K., 2025. Climate and anthropogenic activities control the concentrations of copper, zinc, cadmium and chromium in global inland waters. Commun. Earth Environ. 6 (1), 520.

Kar, S., 2022. Geochemical characteristics of mineral elements: arsenic, fluorine, lead, nitrogen, and carbon. In: Structure and Functions of Pedosphere. Springer Nature Singapore, Singapore, pp. 209–254.

Khan, A.M., Bakar, N.K.A., Bakar, A.F.A., Ashraf, M.A., 2017. Chemical speciation and bioavailability of rare earth elements (REEs) in the ecosystem: a review. Environ. Sci. Pollut. Res. 24 (29), 22764–22789.

Kim, J.J., Kim, Y.S., Kumar, V., 2019. Heavy metal toxicity: an update of chelating therapeutic strategies. J. Trace Elem. Med. Biol. 54, 226–231.

Korotkov, S.M., 2023. Mitochondrial oxidative stress is the general reason for apoptosis induced by different-valence heavy metals in cells and mitochondria. Int. J. Mol. Sci. 24 (19), 14459.

Krawic, C., Zhitkovich, A., 2023. Chemical mechanisms of DNA damage by carcinogenic chromium (VI). In: Advances in Pharmacology, vol. 96. Academic Press, pp. 25–46.

Kumar, A., Singh, N., Pandey, R., Gupta, V.K., Sharma, B., 2018. Biochemical and molecular targets of heavy metals and their actions. In: Biomedical Applications of Metals. Springer International Publishing, Cham, pp. 297–319.

Lachowicz, J.I., Lecca, L.I., Meloni, F., Campagna, M., 2021. Metals and metal-nanoparticles in human pathologies: from exposure to therapy. Molecules. 26 (21), 6639.

Li, H., Santos, F., Butler, K., Herndon, E., 2021. A critical review on the multiple roles of manganese in stabilizing and destabilizing soil organic matter. Environ. Sci. Technol. 55 (18), 12136–12152.

Li, T., Roberts, R., Liu, Z., Tong, W., 2023. TransOrGAN: an artificial intelligence mapping of rat transcriptomic profiles between organs, ages, and sexes. Chem. Res. Toxicol. 36 (6), 916–925.

Lin, X., Chen, T., 2023. A review of in vivo toxicity of quantum dots in animal models. Int. J. Nanomed. 18, 8143–8168.

Liu, L., Wang, J., Zhai, J., Yan, D., Lin, Z., 2024. Regional disparities and technological approaches in heavy metal remediation: a comprehensive analysis of soil contamination in Asia. Chemosphere. 366, 143485.

López-Armada, M.J., Fernández-Rodríguez, J.A., Blanco, F.J., 2022. Mitochondrial dysfunction and oxidative stress in rheumatoid arthritis. Antioxidants. 11 (6), 1151.

Lu, C., Yang, T., Meng, X., Yang, X., 2025. Toxicodynamics of chemical mixtures exposure in the organism body. Toxicol. Assess. Comb. Chem. Environ. 18, 29–46.

Maćkiewicz, E., Pawlaczyk, A., Szynkowska, M.I., 2018. Trace elements in the environment–law, regulations, monitoring and biomonitoring methods. Recent Adv. Trace Elem. 18, 61–104.

Mahimairaja, S., Bolan, N.S., Adriano, D.C., Robinson, B., 2005. Arsenic contamination and its risk management in complex environmental settings. Adv. Agron. 86, 1–82.

Marrocco, I., Altieri, F., Peluso, I., 2017. Measurement and clinical significance of biomarkers of oxidative stress in humans. Oxid. Med. Cell. Longev. 2017 (1), 6501046.

Martínez-Alcalá, I., Bernal, M.P., 2020. Environmental impact of metals, metalloids, and their toxicity. Metalloids Plants: Adv. Future Prospect. 18, 451–488.

Mititelu, M., Neacşu, S.M., Busnatu, Ş.S., Scafa-Udrişte, A., Andronic, O., Lăcraru, A.E., Olteanu, G., 2025. Assessing heavy metal contamination in food: implications for human health and environmental safety. Toxics. 13 (5), 333.

Molina-Villalba, I., Lacasaña, M., Rodríguez-Barranco, M., Hernández, A.F., Gonzalez-Alzaga, B., Aguilar-Garduño, C., Gil, F., 2015. Biomonitoring of arsenic, cadmium, lead, manganese and mercury in urine and hair of children living near mining and industrial areas. Chemosphere. 124, 83–91.

More, S.J., Bampidis, V., Benford, D., Bragard, C., Halldorsson, T.I., Leblanc, J.C., EFSA Scientific Committee, 2023. Re-evaluation of the existing health-based guidance values for copper and exposure assessment from all sources. EFSA J. 21 (1), e07728.

Moubarak, M.M., Pagano Zottola, A.C., Larrieu, C.M., Cuvellier, S., Daubon, T., Martin, O.C., 2024. Exploring the multifaceted role of NRF2 in brain physiology and cancer: a comprehensive review. Neurooncol. Adv. 6 (1), vdad160.

Muchowska, K.B., Varma, S.J., Chevallot-Beroux, E., Lethuillier-Karl, L., Li, G., Moran, J., 2017. Metals promote sequences of the reverse Krebs cycle. Nat. Ecol. Evol. 1 (11), 1716–1721.

Muhammad, F., Nguyen, T.D.T., Raza, A., Akhtar, B., Aryal, S., 2017. A review on nanoparticle-based technologies for biodetoxification. Drug Chem. Toxicol. 40 (4), 489–497.

Nieder, R., Benbi, D.K., Reichl, F.X., 2018. Role of potentially toxic elements in soils. In: Soil Components and Human Health. Springer Netherlands, Dordrecht, pp. 375–450.

Norris, D.O., Hobbs, S.L., 2020. The HPA axis and functions of corticosteroids in fishes. In: Fish Endocrinology, vol. 2. CRC Press. pp. 721–765.

Obert, L.A., Elmore, S.A., Ennulat, D., Frazier, K.S., 2021. A review of specific biomarkers of chronic renal injury and their potential application in nonclinical safety assessment studies. Toxicol. Pathol. 49 (5), 996–1023.

Oros, A., Coatu, V., Damir, N., Danilov, D., Ristea, E., Lazar, L., 2025. Molecular mechanisms and biomarker-based early-warning indicators of heavy metal toxicity in marine fish. Fishes. 10 (7), 339.

Padoan, F., Piccoli, E., Pietrobelli, A., Moreno, L.A., Piacentini, G., Pecoraro, L., 2024. The role of zinc in developed countries in pediatric patients: a 360° view. Biomolecules. 14 (6), 718.

Qu, F., Zheng, W., 2024. Cadmium exposure: mechanisms and pathways of toxicity and implications for human health. Toxics. 12 (6), 388.

Rai, S., Guin, M., De, A., Singh, N.B., 2022. Functionalized nanomaterials: basics, properties and applications. In: Functionalized Nanomaterials for Corrosion Mitigation: Synthesis, Characterization, and Applications. American Chemical Society. pp. 27–66.

Ranaweera, D., Kumarasinghe, U., Senanayake, C., Dassanayake, R.S., Bandara, P.C., Koliyabandara, P.A., 2023. Biogeochemistry: essential link between geosphere and biosphere. Med. Geol.: En Route One Health 18, 37–54.

Raza, A., Tabassum, J., Zahid, Z., Charagh, S., Bashir, S., Barmukh, R., Varshney, R.K., 2022. Advances in "omics" approaches for improving toxic metals/metalloids tolerance in plants. Front. Plant Sci. 12, 794373.

Reinhold, A.K., Rittner, H.L., 2017. Barrier function in the peripheral and central nervous system—a review. Pflugers Arch. Eur. J. Physiol. 469 (1), 123–134.

Rerknimitr, P., Kantikosum, K., Chottawornsak, N., Tangkijngamvong, N., Kerr, S.J., Prueksapanich, P., Panchaprateep, R., 2019. Chronic occupational exposure to lead leads to significant mucocutaneous changes in lead factory workers. J. Eur. Acad. Dermatol. Venereol. 33 (10), 1993–2000.

Rieder, F., Nagy, L.E., Maher, T.M., Distler, J.H., Kramann, R., Hinz, B., Prunotto, M., 2025. Fibrosis: cross-organ biology and pathways to development of innovative drugs. Nat. Rev. Drug Discov. 24, 1–27.

Ro, S.H., Bae, J., Jang, Y., Myers, J.F., Chung, S., Yu, J., Song, H.S., 2022. Arsenic toxicity on metabolism and autophagy in adipose and muscle tissues. Antioxidants. 11 (4), 689.

Saidon, N.B., Szabó, R., Budai, P., Lehel, J., 2024. Trophic transfer and biomagnification potential of environmental contaminants (heavy metals) in aquatic ecosystems. Environ. Pollut. 340, 122815.

Sanders, B.M., Goering, P.L., Jenkins, K., 2023. The role of general and metal-specific cellular responses in protection and repair of metal-induced damage. stress proteins and metallothioneins. In: Toxicology of Metals, vol. I. CRC Press. pp. 165–187.

Santonen, T., Schoeters, G., Nordberg, M., 2022. Biological monitoring of metals and biomarkers. In: Handbook on the Toxicology of Metals, vol. 17. Academic Press. pp. 217–235.

Schrenk, D., Bignami, M., Bodin, L., Chipman, J.K., Del Mazo, J., Nielsen, E., EFSA Panel on Contaminants in the Food Chain (CONTAM), 2020. Update of the risk assessment of nickel in food and drinking water. EFSA J. 18 (11), e06268.

Seyfried, T.N., Chinopoulos, C., 2021. Can the mitochondrial metabolic theory explain better the origin and management of cancer than can the somatic mutation theory? Metabolites. 11 (9), 572.

Shaheen, S.M., Tsadilas, C.D., 2018. Influence of phosphates on fractionation, mobility, and bioavailability of soil metal (loid) s. In: Phosphate in Soils. CRC Press. pp. 186–219.

Skalnaya, M.G., Skalny, A.V., 2018. Essential Trace Elements in Human Health: A Physician's View, vol. 224. Publishing House of Tomsk State University, Tomsk, pp. 1–222.

Soladogun, A.S., Zhang, L., 2024. The neural palette of heme: altered heme homeostasis underlies defective neurotransmission, increased oxidative stress, and disease pathogenesis. Antioxidants. 13 (12), 1441.

Sonke, J.E., Angot, H., Zhang, Y., Poulain, A., Björn, E., Schartup, A., 2023. Global change effects on biogeochemical mercury cycling. Ambio. 52 (5), 853–876.

Srivastava, S., 2016. Emerging therapeutic roles for NAD+ metabolism in mitochondrial and age-related disorders. Clin. Transl. Med. 5 (1), 25.

Sukumaran, P., Nascimento Da Conceicao, V., Sun, Y., Ahamad, N., Saraiva, L.R., Selvaraj, S., Singh, B.B., 2021. Calcium signaling regulates autophagy and apoptosis. Cells. 10 (8), 2125.

Sun, Q., Li, Y., Shi, L., Hussain, R., Mehmood, K., Tang, Z., Zhang, H., 2022. Heavy metals induced mitochondrial dysfunction in animals: molecular mechanism of toxicity. Toxicology. 469, 153136.

Tyagi, S., Dhiman, V.K., Dhiman, V.K., Pandey, H., Singh, D., Sharma, A., Saharan, B.S., 2024. Plant defense strategies and biomarkers against heavy metal-induced stress: a comprehensive review. ACS Agric. Sci. Technol. 4 (2), 129–143.

Umapathi, A., Kumawat, M., Daima, H.K., 2022. Engineered nanomaterials for biomedical applications and their toxicity: a review. Environ. Chem. Lett. 20 (1), 445–468.

Unsal, V., Dalkıran, T., Çiçek, M., Kölükçü, E., 2020. The role of natural antioxidants against reactive oxygen species produced by cadmium toxicity: a review. Adv. Pharm. Bull. 10 (2), 184.

Usmani, S.M., Bremer-Hoffmann, S., Cheyns, K., Cubadda, F., Dumit, V.I., Escher, S.E., Haase, A., 2024. Review of new approach methodologies for application in risk assessment of nanoparticles in the food and feed sector: status and challenges. EFSA Support. Publ. 21 (9), 8826E.

Velugolu, V.S.K., Kumar, P., 2025. The role of chelation therapy in heavy metal detoxification. In: Heavy Metal Toxicity and Neurodegeneration. Academic Press. pp. 449–459.

Vijiyakumar, N., Prince, S.E., 2024. A comprehensive review of cadmium-induced toxicity, signalling pathways, and potential mitigation strategies. Toxicol. Environ. Health Sci. 17, 1–16.

Wise, S.S., Wise, J.P., 2019. Metal carcinogenesis and DNA damage: a case study using hexavalent chromium. In: Carcinogens, DNA Damage and Cancer Risk: Mechanisms of Chemical Carcinogenesis. pp. 171–208.

Wu, X., Cobbina, S.J., Mao, G., Xu, H., Zhang, Z., Yang, L., 2016. A review of toxicity and mechanisms of individual and mixtures of heavy metals in the environment. Environ. Sci. Pollut. Res. 23 (9), 8244–8259.

Zhang, B., Zhang, H., He, J., Zhou, S., Dong, H., Rinklebe, J., Ok, Y.S., 2023. Vanadium in the environment: biogeochemistry and bioremediation. Environ. Sci. Technol. 57 (39), 14770–14786.

Zhang, W.R., Parikh, C.R., 2019. Biomarkers of acute and chronic kidney disease. Annu. Rev. Physiol. 81 (1), 309–333.

Zhao, F.J., Tang, Z., Song, J.J., Huang, X.Y., Wang, P., 2022. Toxic metals and metalloids: uptake, transport, detoxification, phytoremediation, and crop improvement for safer food. Mol. Plant 15 (1), 27–44.

Zhou, H., Peng, J., Duan, X., Yin, H., Huang, B., Zhou, C., Lai, B., 2023. Redox-active polymers as robust electron-shuttle co-catalysts for fast Fe3+/Fe2+ circulation and green Fenton oxidation. Environ. Sci. Technol. 57 (8), 3334–3344.

Zhou, Y., Ding, D., Zhao, Y., Li, Q., Jiang, D., Lv, Z., Deng, S., 2024. Determining priority control toxic metal for different protection targets based on source-oriented ecological and human health risk assessment around gold smelting area. J. Hazard. Mater. 468, 133782.

Zitoun, R., Marcinek, S., Hatje, V., Sander, S.G., Völker, C., Sarin, M., Omanović, D., 2024. Climate change driven effects on transport, fate and biogeochemistry of trace element contaminants in coastal marine ecosystems. Commun. Earth Environ. 5 (1), 560.

Chapter 3

Geochemical and anthropogenic sources of metal contaminants

Akshay Botle[a], Sayli Salgaonkar[a], Rahul Tiwari[b], Divyanka Thakur[a], and Gayatri Barabde[a]

[a]*Department of Environmental Science, The Institute of Science, Dr. Homi Bhabha State University, Mumbai, India*

[b]*Department of Chemistry Institute of Basic Science, Dr B. R. Ambedkar University, Agra, India*

3.1 Introduction

The environmental impact of various toxins has been investigated in numerous studies (Botle et al., 2023; Taghavi et al., 2022). The environment is polluted with chemicals in higher concentrations than elsewhere. Industrialization has grown quickly over the past 100 years (Ali et al., 2023). Environmental matrices contain toxins that can harm terrestrial and aquatic life (Ali et al., 2021). The primary environmental contaminants are organic and inorganic. Mills that generate paint, paper, textiles, and other products release organic pollutants like methylene blue. Major pollutants include "polycyclic aromatic hydrocarbons (PAHs)", "pesticides", "bisphenol A", "phthalate esters", "per-fluorinated compounds", "organic phosphate flame retardants", "micro-nanoplastics", and others (Ahmad et al., 2021; Ali et al., 2018; Clarke and Smith, 2011; Salgaonkar et al., 2024) (F.; Botlee et al., 2024). Moreover, nonbiodegradable inorganic pollutants cannot be easily eliminated from the environment (Taghavi et al., 2022). Radionuclides and heavy metal (HM) ions are inorganic pollutants, which harm the environment and living beings due to their carcinogenicity and toxicity (Bakshe and Jugade, 2023). Some metals, especially nanoscale ones, are poisonous at the smallest concentrations, whereas others are dangerous at critical concentrations (Ajdary et al., 2018; Ma et al., 2015; Sharma, 2015).

"HMs" are crucial to life but hazardous when they accumulate in living beings (Ponce-Hernández et al., 2025). A "HM" is a metal or metalloid with an atomic density (>4 g/cm^3), five times that of water (Iqbal et al., 2024). HMs are toxic metalloids and chemical components (Ali et al., 2023; Botle et al., 2025a). Three classes of metals and metalloid ions exist. Pb, Hg, and Cd are harmful at low quantities, consisting of the first group (Zaynab et al., 2022).

The Metallome in Motion. https://doi.org/10.1016/B978-0-443-44299-5.00002-X

The second group consists of Sb, As, Bi, In, and Tl, which are less harmful, while the third group includes Co, Cu, Zn, Fe, and Se, which are essential and only toxic above a specific concentration (Odobašić et al., 2019). Toxic lighter metals and metalloids include Al, Se, and As (Arora, 2019). Cu, Co, Fe, Ni, Au, Mn, Pd, Ag, Mo, Zn, Pt, and W are naturally occurring HMs that are less harmful (Roy et al., 2024), while As, Cd, Hg, Cr, and Pb are harmful (Nagajyoti et al., 2010). Environmental bioaccumulation, chronic toxicity, and nonbiodegradability make HMs dangerous environmental contaminants. Food chains can transmit and biomagnify HMs, endangering human health (Zaynab et al., 2022).

HMs cannot be chemically or biologically reduced like organic contaminants. They can only be converted into less hazardous species, such as Hg^{2+} to Hg°, As^{3+} to As^{5+}, and Cr^{6+} to Cr^{3+} (Priyadarshanee and Das, 2021). As a result, effective monitoring and surveillance of marine HM concentrations are also desired (Ahmed et al., 2015). HM concentrations originate from environmental sources, and their distribution is causing impacts on national, regional, and local levels (Ma et al., 2019). Most organisms' lives are significantly influenced by the bioaccumulation patterns of HMs such as As, Cu, Cr, Cd, Hg, Co, and Ni (Z. (Rahman and Singh, 2019). Examples of HM contamination limits (mg/L): Cd 0.005, Cr 0.1, Sb 0.006, As 0.05, Pb 0.015, Hg 0.002, Se 0.05 (Rasheed et al., 2022). Toxic HM concentrations harm ecological niches, nutrition, evolution, and ecology (Ponce-Hernández et al., 2025). Five million sites worldwide contain 0.5 billion hectares of soil tainted with metals or metalloids like Hg, Cu, Cr, Cd, Zn, As, Se, Pb, Ni, and Co (Li et al., 2019). However, surface water bodies worldwide have exceeded WHO standards for metals and metalloids such as As, Cr, Ni, Co, Cd, and Mn. As a result, the term HM has been highly discussed among the scientific community (Ponce-Hernández et al., 2025). The pervasive presence of HMs is intriguing (Munir et al., 2021). Due to their widespread usage, toxic metals pollute the environment (Duruibe et al., 2007). Large amounts of toxic metals occur in the environment. HMs in the human skeleton and fatty tissues deplete nutrients and cause cardiac, gastric, central nervous system deficits, neurodevelopmental, immune, reproductive, hepatocellular, renal, hematological, and intrauterine retardation (El-Kady and Abdel-Wahhab, 2018). Thus, this chapter explores geochemical (natural) and anthropogenic (human-induced) sources of metal contamination in the environment, highlights key pathways of metal transport and transformation, and their ecological implications, such as bioaccumulation, biomagnification, and toxicity to biota. It also determines analytical tools and techniques and mitigation and management strategies, such as source control and re-use.

3.2 Geochemical sources of metal contamination

3.2.1 Natural weathering of rocks and minerals

The geochemistry of elements during rock weathering significantly affects soil and sediment formation, evolution, and chemical composition. The fundamental minerals in bedrock break down during chemical weathering, activating and redistributing several elements (Nesbitt and Wilson, 1992; Wu et al., 2021). Metals enter the environment via geochemical processes, including rock and mineral weathering. The breakdown and modification of parent rocks, such as basalts, granites, and ultramafic lithologies, mobilize and transfer trace elements and HMs to soils, sediments, and waterways (Li et al., 2019). The chemical disintegration of minerals releases some of their component elements in soluble forms and generates new (secondary) minerals via chemical interactions between weathering products (Alloway, 2012). Parent material, soil formation methods, environment, and physical-chemical qualities controlled how soil weathering affected HM distribution (Cao and Ikeda, 2000; Nosrati and Collins, 2019). For instance, soil HMs came mostly from parent rock components. However, weathering rate and degree depended on source rock mineral composition, which diluted and enriched soil metals (Zhang and Wang, 2020).

Over 99% of the Earth's crust comprises 10 "major" elements: oxygen, silicon, aluminum, iron, calcium, sodium, potassium (K), magnesium (Mg), phosphorus, and titanium (Ti). The periodic table's remaining elements are called "trace elements" and make up just 1% of the Earth's crust (Alloway, 2012). Identifying human and natural influences on sediment element content is crucial (Loring and Rantala, 1992; Selvaraj et al., 2010). Sedimentary geochemical composition is vital for environmental monitoring and ecosystem evaluation because it is sensitive and dependable at recording natural and anthropogenic components at detectable quantities. Thus, sediment and sedimentary rock geochemistry may reveal weathering patterns and contamination sources (Li et al., 2019). Sulfide deposits and other weathering products pollute ecosystems with HMs (Wu et al., 2021). Basalt contains readily weathered primary mafic silicate minerals such as biotite, olivine, pyroxene, hornblende, feldspar, and glassy groundmass. Transition metals, including Cu, Mn, Pb, V, Co, Zn, Cr, and Ni, are abundant in these minerals (Alloway, 2012; Gislason and Arnórsson, 1993). Since basalt weathers faster than acidic intrusive rocks, soluble components like Mg, Ca and Na are swiftly leached, enriching Fe, Al, and Si (Chorover et al., 2004; Eggleton et al., 1987). Thus, basalt weathering creates fertile soils rich in Fe–Al oxides, but transition metal elements like Co, Cr, Zn, Mn, Ni, and V might pose an environmental problem. Kinetic variables like temperature and runoff govern rock weathering, and the geochemical behavior of transition elements in basalt-weathered soil and sediments has been studied (Wu et al., 2021).

3.2.2 Volcanic activity

More than 2.9 crore people reside within 10 km of active volcanoes, and around 80 crore dwell within 100 km (2011 population statistics), potentially exposing them to environmental and air pollution concerns from gas- and particulate-rich eruptions (Ilyinskaya et al., 2021). HM tainting from volcanic eruptions and associated phenomena is released in gaseous form and dispersed into the atmosphere and oceans (Torres et al., 2023) or deposited on the ground through pyroclastic or ash erosion and weathering. Volcanic activity demonstrates substantial crustal displacement and the Earth's dynamic behavior (Fabricio Neta et al., 2018). Although volcanic eruptions are short-lived, their ash and pyroclastic debris may persist in the surrounding environment for months, decades, or even millions of years, affecting areas hundreds of kilometers away (Ma et al., 2019).

Soil, the major biogeochemical system component, acts as both a source and a sink for contaminants (Pinto et al., 2015). Thus, it helps store and circulate contaminants (Forghani et al., 2019). Environmental and parent rock parameters affect pedological processes (Grison et al., 2015). The parent material determines the soil's metal concentration (Zhang et al., 2018), and most metals accumulate after decomposition and volcanic activity (Adumitroaei et al., 2018), resulting in high baseline metal concentrations in volcanic soil (Memoli et al., 2018). Ash and pyroclastic debris from significant volcanic eruptions include nutrients such as calcium, magnesium, phosphorus, nitrogen, sodium, and potassium, as well as poisonous elements and metalloids (Ermolin et al., 2018). Cu, Fe, Mn, and Zn, which are needed for plant biology, may be disseminated by volcanic ash, but excess quantities can disrupt physiological processes and induce toxicity. The biosphere may also collect nonessential hazardous elements, including Hg, Pb, As, and Cd, in volcanic ash (Carrera-Beltrán et al., 2024).

3.3 Anthropogenic sources of metal contamination

Industrialization has increased soil, water, and air pollution in recent years. HM tainting occurrences have grown dramatically, resulting in large amounts of HMs entering the environment quickly and causing substantial harm (Vareda et al., 2019). HMs are one of the most harmful contaminants in air, water, and soil and are difficult to biodegrade (He et al., 2019). They primarily arise from HM mining and processing, industrial and car waste discharged into rivers, or penetrating the soil through rain. Inhalation, nutrition, and skin contact may transfer HMs from the environment into the food chain and back into the body, posing a serious health risk (Jin et al., 2020). Anthropogenic sources of HMs are presented in (Fig. 3.1).

3.3.1 Mining and smelting operations

The increased usage of complex metals has raised environmental and toxicological concerns (Egorova and Ananikov, 2017). Rapid mining expansion has worsened landscape alterations and environmental contamination (Demková et al., 2017). Ma et al. (2015) reported that excessive mineral extraction has accumulated waste in piles or tailings. Tailings ponds, waste rock dumps, open pits, and other mining facilities harm the land during metal ore extraction and enrichment (Kapusta and Sobczyk, 2015). Mining, transportation, and mineral

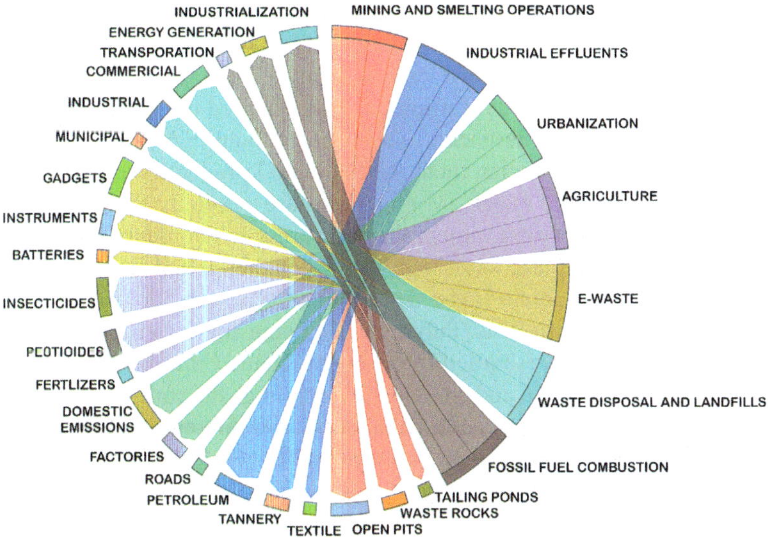

FIG. 3.1 Anthropogenic sources of HM's.

concentration release contaminants, including trace elements, into the environment, compromising the productivity, ecology, and habitat security of mining areas (Li et al., 2019). The metallurgical industry, particularly smelting, impacts the environment through airborne emissions from point sources. Researchers aim to understand stress-induced environmental changes along the pollution gradient (Kapusta and Sobczyk, 2015). Likewise, gold mining wastes originate from metallurgical extraction, mineral processing, and mining. Mineral processing, or beneficiation, uses chemical, physical, and occasionally microbiological methods to separate and concentrate ore minerals. Metallurgical extraction disrupts the crystallographic bonds of ore minerals to recover the required element or compound (Fashola et al., 2016).

Inactive mines often abandon large amounts of waste, including tailings, which are byproducts of mineral ore extraction. These accumulate in steep stockpiles prone to erosion and may pollute the surrounding area (Bori et al., 2016). The primary sources of HM pollution in soil are nonferrous metal mining and smelting (Xing et al., 2020), affecting nearby farmlands (Li et al., 2020). Past Zn and Pb mining and smelting in southern China discharged many trace elements into soil, water, and river sediments, including Pb, Cd, As, and others (Adnan et al., 2024). A study of soils in numerous Chinese cities found that many were contaminated with different HM species (Bi et al., 2020). This activity generates plenty of waste (Fashola et al., 2016). Mining waste includes tailings and overburden rocks. Tailings, a processing fluid from concentrators or mills, remain after mineral, economic metal, or mineral fuel extraction (Hudson-Edwards et al., 2001).

Rocks with high metal content but uneconomical for mining are classified as overburden materials. Mining waste, such as overburden rocks and tailings, causes the most environmental harm (Egli et al., 2017; Khorasanipour et al., 2012). Tailings are fine-grained debris resulting from ore beneficiation. Most authorities prefer to dump tailings near mining sites since transporting or treating them raises mineral production costs. Tailings are rich in unextracted metals. Mining holes are generally filled with overburden boulders. Open-pit miners throw overburden boulders directly into the holes, exposing them to air and water. Weathered and fine overburden rock particles may contain HMs. Openly dumped overburden boulders pollute the ecosystem with HMs (Punia, 2021). Punia and Siva Siddaiah (2017) found that soil near overburden rocks in the Khetri Cu mine area, India, is heavily polluted with Cu and contains several times the concentration of the global average shale, upper continental crust, and reference values from the exact location. Various abandoned mines and the HMs released from them are reported in Table 3.1.

Smelting is the principal source of anthropogenic HM pollution in soil and groundwater. Three global concerns about soil HM pollution at smelting sites include severe contamination, complex sources, and cleanup challenges (Khan et al., 2021; Kumar et al., 2021). Global studies demonstrate elevated hazardous HM levels in soils around smelting facilities (Xu et al., 2021b). Numerous investigations have revealed that HMs such as Sb, As, Cd, Mn, Cu, Pb, Hg, and Zn, often found in smelter soils globally, pose a significant concern (Zeng et al., 2023). In the late 1980s, a global inventory found that mining and smelting operations released around "356–857 × 10^6 kg Pb" and "557–1360 × 10^6 kg Zn" into the environment annually (Adnan et al., 2024). In 2018, China produced almost 58 million tonnes of nonferrous metals, including "5.11 million tonnes" of Pb and "9.03 million tonnes" of Zn (Luo et al., 2023). Smelting is essential for metal extraction and recovery. Metallurgists use sophisticated chemical processes and thermodynamic assessments to optimize metal recovery from ores and secondary resources, such as smelting dust, which includes both valuable and harmful substances (Liu et al., 2023). The smelting process releases large volumes of HM-containing waste gases, which may cause pollution (Lyu et al., 2017). Uncontrolled smelting waste discharge and hazardous liquid leaks during long-term manufacturing also increase HM emissions (Luo et al., 2022; Tang et al., 2019). Toxicity and harsh deterioration of HM-contaminated soil and groundwater ecosystems mean they require a long time to recover (Yang et al., 2020).

3.3.2 Industrial effluents and manufacturing processes

Industrial HM discharge pollutes the environment and endangers humans and ecosystems (Oladimeji et al., 2024). Rapid chemical industry expansion has caused environmental and human problems (Shrestha et al., 2021). Large

TABLE 3.1 Various abandoned mines across the globe and the pollutants released from them.

Sr.no	Location	Mine name	Status	Pollutants detected	Reference
1.	Gulf Creek, Australia	Gulf Creek Mine	Abandoned	Zn, Fe, Pb, As, Ag, Cu, and Cd	(Lottermoser et al., 1999)
2.	SE Queensland, Australia	Mount Perry Mine	Abandoned	Fe, As, Ag, Au, Mo, Pb, Cu, and Mn	(Ashley et al., 2003)
3.	Howe Sound British Columbia, Canada	Britannia Mine	Abandoned	Zn and Cu	(Grout and Levings, 2001)
4.	Wanshan district, Guizhou province, China	Wanshan Mine	Abandoned	Hg	(Qiu et al., 2005)
5	Salsigne, France	Salsigne Mining Area	Abandoned	Zn, Pb, Cu, Cd, As, and Ni	(Pérez and Valiente, 2005)
6	Raniganj, India	Raniganj Coalfield	Abandoned	Ni, Cu, Cr, Pb, As, Co, Zn, and Cd	(De and Mitra, 2004)
7	Ingurtosu, Sardinia, Italy	Ingurtosu mine	Abandoned	Cu, Zn, Ni, Pb, Cd	(Podda et al., 2000; Zuddas and Podda, 2005).
8	Mount TeAroha, New Zealand	Tui Mine	Abandoned	Au, Cu, Zn, Pb, Ag, and Cd	(Morrell et al., 1996)
9	Baixo Alentejo, Portugal	Aljustrel Mine	Abandoned	Hg, Ni, Mo, Fe, Cd, and Pb	(Sánchez-Chardi et al., 2007).
10	Johannesburg, South Africa	Witwatersrand region	Abandoned	Cu, Co, Cr, Zn, Ni, and Pb	(Naicker et al., 2003)
11	Frongoch, west Wales, UK	Frongoch Mine.	Abandoned	Cd, Pb, and Zn	(Milton et al., 2003)
12	Midland province, Zimbabwe	–	Abandoned	Au, Sb, Zn, Pb, Cu, Se, Ni, and As	(Meck et al., 2006)
13	Agrokipia, Cyprus	Agrokipia	Abandoned	Ag, Cd, Zn, Cu, Pb, and Cr	(Hadjipanagiotou et al., 2020)
14	Lasail, Sohar, northern Oman	Lasail Mine	Abandoned	Fe, As, Cu, Hg, and Zn	(Palanivel and Victor, 2020)
15	Mamut,Sabah, Malaysia	Mamut Copper Mine	Abandoned	Pb, Al, Cu, Cd, Ni, Zn, and Mn	(van der Ent and Edraki, 2018)

amounts of wastewater tainted with HMs, which are highly soluble in water, threaten all living things. Cr, Pt, Sn, Ag, Pb, Cd, Cu, V, Ti, Ni, and Zn are the most common contaminants contributing to this problem, with several industries being responsible (Li et al., 2019; Jaishankar et al., 2014; Kim et al., 2019). These metals are found in water ecosystems due to industrial processes such as textile and tannery operations, battery manufacturing, wood processing, petroleum refining, mining, electroplating, and metal plating (Botle et al., 2025b; Oladimeji et al., 2024; Botle et al., 2024b). Inorganic pigment manufacturing produces pigments with Cr compounds and Cd sulfide; petroleum refining produces conversion catalysts contaminated with Cr, Ni, and V; photographic operations produce film with high concentrations of Ag; and ferrocyanide is also a byproduct (Barakat, 2011).

HMs in the chemical processing industry arise from raw materials, industrial operations, incorrect chemical waste disposal, subterranean petrol pipe breaks, and chemical plant discharges. As, Al, Cd, Cu, Cr, Hg, Ni, Pb, Zn, and Fe are primary HMs in these sectors (Rahman et al., 2022). The minerals, gemstones, and metals needed to make many items come from mining and ore processing. Metals are mined for several vital uses (Oladimeji et al., 2024). Mineral processing and metallurgy produce HMs like Cu, Mn, As, Al, Cd, Ni, Hg, Pb, Zn, and Cr (Fashola et al., 2016). In textile dyes, HMs, aromatic compounds, and nonbiodegradable ingredients are present (Kant, 2011; Adane et al., 2021). Gold, Cr, Ni, Zn, and Ag are used in electroplating to preserve and polish items. The jewelry, automotive, electronics, aerospace, and industrial industries employ this procedure to increase corrosion resistance, appearance, and electrical conductivity. Operations may produce wastewater with significant quantities of harmful HMs (Celary and Sobik-Szołtysek, 2014; Rahman et al., 2021; Rajoria et al., 2022). Paper production processes like washing, pulp bleaching, wood digestion, and dewatering release organic and inorganic substances, lignin, tannins, resins, and HMs along with their effluents (Singh and Chandra, 2019). Petroleum refineries create V, Ni, and Cr-containing effluents from conversion catalysts, while photographic activities produce Ag and ferrocyanide-rich films (Shrestha et al., 2021).

3.3.3 Urbanization and infrastructure development

Intensive urbanization, a global issue, leads to pollution of the urban environment with nonbiodegradable, toxic pollutants that accumulate in high concentrations, particularly in urban soils and plants (Tešić et al., 2022). HMs have been extracted directly or with related minerals from the Earth's crust for rapid industrialization and urbanization. As tiny components of fossil fuels and industrial products, these metals accumulate in the biosphere, increasing HM concentrations in soil, water, and the atmosphere (Bai et al., 2016). Urban soil, water, sediment, highway dust, and animals contain HMs resulting from rapid industrialization and urbanization (Swain, 2024).

Society needs infrastructure to provide basic services and build the economy. Rapid infrastructural growth sometimes pollutes the environment. The demand for infrastructure, including transportation networks, energy facilities, industrial zones, and urban settlements, skyrockets as populations rise and urbanization intensifies. These advances aim to increase living standards and economic success. However, they typically involve natural resource extraction and consumption, land use changes, and pollution emissions into the air, water, and soil (Rathoure, 2024). Global building is experiencing a golden era due to significant economic growth and urbanization. This has generated a lot of construction waste (Wu et al., 2022). The United States generates 700 million tonnes of construction waste annually, whereas the EU produces over 800 million tonnes (Wu et al., 2019). South Korea accounts for 49.9% of global construction waste (Wu et al., 2022).

Urbanization has increased people's well-being but has created substantial environmental issues (Bing et al., 2021; Liang et al., 2019). In particular, soil HM contamination threatens worldwide environmental health. HMs pollute five million locations in China, Europe, Australia, and America, and 0.12 million acres of land in China per year (Zheng et al., 2023). Metal emissions are concentrated in cities. Urbanized and peri-urban regions emit HMs mainly from roads and factories (Bai et al., 2016). Human-induced sources primarily contribute to urban HM contamination (Tešić et al., 2022). L'opez and Lobo (2014) discovered typical building waste contaminants in the leachate in a European construction waste dump.(Zhang et al., 2017) conducted leachate studies on a construction waste dump to see how sulfide content affected As leaching but found no linear link. Urban soils and road dusts contain HMs from various sources, such as domestic emissions, traffic emissions, atmospheric deposition, and industrial emissions (Tešić et al., 2022). HMs in urban ecosystems affect environmental quality (Borgogno-Mondino et al., 2015).

3.3.4 Agricultural practices and agrochemicals

Agriculture uses agrochemicals to preserve crops, boost growth, and provide soil nutrients. These chemicals include insecticides, plant growth regulators, fertilizers, and soil conditioners. Animal husbandry also uses certain chemicals (Mandal et al., 2020). Agrochemicals used in traditional agriculture for pest control and crop yield significantly affect beneficial nontarget species and human health (Gill and Garg, 2014; Müller, 2018; Kim et al., 2017). Residual persistence, bioaccumulation, and active component toxicity determine agroecosystem exposure risks at various trophic levels (Naccarato et al., 2020). Crop growth and development are enhanced with agrochemicals, increasing yield. Various phosphatic and micronutrient fertilizers contain hazardous metals (Aktaruzzaman et al., 2024).

Chemical fertilizers, primarily inorganic ones, are essential for crop productivity. In 2019, around 220 million tonnes of commercial fertilizers and liming ingredients were applied globally, primarily on farms (Rashid et al., 2023). Due to HMs accumulating in soil and plant absorption, environmental pollution has been rising rapidly, disrupting agriculture (Alengebawy et al., 2021). Long-term fertilizer usage causes HMs to accumulate in agricultural soils, reducing soil fertility as well as plant development and production (Ai et al., 2020). Recent worldwide pesticide consumption is 2 million tonnes, including 17.5% fungicides, 29.5% insecticides, 47.5% herbicides, and 5.5% other pesticides (De et al., 2014; Ma et al., 2019; Sharma et al., 2019). China consumes the most pesticides worldwide, followed by Brazil, France, Thailand, the United States, and India, as well as Canada, Italy, Argentina, and Japan. Agriculture consumes 85% of pesticide output worldwide (Alengebawy et al., 2021).

Phosphate (P) fertilizers with the highest concentration of HM contaminants are P fertilizers (Rashid et al., 2023). In superphosphate fertilizers, Ni, Cu, Cr, Pb, Cd, Zn, and Co may act as pollutants. In soil with and without P fertilizer additions, Zn concentrations were greater in the modified soil and the growing plants (Thomas et al., 2012). P fertilizers consistently enhance soil Cd (Järup, 2003; Zhuang et al., 2020; Mar et al., 2012). In addition to P fertilizers, iron, Cu, and Zn sulfates may include HM pollutants like Pb (Atafar et al., 2010; Satarug et al., 2003; Gimeno-García et al., 1996). Several agricultural fungicides and insecticides have high HM element concentrations in their active components (Rashid et al., 2023). REE-enriched fertilizers boost seed germination, plant resistance, root development, chlorophyll content, and agricultural production (Naccarato et al., 2020). Toxicological investigations showed that REEs in soil may enter the food chain via plant absorption, influencing food quality and human health (Carpenter et al., 2015; Huang and Jin, 2008; Huang et al., 2019; Naccarato et al., 2020).

3.3.5 Waste disposal and landfills

A dump is a ground hole used to bury waste (Gavrilescu et al., 2015). Landfills are correctly planned and built into or on top of the earth (Siddiqua et al., 2022). Most nations use landfills to dispose of municipal solid waste (MSW) landfill sites since it is the most straightforward and cost-effective approach (Madon et al., 2019). The most common form of MSW disposal is landfills, which accept large volumes of municipal, commercial, and industrial trash (Chakraborty et al., 2022; Hama Aziz et al., 2023; Parvin and Tareq, 2021). Landfills isolate trash from the environment (Siddiqua et al., 2022). Controlled landfills bury garbage in an engineered way, separate it from groundwater, and keep it dry (Indelicato et al., 2017). One metric tonne of landfill MSW produces 0.2 m^3 of leachate. Moisture content, landfill age, site hydrology, meteorological conditions, and waste stabilization affect leachate quality and quantity. They are the biggest polluters around the landfill (Gworek et al., 2016). Protection of landfill bottoms prevents contamination of subsurface water. End-of-day garbage should be covered with dirt. This prevents animals and insects from digging up garbage. It also reduces air pollution caused by odors (Siddiqua et al., 2022).

Over 100,000 active, closed, and abandoned landfills exist worldwide, including over 150,000 in Europe and 20,000 in China. However, waste disposal has generated environmental difficulties in both industrialized and developing nations. The Statistics Yearbook 2018 reports 657 sanitary landfills in China, a typical developing nation, with a daily treatment capacity of 3.5 million tonnes (Wang et al., 2022). Leachate, a black, foul-smelling liquid generated when rainfall mixes with decaying garbage, is a significant landfill concern. Complex organic and inorganic components, including toxic metals, constitute leachate (Adu and Aneke, 2025). Because landfills are usually located near riverbanks, waste and contamination may enter the aquatic environment. Waste disposal and treatment are challenging in underdeveloped countries due to a lack of technology and infrastructure (Sulistyowati et al., 2023). Due to their migration into soils and waterways, landfill leachate HMs such as Hg, Zn, Cu, Pb, As, Cd, and Cr are a significant concern (Adu and Aneke, 2025). Cr, Cu, Cd, As, Zn, Pb, and Hg dominate waste disposal leachate (Chu et al., 2019). Ceramics, light bulbs, consumer electronics, landfilled batteries, and glass contribute to the production of these HMs (Iravanian and Ravari, 2020). According to (Ogunbanjo et al., 2016), landfill soil was highly Cd-polluted. HMs in landfill soil may pose ecological and human health risks (Aydi, 2015; Khan et al., 2017; Liu et al., 2021). Due to excessive Hg and As levels, landfill soil was deemed ecologically risky (Obiri-Nyarko et al., 2021).

3.3.6 Fossil fuel combustion and vehicular emissions

Poor air quality, particularly in cities, is caused by human activity. The WHO 2014 study estimated that seven million urban people died from air pollution in 2012 (Ogunkunle and Ahmed, 2021). Inorganic and organic metals may be released into the air by burning fossil fuels, depending on the fuel type and manner. A few HMs may catalyze the atmospheric conversion of primary air pollutants into secondary compounds. Chemical processes may turn primary pollutants, including aerosols, ozone, acids, and peroxynitrate, into secondary contaminants (Putros and Khadim, 2024). Vehicle traffic is a significant cause of air pollution due to population growth, urban expansion, and an excessive global vehicle fleet. From 2000 to 2018, vehicle output grew by 34% and truck production by 128% (Salazar-Rojas et al., 2023).

Due to industry growth, increased transportation use, rapid urbanization, booming construction, rapid economic growth, and increased energy demands, air pollution in Indian cities has worsened (Botle et al., 2020). Infrastructure development drives economic growth in this area, which is mainly powered by fossil fuels. India's 5.89 million kilometers of roads carry 64.5% of commodities and 90% of passengers (Mohanraj et al., 2024). Karthick et al. (2022)

state that transportation has been crucial to human civilization for millennia. However, the global transportation network depends mainly on fossil fuels, raising carbon emissions (CEs). Thus, reducing CEs and promoting sustainable transportation are rising concerns. Metals discharged into the atmosphere by traffic operations pose severe health risks via soil, dust, skin contact, or inhalation (Tiwari et al., 2023b). Numerous risk assessment studies have examined the toxicity and health effects of metals and particulate matter (PM) in the air on humans worldwide (Tiwari et al., 2023a). Similarly, cars contaminate roadside habitats with several pollutants (Alexander, 2015). HMs are present in fuel tank walls, fuels, engines, vehicle components, catalytic converters, brake pads, tires, and road surface materials. Traffic contributes to roadside soil pollution owing to the long-term deposition of HMs. Tiwari et al. (2022) used principal component analysis (PCA) to allocate metal sources and found that vehicle emissions accounted for 33.6% of the variation in Al, Ca, Cr, Cu, Fe, and Ni loading. Geogenic roadway dust may include natural HMs in addition to traffic-related sources. The HM content of roadside silt is heterogeneous and seems to be influenced by background emissions and road conditions (Mohanraj et al., 2024).

3.3.7 Electronic waste

Global technology and urbanization continue to replace personal, household, medical, and agricultural tasks with machines. This drives the worldwide demand and supply of high-tech electronics, including computers, phones, and other gadgets. Most wealthy nations manufacture these gadgets with a predetermined shelf life (Owonikoko and Alimba, 2024). When broken, outmoded, or replaced by new or advanced items, they are usually relocated to poor nations to avoid the expensive disposal and recycling costs in rich countries. The United Nations University's worldwide e-waste monitoring team predicted that 50 million metric tonnes of electronics are thrown away annually, indicating a worldwide growth in e-waste (Forti et al., 2020). E-waste comes from obsolete or unusable electronics (Okeke et al., 2024). Common solid trash like e-waste is recyclable (Wang et al., 2024). Liquid crystal display, cathode ray tube televisions, air conditioners, washing machines, refrigerators, and other e-waste comprise plastic, metals, and glass. Experts are studying it due to its vast amount, difficulty in recycling, and environmental impact. Global e-waste generation is 50 million tonnes per year, and officially recorded collection and recycling were 17.4% higher than in 2019 (Wang et al., 2024). China is one of the top electrical and electronic equipment makers and users, generating 11.17 million tonnes of e-waste in 2019 (Tian et al., 2022).

The fastest-growing type of trash and the richest secondary source of HMs is e-waste. The globe produced a record "62 million tonnes" of e-waste in 2022, up 15.7% from 2019. Formal e-waste collection and recycling have only risen by 5% since 2019, reaching 22.3% in 2022. In 2022, e-waste included "31 million tonnes" of metals and "17 million tonnes" of plastic (Forti et al., 2020; Golzar-Ahmadi et al., 2024). Most countries classify e-waste as hazardous waste because it contains toxic metals like As, Cd, barium, beryllium, Cr, Zn, Ni, Hg, indium, Cu, and Pb, which harm humans and the environment (Robinson, 2009; De Oliveira et al., 2021). Computers and laptops contain Zn, As, Cd, Cu, Pb, and Cr; phones and chargers contain Cu, Pb, Hg, and Ni; televisions contain Pb, Cd, and Zn; and lighting contains Se, Hg, and As (Adu and Aneke, 2025). Despite growing awareness, only 17.4% of worldwide e-waste is recycled, leaving the rest in landfills and worsening HM contamination (Chakraborty et al., 2022; Edokpayi et al., 2016; Wang et al., 2022). Africa produces less than 1% of global e-waste, whereas Asia and America create the most. E-waste enters Africa via Nigeria, Tunisia, Ghana, and South Africa, with Nigeria leading the way (Wang et al., 2024). Studies in China, Malaysia, Bangladesh, and India show that HM pollution is a global issue, with e-waste contributing alarmingly, highlighting the need for better waste management to reduce HM leaching (Adu and Aneke, 2025).

3.4 Environmental pathways and transformation

3.4.1 Air–water–soil interactions

The hydrosphere, lithosphere, and atmosphere are all potential entry points for pollutants into the ecosystem. Anthropogenic activity is a major source of contaminants entering the ecosystem, in addition to the natural pathways mentioned before, such as volcanic activity and rock weathering. Direction, temperature, air mass circulation, surface water movement, and wind speed all affect the movement of HMs and other pollutants. In addition to these, other elements, including the partition coefficient, polarity, vapor pressure, and molecular stability, affect how the contaminants are distributed and transported (Briffa et al., 2020). These elements of the environment—air (temperature, wind speed, light intensity, etc.), water (depth, flow rate, temperature, pH, etc.), soil (organic, inorganic, etc.), and biota (flora, fauna, size, etc.)—all have unique characteristics. Chemicals often enter and diffuse into the environment primarily through the air and water. Chemical contamination pathways include soil and biota in addition to air and water (Pachana et al., 2010).

Every element of the environment contains HMs, which can be transported from one medium to another. Aerosols containing HMs are found in the atmosphere. Following that, these aerosols are naturally deposited in soil, water, and biota via precipitation and sedimentation processes. Atmospheric deposition is a significant pathway by which metals penetrate other components of the environment. The HM behavior during atmospheric transport depends on its particle size distribution and climatic circumstances. The possible toxicity of HMs and their buildup in aquatic settings make HM contamination a major issue. HMs are absorbed into sediments after being discharged into waterbodies. The species residing in these habitats begin to accumulate the metals at an unpredictable rate following metal adsorption on the sediments. Crops cultivated in contaminated soil collect HMs when they are adsorbed to soil particles. Therefore, through the food chain, HMs from the soil have an impact on people. The two methods by which biota absorb metals are through foliar and root uptake. All elements of the environment, including soil, water, air, and biota, are contaminated by HMs, which have an impact on human health since they can enter the body through the food chain, drinking water, or skin contact (Aithani and Kushawaha, 2023).

3.4.2 Metal speciation and complexation

Features of an element's physical and chemical form are referred to as speciation. The following factors help define speciation: "oxidation state, stoichiometry, coordination (including the quantity and kind of ligands), physical state", or connection with other phases. These characteristics are essential in evaluating toxicity because they control how an element behaves chemically in both environmental and human organs (Reeder et al., 2006). A metal's solubility, absorption behavior, and, in many cases, toxicity are all influenced by the chemical and physical characteristics that characterize speciation. Uptake behavior and solubility influence the metal's mobility in the environment and hence constrain pathways of exposure to species, including humans. The speciation of a metal has a direct impact on absorption via a physiological membrane upon exposure, allowing for systemic circulation entrance. However, biological fluids (such as gut or lung fluids) may undergo a speciation change before any absorption takes place, which could impact absorption and ensuing toxicity. Detoxification procedures within organ systems can affect transport, excretion, and storage, in addition to changing speciation and toxicity (Plumlee et al., 2006).

A metal's oxidation state or ligand interactions may greatly affect its behavior. Each species has a unique behavior, making stability and responsiveness generalizations impossible. A complex is a molecule with a core atom or ion—a metalloid—bonded to surrounding atoms or molecules in a specific geometric configuration. These neighboring atoms or molecules are called ligands. They might be organic or inorganic (Martinez-Guijarro et al., 2021). The adsorption of the complexed ions differs from that of the free ions due to the production of charged species (positive, negative, or neutral) during the formation of complexes with the metal(loid) ions. For example, the following differently charged species are produced when $Cd2^+$ complexes with the chloride ligand: Cd^{2+}, $CdCl^+$, $CdCl_2°$, $CdCl_3^-$ (Draszawka-Bołzan, 2015). Because of their propensity to form covalent connections, metalloids exhibit toxicological characteristics. The formation of covalent bonds with organic groups is one of their two main actions. Thus, when they connect to nonmetallic cellular macromolecule components, they may generate lipophilic ions and compounds and cause injury. Because metalloids are lipophilic, their ecological distribution and toxicity vary from basic ionic forms. Lipophilic compounds include deadly methylated As and tributyltin oxide. Pb and Hg bind to protein sulfhydryl groups as examples of binding to nonmetallic elements (Briffa et al., 2020).

3.4.3 Transport mechanisms

HM pollution mainly arises from the effluents of industrial units (Srivastava and Majumder, 2008). Water resources are being irrigated by effluents from fertilizer and paper mills, which introduce HMs, cyanides, ammonia, and other alkalis (Basta and Gradwohl, 2007; Guven and Akinci, 2008). Significant concentrations of HM ions can be found in the wastewater from leather, film and photography, galvanometry, mining, electroplating, metal cleaning, and dye and pigment industries (Naidu and Bolan, 2008). Since HMs like Pb, Cd, and As are among the PM in traffic emissions, roads and cars, in addition to industries, significantly contribute to the environmental load of HMs (Sun et al., 2001). Metals typically reach the aquatic environment from geological erosion, human activity, or atmospheric deposition brought on by mining activities, urban sewage, and industrial waste (Gautam et al., 2016). Metals also reach the aquatic environment from atmospheric deposition, geological milieu erosion, or human activity caused by mining waste, household sewage, and industrial effluents (Timothy and Tagui Williams, 2019). HM mobilization in the environment by anthropogenic sources has become an essential mechanism in the geochemical cycling of these metals (Li et al., 2004). Large amounts of HMs are dumped into the environment, plants, and soil by stationary and mobile sources in industrial areas, surpassing the levels of natural emissions (Bilos et al., 2001). The air quality may be impacted by dust and other airborne particles produced by HMs in the soil. Inhalation of substantial amounts of HM particles for prolonged periods may elevate the metals' load on the human body and pose a health risk (Gray et al., 2003).

Soils have been polluted by metals deposited on roads and in factories, as well as by automobiles and industry. Old orchards that used arsenic-containing insecticides, fields that received sewage or municipal sludge, areas near mining waste, regions where chemicals may have been discarded, and areas downwind from industrial sites can all contaminate soils. These metals also accumulate when humans and animals, particularly cattle, consume plants and crops near highways and factories. Traffic pollution is a major source of soil contamination because HMs accumulate. As a result, emerging nations are paying more attention to local contamination brought on by transportation activities (Princewill-Ogbonna and Ogbonna, 2011). Pb, Cd, Zn, and Ni are found in fuel as antiknock additives and are released by high traffic on roads (Atayese et al., 2008). Soil pollution has resulted from the deposition of metals produced by vehicles and the movement of metals deposited on the road surface by air and runoff water

(Ogbonna and Okezie, 2011). However, soil not only serves as a growing medium for plants or a pool for the removal of unwanted elements, but it also transmits numerous toxins to the atmosphere, groundwater, surface water, and food (Addo et al., 2012). Therefore, soil pollution may pose a health risk to people not only by affecting the cleanliness of food and drinking water but also by affecting the quality of the air, particularly the enriched trace metal content of airborne particles that originate from soil.

3.5 Metal contamination in food chains and ecosystems

3.5.1 Bioaccumulation and biomagnification potential

All of the imbalances brought about by previous or current human-caused pollution inputs from urban and industrial processes may supplement and occasionally even exceed those resulting from natural geological causes. Therefore, biological systems, which are continuously synthesizing, altering, and decomposing organic and inorganic chemical species, appear to be more affected by man-made environmental influences in many circumstances. The food chain, the most basic illustration of producer-consumer connections in an ecosystem, contains trace mineral elements in every link. Although the needs for macronutrients are satisfied, the essential elements in people, animals, and plants are needed in trace amounts as catalysts for metabolic processes and for the best possible growth, productivity, and health (Szynkowska et al., 2018). Animals and humans may absorb them via the food chain, drinking water, or air. Human activity redistributes and reorganizes Earth's crustal materials to a degree that might have catastrophic environmental effects. Since no element can be created or destroyed, humans' contribution to pollution is limited to creating new paths for elements to distribute. First, metals may enter food chains from seawater solutions via marine animals' permeable membranes. Nonreactive metals are insoluble chemical compounds, whereas reactive metals bond to sediments, making them indestructible and stored in ecosystems (Langston and Bebianno, 2013).

Some of these chemicals are transportable, while others accumulate in plant and animal cells. Bioaccumulation in living organisms is sometimes called "biomagnification" or "bioaccumulation". Biota may accumulate trace elements. Bioaccumulation is the net accumulation of a trace element in a target tissue or organism after exposure. Trace elements ingested by the organism or adsorbed to surfaces might bioaccumulate in a tissue or throughout the body. Environmental sources of trace element bioaccumulation include air, water, solid phases, and food (McGeer, 2004). Biomagnification occurs when diet-based bioaccumulation raises an organism's concentration within a food chain. Biomagnification may be assessed on a whole-body, tissue/organ-specific, or lipid-content basis. Biomagnification for trace elements on a tissue- and organ-specific basis is difficult since trace element disposal in organs, including the liver, kidney, and brain, varies by species. This may misrepresent food chain biomagnification (Gray, 2002; McGeer, 2004).

Trace elements can be found in soil as part of the soil material or minerals, precipitated with other compounds, dissolved in the soil solution, sorbed on exchange sites, complexed with organic and inorganic ligands, or present in microorganisms, plants, and animals. Chelation, adsorption–desorption, and precipitation–dissolution influence soil trace element mobility and availability. Many man-made sources discharge trace elements into the industrial environment (He et al., 2005). Consequently, this may result in elevated levels of trace elements in the surrounding environment. Moreover, metal pollution threatens aquatic ecosystems. Metals accumulate in ecosystems because their reactive forms bond to sediments, and their nonreactive counterparts are insoluble oxides and salts. In contrast, organic chemicals may be converted into carbon dioxide and water and eliminated from the environment. They may enter food chains directly from saltwater solutions once they reach marine organisms' permeable membranes. These pollutants may cause damage for decades after leaving the environment following a pollution catastrophe (Langston and Bebianno, 2013).

3.5.2 Interaction with biota and microbial communities

Due to their abundance, long biological half-life, and persistence, HMs disrupt the ecosystem. The behavior of metal pollution in an ecosystem depends on its chemical properties, abiotic factors, and biotic interactions. These may cause bioaccumulation, degradation, or phase changes, all of which are harmful. The environment is primarily affected by HM biomagnification in biological tissues. HM pollution begins with phytoplankton absorption. Secondary consumers eat primary producers and primary consumers, whereas primary consumers eat phytoplankton. Higher consumers and apex predators are affected as we ascend the trophic chain. Animals accumulate HMs in the kidney, liver, and reproductive organs. High soil HM concentrations limit soil microbial biomass, diversity, and activity. However, certain soil bacteria can clear away HM contamination. Their bodies can utilize and tolerate HMs due to physiological mechanisms. They also make HMs accessible in the rhizospheres of phytoremediation plants (Abdu et al., 2017).

Ecotoxicological research has connected HM toxicity to microbial diversity, structure, and population fluctuations. Some HMs act as electron acceptors or donors for soil microorganisms during metabolism. In this case, bacteria utilize a lot of metal without sustaining damage. These metals include Cr, V, As, Se, Cu, iron, Mn, and others with different oxidation states. Even though soil bacteria require HMs, microorganisms are particularly susceptible to HM stress. High metal contamination causes organic matter to accumulate at the soil's surface layer, preventing soil microorganisms from functioning effectively (Abdu et al., 2017).

3.5.3 Impact on soil health, water quality, and biodiversity

HM contamination of soil is one of the biggest concerns in the developed world (Hinojosa et al., 2004). Because they alter the microbial community that produces enzymes, HMs have an indirect impact on soil enzymatic activity (Huang and Bing, 2009). HMs affect soil biota by interfering with microbial processes and lowering soil microorganism numbers and activity. On the other hand, the long-term effects of HMs might improve the tolerance of fungi, such as arbuscular mycorrhizal fungi, and bacterial communities, which can be crucial for the recovery of damaged ecosystems (Mora et al., 2005). According to Karaca et al. (2010), because the enzymes in the soil system have varying chemical affinities, different metals have diverse effects on enzyme activity.

HMs alter soil structure by decreasing aggregate formation and stability. Maintaining soil porosity, water penetration, and structure requires aggregates. HMs, including Cd, Pb, and Cu, destabilize aggregates, constricting soil. Soil texture may be affected by HM accumulation and particle size dispersion. Metals like Ni and Zn change clay, silt, and sand proportions, thereby affecting soil texture. HM contamination reduces soil porosity, impacting nutrient, water, and air movement. HMs like Cr, Cd, and Pb clog soil pores, decreasing water percolation and root development. HMs may also affect soil water retention. Reduced pore interconnectivity and soil porosity lower water storage and enhance discharge at high HM concentrations. Cu and Zn accumulation reduces soil water retention, increasing runoff and reducing plant water availability. HM contamination accelerates soil erosion. HM accumulation in topsoil weakens soil aggregate stability, increasing the risk of wind and water erosion (Angon et al., 2024). Numerous authorities' conclusions on dangerous metal pollution have raised concerns worldwide. HMs have long been considered major water pollutants due to their toxicity and tendency to induce cancer and mutagenesis in animals. They are among the most common, highly toxic, and persistent pollutants. Although all HMs are detrimental, Pb, Cd, and Hg are perhaps the most dangerous (Singh et al., 2014). Aquatic organisms may accumulate HMs via sediments, soil erosion and runoff, airborne dust and aerosols, and waste water discharges (Goodwin et al., 2003). The aquatic ecosystem progressively releases HMs from sediments into the overlying water. Aquatic sediments are a major source of HMs. In rivers, lakes, and coastal regions, polluted sediments may directly infect fish and other biota, endangering human and environmental health. These metals accumulate in aquatic organisms and enter the food chain, where humans absorb them. Adsorption and accumulation depend on these elements' content, water physiochemistry, body distribution, and metal

TABLE 3.2 Effects of HMs on ecosystems.

Ecosystem	Impacts
Soil	• Influence on soil biology and biochemistry, organic matter, pH, and clay content • Modify the microbial community to indirectly change the enzymatic performance of the soil • Damage soil biota by altering vital microbial functions, lowering biotic populations, and reducing activity
Plants	• Risk to human and animal health due to HM uptake by plants and their bioaccumulation in the food chain • Chlorosis, yield depression, poor plant growth, and even decreased nutrient uptake, metabolic problems, and a decreased capacity to fix molecular nitrogen in leguminous plants are all consequences of phytotoxicity • Delay in seed germination
Aquatic environment	• Genration of Reactive Oxygen Species • Fish exposed to HMs develop particular enzymes that alter metabolism, leading to cellular toxicity, necrosis, and eventually tissue death • Results in severe liver and kidney atrophy, along with histological alterations
Humans	• Nausea, vomiting, muscular weakness, abdominal cramps, and dyspnea • Death and pulmonary edema are the outcomes of excessive exposure • Effects on the kidneys and lungs, such as bronchiolitis, alveolitis, and emphysema • Anosmia, cancer, heart failure, cerebrovascular infarction, osteoporosis, emphysema, proteinuria, cataracts, and other clinical problems • Growth and reproduction problems

physiological effects (Singh et al., 2017). Detailed effects of HMs on ecosystems are provided in (Table 3.2).

3.6 Analytical tools and techniques for source identification

3.6.1 Geochemical fingerprinting and isotope analysis

In order to identify certain geological reservoirs on Earth, geochemical fingerprints are utilized. This involves characterizing the many habitats that contribute to the formation of a rock of interest. Specifically, geochemical fingerprints can be used to distinguish different types of water, document processes that

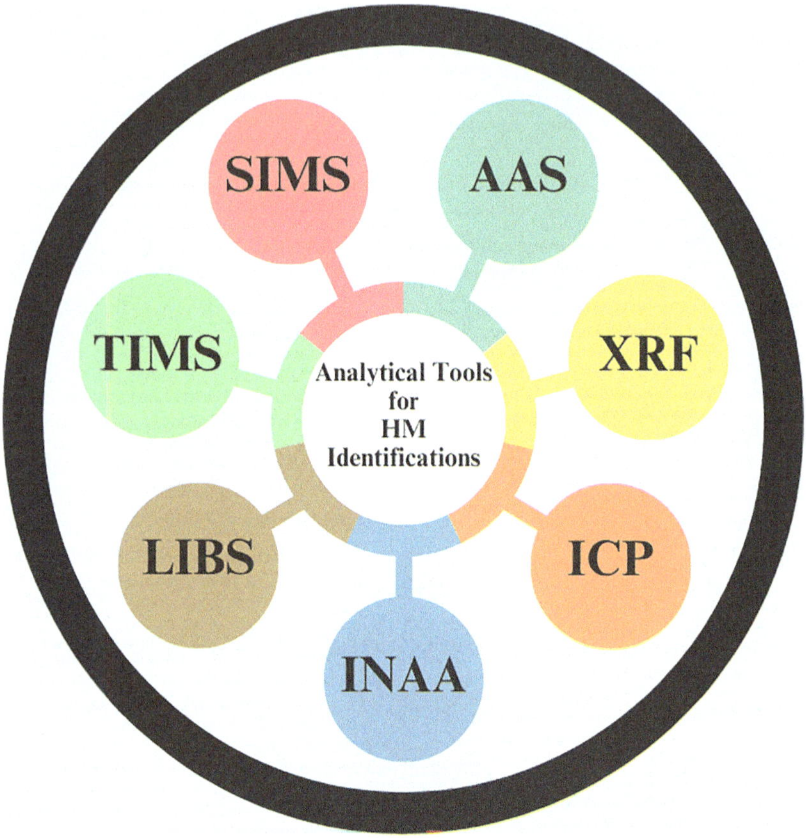

FIG. 3.2 Analytical tools used for the identification of HMs.

took place during the Earth's very early history, differentiate between different mantle reservoirs, characterize changes in the redox state (oxic/anoxic), characterize the evolution of the atmosphere and ocean, identify biosignatures, clarify the origin of clastic sediments, characterize magmatic rocks from different geotectonic settings, clarify impact events, and illustrate anthropogenic imprints (Hoefs, 2010). The analytical tools used for the identification of HMs are explained in Fig. 3.2.

From small scales to global scales, such as large mantle reservoirs like the DUPAL radiogenic isotope anomaly in the southern hemisphere, and from short events to slow, long-lasting events, all spatial and temporal scales exhibit geochemical fingerprints in the form of distinctive chemical signatures (Duprè, 1983). A geochemical fingerprint should ideally be able to identify a sample's origin while ruling out other possible sources.

Among the most often used and reasonably priced analytical methods, "atomic absorption spectrophotometer (AAS)" is accessible in numerous geological labs worldwide. "Acetylene-nitrous oxide (2950°C)" and "Air-acetylene (2150°C–2300°C)" are the two most popular oxidant-fuel combinations used in "AAS," most often to determine various elemental groups. In the most advanced systems, liquefied petroleum gas, which is readily available everywhere, and a special burner are used to analyze some of the most easily ionizable elements, including Na, K, Mg, Co, Ni, Cu, Ag, Au, Zn, Cd, and Pb (V et al., 2023).

Geological samples are analyzed using both "wavelength dispersive x-ray fluorescence (WD-XRF)" and "energy dispersive x-ray fluorescence (ED-XRF)". While the "WD-XRF" measures the elements "Be to U" one after the other, the "ED-XRF" may measure the concentrations of all elements "Na to U" by obtaining the energy-dispersive spectrum simultaneously. Because of its better resolution, "WD-XRF" may be used to analyze more complex materials like rocks and soils. In addition, "WD-XRF" offers maximum sensitivity, making it possible to measure even a few common trace elements in rock samples (Balaram, 2021).

Minor, major, and trace elements in a range of geological materials can be accurately determined using the potent multielement analytical method known as "Inductively Coupled Plasma Optical Emission Spectrophotometer (ICP-OES)". When examined in a glove box, the current high-resolution ICP-OES can measure radioactive plutonium (Pu) isotopes in nuclear samples (Krachler et al., 2016).

The process of turning stable atomic nuclei into radioactive nuclei by irradiating them with a neutron flux in a nuclear reactor, and then measuring the radiation emitted by these radioactive nuclei, is the foundation of instrumental neutron activation analysis (INAA). Major, minor, and multiple groups of trace elements, such as rare earth elements (REEs) and platinum group elements (PGEs), in various geological materials can be analyzed qualitatively and quantitatively using this method (Balaram, 2021).

Even at ng/ml levels, elemental concentrations ranging from Li to U in various rock types can be analyzed using microwave plasma atomic emission spectrometry (MP-AES). In order to better understand how the recent extreme events affected the quality of water and sediment, (Franchi et al., 2020) used MP-AES to analyze HMs in sediments and to detect flood-drought cycle records retained in the sediments of the Notwane reservoir, Botswana.

One effective analytical method for the elemental characterization of many materials, including geological samples, is "Laser-induced breakdown spectrometry (LIBS)" (Buckley, 2021). LIBS excites the elemental constituents of a solid, liquid, or gas sample by applying a highly concentrated, intense laser beam to its surface. Both qualitative and quantitative information about a specific element in a sample can be obtained by selecting an emission spectral line that is free of interference. One of the main benefits of LIBS is its capacity to identify and determine lighter elements, such as C, B, Be, and Li, which the XRF approach cannot (Anabitarte García et al., 2012). Based on the chemical makeup of a specific mineral or rock, LIBS is a very useful analytical method for geochemical fingerprinting investigations.

The C, N, S, and O isotope ratios in plant materials, soils, sediments, and gases are usually measured using isotope ratio mass spectrometry (IRMS). An elemental analyzer is used for bulk C, N, S, etc., testing. The N isotope composition of nitrogen may reveal its origin and destiny. Nitrogen is present in air, water, and soil as NH_4, N_2O, NOx, and HNO_3. Nitrogen is a particular biomarker of life in the geological record since the nitrogen cycle relies on biological activity on Earth. The dynamic pumping mode of the IRMS analyses nitrogen isotopes using N_2 as an analyte and an electron-impact gas source. Nitrogen is quantitatively extracted from its matrix, converted into N_2 gas, purified (usually by offline vacuum extraction), and analyzed (V et al., 2023).

As a typical technique for determining radioisotope and stable isotope composition and concentration, the Thermal Ionization Mass Spectrometer (TIMS) has been used since the 1980s. This method employs ion-exchange techniques to extract the elements whose isotopic compositions must be estimated from other rock or mineral sample components. After purifying the liquid sample, a metal filament is heated to evaporate the solvent. TIMS utilizes a magnetic sector mass spectrometer for quantitative separation and detection, but a multicollector device may detect many isotopes and provide high-precision ratio measurements (Li et al., 2011).

One method for analyzing the composition of solids is secondary-ion mass spectrometry (SIMS). This method ejects ions of opposite charge from the solid material's surface by sputtering it with a focused primary ion beam (Cs^+ or O^-). The surface's elemental, isotopic, or molecular makeup is then ascertained by analyzing the released secondary ions. The SIMS technique was used to determine the carbon isotopes and trace elements in the zircon samples in the historic

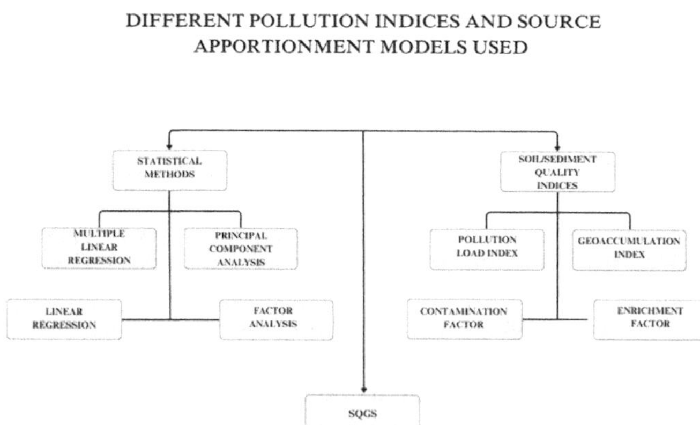

FIG. 3.3 Different pollution indices and source apportionment models used.

finding of microfossils preserved in Archean rocks that date back about 4.1 billion years (Bell et al., 2015).

3.6.2 Pollution indices and source apportionment models

Numerous methods for evaluating pollution have been created, accounting for the impacts of different kinds of human activity, such as traffic, industry, and agriculture. Some techniques are based on an element's accessible or reactive pool, in addition to overall concentrations. Different indices and models used are described in (Fig. 3.3).

Sediment/soil quality guidelines (SQGs) are the most straightforward method for evaluating the level of HM contamination in sediments and soils. These recommendations include a range of HM concentration values that must be evaluated. These numbers may be regarded as the HM threshold concentrations at which harmful biological consequences occur. By comparing the concentrations provided by SQGs with the measured concentrations, HM contamination can be easily evaluated. Typically, these values can be obtained through bioassay tests in addition to background concentrations (Burton, 2002; Canadian Council of Ministers of the Environment, 2002).

The statistical link between geochemical characteristics has been extensively used to measure background values and contamination levels using statistical methods such as multiple linear regression, factor analysis, PCA, and linear regression (De Saedeleer et al., 2010; Ho et al., 2010).

Using a data set of 600 arable soil samples and the correlations between HMs clay, and organic matter content, (De Temmerman et al., 2003) determined that the northern part of Belgium was contaminated based on results that were outside the usual range. It is also proposed that isotopic ratios (of Pb, Cd, Cr, Cu, and Zn isotopes) provide a sensitive way to differentiate between the anthropogenic portions of these metals and their geological background (Hoefs, 2010).

The computation of environmental quality indicators (soil/sediment quality indices) is the foundation of quantitative approaches. These techniques are thought to be a useful way to turn unprocessed environmental data into general knowledge for nonspecialists. Decision-makers can use this transformation to rank and prioritize polluted locations for additional research (Dung et al., 2013). The pollution load index (PLI), enrichment factor, contamination factor (CF), and geoaccumulation index (Igeo) are the indicators that are employed. Muller (1969) developed the Igeo, which makes it possible to determine and categorize the contamination level of sediments and soils into seven levels, ranging from severely polluted to unpolluted. Igeo is a quantitative indicator of HM contamination in sediments and soils, but it ignores grain size and geochemical variability and understates contamination due to its artificial numerical factor (1.5). Shale, sedimentary rock, continental crust, upper continental crust, etc., are often used as enrichment factor references. Using different normalization factors and background data from various methods, several studies have used this indicator.

The PLI measures soil and sediment HM contamination. This indicator was designed for soils but is now utilized for sediments. An integrated index includes all researched HMs. This index is simple enough for nonscientists to grasp and allows comparison of contamination levels since it includes all of the metals under consideration. CF is the ratio of a sample's HM concentration to its reference or background concentration. The contamination status of a single HM in the sample location is assessed by comparing their CF (Dung et al., 2013).

3.6.3 Global information systems and remote sensing in source mapping

Global Information System (GIS) software can study river HM contamination by collecting data on HM concentrations in water, sediments, and suspended particles. A large volume of data that is challenging to manage on paper can be handled more easily with GIS software. Land use maps, HM concentrations in the surveyed area, drainage pattern layers, and geochemical maps of HMs are all digitized using GIS software. Information about the causes of HM pollution in water and its detrimental impacts on urban areas, agricultural areas, and other land units can be obtained with the aid of GIS. Values associated with spatiotemporal or spatial processes can be predicted and analyzed using geostatistics. The main purposes of geostatistical techniques are to interpolate values for regions where samples were not collected and to explain spatial patterns (Sharma et al., 2021).

In past years, remote sensing methods have drawn a lot of interest for mapping harmful metals. To recognize the sources of soil hazardous metals, remote sensing is essential (Melendez-Pastor et al., 2011). At low to moderate concentrations, toxic HMs have a featureless appearance and attach easily to minerals and organic matter. Remote sensing spectra prove useful for mapping the dispersal of hazardous HMs in soil because they provide information on Feoxides, clays, and organic matter in vegetation cover or soils (Peng et al., 2015). Advanced remote sensing techniques have been used to quickly and affordably study HM pollution in soil. By using "space-supported hyperspectral sensors", models are created that help map HM concentrations over a large area. On agricultural and residential properties, floods spread pollutants, which remain there for many years until soil erosion removes them. HMs in contaminated soils have a negative impact on the environment, food, and human health (Foulds et al., 2014). Remote sensing is essential for identifying and treating HM-polluted soils due to urbanization and a lack of high-quality food. Remote sensing quickly assesses HM contamination danger. Traditional soil sampling, chemical digestion, and interpolation methods for estimating HMs for geographical risk maps are expensive and time-consuming (Zhang et al., 2012). In HM soil pollution research, advanced hyperspectral remote sensing techniques are commonly used because they provide a quicker, more reasonable, and more inclusive picture of pollution. Soil pollution can be mapped using continuous, information-rich spectra from hyperspectral imaging.

3.7 Mitigation strategies and management approaches

3.7.1 Source control and sustainable mining

The growth-centered strategy promoted by the Rio Earth Summit is followed by the mining industry's use of sustainability language. The literature demonstrates how mining can support sustainable development by emphasizing positive effects on the economy, environment, and community. Two crucial areas are not sufficiently covered by these pillars (the triple bottom line) in a mining environment, nevertheless. One is safety, which is perhaps the most important factor in the mining industry. A focus on the methods used to extract the mineral resource itself is the second aspect that is lacking. If mine managers then concentrate on the following five areas—safety, environment, economy, efficiency, and community—they will be on track to create a sustainable mining operation. Safety should be the top priority in a mining operation for both moral and commercial reasons. A dedication to risk management, proper attitudes and behaviors, the necessity of reporting systems, an emphasis on education and training, and attention to procedures and equipment are all traits of safe mines. A mine cannot be viable unless it is profitable. Mine managers want to maximize income while minimizing expenses in order to sustainably create profit for as long as feasible.

In addition, this will maximize the fair advantages for all parties involved, including shareholders, workers, businesses, communities that rely on mining, and governments that profit from taxes and royalties. Reduced labor costs, fewer labor disputes, higher retention rates, reduced health care costs, reduced production costs, less regulatory burden, reduced closure costs, lower borrowing costs, lower insurance costs, and better investor relations are all examples of how a mining company's economic performance will improve if it incorporates sustainable development into its operations. In addition, a mine must manage and extract resources efficiently. To maximize resource extraction, geologists, metallurgists, and mining engineers work together. There are many instances of nonsustainable mining methods, such as "high grading" the ore body, which involves extracting only the best material for immediate profit. It makes perfect commercial sense for mine sites to implement cutting-edge environmental management techniques. Long-term liabilities like acid mine drainage could arise if environmental values are not protected throughout the design and operation phases. Last but not least, a mine needs a "social license to operate." Opposition and conflict may arise if the community is not involved and supportive of a mining activity. Corporation-run mining activities have frequently been interrupted recently, especially by local artisanal and small-scale miners who were mining frequently prior to the start of the larger-scale operations (Laurence, 2011).

3.7.2 Remediation technologies

Some remediation approaches, such as soil washing, soil thermal desorption, phytoremediation, and others, have been developed in light of the severity and widespread nature of HM-contaminated sites. Thermal desorption is a process in which contaminants are extracted from the soil using direct or indirect heating (Teng et al., 2020). The high efficiency, short treatment cycle, lack of secondary contamination, high safety, and recycling of soil and pollutants are all benefits of this approach (Zhao et al., 2019). However, thermal desorption is only effective for removing volatile contaminants and is constrained by the need for costly equipment and a prolonged desorption period.

To lower the amount of HMs in the soil, uncontaminated soil must be substituted for contaminated soil. This is possible for small amounts of highly polluted shallow soil in a small area. Total soil exchange, subsurface topsoil replacement, partial soil exchange, and the technique of overlaying fresh soil to lower the concentration of soil contaminants are the primary steps in soil remediation (Song et al., 2022). Because of its high efficiency, low cost, ease of use, and comprehensive processing, chemical leaching has drawn a lot of attention (Hu et al., 2021). Chemical leaching dissolves HMs from soil by infusing extraction solutions, including chelators, bases, salts, acids, or surfactants. Chemical leaching effectiveness depends on soil texture, leaching agents, organic matter content, pH, time, concentration, solid–liquid ratio, and HMs. The main leaching agents include acids, bases, salts, chelating agents, and surfactants (Marques et al., 2013). By injecting inorganic substances, the complexes that have developed between HMs and functional groups on the soil surface are broken down by ion exchange, complexation, or acidolysis, which extracts the metals.

The transformation of HMs into less hazardous, immobile, and insoluble forms is known as stabilization. It has been demonstrated that stabilization is an inexpensive, practical, and efficient remediation technique (Xu et al., 2021a). Inorganic, organic, and organic–inorganic composite stabilizers are injected into soil to stabilize HMs. Cation exchange, complexation, precipitation, physisorption, and electrostatic interaction stabilize soil HMs with alkaline materials such as cement, lime, fly ash, steel slag, and blast furnace slag. Lime, the earliest and most frequently used stabilizer, improves soil pH and reduces HM solubility (Xu et al., 2021a).

HM mobility, toxicity, and environmental availability are all decreased via chemical oxidation or reduction (Marques et al., 2013). It is possible to successfully eliminate HMs, especially redox-sensitive metals or metalloids (Liang et al., 2022). Chemical redox is comparatively faster and more efficient; however, it can occasionally be constrained by cost and the potential for secondary contamination. The change in shared electron pairs or the gain or loss of electrons are the fundamental components of the redox reaction. Physical and chemical features of the soil, HM characteristics, concentrations of HMs and oxidants/reductants, pH, and temperature are the main elements influencing the oxidation/reduction process (Song et al., 2022).

"Phytoextraction", "Phytostabilization", "Phytotransformation", and "Phytovolatilization" are the four main categories of phytoremediation. The types of soil and plants, the makeup of rhizosphere microorganisms, and the intricate relationship between the geochemical forms of pollutants should all be taken into consideration when choosing a phytoremediation approach in practice (Wang et al., 2020). Phytostabilization is defined as the process of lowering the bioavailability of HMs and stopping their off-site movement by immobilizing or inactivating them in-situ. Phytostabilization is mostly applied at contaminated, abandoned sites, including sewage treatment plants, urban landfills, and mine wastelands. The process by which HMs are eliminated through plant transpiration is known as phytovolatilization. Plant roots take up HMs from the soil, move them through the xylem, transform them into volatile forms, and then release them into the atmosphere through stomata (Zhang et al., 2013). Phytovolatilization was the primary process that removed Hg, As, and Se from the soil. Utilizing unique plants with a potent enrichment capacity, phytoextraction transports and stores HMs in the aboveground portion of the plant before harvesting them to remove them from the contaminated soil. The secret to phytoextraction is the identification and screening of hyperaccumulator plants.

Microbial remediation is the biological activity of microorganisms that absorb or convert HMs into low-toxicity compounds. Bioleaching, biosorption, biomineralization, biovolatilization, and bioaccumulation are the primary mechanisms involved in microbial remediation for soil contaminated with HMs (Verma and Kuila, 2019). Microorganisms affect soil HM transport and transformation. Microorganisms reduce the toxicity of As and Cr by oxidizing As^{3+} to As^{5+} and reducing Cr^{6+} to Cr^{3+}. Hg-resistant microorganisms convert soil methylmercury to elemental Hg (Song et al., 2022).

3.7.3 Policy and regulatory frameworks

Stricter laws should be passed by lawmakers, who should also mandate that hazardous waste containing HMs be disposed of and treated properly, monitor and control HM pollution from shipbreaking yards and industrial operations, and fund public awareness campaigns and educational initiatives on HM toxicity. Incorporating lessons on HM toxicity and its health effects into school curricula, creating materials specifically tailored to various age groups and stakeholders, and working with health professionals to plan teacher workshops and training sessions are all critical tasks performed by educators. In high-risk groups, such as e-waste scavengers, health professionals should perform routine physical examinations and blood tests for HMs; offer direction and assistance for the treatment and management of HM poisoning cases; and collaborate with educators and legislators to develop and distribute educational materials on HM toxicity. We can endeavor to lessen the threats that HM contamination poses to the community's health and environment by implementing these steps to close the knowledge and awareness gaps (Maghchiche and Meghchiche, 2024). The efficiency of national initiatives to reduce HM pollution can be increased by taking part in international agreements and partnerships. Researching phytoremediation and bioremediation may provide sustainable solutions for polluted sites. Using eco-friendly goods and better industrial practices may reduce HM emissions. This entails encouraging firms to adopt waste-reduction best practices (Udongwo, 2023).

Several worldwide treaties and protocols address HM contamination. The 1979 Convention on Long-Range Transboundary Air Pollution (CLRTAP) aims to avoid and progressively decrease air pollution, especially long-range transboundary air pollution, while protecting the environment. CLRTAP accepted the HMs Protocol in Aarhus, Denmark, in 1998. This pact mandates parties to reduce Hg, Pb, and Cd emissions below 1990 levels. It mandates the phaseout of leaded petrol and imposes strict stationary source emission limits. Another major international agreement to protect the environment and human health from Hg and its compounds is the Minamata Convention on Hg, which is legally binding. The 2013 convention addresses Hg's supply, commerce, usage in products and processes, emissions, releases, and disposal. In addition, the goal of the 1992 Basel Convention on the Control of Transboundary Movements of Hazardous Wastes and Their Disposal is to stop the movement of hazardous wastes, especially HMs, to poorer nations. The fact that more than 170 nations have ratified the treaty highlights its importance on a worldwide scale.

3.8 Conclusion

HMs are toxic, persistent, and irreversible environmental contaminants. When HMs are employed recklessly to improve soil productivity, they accumulate and harm plants and soil. Industrial waste poured into rivers, seas, and oceans harms aquatic ecosystems, causing various abnormalities in fish and aquatic animals. Metals may accumulate in the tissues of fish and aquatic plants. This can be prevented by advancing industrial and technical technologies while developing and implementing effective pollution treatment methods. In conclusion, understanding and managing HM pollution have improved, but more research is needed to enhance cleaning procedures and regulatory frameworks. Future endeavors should focus on improving monitoring systems, promoting sustainable industrial practices, and fostering international collaboration to mitigate the impacts of HM pollution on aquatic ecosystems and human health.

References

Abdu, N., Abdullahi, A.A., Abdulkadir, A., 2017. Heavy metals and soil microbes. Environ. Chem. Lett. 15 (1), 65–84. doi:10.1007/s10311-016-0587-x.

Adane, T., Adugna, A.T., Alemayehu, E., 2021. Textile industry effluent treatment techniques. J. Chem. 2021, 1–14. doi:10.1155/2021/5314404.

Addo, M.A., Darko, E.O., Gordon, C., Nyarko, B.J.B., Gbadago, J.K., Nyarko, E., Affum, H.A., Botwe, B.O., 2012. Evaluation of heavy metals contamination of soil and vegetation in the vicinity of a cement factory in the Volta Region, Ghana. https://ugspace.ug.edu.gh/items/398a78bd-6499-4c7c-9b6e-e84680d7015e.

Adnan, M., Xiao, B., Ali, M.U., Xiao, P., Zhao, P., Wang, H., Bibi, S., 2024. Heavy metals pollution from smelting activities: a threat to soil and groundwater. Ecotoxicol. Environ. Saf. 01476513. 274, 116189. doi:10.1016/j.ecoenv.2024.116189.

Adu, J.T., Aneke, F.I., 2025. Evaluation of heavy metal contamination in landfills from e-waste disposal and its potential as a pollution source for surface water bodies. Results in Engineering. 25 (25901230) Available from: https://www.sciencedirect.com/science/journal/25901230. doi:10.1016/j.rineng.2025.104431.

Adumitroaei, M.V., Iancu, G.O., Răţoi, B.G., Doru, C.S., Sandu, C.M., 2018. Spatial distribution and geochemistry of major and trace elements from mohoş peatland, harghita mountains, Romania. Holocene. 14770911. 28 (12), 1936–1947. Available from: http://hol.sagepub.com/. doi:10.1177/0959683618798174.

Ahmad, W., Khan, A., Ali, N., Khan, S., Uddin, S., Malik, S., Ali, N., Khan, H., Khan, H., Bilal, M., 2021. Photocatalytic degradation of crystal violet dye under sunlight by chitosan-encapsulated ternary metal selenide microspheres. Environ. Sci. Pollut. Res. 0944-1344. 28 (7), 8074–8087. doi:10.1007/s11356-020-10898-7.

Ahmed, M.K., Shaheen, N., Islam, M.S., Habibullah-al-Mamun, M., Islam, S., Mohiduzzaman, M., Bhattacharjee, L., 2015. Dietary intake of trace elements from highly consumed cultured fish (*Labeo rohita, Pangasius pangasius* and *Oreochromis mossambicus*) and human health risk implications in Bangladesh. Chemosphere. 18791298. 128, 284–292. Available from: https://www.elsevier.com/locate/chemosphere. doi:10.1016/j.chemosphere.2015.02.016.

Ai, P., Jin, K., Alengebawy, A., Elsayed, M., Meng, L., Chen, M., Ran, Y., 2020. Effect of application of different biogas fertilizer on eggplant production: analysis of fertilizer value and risk assessment. Environ. Technol. Innov. 23521864. 19, 101019. doi:10.1016/j.eti.2020.101019.

Aithani, D., Kushawaha, J., 2023. Heavy metals contamination in environment. In: Selvasembian, R., Thokchom, B., Singh, P., Jawad, A.H., Gwenzi, W. (Eds.), Remediation of Heavy Metals: Sustainable Technologies and Recent Advances. Wiley, India, pp. 15–30. Available from: https://onlinelibrary.wiley.com/doi/book/10.1002/9781119853589. doi:10.1002/9781119853589.ch2.

Ajdary, M., Moosavi, M.A., Rahmati, M., Falahati, M., Mahboubi, M., Mandegary, A., Jangjoo, S., Mohammadinejad, R., Varma, R.S., 2018. Health concerns of various nanoparticles: a review of their in vitro and in vivo toxicity. Nanomaterials. 20794991. 8 (9). Available from: http://www.mdpi.com/2079-4991/8/9/634/pdf. doi:10.3390/nano8090634.

Aktaruzzaman, M., Zakir, H.M., Quadir, Q.F., Rashid, M.H., Supti Mallick, P.B., Nayeem, S.M.M.R., 2024. Toxic heavy metals content in different agrochemicals available in markets of Bangladesh and their loads to the agricultural lands. Environ. Monit. Assess. 0167-6369. 196 (11). doi:10.1007/s10661-024-13212-x.

Alengebawy, A., Abdelkhalek, S.T., Qureshi, S.R., Wang, M.Q., 2021. Heavy metals and pesticides toxicity in agricultural soil and plants: ecological risks and human health implications. Toxics. 23056304. 9 (3), 1–34. Available from: https://www.mdpi.com/2305-6304/9/3/42/pdf. doi:10.3390/toxics9030042.

Alexander, P., 2015. Assessment of heavy metals in roadside surface soil and vegetation along Mubi – michika Major Road in Adamawa State, Nigeria. Int. J. Appl. Sci. Biotechnol. 2091-2609. 3 (3), 545–551. doi:10.3126/ijasbt.v3i3.12934.

Ali, F., Ibrahim, M., Khan, F., Bibi, I., Shah, S.W.H., 2018. Binding affinities of cationic dyes in the presence of activated charcoal and anionic surfactant in the premicellar region. Mater. Res. Express. 20531591. 5 (3). Available from: http://iopscience.iop.org/article/10.1088/2053-1591/aab565/pdf. doi:10.1088/2053-1591/aab565.

Ali, N., Hassan Riead, M.D.M., Bilal, M., Yang, Y., Khan, A., Ali, F., Karim, S., Zhou, C., Wenjie, Y., Sher, F., Iqbal, H.M.N., 2021. Adsorptive remediation of environmental pollutants using magnetic hybrid materials as platform adsorbents. Chemosphere. 00456535. 284, 131279. doi:10.1016/j.chemosphere.2021.131279.

Ali, Z., Ullah, R., Tuzen, M., Ullah, S., Rahim, A., Saleh, T.A., 2023. Colorimetric sensing of heavy metals on metal doped metal oxide nanocomposites: a review. Trends in Environmental Analytical Chemistry. 22141588. 37, e00187. doi:10.1016/j.teac.2022.e00187.

Alloway, B.J., 2012. Heavy Metals in Soils: Trace Metals and Metalloids in Soils and Their Bioavailability, Vol. 22. Springer Science & Business Media. https://books.google.com/books?hl=en&lr=&id=Soovc_GOk48C&oi=fnd&pg=PR5&dq=Alloway,+B.J.,+2013.+Heavy

+Metals+In+Soils,+22.+Springer,+Dordrecht.&ots=RI6OTVmmwL&sig=wKyK4sHIbYxTmnxxVjCeqMckfB4.

Anabitarte García, F., Cobo García, A., López Higuera, J.M., 2012. *Laser-induced breakdown spectroscopy: fundamentals, applications, and challenges*. https://repositorio.unican.es/xmlui/handle/10902/2577.

Angon, P.B., Islam, M.S., KC, S., Das, A., Anjum, N., Poudel, A., Suchi, S.A., 2024. Sources, effects and present perspectives of heavy metals contamination: soil, plants and human food chain. Heliyon. 24058440. 10 (7). Available from: https://www.sciencedirect.com/science/journal/24058440. doi:10.1016/j.heliyon.2024.e28357.

Arora, R., 2019. Adsorption of heavy metals–a review. Mater. Today Proc. 18, 4745–4750. https://www.sciencedirect.com/science/article/pii/S221478531932646X.

Ashley, P.M., Lottermoser, B.G., Chubb, A.J., 2003. Environmental geochemistry of the Mt Perry copper mines area,SE Queensland, Australia. Geochemistry: Exploration, Environment, Analysis 3 (4), 345–357. doi:10.1144/1467-7873/03-014.

Atafar, Z., Mesdaghinia, A., Nouri, J., Homaee, M., Yunesian, M., Ahmadimoghaddam, M., Mahvi, A.H., 2010. Effect of fertilizer application on soil heavy metal concentration. Environmental Monitoring and Assessment 160 (1), 83–89. https://idp.springer.com/authorize/casa?redirect_uri=https://link.springer.com/article/10.1007/s10661-008-0659-x&casa_token=kYoBsoVzcEMAAAAA:zx5OHsNzaK-sK0sRLVZ_jP3wBmrj_-gSrHaNhWCN-Z12ihLmRQIH8-NWRk-pFeWATsF1nD–G-_O7F_LO.

Atayese, M.O., Eigbadon, A.I., Adesodun, J.K., 2008, Heavy metal contamination of Amaranthus grown along major highways in Lagos, Nigeria. Afr. Crop Sci. J. 16 (4). https://www.ajol.info/index.php/acsj/article/view/54390.

Aydi, A., 2015. Assessment of heavy metal contamination risk in soils of landfill of Bizerte (Tunisia) with a focus on application of pollution indicators. Environ. Earth Sci. 1866-6280. 74 (4), 3019–3027. doi:10.1007/s12665-015-4332-8.

Bai, Y., Wang, M., Peng, C., Alatalo, J.M., 2016. Impacts of urbanization on the distribution of heavy metals in soils along the Huangpu River, the drinking water source for Shanghai. Environ. Sci. Pollut. Res. 16147499. 23 (6), 5222–5231. Available from: http://www.springerlink.com/content/0944-1344. doi:10.1007/s11356-015-5745-3.

Bakshe, P., Jugade, R., 2023. Phytostabilization and rhizofiltration of toxic heavy metals by heavy metal accumulator plants for sustainable management of contaminated industrial sites: a comprehensive review. J. Hazard. Mater. Adv. 27724166. 10, 100293. doi:10.1016/j.hazadv.2023.100293.

Balaram, V., 2021. Current and emerging analytical techniques for geochemical and geochronological studies. Geol. J. 0072-1050. 56 (5), 2300–2359. doi:10.1002/gj.4005.

Barakat, M.A., 2011. New trends in removing heavy metals from industrial wastewater. Arab. J. Chem. 18785352. 4 (4), 361–377. doi:10.1016/j.arabjc.2010.07.019.

Basta, N., Gradwohl, R., 2007. Estimation of Cd, Pb, and Zn Bioavailability in smelter-contaminated soils by a sequential extraction procedure. Journal of Soil Contamination. 1058-8337. 9 (2), 149–164. doi:10.1080/10588330008984181.

Bell, E.A., Boehnke, P., Harrison, T.M., Mao, W.L., 2015. Potentially biogenic carbon preserved in a 4.1 billion-year-old zircon. Proc. Natl. Acad. Sci. USA 10916490. 112 (47), 14518–14521. Available from: http://www.pnas.org/content/112/47/14518.full.pdf. doi:10.1073/pnas.1517557112.

Bi, X., Zhang, M., Wu, Y., Fu, Z., Sun, G., Shang, L., Li, Z., Wang, P., 2020. Distribution patterns and sources of heavy metals in soils from an industry undeveloped city in Southern China. Ecotoxicol. Environ. Saf. 01476513. 205, 111115. doi:10.1016/j.ecoenv.2020.111115.

Bilos, C., Colombo, J.C., Skorupka, C.N., Presa, M.J.R., 2001. Sources, distribution and variability of airborne trace metals in La Plata City area, Argentina. Environ. Pollut. 02697491. 111 (1), 149–158. doi:10.1016/S0269-7491(99)00328-0.

Bing, H., Qiu, S., Tian, X., Li, J., Zhu, H., Wu, Y., Zhang, G., 2021. Trace metal contamination in soils from mountain regions across China: spatial distribution, sources, and potential drivers. Soil Ecol. Lett.

3 (3), 189–206. https://idp.springer.com/authorize/casa?redirect_uri=https://link.springer.com/article/10.1007/s42832-021-0080-8&casa_token=R9yQV3Nl2VYAAAAA:GCQDdCcZT-pqdX-bx4kCFSTF_XIu8glmZ7gcIkfP2siUpDkUf0lIPnB-7lkn4GZ2WAYOGDKRFUQVEvMYt.

Borgogno-Mondino, E., Fabietti, G., Ajmone-Marsan, F., 2015. Soil quality and landscape metrics as driving factors in a multi-criteria GIS procedure for peri-urban land use planning. Urban For. Urban Green. 14 (4), 743–750. https://www.sciencedirect.com/science/article/pii/S1618866715000977.

Bori, J., Vallès, B., Navarro, A., Riva, M.C., 2016. Geochemistry and environmental threats of soils surrounding an abandoned mercury mine. Environ. Sci. Pollut. Res. 16147499. 23(13), 12941–12953. Available from: http://www.springerlink.com/content/0944-1344. doi:10.1007/s11356-016-6463-1.

Botle, A., Salgaonkar, S., Barabde, G., Herlekar, M., 2024a. Abatement of pharmaceutical compounds in wastewater using green nanomaterials: an eco-friendly alternative to conventional nanomaterials. In: Bhat, S.A., Kumar, V., Li, F., Verma, P., Eds. Detection and Treatment of Emerging Contaminants in Wastewater. IWA Publishing, pp. 227–251. doi:10.2166/9781789063752_0227.

Botle, A., Salgaonkar, S., Barabde, G., Tiwari, R., 2025a. Health Concerns and Issues Associated with Toxic Heavy Metals Global Perspectives of Toxic Metals in Bio Environs: Volume 1: Environmental Impact, Ecotoxicology, Health Concerns, and Modelling. Springer Science+Business Media, India, pp. 161–193. doi:10.1007/978-3-031-89725-2_7.

Botle, A., Salgaonkar, S., Tiwari, R., Ambadekar, S., Barabde, G.R., 2023. Brief status of contamination in surface water of rivers of India by heavy metals: a review with pollution indices and health risk assessment. Environ. Geochem. Health. 15732983. 45 (6), 2779–2801. Available from: https://www.springer.com/journal/10653. doi:10.1007/s10653-022-01463-x.

Botle, A., Salgaonkar, S., Tiwari, R., Barabde, G., 2024b. Unveiling heavy metal pollution dynamics in sediments of river Ulhas, Maharashtra, India: a comprehensive analysis of anthropogenic influence, pollution indices, and health risk assessment. Environ. Geochem. Health 46 (10), 419. doi:10.1007/s10653-024-02208-8.

Botle, A., Salgaonkar, S., Tiwari, R., Barabde, G., 2025b. Heavy metal pollution in River Ulhas, Maharashtra, India: unraveling contamination dynamics through pollution indices, multivariate analysis, and health risk assessment. Int. J. Environ. Res. 19 (3), 88. doi:10.1007/s41742-025-00754-2.

Botle, A., Singhal, R.K., Basu, H., Manisha, V., Masih, J., 2020. Health risk assessment of heavy metals associated with Coarse and Quasi-accumulative airborne particulate matter in Mumbai City situated on the Western Coast of India. Environ. Technol. Innov. 23521864. 19, 100857. doi:10.1016/j.eti.2020.100857.

Briffa, J., Sinagra, E., Blundell, R., 2020. Heavy metal pollution in the environment and their toxicological effects on humans. Heliyon 6 (9), e04691. doi:10.1016/j.heliyon.2020.e04691.

Buckley, S., 2021. Geochemical analysis using laser-induced breakdown spectroscopy. Spectroscopy (Santa Monica). 08876703. 36 (10), 9–15. Available from: https://www.spectroscopyonline.com/view/geochemical-analysis-using-laser-induced-breakdown-spectroscopy. doi:10.56530/spectroscopy.az2280i6.

Burton, G.A., 2002. Sediment quality criteria in use around the world. Limnology 3 (2), 65–75. doi:10.1007/s102010200008.

Canadian Council of Ministers of the Environment, 2002. Canadian Environmental Quality Guidelines, Vol. 2. Canadian Council of Ministers of the Environment.

Cao, H., Ikeda, S., 2000. Exposure assessment of heavy metals resulting from farmland application of wastewater sludge in Tianjin, China: the examination of two existing national standards for soil and farmland-used sludge. Risk Anal. 0272-4332. 20 (5), 613–626. doi:10.1111/0272-4332.205056.

Carpenter, D., Boutin, C., Allison, J.E., Parsons, J.L., Ellis, D.M., 2015. Uptake and effects of six rare earth elements (REEs) on selected native and crop species growing in contaminated soils. Plos One. 19326203. 10 (6). Available from: http://www.plosone.org/article/fetchObject.action?uri=info:doi/10.1371/journal.pone.0129936&representation=PDF. doi:10.1371/journal.pone.0129936.

Carrera-Beltrán, L., Gavilanes-Terán, I., Idrovo-Novillo, J., Valverde, V.H., Rodríguez-Pinos, A., Paredes, C., Signes-Pastor, A.J., Carbonell-Barrachina, Á.A., 2024. Environmental pollution by heavy metals within the area influenced by the Tungurahua volcano eruption – ecuador. Ecotoxicol. Environ. Saf. 10902414. 270. Available from: https://www.sciencedirect.com/science/journal/01476513. doi:10.1016/j.ecoenv.2023.115919.

Celary, P., Sobik-Szołtysek, J., 2014. Vitrification as an alternative to landfilling of tannery sewage sludge. Waste Manag. 0956053X. 34 (12), 2520–2527. doi:10.1016/j.wasman.2014.08.022.

Chakraborty, S.C., Qamruzzaman, M., Zaman, M.W.U., Alam, M.M., Hossain, M.D., Pramanik, B.K., Nguyen, L.N., Nghiem, L.D., Ahmed, M.F., Zhou, J.L., Md. Ibrahim.H., M., Hossain, M.A., Johir, M.A.H., Ahmed, M.B., Sithi, J.A., Zargar, M., Moni, M.A., 2022. Metals in e-waste: occurrence, fate, impacts and remediation technologies. Process Saf. Environ. Prot. 09575820. 162, 230–252. doi:10.1016/j.psep.2022.04.011.

Chorover, J., Amistadi, M.K., Chadwick, O.A., 2004. Surface charge evolution of mineral-organic complexes during pedogenesis in Hawaiian basalt. Geochim. Cosmochim. Acta 68 (23), 4859–4876. https://www.sciencedirect.com/science/article/pii/S0016703704004429.

Chu, Z., Fan, X., Wang, W., Huang, W.-C., 2019. Quantitative evaluation of heavy metals' pollution hazards and estimation of heavy metals' environmental costs in leachate during food waste composting. Waste Manag. 0956053X. 84, 119–128. doi:10.1016/j.wasman.2018.11.031.

Clarke, B.O., Smith, S.R., 2011. Review of 'emerging' organic contaminants in biosolids and assessment of international research priorities for the agricultural use of biosolids. Environ. Int. 18736750. 37 (1), 226–247. Available from: https://www.elsevier.com/locate/envint. doi:10.1016/j.envint.2010.06.004.

De Oliveira, R.P., Benvenuti, J., Espinosa, D.C.R., 2021. A review of the current progress in recycling technologies for gallium and rare earth elements from light-emitting diodes. Renew. Sustain. Energy Rev. 145, 111090. https://www.sciencedirect.com/science/article/pii/S1364032121003786.

De Saedeleer, V., Cappuyns, V., De Cooman, W., Swennen, R., 2010. Influence of major elements on heavy metal composition of river sediments. Geol. Belg. 13748505. 13 (3), 257–267. Available from: http://popups.ulg.ac.be/Geol/docannexe.php?id=3029.

De Temmerman, L., Vanongeval, L., Boon, W., Hoenig, M., Geypens, M., 2003. Heavy metal content of arable soils in Northern Belgium. Water, Air, and Soil Pollution. 0049-6979. 148 (1-4), 61–76. doi:10.1023/a:1025498629671.

De, A., Bose, R., Kumar, A., Mozumdar, S., 2014. Targeted Delivery of Pesticides Using Biodegradable Polymeric Nanoparticles SpringerBriefs in Molecular Science. Springer, India. doi:10.1007/978-81-322-1689-6.

De, S., Mitra, A.K., 2004. Mobilization of heavy metals from mine spoils in a part of Raniganj coalfield, India: causes and effects. Environ. Geosci. 10759565. 11 (2), 65–76. Available from: http://archives.datapages.com/data/browse/environmental-geosciences-deg/. doi:10.1306/eg.10010303007.

Demková, L., Jezný, T., Bobuľská, L., 2017. Assessment of soil heavy metal pollution in a former mining area—Before and after the end of mining activities. Soil Water Res. 12 (4), 229–236. doi:10.17221/107/2016-swr.

Draszawka-Bołzan, B., 2015. Heavy metals in soils. World News Nat. Sci. 2, 20–37.

Dung, T.T.T., Cappuyns, V., Swennen, R., Phung, N.K., 2013. From geochemical background determination to pollution assessment of heavy metals in sediments and soils. Rev. Environ. Sci. Biotechnol. 15691705. 12 (4), 335–353. doi:10.1007/s11157-013-9315-1.

Duprè, B., 1983. Pb-Sr isotopic variation in Indian Ocean basalts and mixing phenomena. Nature 303, 536–538.

Duruibe, J.O., Ogwuegbu, M.O.C., Egwurugwu, J.N., 2007. Heavy metal pollution and human biotoxic effects. Int. J. Phys. Sci. 2 (5), 112–118. https://academicjournals.org/article/article1380209337_Duruibe%20et%20al.pdf/1000.

Edokpayi, J., Odiyo, J., Popoola, O., Msagati, T., 2016. Assessment of trace metals contamination of surface water and sediment: a case study of Mvudi River, South Africa. Sustainability. 2071-1050. 8 (2), 135. doi:10.3390/su8020135.

Eggleton, R.A., Foudoulis, C., Varkevisser, D., 1987. Weathering of basalt: changes in rock chemistry and mineralogy. Clays and Clay Minerals 35 (3), 161–169. https://www.cambridge.org/core/journals/clays-and-clay-minerals/article/weathering-of-basalt-changes-in-rock-chemistry-and-mineralogy/89F141DFFF591C96F031EF387806A5AB.

Egli, M., Berger, A., Kündig, R., Krebs, R., de Castro Portes, R., Berger, R., Widmer, R., 2017. The long-term interaction of mine tailings with soils and the wider environment: examples from Mont Chemin, Switzerland. J. Geochem. Explor. 03756742. 182, 53–69. doi:10.1016/j.gexplo.2017.08.011.

Egorova, K.S., Ananikov, V.P., 2017. Toxicity of metal compounds: knowledge and myths. Federation Organometallics. 15206041. 36 (21), 4071–4090. Available from: http://pubs.acs.org/loi/orgnd7. doi:10.1021/acs.organomet.7b00605.

El-Kady, A.A., Abdel-Wahhab, M.A., 2018. Occurrence of trace metals in foodstuffs and their health impact. Trends in Food Science and Technology. 09242244. 75, 36–45. Available from: http://www.elsevier.com/wps/find/journaldescription.cws_home/601278/description#description. doi:10.1016/j.tifs.2018.03.001.

Ermolin, M.S., Fedotov, P.S., Malik, N.A., Karandashev, V.K., 2018. Nanoparticles of volcanic ash as a carrier for toxic elements on the global scale. Chemosphere. 18791298. 200, 16–22. Available from: http://www.elsevier.com/locate/chemosphere. doi:10.1016/j.chemosphere.2018.02.089.

Fabricio Neta, A.D.B., Do Nascimento, C.W.A., Biondi, C.M., van Straaten, P., Bittar, S.M.B., 2018. Natural concentrations and reference values for trace elements in soils of a tropical volcanic archipelago. Environ. Geochem. Health. 15732983. 40 (1), 163–173. Available from: https://www.wkap.nl/journalhome.htm/0269-4042. doi:10.1007/s10653-016-9890-5.

Fashola, M., Ngole-Jeme, V., Babalola, O., 2016. Heavy metal pollution from gold mines: environmental effects and bacterial strategies for resistance. Int. J. Environ. Res. Public Health 13 (11), 1047. doi:10.3390/ijerph13111047.

Forghani, G., Kelm, U., Mazinani, V., 2019. Spatial distribution and chemical partitioning of potentially toxic elements in soils around Khatoon-Abad Cu Smelter, SE Iran. J. Geochem. Explor. 196, 66–80. https://www.sciencedirect.com/science/article/pii/S0375674218300669.

Forti, V., Balde, C.P., Kuehr, R., Bel, G., 2020. The global E-waste monitor 2020: quantities, flows and the circular economy potential. https://collections.unu.edu/view/UNU:7737.

Foulds, S.A., Brewer, P.A., Macklin, M.G., Haresign, W., Betson, R.E., Rassner, S.M.E., 2014. Flood-related contamination in catchments affected by historical metal mining: an unexpected and emerging hazard of climate change. Sci. Total Environ. 00489697. 476-477, 165–180. doi:10.1016/j.scitotenv.2013.12.079.

Franchi, F., Ahad, J.M.E., Geris, J., Jhowa, G., Petros, A.K., Comte, J.C., 2020. Modern sediment records of hydroclimatic extremes and associated potential contaminant mobilization in semi-arid environments: lessons learnt from recent flood-drought cycles in southern Botswana. J. Soils Sediments. 16147480. 20 (3), 1632–1650. Available from: http://www.springerlink.com/content/1439-0108. doi:10.1007/s11368-019-02454-9.

Gautam, P.K., Gautam, R.K., Banerjee, S., Chattopadhyaya, M.C., Pandey, J.D., 2016. Heavy Metals in the Environment: Fate, Transport, Toxicity and Remediation Technologies Heavy Metals: Sources, Toxicity and Remediation Techniques. Nova Science Publishers, Inc, India, 101–130. Available from: https://www.novapublishers.com/catalog/product_info.php?products_id=57531.

Gavrilescu, M., Demnerová, K., Aamand, J., Agathos, S., Fava, F., 2015. Emerging pollutants in the environment: present and future challenges in biomonitoring, ecological risks and bioremediation. New Biotechnol. 18716784. 32 (1), 147–156. doi:10.1016/j.nbt.2014.01.001.

Gill, H.K., Garg, H., 2014. Pesticide: environmental impacts and management strategies. Pesticides-Tox. Asp. 8 (187), 10–5772. https://books.google.com/books?hl=en&lr=&id=PiShDwAAQBAJ&oi=fnd&pg=PA187&dq=Gill,+H.K.,+Garg,+H.,+2014.+Pesticides:+environmental+impacts+and+management+strategies.+In:+Larramendy,+M.L.,+Soloneski,+S.+(Eds.),+Pesticides+-+Toxic+Aspects.+InTech,+Rijeka&ots=B_pI3-e_UQ&sig=d9cDxl64vU-t4zmGJFct1bcFMxE.

Gimeno-García, E., Andreu, V., Boluda, R., 1996. Heavy metals incidence in the application of inorganic fertilizers and pesticides to rice farming soils. Environ. Pollut. 92 (1), 19–25. https://www.sciencedirect.com/science/article/pii/0269749195000909.

Gislason, S.R., Arnórsson, S., 1993. Dissolution of primary basaltic minerals in natural waters: saturation state and kinetics. Chem. Geol. 00092541. 105 (1-3), 117–135. doi:10.1016/0009-2541(93)90122-Y.

Golzar-Ahmadi, M., Bahaloo-Horeh, N., Pourhossein, F., Norouzi, F., Schoenberger, N., Hintersatz, C., Chakankar, M., Holuszko, M., Kaksonen, A.H., 2024. Pathway to industrial application of heterotrophic organisms in critical metals recycling from e-waste. Biotechnology Advances. 07349750. 77, 108438. doi:10.1016/j.biotechadv.2024.108438.

Goodwin, T.H., Young, A.R., Holmes, M.G.R., Old, G.H., Hewitt, N., Leeks, G.J.L., Packman, J.C., Smith, B.P.G., 2003. The temporal and spatial variability of sediment transport and yields within the Bradford Beck catchment, West Yorkshire. Sci. Total Environ. 00489697. 314-316, 475–494. https://www.elsevier.com/locate/scitotenv. doi:10.1016/S0048-9697(03)00069-X.

Gray, C.W., McLaren, R.G., Roberts, A.H., 2003. Atmospheric accessions of heavy metals to some New Zealand pastoral soils. Sci. Total Environ. 305 (1–3), 105–115.

Grison, H., Petrovsky, E., Stejskalova, S., Kapicka, A., 2015. Magnetic and geochemical characterization of A ndosols developed on basalts in the M assif C entral, F rance. Geochem. Geophys. Geosyst. 1525-2027. 16 (5), 1348–1363. doi:10.1002/2015gc005716.

Grout, J.A., Levings, C.D., 2001. Effects of acid mine drainage from an abandoned copper mine, Britannia Mines, Howe Sound, British Columbia, Canada, on transplanted blue mussels (Mytilus edulis). Mar. Environ. Res. 01411136. 51 (3), 265–288. doi:10.1016/s0141-1136(00)00104-5.

Guven, D.E., Akinci, G., 2008. Heavy metals partitioning in the sediments of Izmir Inner Bay. J. Environ. Sci. 10010742. 20 (4), 413–418. doi:10.1016/S1001-0742(08)62072-0.

Gworek, B., Dmuchowski, W., Koda, E., Marecka, M., Baczewska, A., Brągoszewska, P., Sieczka, A., Osiński, P., 2016. Impact of the municipal solid waste łubna landfill on environmental pollution by heavy metals. Water. 2073-4441. 8 (10), 470. doi:10.3390/w8100470.

Hadjipanagiotou, C., Christou, A., Zissimos, A.M., Chatzitheodoridis, E., Varnavas, S.P., 2020. Contamination of stream waters, sediments, and agricultural soil in the surroundings of an abandoned copper mine by potentially toxic elements and associated environmental and potential human health–derived risks: a case study from Agrokipia, Cyprus. Environ. Sci. Pollut. Res. 16147499. 27 (33), 41279–41298. Available from: https://link.springer.com/journal/11356. doi:10.1007/s11356-020-10098-3.

Hama Aziz, K.H., Mustafa, F.S., Omer, K.M., Hama, S., Hamarawf, R.F., Rahman, K.O., 2023. Heavy metal pollution in the aquatic environment: efficient and low-cost removal approaches to eliminate their toxicity: a review. RSC Adv. 20462069. 13 (26), 17595–17610. Available from: http://pubs.rsc.org/en/journals/journal/ra. doi:10.1039/d3ra00723e.

He, J., Yang, Y., Christakos, G., Liu, Y., Yang, X., 2019. Assessment of soil heavy metal pollution using stochastic site indicators. Geoderma. 00167061. 337, 359–367. doi:10.1016/j.geoderma.2018.09.038.

He, Z.L., Yang, X.E., Stoffella, P.J., 2005. Trace elements in agroecosystems and impacts on the environment. Journal of Trace Elements in Medicine and Biology 19 (2–3), 125–140.

Hinojosa, M.B., Carreira, J.A., García-Ruíz, R., Dick, R.P., 2004. Spain Soil moisture pre-treatment effects on enzyme activities as indicators of heavy metal-contaminated and reclaimed soils. Soil Biol. Biochem. 00380717. 36 (10), 1559–1568. doi:10.1016/j.soilbio.2004.07.003.

Ho, H.H., Swennen, R., Van Damme, A., 2010. Distribution and contamination status of heavy metals in estuarine sediments near Cua Ong Harbor, Ha Long Bay, Vietnam. Geol. Belg. https://popups.uliege.be/1374-8505/index.php?id=2844.

Hoefs, J., 2010. Geochemical fingerprints: a critical appraisal. Eur. J. Mineral. 0935-1221. 22 (1), 3–15. doi:10.1127/0935-1221/2010/0022-1997.

Hu, W., Niu, Y., Zhu, H., Dong, K., Wang, D., Liu, F., 2021. Remediation of zinc-contaminated soils by using the two-step washing with citric acid and water-soluble chitosan. Chemosphere. 00456535. 282, 131092. doi:10.1016/j.chemosphere.2021.131092.

Huang, S.-H., Bing, P., 2009. Chromium accumulation, microorganism population and enzyme activities in soils around chromium-containing slag heap of steel alloy factory. Trans. Nonferrous Met. Soc. China 19 (1), 241–248.

Huang, S.-W., Jin, J.-Y., 2008. Status of heavy metals in agricultural soils as affected by different patterns of land use. Environmental Monitoring and Assessment 139 (1), 317–327. https://idp.springer.com/authorize/casa?redirect_uri=https://link.springer.com/article/10.1007/s10661-007-9838-4&casa_token=XvN0KtWSaSIAAAAA:_S3cg2LeeZfhvlJsxu49nwXFL0nhxhnd_8bqIpPF78Cp4UyWhq7SuoSJ1tMcqSmQWo0BgymErBW_DW6s.

Huang, Y., Wang, L., Wang, W., Li, T., He, Z., Yang, X., 2019. Current status of agricultural soil pollution by heavy metals in China: a meta-analysis. Sci. Total Environ. 00489697. 651 (Pt 2), 3034–3042. doi:10.1016/j.scitotenv.2018.10.185.

Hudson-Edwards, K.A., Macklin, M.G., Miller, J.R., Lechler, P.J., 2001. Sources, distribution and storage of heavy metals in the Río Pilcomayo, Bolivia. J. Geochem. Explor. 03756742. 72 (3), 229–250. doi:10.1016/S0375-6742(01)00164-9.

Ilyinskaya, E., Mason, E., Wieser, P.E., Holland, L., Liu, E.J., Mather, T.A., Edmonds, M., Whitty, R.C.W., Elias, T., Nadeau, P.A., Schneider, D., McQuaid, J.B., Allen, S.E., Harvey, J., Oppenheimer, C., Kern, C., Damby, D., 2021. Rapid metal pollutant deposition from the volcanic plume of Kīlauea, Hawai'i. Commun. Earth Environ. 26624435. 2 (1). Available from: https://www.nature.com/commsenv/. doi:10.1038/s43247-021-00146-2.

Indelicato, S., Orecchio, S., Avellone, G., Bellomo, S., Ceraulo, L., Di Leonardo, R., Di Stefano, V., Favara, R., Candela, E.G., Pica, L.L., Morici, S., Pecoraino, G., Pisciotta, A., Scaletta, C., Vita, F., Vizzini, S., Bongiorno, D., 2017. Effect of solid waste landfill organic pollutants on groundwater in three areas of Sicily (Italy) characterized by different vulnerability. Environ. Sci. Pollut. Res. 16147499. 24 (20), 16869–16882. Available from: http://www.springerlink.com/content/0944-1344. doi:10.1007/s11356-017-9198-8.

Iqbal, A., Cevik, E., Mustafa, A., Qahtan, T.F., Zeeshan, M., Bozkurt, A., 2024. Emerging developments in polymeric nanocomposite membrane-based filtration for water purification: a concise overview of toxic metal removal. Chem. Eng. J. 13858947. 481, 148760. doi:10.1016/j.cej.2024.148760.

Iravanian, A., Ravari, S.O., 2020. Types of contamination in landfills and effects on the environment: a review study. IOP Conf. Ser. Earth Environ. Sci. 1755-1307. 614 (1), 012083. doi:10.1088/1755-1315/614/1/012083.

J.S, G., 2002. Biomagnification in marine systems: the perspective of an ecologist. Mar. Pollut. Bull. 0025326X. 45 (1-12), 46–52. doi:10.1016/S0025-326X(01)00323-X.

Jaishankar, M., Tseten, T., Anbalagan, N., Mathew, B.B., Beeregowda, K.N., 2014. Toxicity, mechanism and health effects of some heavy metals. Interdiscip. Toxicol. 13379569. 7 (2), 60–72. Available from: http://versita.com/science/medicine/it/. doi:10.2478/intox-2014-0009.

Järup, L., 2003. Hazards of heavy metal contamination. Br. Med. Bull. 68 (1), 167–182. https://academic.oup.com/bmb/article-abstract/68/1/167/421303.

Jin, M., Yuan, H., Liu, B., Peng, J., Liping, X., Yang, D., 2020. Review of the distribution and detection methods of heavy metals in the environment. Anal. Methods. 1759-9660. 12 (48), 5747–5766. doi:10.1039/d0ay01577f.

Kant, R., 2011. Textile dyeing industry an environmental hazard. https://www.scirp.org/html/4-8301582_17027.htm.

Kapusta, P., Sobczyk, Ł., 2015. Effects of heavy metal pollution from mining and smelting on enchytraeid communities under different land management and soil conditions. Sci. Total Environ. 00489697. 536, 517–526. doi:10.1016/j.scitotenv.2015.07.086.

Karaca, A., Cetin, S.C., Turgay, O.C., Kizilkaya, R., 2010. Effects of heavy metals on soil enzyme activities. In: Soil Heavy Metals, Vol. 19. Springer, Berlin Heidelberg, pp. 237–262. doi:10.1007/978-3-642-02436-8_11.

Karthick, L., Stephen Leon, J., Ravi, R., Michel, J., Jagadish, C.A., 2022. Vehicle safety system for two wheeler – a critical review. Mater. Today Proc. 22147853. 52, 1594–1597. doi:10.1016/j.matpr.2021.11.258.

Khan, K.Y., Ali, B., Cui, X., Feng, Y., Yang, X., Stoffella, P.J., 2017. Impact of different feedstocks derived biochar amendment with cadmium low uptake affinity cultivar of pak choi (*Brassica rapa* ssb. *Chinensis* L.) on phytoavoidation of Cd to reduce potential dietary toxicity. Ecotoxicol. Environ. Saf. 141, 129–138. https://www.sciencedirect.com/science/article/pii/S0147651317301537.

Khan, S., Naushad, M., Lima, E.C., Zhang, S., Shaheen, S.M., Rinklebe, J., 2021. Global soil pollution by toxic elements: current status and future perspectives on the risk assessment and remediation strategies – a review. J. Hazard. Mater. 03043894. 417, 126039. doi:10.1016/j.jhazmat.2021.126039.

Khorasanipour, M., Tangestani, M.H., Naseh, R., Hajmohammadi, H., 2012. Chemical fractionation and contamination intensity of trace elements in stream sediments at the sarcheshmeh porphyry copper mine, SE Iran. Mine Water Environ. 1025-9112. 31 (3), 199–213. doi:10.1007/s10230-012-0198-0.

Kim, -J.-J., Kim, Y.-S., Kumar, V., 2019. Heavy metal toxicity: an update of chelating therapeutic strategies. Journal of Trace Elements in Medicine and Biology 54, 226–231. doi:10.1016/j.jtemb.2019.05.003.

Kim, K.-H., Kabir, E., Jahan, S.A., 2017. Exposure to pesticides and the associated human health effects. Sci. Total Environ. 575, 525–535. https://www.sciencedirect.com/science/article/pii/S004896971631926X.

Krachler, M., Alvarez-Sarandes, R., Rasmussen, G., 2016. High-resolution inductively coupled plasma optical emission spectrometry for^{234} U/^{238} Pu age dating of plutonium materials and comparison to sector field inductively coupled plasma mass spectrometry. Analytical Chemistry 88 (17), 8862–8869. doi:10.1021/acs.analchem.6b02472.

Kumar, M., Seth, A., Singh, A.K., Rajput, M.S., Sikandar, M., 2021. Remediation strategies for heavy metals contaminated ecosystem: a review. Environ. Sustain. Indic. 26659727. 12. Available from: www.journals.elsevier.com/environmental-and-sustainability-indicators. doi:10.1016/j.indic.2021.100155.

Langston, W.J., Bebianno, M.J., 2013. Metal Metabolism in Aquatic Environments, Vol. 7. Springer Science & Business Media. https://books.google.com/books?hl=en&lr=&id=9nsoBgAAQBAJ&oi=fnd&pg=PR11&dq=Langston+WJ,+Bebianno+MJ,+editors.+Metal+metabolism+in+aquatic+environment.+London:+Chapman+%26+Hall%3B+1998.&ots=zqhekbGWiM&sig=0GbrgG8DNdC9cyOiflulWqPlkLs.

Laurence, D., 2011. Establishing a sustainable mining operation: an overview. J. Clean. Prod. 09596526. 19 (2-3), 278–284. doi:10.1016/j.jclepro.2010.08.019.

Li, C.F., Li, X.H., Li, Q.L., Guo, J.H., Li, X.H., 2011. Directly determining 143Nd/ 144Nd isotope ratios using thermal ionization mass spectrometry for geological samples without separation of Sm-Nd. J. Anal. At. Spectrom. 13645544. 26 (10), 2012–2022. doi:10.1039/c0ja00081g.

Li, C., Zhou, K., Qin, W., Tian, C., Qi, M., Yan, X., Han, W., 2019. A review on heavy metals contamination in soil: effects, sources, and remediation techniques. Soil Sediment Contam. 1532-0383. 28 (4), 380–394. doi:10.1080/15320383.2019.1592108.

Li, L., Zhang, Y., Ippolito, J.A., Xing, W., Qiu, K., Yang, H., 2020. Lead smelting effects heavy metal concentrations in soils, wheat, and potentially humans. Environ. Pollut. 02697491. 257, 113641. doi:10.1016/j.envpol.2019.113641.

Li, X., Lee, S.-L., Wong, S.-C., Shi, W., Thornton, I., 2004. The study of metal contamination in urban soils of Hong Kong using a GIS-based approach. Environ. Pollut. 02697491. 129 (1), 113–124. doi:10.1016/j.envpol.2003.09.030.

Liang, L., Wang, Z., Li, J., 2019. The effect of urbanization on environmental pollution in rapidly developing urban agglomerations. J. Clean. Prod. 237, 117649. https://www.sciencedirect.com/science/article/pii/S0959652619324990.

Liang, W., Wang, G., Peng, C., Tan, J., Wan, J., Sun, P., Li, Q., Ji, X., Zhang, Q., Wu, Y., Zhang, W., 2022. Recent advances of carbon-based nano zero valent iron for heavy metals remediation in soil and water: a critical review. J. Hazard. Mater. 03043894. 426, 127993. doi:10.1016/j.jhazmat.2021.127993.

Liu, B., Zhang, L., Wang, Q., 2021. Demand gap analysis of municipal solid waste landfill in Beijing: based on the municipal solid waste generation. Waste Manag. 134, 42–51. https://www.sciencedirect.com/science/article/pii/S0956053X21004323.

Liu, X., Wu, F., Qu, G., Zhang, T., He, M., 2023. Recycling and reutilization of smelting dust as a secondary resource: a review. J. Environ. Manag. 03014797. 347, 119228. doi:10.1016/j.jenvman.2023.119228.

López, A., Lobo, A., 2014. Emissions of C&D refuse in landfills: a European case. Waste Manag. 34 (8), 1446–1454. doi:10.1016/j.wasman.2014.04.004.

Loring, D.H., Rantala, R.T.T., 1992. Manual for the geochemical analyses of marine sediments and suspended particulate matter. Earth-Science Reviews. 00128252. 32 (4), 235–283. doi:10.1016/0012-8252(92)90001-a.

Lottermoser, B.G., Ashley, P.M., Lawie, D.C., 1999. Environmental geochemistry of the Gulf Creek copper mine area, north-eastern New South Wales, Australia. Environ. Geol. 39 (1), 61–74. doi:10.1007/s002540050437.

Luo, X., Wu, C., Lin, Y., Li, W., Deng, M., Tan, J., Xue, S., 2023. Soil heavy metal pollution from Pb/Zn smelting regions in China and the remediation potential of biomineralization. J. Environ. Sci. 10010742. 125, 662–677. doi:10.1016/j.jes.2022.01.029.

Luo, Y., Zheng, Z., Wu, P., Wu, Y., 2022. Effect of different direct revegetation strategies on the mobility of heavy metals in artificial zinc smelting waste slag: implications for phytoremediation. Chemosphere. 00456535. 286 (Pt 1), 131678. doi:10.1016/j.chemosphere.2021.131678.

Lyu, Y., Zhang, K., Chai, F., Cheng, T., Yang, Q., Zheng, Z., Li, X., 2017. Atmospheric size-resolved trace elements in a city affected by non-ferrous metal smelting: indications of respiratory deposition and health risk. Environ. Pollut. 02697491. 224, 559–571. doi:10.1016/j.envpol.2017.02.039.

Ma, L., Sun, J., Yang, Z., Wang, L., 2015. Heavy metal contamination of agricultural soils affected by mining activities around the Ganxi River in Chenzhou, Southern China. Environmental Monitoring and Assessment. 0167-6369. 187 (12). doi:10.1007/s10661-015-4966-8.

Ma, Q., Han, L., Zhang, J., Zhang, Y., Lang, Q., Li, F., Han, A., Bao, Y., Li, K., Alu, S., 2019. Environmental Risk Assessment of Metals in the Volcanic Soil of Changbai Mountain. Int. J. Environ. Res. Public Health. 1660-4601. 16 (11), 2047. doi:10.3390/ijerph16112047.

Madon, I., Drev, D., Likar, J., 2019. Long-term risk assessments comparing environmental performance of different types of sanitary landfills. Waste Manag. 96, 96–107. https://www.sciencedirect.com/science/article/pii/S0956053X19304477.

Maghchiche, A., Meghchiche, N., 2024. Current awareness and knowledge of heavy metals. African Journal of Environmental Sciences and Renewable Energy. 3027-2114. 16 (1), 17–29. doi:10.62154/ajesre.2024.016.010373.

Mandal, A., Sarkar, B., Mandal, S., Vithanage, M., Patra, A.K., Manna, M.C., 2020. Impact of agrochemicals on soil health. In: Agrochemicals Detection, Treatment and Remediation. Elsevier, pp. 161–187. https://www.sciencedirect.com/science/article/pii/B9780081030172000076.

Mar, S.S., Okazaki, M., Motobayashi, T., 2012. The influence of phosphate fertilizer application levels and cultivars on cadmium uptake by Komatsuna (*Brassica rapa*L. var.*perviridis*). Soil Science and Plant Nutrition 58 (4), 492–502. doi:10.1080/00380768.2012.704394.

Marques, A.P., Rangel, A.O., Castro, P.M., 2013. Erratum: remediation of heavy metal contaminated soils: an overview of site remediation techniques (Critical Reviews in Environmental Science and Technology (2011) 41:10 (879–914). Crit. Rev. Environ. Sci. Technol. 43 (15), 1740.

Martinez-Guijarro, R., Pachés, M., Romero, I., Aguado, D., 2021. Sources, mobility, reactivity, and remediation of heavy metal(loid) pollution: a review. Advances in Environmental and Engineering Research. 27666190. 02 (04), 1–33. doi:10.21926/aeer.2104033.

McGeer, J., 2004. Issue paper on the bioavailability and bioaccumulation of metals. US Environmental Protection Agency. https://books.google.com/books?hl=en&lr=&id=Bsk7Tosoq7sC&oi=fnd&pg=PA1&dq=US+Environmental+Protection+Agency.+McGeer+J,+Henningsen+G,+Lanno+R,+Fisher+N,+Sappington+K,+Drexler+J.+Issue+paper+on+the+bioavailability+and+bioaccumulation+of+metals.+Washington%3B+2004&ots=_VGnFh38Di&sig=C7Ehrt2c0rNeOYLiv23kSZVXOXg.

Meck, M., Love, D., Mapani, B., 2006. Zimbabwean mine dumps and their impacts on river water quality – a reconnaissance study. Phys. Chem. Earth A/B/C 31 (15), 797–803. doi:10.1016/j.pce.2006.08.029.

Melendez-Pastor, I., Navarro-Pedreño, J., Gómez, I., Almendro-Candel, M.B., 2011. The use of remote sensing to locate heavy metal as source of pollution. Advances in Environmental Research 7, 217–234. Available from: http://www.novapublishers.org/catalog/product_info.php?products_id=29755.

Memoli, V., Eymar, E., García-Delgado, C., Esposito, F., Panico, S.C., De Marco, A., Barile, R., Maisto, G., 2018. Soil element fractions affect phytotoxicity, microbial biomass and activity in volcanic areas. Sci. Total Environ. 00489697. 636, 1099–1108. doi:10.1016/j.scitotenv.2018.04.327.

Milton, A., Cooke, J.A., Johnson, M.S., 2003. Accumulation of lead, zinc, and cadmium in a wild population of *Clethrionomys glareolus* from an abandoned lead mine. Arch. Environ. Contam. Toxicol. 44 (3), 0405–0411. doi:10.1007/s00244-002-2014-5.

Mohanraj, R., Akil Prasath, R.V., Balaramdas, K.R., Amjad, K.T., 2024. Bioavailable fractions of heavy metals in the road dust during infrastructure construction at urban Coimbatore and its potential health implications, India. Environ. Geochem. Health. 15732983. 46 (8). Available from: https://www.springer.com/journal/10653. doi:10.1007/s10653-024-02040-0.

Mora, A.P.D., Ortega-Calvo, J.J., Cabrera, F., Madejón, E., 2005. Changes in enzyme activities and microbial biomass after "in situ" remediation of a heavy metal-contaminated soil. Appl. Soil Ecol. 09291393. 28 (2), 125–137. doi:10.1016/j.apsoil.2004.07.006.

Morrell, W.J., Stewart, R.B., Gregg, P.E.H., Bolan, N.S., Horne, D., 1996. An assessment of sulphide oxidation in abandoned base-metal tailings, Te Aroha, New Zealand. Environ. Pollut. 94 (2), 217–225. doi:10.1016/S0269-7491(96)00059-0.

Müller, C., 2018. Impacts of sublethal insecticide exposure on insects — facts and knowledge gaps. Basic Appl. Ecol. 14391791. 30, 1–10. doi:10.1016/j.baae.2018.05.001.

Muller, G., 1969. Index of geoaccumulation in sediments of the Rhine River. https://www.sid.ir/paper/618491/fa.

Munir, N., Jahangeer, M., Bouyahya, A., El Omari, N., Ghchime, R., Balahbib, A., Aboulaghras, S., Mahmood, Z., Akram, M., Ali Shah, S.M., Mikolaychik, I.N., Derkho, M., Rebezov, M., Venkidasamy, B., Thiruvengadam, M., Shariati, M.A., 2021. Heavy metal contamination of natural foods is a serious health issue: a review. Sustainability 14 (1), 161. doi:10.3390/su14010161.

Naccarato, A., Tassone, A., Cavaliere, F., Elliani, R., Pirrone, N., Sprovieri, F., Tagarelli, A., Giglio, A., 2020. Agrochemical treatments as a source of heavy metals and rare earth elements in agricultural soils and bioaccumulation in ground beetles. Sci. Total Environ. 00489697. 749, 141438. doi:10.1016/j.scitotenv.2020.141438.

Nagajyoti, P.C., Lee, K.D., Sreekanth, T.V.M., 2010. Heavy metals, occurrence and toxicity for plants: a review. Environ. Chem. Lett. 8 (3), 199–216. doi:10.1007/s10311-010-0297-8.

Naicker, K., Cukrowska, E., McCarthy, T.S., 2003. Acid mine drainage arising from gold mining activity in Johannesburg, South Africa and environs. Environ. Pollut. 122 (1), 29–40. doi:10.1016/S0269-7491(02)00281-6.

Naidu, R., Bolan, N.S., 2008. Contaminant chemistry in soils: key concepts and bioavailability. Developments in Soil Science 32, 9–37.

Nesbitt, H.W., Wilson, R.E., 1992. Recent chemical weathering of basalts. American Journal of Science 292 (10), 740–777. https://ajsonline.org/article/60583-recent-chemical-weathering-of-basalts.

Nosrati, K., Collins, A.L., 2019. A soil quality index for evaluation of degradation under land use and soil erosion categories in a small mountainous catchment, Iran. J. Mt. Sci. 19930321. 16 (11), 2577–2590. Available from: http://www.springer.com/west/home?SGWID=4-102-70-173618726-0&changeHeader=true. doi:10.1007/s11629-019-5567-8.

Obiri-Nyarko, F., Duah, A.A., Karikari, A.Y., Agyekum, W.A., Manu, E., Tagoe, R., 2021. Assessment of heavy metal contamination in soils at the Kpone landfill site, Ghana: implication for ecological and health risk assessment. Chemosphere. 18791298. 282. Available from: https://www.elsevier.com/locate/chemosphere. doi:10.1016/j.chemosphere.2021.131007.

Odobašić, A., Šestan, I., Begić, S., 2019. Biosensors for determination of heavy metals in waters. In: Biosensors for Environmental Monitoring. IntechOpen. https://books.google.com/books?hl=en&lr=&id=zzf8DwAAQBAJ&oi=fnd&pg=PA139&dq=Odoba%C5%A1ic%C2%B4+,+A.,+%C5%A0estan,+I.,+Begic%C2%B4+,+S.,+2019.+Biosensors+for+determination+of+heavy+metals+in+waters.+Biosensors+for+Environmental+Monitoring.+IntechOpen&ots=mvFClUEzcX&sig=54bxV_wpurWKcMF1Ezf66B34zdc.

Ogbonna, P.C., Okezie, N., 2011. Heavy metal level and macronutrient contents of roadside soil and vegetation in Umuahia, Nigeria. Terrest. Aquat. Environ. Toxicol. 5 (1), 35–39.

Ogunbanjo, O., Onawumi, O., Gbadamosi, M., Ogunlana, A., Anselm, O., 2016. Chemical speciation of some heavy metals and human health risk assessment in soil around two municipal dumpsites in Sagamu, Ogun state, Nigeria. Chem. Speciat. Bioavailab. 0954-2299. 28 (1-4), 142–151. doi:10.1080/09542299.2016.1203267.

Ogunkunle, O., Ahmed, N.A., 2021. Overview of biodiesel combustion in mitigating the adverse impacts of engine emissions on the sustainable human–environment scenario. Sustainability. 2071-1050. 13 (10), 5465. doi:10.3390/su13105465.

Okeke, E.S., Enochoghene, A., Ezeudoka, B.C., Kaka, S.D., Chen, Y., Mao, G., ThankGodEze, C., Feng, W., Wu, X., 2024. A review of heavy metal risks around e-waste sites and comparable municipal dumpsites in major African cities: recommendations and future perspectives. Toxicology. 18793185. 501. Available from: https://www.sciencedirect.com/science/journal/0300483X. doi:10.1016/j.tox.2023.153711.

Oladimeji, T.E., Oyedemi, M., Emetere, M.E., Agboola, O., Adeoye, J.B., Odunlami, O.A., 2024. Review on the impact of heavy metals from industrial wastewater effluent and removal technologies. Heliyon. 24058440. 10 (23), e40370. doi:10.1016/j.heliyon.2024.e40370.

Owonikoko, W.M., Alimba, C.G., 2024. Systematic literature review of heavy metal contamination of the Nigerian environment from e-waste management: associated health and carcinogenic risk assessment. Toxicology. 0300483X. 505, 153811. doi:10.1016/j.tox.2024.153811.

Pachana, K., Wattanakornsiri, A., Nanuam, J., 2010. Heavy metal transport and fate in the environmental compartments. NU Sci. J. 7 (1), 1–11.

Palanivel, T.M., Victor, R., 2020. Contamination assessment of heavy metals in the soils of an abandoned copper mine in Lasail, Northern Oman. Int. J. Environ. Stud. 10290400. 77 (3), 432–446. Available from: https://www.tandf.co.uk/journals/titles/00207233.asp. doi:10.1080/00207233.2019.1644030.

Parvin, F., Tareq, S.M., 2021. Impact of landfill leachate contamination on surface and groundwater of Bangladesh: a systematic review and possible public health risks assessment. Appl. Water Sci. 21905495. 11 (6). Available from: https://www.springer.com/journal/13201. doi:10.1007/s13201-021-01431-3.

Peng, Y., Xiong, X., Adhikari, K., Knadel, M., Grunwald, S., Greve, M.H., 2015. Modeling soil organic carbon at regional scale by combining multi-spectral images with laboratory spectra.

PLoS ONE. 19326203. 10 (11). Available from: http://www.plosone.org/article/fetchObject.action?uri=info:doi/10.1371/journal.pone.0142295&representation=PDF. doi:10.1371/journal.pone.0142295.

Pérez, G., Valiente, M., 2005. Determination of pollution trends in an abandoned mining site by application of a multivariate statistical analysis to heavy metals fractionation using SM&T-SES. J. Environ. Monit. 14640325. 7 (1), 29–36. doi:10.1039/b411316k.

Pinto, M.C., da Silva, E.F., Silva, M., Melo-Gonçalves, P., 2015. Heavy metals of Santiago Island (Cape Verde) top soils: estimated background value maps and environmental risk assessment. Journal of African Earth Sciences 101, 162–176. https://www.sciencedirect.com/science/article/pii/S1464343X14003197.

Plumlee, G.S., Morman, S.A., Ziegler, T.L., 2006. The toxicological geochemistry of earth materials: an overview of processes and the interdisciplinary methods used to understand them. Reviews in Mineralogy and Geochemistry 64 (1), 5–57.

Podda, F., Zuddas, P., Minacci, A., Pepi, M., Baldi, F., 2000. Heavy metal coprecipitation with hydrozincite [Zn 5 (CO 3) 2 (OH) 6] from mine waters caused by photosynthetic microorganisms. Applied and Environmental Microbiology. 0099-2240. 66 (11), 5092–5098. doi:10.1128/aem.66.11.5092-5098.2000.

Ponce-Hernández, A., Carranza-Álvarez, C., Ceballos-Maldonado, J.G., Rubio-Gómez, J.A., Martínez-Soto, D., 2025. Overview of the heavy metal contamination in Mexico: sources of the contamination and issues in human health. Environ. Geochem. Health. 15732983. 47 (3). Available from: https://www.springer.com/journal/10653. doi:10.1007/s10653-025-02390-3.

Princewill-Ogbonna, I.L., Ogbonna, P.C., 2011. Heavy metal content in soil and medicinal plants in high traffic urban area. https://www.cabidigitallibrary.org/doi/full/10.5555/20113189788.

Priyadarshanee, M., Das, S., 2021. Biosorption and removal of toxic heavy metals by metal tolerating bacteria for bioremediation of metal contamination: a comprehensive review. Journal of Environmental Chemical Engineering. 22133437. 9 (1), 104686. doi:10.1016/j.jece.2020.104686.

Punia, A., 2021. Role of temperature, wind, and precipitation in heavy metal contamination at copper mines: a review. Environ. Sci. Pollut. Res. 0944-1344. 28 (4), 4056–4072. doi:10.1007/s11356-020-11580-8.

Punia, A., Siva Siddaiah, N., 2017. Assessment of heavy metal contamination in groundwater of Khetri Copper Mine Region, India and health risk assessment. Asian J. Water Environ. Pollut. 14 (4), 9–19. doi:10.3233/ajw-170032.

Putros, M.D., Khadim, H.J., 2024. Assessment of heavy metal contamination in soils adjacent to fossil fuel power plants in Iraq: a mini-review. Al-Salam J. Eng. Technol. 2790-4822. 4 (1), 27–35. doi:10.55145/ajest.2025.04.01.003.

Qiu, G., Feng, X., Wang, S., Shang, L., 2005. Mercury and methylmercury in riparian soil, sediments, mine-waste calcines, and moss from abandoned Hg mines in east Guizhou province, Southwestern China. Appl. Geochem. 08832927. 20 (3), 627–638. doi:10.1016/j.apgeochem.2004.09.006.

Rahman, M.L., Wong, Z.J., Sarjadi, M.S., Soloi, S., Arshad, S.E., Bidin, K., Musta, B., 2021. Heavy metals removal from electroplating wastewater by waste fiber-based poly(Amidoxime) ligand. Water (Switzerland). 20734441. 13 (9). Available from: https://www.mdpi.com/2073-4441/13/9/1260/pdf. doi:10.3390/w13091260.

Rahman, S.U., Yasin, G., Nawaz, M.F., Cheng, H., Azhar, M.F., Riaz, L., Javed, A., Lu, Y., 2022. Evaluation of heavy metal phytoremediation potential of six tree species of Faisalabad city of Pakistan during summer and winter seasons. J. Environ. Manag. 03014797. 320, 115801. doi:10.1016/j.jenvman.2022.115801.

Rahman, Z., Singh, V.P., 2019. The relative impact of toxic heavy metals (THMs) (arsenic (As), cadmium (Cd), chromium (Cr)(VI), mercury (Hg), and lead (Pb)) on the total environment: an overview. Environmental Monitoring and Assessment. 15732959. 191 (7). Available from: https://link.springer.com/journal/10661. doi:10.1007/s10661-019-7528-7.

Rajoria, S., Vashishtha, M., Sangal, V.K., 2022. Treatment of electroplating industry wastewater: a review on the various techniques. Environ. Sci. Pollut. Res. 29 (48), 72196–72246. doi:10.1007/s11356-022-18643-y.

Rasheed, T., Kausar, F., Rizwan, K., Adeel, M., Sher, F., Alwadai, N., Alshammari, F.H., 2022. Two dimensional MXenes as emerging paradigm for adsorptive removal of toxic metallic pollutants from wastewater. Chemosphere. 00456535. 287 (Pt 3), 132319. doi:10.1016/j.chemosphere.2021.132319.

Rashid, A., Schutte, B.J., Ulery, A., Deyholos, M.K., Sanogo, S., Lehnhoff, E.A., Beck, L., 2023. Heavy metal contamination in agricultural soil: environmental pollutants affecting crop health. Agronomy. 20734395. 13 (6). Available from: https://www.mdpi.com/journal/agronomy/. doi:10.3390/agronomy13061521.

Rathoure, A.K., 2024, Understanding pollution pathways and infrastructure impacts. Octa J. Environ. Res. 12 (2). https://www.sciencebeingjournal.com/sites/default/files/01%20 20240404_1202_AK01.pdf.

Reeder, R.J., Schoonen, M.A.A., Lanzirotti, A., 2006. Metal speciation and its role in bioaccessibility and bioavailability. Reviews in Mineralogy and Geochemistry 64 (1), 59–113. doi:10.2138/rmg.2006.64.3.

Robinson, B.H., 2009. E-waste: an assessment of global production and environmental impacts. Sci. Total Environ. 00489697. 408 (2), 183–191. doi:10.1016/j.scitotenv.2009.09.044.

Roy, R., Samanta, S., Pandit, S., Naaz, T., Banerjee, S., Rawat, J.M., Chaubey, K.K., Saha, R.P., 2024. An overview of bacteria-mediated heavy metal bioremediation strategies. Appl. Biochem. Biotechnol. 15590291. 196 (3), 1712–1751. Available from: https://www.springer.com/journal/12010. doi:10.1007/s12010-023-04614-7.

Salazar-Rojas, T., Cejudo-Ruiz, F.R., Gutiérrez-Soto, M.V., Calvo-Brenes, G., 2023. Assessing heavy metal pollution load index (PLI) in biomonitors and road dust from vehicular emission by magnetic properties modeling. Environ. Sci. Pollut. Res. 16147499. 30 (39), 91248–91261. Available from: https://www.springer.com/journal/11356. doi:10.1007/s11356-023-28758-5.

Salgaonkar, S., Botle, A., Barabde, G., Herlekar, M., 2024. Micro-nanoplastics from stormwater runoffs to water bodies: an in-depth investigationIn: Bhat, S.A., Kumar, V., Li, F., Kumar, S. (Eds.), Management of Micro and Nano-plastics in Soil and Biosolids. Springer Nature, Switzerland, pp. 95–117. doi:10.1007/978-3-031-51967-3_4.

Sánchez-Chardi, A., Marques, C.C., Nadal, J., da Luz Mathias, M., 2007. Metal bioaccumulation in the greater white-toothed shrew, Crocidura russula, inhabiting an abandoned pyrite mine site. Chemosphere. 00456535. 67 (1), 121–130. Available from: https://www.elsevier.com/locate/chemosphere doi:10.1016/j.chemosphere.2006.09.009.

Satarug, S., Baker, J.R., Urbenjapol, S., Haswell-Elkins, M., Reilly, P.E.B., Williams, D.J., Moore, M.R., 2003. Australia A global perspective on cadmium pollution and toxicity in non-occupationally exposed population. Toxicol. Lett. 137 (1-2), 65–83. doi:10.1016/S0378-4274(02)00381-8.

Selvaraj, K., Parthiban, G., Arthur Chen, C.T., Lou, J.Y., 2010. Anthropogenic effects on sediment quality offshore southwestern Taiwan: assessing the sediment core geochemical record. Cont. Shelf Res. 02784343. 30 (10-11), 1200–1210. doi:10.1016/j.csr.2010.03.010.

Sharma, A., Kumar, V., Shahzad, B., Tanveer, M., Sidhu, G.P.S., Handa, N., Kohli, S.K., Yadav, P., Bali, A.S., Parihar, R.D., Dar, O.I., Singh, K., Jasrotia, S., Bakshi, P., Ramakrishnan, M., Kumar, S., Bhardwaj, R., Thukral, A.K., 2019. Worldwide pesticide usage and its impacts on ecosystem. SN Appl. Sci. 1 (11). doi:10.1007/s42452-019-1485-1.

Sharma, V.K., Filip, J., Zboril, R., Varma, R.S., 2015. Natural inorganic nanoparticles–formation, fate, and toxicity in the environment. Chemical Society Reviews 44 (23), 8410–8423. https://pubs.rsc.org/en/content/articlehtml/2015/cs/c5cs00236b.

Sharma, V., Sharma, M., Pandita, S., Kour, J., Sharma, N., 2021. Application of geographic information system and remote sensing in heavy metal assessment. In: Heavy Metals in the Environment. Elsevier, pp. 191–204. doi:10.1016/B978-0-12-821656-9.00011-0.

Shrestha, R., Ban, S., Devkota, S., Sharma, S., Joshi, R., Tiwari, A.P., Kim, H.Y., Joshi, M.K., 2021. Technological trends in heavy metals removal from industrial wastewater: a review. Journal of Environmental Chemical Engineering. 22133437. 9 (4). Available from: http://www.journals.elsevier.com/journal-of-environmental-chemical-engineering/. doi:10.1016/j.jece.2021.105688.

Siddiqua, A., Hahladakis, J.N., Al-Attiya, W.A.K.A., 2022. An overview of the environmental pollution and health effects associated with waste landfilling and open dumping. Environ. Sci. Pollut. Res. 29 (39), 58514–58536. doi:10.1007/s11356-022-21578-z.

Singh, A.K., Chandra, R., 2019. Pollutants released from the pulp paper industry: aquatic toxicity and their health hazards. Aquat. Toxicol. 0166445X. 211, 202–216. doi:10.1016/j.aquatox.2019.04.007.

Singh, A., Singh, D., Yadav, H., 2017. Impact and assessment of heavy metal toxicity on water quality, edible fishes and sediments in lakes: a review. Trends Biosci. 10 (8), 1551–1560.

Singh, A., Singh, J., Singh, A., Singh, R., 2014, Biomedical waste management and their possible health risks with controlling measures in the Bareilly City, UP, India. Octa J. Environ. Res. 2 (4). https://www.nswai.org/docs/BIOMEDICAL%20WASTE%20MANAGEMENT%20AND%20THEIR%20POSSIBLE%20HEALTH%20RISKS.pdf.

Song, P., Xu, D., Yue, J., Ma, Y., Dong, S., Feng, J., 2022. Recent advances in soil remediation technology for heavy metal contaminated sites: a critical review. Sci. Total Environ. 00489697. 838 (Pt 3), 156417. doi:10.1016/j.scitotenv.2022.156417.

Srivastava, N.K., Majumder, C.B., 2008. Novel biofiltration methods for the treatment of heavy metals from industrial wastewater. J. Hazard. Mater. 03043894. 151 (1), 1–8. doi:10.1016/j.jhazmat.2007.09.101.

Sulistyowati, L., Nurhasanah, N., Riani, E., Cordova, M.R., 2023. Heavy metals concentration in the sediment of the aquaticenvironment caused by the leachate discharge from a landfill. Glob. J. Environ. Sci. Manag. 23833866. 9 (2), 323–336. Available from: https://www.gjesm.net/. doi:10.22034/gjesm.2023.02.11.

Sun, B., Zhao, F.J., Lombi, E., McGrath, S.P., 2001. Leaching of heavy metals from contaminated soils using EDTA. Environ. Pollut. 02697491. 113 (2), 111–120. doi:10.1016/s0269-7491(00)00176-7.

Swain, C.K., 2024. Environmental pollution indices: a review on concentration of heavy metals in air, water, and soil near industrialization and urbanisation. Discover Environment. 27319431. 2 (1). Available from: https://link.springer.com/journal/44274. doi:10.1007/s44274-024-00030-8.

Szynkowska, M.I., Pawlaczyk, A., Maćkiewicz, E., 2018. Bioaccumulation and biomagnification of trace elements in the environment. In: Chojnacka, K., Saeid, A., Eds. Recent Advances in Trace Elements (first ed.). Wiley, pp. 251–276. doi:10.1002/9781119133780.ch13.

Taghavi, R., Rostamnia, S., Farajzadeh, M., Karimi-Maleh, H., Wang, J., Kim, D., Jang, H.W., Luque, R., Varma, R.S., Shokouhimehr, M., 2022. Magnetite metal-organic frameworks: applications in environmental remediation of heavy metals, organic contaminants, and other pollutants. Inorg. Chem. 1520510X. 61 (40), 15747–15783. Available from: http://pubs.acs.org/journal/inocaj. doi:10.1021/acs.inorgchem.2c01939.

Tang, L., Tang, C., Xiao, J., Zeng, P., Tang, M., Wang, Z., Zhang, Z., 2019. A cleaner process for lead recovery from lead-containing hazardous solid waste and zinc leaching residue via reducing-matting smelting. J. Clean. Prod. 09596526. 241, 118328. doi:10.1016/j.jclepro.2019.118328.

Teng, D., Mao, K., Ali, W., Xu, G., Huang, G., Niazi, N.K., Feng, X., Zhang, H., 2020. Describing the toxicity and sources and the remediation technologies for mercury-contaminated soil. RSC Adv. 20462069. 10 (39), 23221–23232. Available from: http://pubs.rsc.org/en/journals/journal/ra. doi:10.1039/d0ra01507e.

Tešić, M., Stojanović, N., Knežević, M., Đunisijević-Bojović, D., Petrović, J., Pavlović, P., 2022. The impact of the degree of urbanization on spatial distribution, sources and levels of heavy metals pollution in urban soils—a case study of the city of Belgrade (Serbia). Sustainability. 2071-1050. 14 (20), 13126. doi:10.3390/su142013126.

Thomas, E.Y., Omueti, J.A.I., Ogundayomi, O., 2012. The effect of phosphate fertilizer on heavy metal in soils and *Amaranthus caudatus*. Agric. Biol. J. N. Am. 3 (4), 145–149. https://www.Sci-Hub.org/ABJNA/PDF/2012/4/ABJNA-3-4-145-149.pdf

Tian, T., Liu, G., Yasemi, H., Liu, Y., 2022. Managing e-waste from a closed-loop lifecycle perspective: china's challenges and fund policy redesign. Environ. Sci. Pollut. Res. 0944-1344. 29 (31), 47713–47724. doi:10.1007/s11356-022-19227-6.

Timothy, N., Williams, E.T., 2019. Environmental Pollution by Heavy Metal: an Overview. Int. J. Environ. Chem. 2640-1452. 3 (2), 72. doi:10.11648/j.ijec.20190302.14.

Tiwari, R., Botle, A., Bhat, S.A., Singh, P.P., Taneja, A., 2022. Chemical characterization and health risk assessement of size segreated PM at world heritage site, Agra. Cleaner Chemical Engineering. 27727823. 3, 100049. doi:10.1016/j.clce.2022.100049.

Tiwari, R., Botle, A., Kumar, R., Singh, P.P., Taneja, A., 2023a. Morphology and health risk assessment of potential toxic elements in size segregated PM at traffic intersection in Northern India. J. Trace Elem. Miner. 4, 100074. doi:10.1016/j.jtemin.2023.100074.

Tiwari, R., Botle, A., Rajouriya, K., Singh, P., Taneja, A., 2023b. Chemical fraction and health effect of size segregate PM at national highway of Northern India. Pollution 9 (4). doi:10.22059/poll.2023.360350.1946.

Torres, P., Llopis, A.L., Melo, C.S., Rodrigues, A., 2023. Environmental impact of cadmium in a volcanic archipelago: research challenges related to a natural pollution source. J. Mar. Sci. Eng. 20771312. 11 (1). Available from: http://www.mdpi.com/journal/jmse. doi:10.3390/jmse11010100.

Udongwo, A., 2023. Monitoring, assessment, and remediation of heavy metal contamination: techniques, strategies, and policy frameworks. Communication in Physical Sciences 10 (3), 250–261.

V, B., M, R., Mir, A.R., 2023. Developments in analytical techniques for chemostratigraphy, chronostratigraphy, and geochemical fingerprinting studies: current status and future trends. J. S. Am. Earth Sci. 129, 104528. doi:10.1016/j.jsames.2023.104528.

van der Ent, A., Edraki, M., 2018. Environmental geochemistry of the abandoned Mamut Copper Mine (Sabah) Malaysia. Environ. Geochem. Health. 0269-4042. 40 (1), 189–207. doi:10.1007/s10653-016-9892-3.

Vareda, J.P., Valente, A.J.M., Durães, L., 2019. Assessment of heavy metal pollution from anthropogenic activities and remediation strategies: a review. J. Environ. Manag. 246, 101–118. doi:10.1016/j.jenvman.2019.05.126.

Verma, S., Kuila, A., 2019. Bioremediation of heavy metals by microbial process. Environ. Technol. Innov. 23521864. 14, 100369. doi:10.1016/j.eti.2019.100369.

Wang, R., Zhan, L., Xu, Z., Liu, Y., 2024. Constructing high-resolution fingerprints and analyzing complex pollution source of electronic waste recycling base. Resour. Conserv. Recycl. 09213449. 202, 107364. doi:10.1016/j.resconrec.2023.107364.

Wang, S., Han, Z., Wang, J., He, X., Zhou, Z., Hu, X., 2022. Environmental risk assessment and factors influencing heavy metal concentrations in the soil of municipal solid waste landfills. Waste Manag. 0956053X. 139, 330–340. doi:10.1016/j.wasman.2021.11.036.

Wang, Y., Luo, Y., Zeng, G., Wu, X., Wu, B., Li, X., Xu, H., 2020. Characteristics and in situ remediation effects of heavy metal immobilizing bacteria on cadmium and nickel co-contaminated soil. Ecotoxicol. Environ. Saf. 01476513. 192, 110294. doi:10.1016/j.ecoenv.2020.110294.

Wu, G., Wang, L., Yang, R., Hou, W., Zhang, S., Guo, X., Zhao, W., 2022. Pollution characteristics and risk assessment of heavy metals in the soil of a construction waste landfill site. Ecological Informatics. 15749541. 70, 101700. doi:10.1016/j.ecoinf.2022.101700.

Wu, H., Zuo, J., Zillante, G., Wang, J., Yuan, H., 2019. Status quo and future directions of construction and demolition waste research: a critical review. J. Clean. Prod. 09596526. 240, 118163. doi:10.1016/j.jclepro.2019.118163.

Wu, W., Qu, S., Nel, W., Ji, J., 2021. The influence of natural weathering on the behavior of heavy metals in small basaltic watersheds: a comparative study from different regions in China. Chemosphere. 00456535. 262, 127897. doi:10.1016/j.chemosphere.2020.127897.

Xing, W., Liu, H., Banet, T., Wang, H., Ippolito, J.A., Liping, L., 2020. Cadmium, copper, lead and zinc accumulation in wild plant species near a lead smelter. Ecotoxicol. Environ. Saf. 01476513. 198, 110683. doi:10.1016/j.ecoenv.2020.110683.

Xu, D.M., Fu, R.B., Liu, H.Q., Guo, X.P., 2021b. Current knowledge from heavy metal pollution in Chinese smelter contaminated soils, health risk implications and associated remediation progress in recent decades: a critical review. J. Clean. Prod. 09596526. 286. Available from: https://www.journals.elsevier.com/journal-of-cleaner-production. doi:10.1016/j.jclepro.2020.124989.

Xu, D.M., Fu, R.B., Wang, J.X., Shi, Y.X., Guo, X.P., 2021a. Chemical stabilization remediation for heavy metals in contaminated soils on the latest decade: available stabilizing materials and associated evaluation methods–A critical review. J. Clean. Prod. 09596526. 321. Available from: https://www.journals.elsevier.com/journal-of-cleaner-production. doi:10.1016/j.jclepro.2021.128730.

Yang, Y., Yang, X., He, M., Christakos, G., 2020. Beyond mere pollution source identification: determination of land covers emitting soil heavy metals by combining PCA/APCS, GeoDetector and GIS analysis. CATENA. 03418162. 185, 104297. doi:10.1016/j.catena.2019.104297.

Zaynab, M., Al-Yahyai, R., Ameen, A., Sharif, Y., Ali, L., Fatima, M., Khan, K.A., Shuangfei, L., 2022. Health and environmental effects of heavy metals. J. King Saud Univ. Sci. 10183647. 34 (1), 101653. doi:10.1016/j.jksus.2021.101653.

Zeng, J., Ke, W., Deng, M., Tan, J., Li, C., Cheng, Y., Xue, S., 2023. A practical method for identifying key factors in the distribution and formation of heavy metal pollution at a smelting site. J. Environ. Sci. 10010742. 127, 552–563. doi:10.1016/j.jes.2022.06.026.

Zhang, B., Wu, D., Zhang, L., Jiao, Q., Qingting, L., 2012. Application of hyperspectral remote sensing for environment monitoring in mining areas. Environ. Earth Sci. 1866-6280. 65 (3), 649–658. doi:10.1007/s12665-011-1112-y.

Zhang, J., Kim, H., Dubey, B., Townsend, T., 2017. Arsenic leaching and speciation in C&D debris landfills and the relationship with gypsum drywall content. Waste Manag. 0956053X. 59, 324–329. doi:10.1016/j.wasman.2016.10.023.

Zhang, Q., Wang, C., 2020. Natural and human factors affect the distribution of soil heavy metal pollution: a review. Water Air Soil Pollut. 231 (7). doi:10.1007/s11270-020-04728-2.

Zhang, S.Y., Sun, G.X., Yin, X.X., Rensing, C., Zhu, Y.G., 2013. Biomethylation and volatilization of arsenic by the marine microalgae *Ostreococcus tauri*. Chemosphere. 18791298. 93 (1), 47–53. Available from: https://www.elsevier.com/locate/chemosphere. doi:10.1016/j.chemosphere.2013.04.063.

Zhang, X., Wei, S., Sun, Q., Wadood, S.A., Guo, B., 2018. Source identification and spatial distribution of arsenic and heavy metals in agricultural soil around Hunan industrial estate by positive matrix factorization model, principle components analysis and geo statistical analysis. Ecotoxicol. Environ. Saf. 01476513. 159, 354–362. doi:10.1016/j.ecoenv.2018.04.072.

Zhao, C., Dong, Y., Feng, Y., Li, Y., Dong, Y., 2019. Thermal desorption for remediation of contaminated soil: a review. Chemosphere. 00456535. 221, 841–855. doi:10.1016/j.chemosphere.2019.01.079.

Zheng, F., Guo, X., Tang, M., Zhu, D., Wang, H., Yang, X., Chen, B., 2023. Variation in pollution status, sources, and risks of soil heavy metals in regions with different levels of urbanization. Sci. Total Environ. 00489697. 866, 161355. doi:10.1016/j.scitotenv.2022.161355.

Zhuang, Z., Mu, H.-Y., Fu, P.-N., Wan, Y.-N., Yu, Y., Wang, Q., Li, H.-F., 2020. Accumulation of potentially toxic elements in agricultural soil and scenario analysis of cadmium inputs by fertilization: a case study in Quzhou county. J. Environ. Manag. 03014797. 269, 110797. doi:10.1016/j.jenvman.2020.110797.

Zuddas, P., Podda, F., 2005. Variations in physico-chemical properties of water associated with bio-precipitation of hydrozincite [Zn5(CO3)2(OH)6] in the waters of Rio Naracauli, Sardinia (Italy). Appl. Geochem. 08832927. 20 (3), 507–517. doi:10.1016/j.apgeochem.2004.09.008.

Chapter 4

Metal bioavailability: Speciation, complexation, and redox dynamics

Sania Gupta and Niharika Shanker
Amity Institute of Food Technology, Amity University, Noida, Uttar Pradesh, India

4.1 Introduction

One of the fundamental ideas in environmental chemistry and ecotoxicology is metal bioavailability. It establishes how much a metal can be absorbed by living organisms and impacts biology in natural systems. Because bioavailability represents the chemically active portion that interacts with biological receptors, it is a more reliable indicator of toxicity and ecological danger than total metal concentrations. Bioavailability in ecotoxicology might mean two different things: Metals that are available for organisms to absorb and incorporate into metabolic processes are referred to as having environmental bioavailability. The term "toxicological bioavailability" refers to the amount of metal that is absorbed and interacts with organs, potentially producing harmful effects. It is necessary to comprehend both viewpoints in order to properly assess risks and manage pollution. In both terrestrial and aquatic settings, metal behavior is controlled by: (1) Speciation: Determines the metals' chemical form (such as free ions, complexes, or particulates), which has a direct impact on toxicity and mobility. (2) Complexation: When metals bond to either inorganic or organic ligands, their transport methods and reactivity are altered. (3) Redox dynamics: Dictates a metal's oxidation state, which impacts its solubility and bioavailability. Metals such as Cu, Zn, and Ni may sequester or release episodically due to redox changes. Environmental factors, including pH, ionic strength, and microbial activity, have a significant impact on these interrelated processes (Magalhães et al., 2015). Ecological danger is frequently overestimated or underestimated in traditional assessments based on total metal concentrations. For instance: Even at high quantities, metals attached to particles might not be bioavailable. Despite being found in small amounts, free metal ions can be extremely hazardous because

The Metallome in Motion. https://doi.org/10.1016/B978-0-443-44299-5.00007-9

of their reactivity. Therefore, models based on speciation, such as the Biotic Ligand Model (BLM) and Free Ion Activity Model, have become more accurate instruments for forecasting bioavailability (Sigg and Xue, 1994). current chapter highlights the necessity of moving beyond equilibrium models and taking kinetic fluxes and dynamic speciation into account. It emphasizes the importance of recognizing how colloids and natural organic matter (NOM) affect metal uptake, occasionally enhancing bioavailability in unexpected ways. In addition, it examines how redox processes mobilize trace metals in wetlands and sediments under varying conditions (VanBriesen et al., 2011).

4.2 Metal speciation

The term "metal speciation" describes how a metal is distributed across various chemical forms in a system, such as free ions, complexes, precipitates, adsorbed species, etc. A metal's mobility, toxicity, bioavailability, and environmental destiny are all determined by its speciation. The concentration of all metals is not enough; speciation identifies the forms that are environmentally mobile or physiologically active.

4.2.1 Types of metal species

- Free ions (e.g., Cu^{2+}, Zn^{2+}): highly bioavailable and often toxic
- Inorganic complexes (e.g., $PbCl^{+}$, $CdSO_4$): moderate bioavailability
- Organic complexes (e.g., Cu-humic acid): often less bioavailable but can enhance transport
- Particulate-bound metals: adsorbed onto clay, oxides, or organic matter—low mobility
- Colloidal forms: intermediate between dissolved and particulate; may be bioavailable to filter feeders

4.2.2 Environmental factors influencing speciation

- pH: Influences complexation and solubility. Reduced pH increases the toxicity and concentration of free ions.
- Redox potential (Eh): Regulates states of oxidation. As an illustration, there are two forms of chromium: the less hazardous Cr(III) and the extremely poisonous and mobile Cr(VI). Iron alternates between Fe^{2+} and Fe^{3+} based on redox circumstances.
- Ionic strength Affects complex stability and activity coefficients. Stable complexes are formed when organic matter binds metals through carboxyl and phenolic groups.
- Ligand availability: The presence of natural organic acids or chelators, such as ethylenediaminetetraacetic acid (EDTA), changes the process of speciation.

4.2.3 Speciation and toxicity

- The species determines the toxicity: Cr(VI) has a cellular absorption and oxidative potential that make it 100–1000× more hazardous than Cr(III). While Cu complexed with organic ligands is less hazardous to phytoplankton, Cu^{2+} is toxic to them.
- Speciation influences the mechanisms of uptake: Ion channels allow the entry of free ions, while complexed forms can either be inaccessible or taken up by endocytosis.

4.2.4 Analytic techniques

The concentrations of free ions are measured by voltammetry. Inductively coupled plasma mass spectrometry (ICP-MS), combined with chromatography, separates and measures species (e.g., Cr(III) vs. Cr(VI)). Bioavailable fractions and labile species are estimated by Diffusive Gradients in Thin Films (DGT). Windermere Humic Aqueous Model (WHAM) and MINTEQ are modeling tools that simulate speciation in different scenarios.

4.3 Complexation mechanisms

In environmental systems, metal complexation is a basic mechanism that controls the toxicity, mobility, and bioavailability of metals. It entails the interaction of metal ions with ligands, which are ions or molecules that can donate electron pairs in order to create coordinate covalent connections. These ligands can be either organic (such as humic compounds, amino acids, or EDTA) or inorganic (such as carbonate, sulfate, or chloride), and the charge, ionic radius, and electronic configuration of the metal all affect how well they attach (Fig. 4.1). The speciation of metals is changed by complexation, which frequently lowers the concentration of free metal ions—usually the most dangerous and bioavailable forms. For example, aquatic organisms are less harmed by copper attached to dissolved organic matter (DOM) than by free Cu^{2+} ions. Not all complexes, meanwhile, are inert; some may help move metals across biological membranes by "ligand-assisted uptake," in which the complex imitates a nutrient or takes advantage of preexisting transport channels (Domingos et al., 2015).

There are kinetic and thermodynamic parameters that control the stability of metal-ligand complexes. Formation constants (log K) measure thermodynamic stability by reflecting the equilibrium favorability of complex formation. Because of the chelate effect, which strengthens binding, ligands with multiple donor atoms, or polydentate ligands, produce more stable complexes. Hexadentate ligands like EDTA, for instance, can be used in analytical chemistry and environmental remediation because they can form extremely stable complexes with metals like Pb^{2+} and Fe^{3+}. In contrast, kinetic stability controls

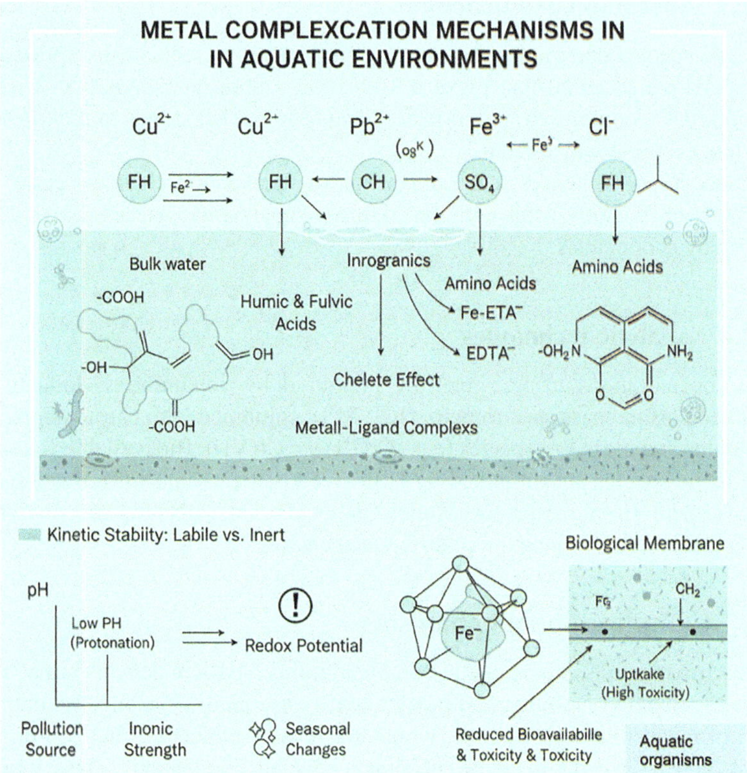

FIG. 4.1 Metal complexation in aquatic systems, showing ligand-controlled metal speciation, stability, and bioavailability under varying environmental conditions.

the rate at which complexes form or dissolve. Inert complexes linger in the environment, while thermodynamically stable complexes that are kinetically labile allow for quick interchange with other ligands (Fortin, 2024).

Ionic strength, redox potential, and pH are examples of environmental factors that have a significant impact on complexation behavior. When ligand donor sites are protonated at low pH, their binding ability decreases, which raises the percentage of free metal ions. On the other hand, a higher pH promotes complex formation and deprotonation. The complexation tendencies and solubilities of Fe^{2+} and Fe^{3+}, for instance, differ, indicating the significance of redox dynamics. Complexation is especially significant in natural streams containing organic materials. Metals like Cu, Zn, and Pb are bound by fulvic and humic acids, which are abundant in carboxyl and phenolic groups. This alters the metals' transit and bioavailability. These relationships are dynamic and subject to change in response to pollution inputs, microbial activity, and seasonal variations (Slaveykova and Wilkinson, 2005).

For the purpose of forecasting metal behavior in ecosystems, creating efficient remediation plans, and developing precise models of metal toxicity, it is essential to comprehend complexation mechanisms. Taking into account ligand competition and environmental factors, complexation equilibria are simulated using programs such as Visual MINTEQ and WHAM. Furthermore, sophisticated methods that assess labile metal species and provide real-time bioavailability insights include voltammetry and DGT. The ecological and toxicological impact of metals in the biosphere is largely shaped by complexation, which is ultimately more than just a fascinating chemical phenomenon (Di Toro et al., 2001).

4.4 Biotic ligand model

Metal toxicity and bioavailability in aquatic environments can be predicted using a mechanistic framework called the BLM. It suggests that toxicity occurs when a metal ion attaches itself to a particular biological receptor, referred to as the biotic ligand, on the surface of aquatic animals, such as the membranes of invertebrates or fish gills. Toxic metal buildup at these receptor sites is estimated by the model, which combines physiological interactions, competitive binding, and chemical speciation. In contrast to conventional models that only include concentrations of total or dissolved metals, the BLM highlights the role of free ion activity as well as the competing effects of other cations, such as Ca2+, Mg2+, Na+, and H+, which can reduce toxicity by sharing binding sites (Erickson, 2013).

4.4.1 Competitive binding and water chemistry

The idea that metal toxicity depends on both the concentration of the metal and the chemistry of the surrounding water is a fundamental component of the BLM. For example, hazardous buildup is less likely in high-hardness waters (rich in Ca^{2+} and Mg^{2+}) because these innocuous cations compete with poisonous metals like Cu^{2+} or Zn^{2+} for binding to the biotic ligand. Dissolved organic carbon (DOC) has the ability to combine with metals, reducing their bioavailability and free ion activity. Another important factor is pH; with higher pH, metals may form less bioavailable hydroxide complexes, whereas at lower pH, higher H^+ concentrations may outcompete metals for ligand sites. The BLM is extremely sensitive to site-specific conditions as a result of these interactions, which enables more precise risk estimates.

4.4.2 Applications and regulatory use

Regulatory organizations, such as the United StatesEnvironmental Protection Agency (EPA), have widely adopted the BLM for establishing water quality standards for metals like copper, silver, and zinc. It is especially helpful in determining site-specific rules that avoid being overly conservative or inadequately protective by reflecting local water chemistry. Software tools that mimic metal speciation and forecast acute toxicity outcomes, such as LC50 values, have integrated the model. These predictions frequently demonstrate strong similarities between modeled and observed toxicity when verified against empirical bioassay data (Niyogi and Wood, 2004).

4.4.3 Limitations and future directions

Even with its advantages, the BLM has drawbacks. It usually deals with exposures to a single metal and makes the assumption that everything is in equilibrium, which might not be the case for dynamic environmental systems. It may also overlook long-term impacts or interactions in metal mixes because it concentrates on acute toxicity. In addition, high-quality input data, such as DOC and competing ion concentrations, are necessary for the model to be accurate. In order to address these shortcomings, scientists are trying to expand the BLM to cover terrestrial applications, combination effects, and chronic toxicity endpoints. Refinement of predictions is also being investigated through hybrid models that include membrane surface potentials and electrostatic interactions.

4.5 Redox dynamics

In environmental systems, especially soils and aquatic sediments, oxidation–reduction conditions fluctuate. This phenomenon is known as redox dynamics. Metal mobility, solubility, and speciation are all significantly impacted by these factors. Metals often undergo oxidation to produce insoluble hydroxides and oxides that precipitate and reduce their bioavailability. Iron and manganese, for instance, are frequently found as comparatively stationary Fe(III) and Mn(IV) oxides, respectively. However, reducing conditions, which are frequently brought on by microbial activity or water saturation, can change these metals into more soluble forms, such as Mn(II) and Fe(II), which increases their mobility and potential toxicity.

4.5.1 Redox-induced speciation shifts

Metals' oxidation state is determined by the redox state of their surroundings, which, in turn, influences how they behave chemically. Under oxidizing conditions, for example, chromium occurs as Cr(VI), a highly mobile and poisonous form. It transforms into Cr(III), which is less poisonous and more prone to precipitate under reducing circumstances. In an analogous manner, copper can transition from Cu(I) to Cu(II), with reduced organic sulfur groups in anoxic soils frequently stabilizing Cu(I). Due to the important role that bacteria play in mediating redox reactions, these changes are both chemical and biological in nature.

4.5.2 Environmental triggers and cycles

Redox fluctuations are common in natural environments, particularly in wetland soils and stream sediments, as a result of variations in water saturation, microbial respiration, and the breakdown of organic matter. Anoxic conditions brought on by oxygen depletion during flooding encourage the reduction of iron and manganese oxides. Through this process, trace metals such as Zn, Co, and Ni may be released into the soil solution. Certain metals, including Cu and Cd, may remain mobile upon reoxidation, such as during drying, depending on their complexation and solid-phase affiliations, while other metals may reprecipitate (Zhang and Furman, 2021).

4.5.3 Interactions with organic matter and sulfides

In addition, redox dynamics affect how metals interact with sulfide minerals and NOM. Microbial sulfate reduction under reducing conditions produces sulfide ions that have the ability to precipitate metals as metal sulfides (such as CuS and CdS), thereby immobilizing them. The degree of sequestration is determined by the thermodynamic stability of these sulfides and the availability of sulfate. By promoting redox reactions and stabilizing reduced metal species through complexation, organic matter can function as both an electron donor and an electron acceptor (Giraldo-Gómez et al., 2021).

4.5.4 Implications for bioavailability and risk

When the redox conditions change, metal bioavailability is quite dynamic. For instance, sulfide precipitation or organic binding may cause Ni and Co to drop during anoxic phases, while bioavailable Zn and Cu may increase. Ecotoxicology, nutrient cycling, and contaminant transportation are all directly impacted by these changes, particularly in agricultural wetlands and floodplain soils. Determining environmental danger, forecasting metal behavior, and creating efficient remediation plans all depend on an understanding of redox dynamics.

4.6 Environmental parameters

Environmental factors play a crucial role in determining how metals behave in natural systems, affecting their biological impact, speciation, and transport. pH is one of the most notable master variables among them. It directly affects the bioavailability of metals by controlling their ionic form and solubility. Increased concentrations of hydrogen ions support the breakdown of metal complexes at low pH, which raises the amounts of free metal ions like Cu^{2+}, Pb^{2+}, and Al^{3+}—forms that are extremely bioavailable and frequently harmful to aquatic life. At higher pH levels, on the other hand, metals tend to precipitate as carbonates or hydroxides, which decreases their toxicity and mobility. Aquatic ecosystems can have their community composition altered by even small pH changes, favoring acid-tolerant species while suppressing sensitive taxa (Allen et al., 1993).

A protective effect against metal toxicity is provided by water hardness, which is determined by the concentration of calcium and magnesium ions. By competing with harmful metals for binding sites on biological membranes, such as fish gills, these cations lower the intake of metals. For instance, competitive inhibition by calcium ions considerably reduces copper toxicity in hard water. Regulatory organizations, such as the United States EPA, recognize this buffering effect and use hardness-adjusted standards for metals like cadmium, zinc, and nickel (Gensemer and Playle, 1999).

Moreover, DOM, especially fulvic and humic acids, has a significant impact on metal bioavailability. Functional groups found in DOM, such as carboxyl, phenolic, and sulfur-containing moieties, bind to metal ions and create stable complexes. By reducing the proportion of free metal ions, these complexes frequently lessen toxicity. A few metal-DOM complexes, however, are nevertheless accessible due to their nature, particularly when utilized by filter feeders or in ligand-assisted absorption mechanisms. Metal behavior in aquatic and soil ecosystems is further complicated by the seasonal and regional variations in DOM quality and quantity (Santore et al., 2001).

Chemical kinetics and biological processes are both impacted by temperature. Elevated temperatures have the potential to improve metal uptake by speeding up microbial metabolism and metal dissolution. Furthermore, temperature affects the solubility of gases like oxygen.

4.7 Biological responses

Numerous biological reactions are displayed by organisms exposed to metals in their surroundings, which are indicative of the metal's speciation as well as the degree of exposure. Understanding how metals interact with living systems and evaluating ecological danger depends heavily on these responses. One of the most popular methods uses biomarkers, which are physiological, molecular, or biochemical signs that indicate exposure to or the effects of toxic metals. Metals such as cadmium, zinc, and copper, for instance, cause the upregulation of metallothioneins, low-molecular-weight proteins high in cysteine that function as both detoxifying agents and exposure biomarkers. Likewise, under metal stress, enzymes like glutathione-S-transferase and superoxide dismutase are frequently increased, signifying oxidative damage and the activation of antioxidant defenses (Amiard et al., 2006).

In contrast, whole species or communities are utilized as bioindicators to track the health of the ecosystem. Bivalves, earthworms, and green algae are among the species that are especially helpful because their tissues accumulate metals in proportion to the quantities in their surroundings. The Mediterranean mussel (*Mytilus galloprovincialis*), for example, has been widely employed to monitor coastal metal contamination because of its sedentary character and high ability for bioaccumulation. In terrestrial settings, plants such as Brassica juncea and Sedum alfredii are also used to monitor and treat heavy metal pollution (Viarengo and Nott, 1993). It's important to remember that bioaccumulation does not always mean toxicity. Numerous species have systems in place to store metals in innocuous forms, such as vacuoles or by binding to phytochelatins. This internal chelation and sequestration minimize interference with essential metabolic processes by lowering the concentration of free ions within cells. Metals are sometimes confined to extracellular polymers or segregated in cell walls, which effectively isolate them from delicate biological components. These tactics are particularly common in species that can survive in contaminated habitats without showing obvious symptoms of stress, such as metal tolerant species and hyperaccumulators (Rainbow, 2002).

The exposure route affects the biological reaction as well. Metals absorbed through the gills or roots may undergo different processing than those acquired by ingestion. Dissolved metal speciation, such as the existence of free ions versus complexed forms, affects the toxicity and absorption efficiency of aquatic species. In terrestrial systems, metal availability and uptake pathways can be altered by microbial interactions in the rhizosphere and root exudates. Environmental factors, metal chemistry, and organismal physiology interact to shape the complex and species-specific biological reactions to metals. Designing successful biomonitoring and remediation plans, as well as creating precise models of metal bioavailability, depends on an understanding of these reactions.

4.8 Analytical techniques

To comprehend environmental mobility, toxicity, and bioavailability, metal speciation must be accurately determined. Metals' interactions with animals and ecosystems are determined by their chemical form, whether they are free ions, complexed, colloidal, or particulate. Total metal concentrations alone cannot predict ecological impact. Speciation analysis methods must, consequently, be sensitive, selective, and able to differentiate between binding partners, coordination environments, and oxidation states (Tercero Espinoza and van den Berg, 2006).

4.8.1 Electrochemical technique

Free metal ions and labile complexes are frequently measured using electrochemical techniques, including Absence of Gradients and Nernstian Equilibrium Stripping (AGNES), scanning stripping chronopotentiometry (SSCP), and anodic stripping voltammetry. Dynamic speciation investigations benefit greatly from these methods' high sensitivity and in situ operation. While SSCP offers kinetic insights into metal–ligand interactions, AGNES, for instance, enables the direct measurement of free ion concentrations without interference from complexed forms (Town et al., 2009).

4.8.2 Chromatographic and spectrometric methods

Exact separation and quantification of metal species are made possible by chromatography in conjunction with mass spectrometry, such as gas chromatography–mass spectrometry and liquid chromatography–ICP-MS (LC-ICP-MS). Since the toxicity of metals like arsenic, selenium, and mercury varies greatly between species, these techniques are very useful for speciation. As(III), As(V), and organoarsenic compounds, for example, can all be distinguished by LC-ICP-MS and have different toxicological profiles. Spectrometric methods, including X-ray fluorescence, atomic absorption spectroscopy, and ICP-MS, are also utilized for speciation and total metal quantification when combined with separation techniques. These tools provide low detection limits and are crucial for biological and environmental material analysis at the trace level (Filella and Town, 2008).

4.8.3 Voltammetry and ligand interaction studies

Particularly helpful for researching redox behavior and metal-ligand complexation are voltammetric techniques. Peak shifts and current responses can be used to derive kinetic parameters, redox transitions, and stability constants. For metals like iron, copper, and chromium—which have different bioavailabilities depending on their oxidation state—this is essential.

4.8.4 Modeling tools and software

Metal behavior under various environmental situations is simulated by chemical speciation models like WHAM, Visual MINTEQ, and ECOSAT to supplement experimental data. Environmental factors, including pH and ionic strength, ligand competition, and equilibrium constants, are all included in these models. Metal fluxes toward biological interfaces can be kinetically modeled using MHEDYN and FLUXY for more dynamic systems, taking reaction and diffusion rates into consideration (Unsworth and van Leeuwen, 2005).

4.8.5 Emerging techniques and innovations

Recent developments in high-resolution mass spectrometry (e.g., Orbitrap and FT-ICR MS), electrochemical sensors, and microfluidic technologies enable ultra-sensitive, portable, and real-time speciation investigations. By allowing the identification of hitherto unreachable species and interactions, these instruments are pushing the boundaries of environmental monitoring and risk assessment.

4.9 Case studies

It needs both theoretical models and actual data from field and lab research to comprehend metal bioavailability in environmental systems. Researchers have shown that the concentration of free Cu^{2+} ions is a more reliable indicator of toxicity than total copper levels in microalgae, which is a well-known example of copper toxicity. Microalgal species like Chlamydomonas reinhardtii showed signs of organelle damage, oxidative stress, and growth suppression in controlled tests when exposed to high levels of free Cu^{2+}. Lipid peroxidation, elevated reactive oxygen species, and reduced photosynthetic efficiency were some of these consequences. It is interesting to note that DOM or humic acids have been demonstrated to lessen copper toxicity by complexing with Cu^{2+} and lowering its toxic impact and bioavailability (Franklin et al., 2000). Another strong argument concerns the uptake of lead in freshwater microalgae, specifically Chlamydomonas reinhardtii, in response to different levels of carbonate. Pb-carbonato complexes have been shown to contribute to lead internalization in ways that are not consistent with free Pb^{2+} concentrations. Particularly in diffusion-limited situations, this points to a potential "piggy-back" transport mechanism in which the cell absorbs entire metal-ligand complexes. In contrast to Chlorella vulgaris, the uptake was noticeably greater in C. reinhardtii, indicating species-specific variations in metal transport routes (Slaveykova and Wilkinson, 2002). According to research on stream sediments and wetland soils, redox dynamics are also essential for metal mobilization. The breakdown of iron and manganese oxides makes metals like Zn, Co, and Ni more soluble under reducing circumstances. In contrast, metals such as copper can be mobilized by oxidizing conditions, usually by oxidizing sulfide-bound forms. One study found that whereas wetland soils had a more complex response, with some metals becoming less accessible over time, stream sediments' trace metal bioaccessibility rose as a result of repeated redox cycling. These results highlight how crucial redox variations are in determining metal speciation and ecological danger (Leclerc and Wilkinson, 2014). The intricacy of metal bioavailability and the requirement for integrated strategies that take chemical speciation, environmental factors, and biological reactions into account are both highlighted by these case studies taken together. The limits of relying exclusively on total metal concentrations for risk assessment are also highlighted, and the predictive ability of models such as the BLM is validated (Gagnon and Saulnier, 2003).

4.10 Challenges and knowledge gaps

Even with major advancements in our understanding of metal bioavailability, environmental risk assessment and forecast accuracy are still constrained by a number of enduring issues and information gaps. Measuring the amounts of free ions in complicated environmental media is one of the biggest challenges. Although free ions are frequently the most hazardous and accessible metals, their measurement is made more difficult by the existence of colloids, competing ligands, and dynamic speciation processes. Although methods like DGT and voltammetry provide partial solutions, they could miss kinetically labile or transient species, particularly in heterogeneous systems like sediments or wastewater effluents. Beyond simple complexation, the role of NOM is another significant gap. The potential of NOM to bind metals and lower toxicity is well known, but new research indicates that, in some circumstances, it may also promote metal uptake. For instance, NOM can change surface characteristics and possibly improve metal transport by adhering to biological membranes. Furthermore, it is possible that certain metal-NOM complexes are bioavailable via "piggy-back" pathways, casting doubt on the notion that complexation necessarily lowers toxicity. Since binding affinities and kinetics differ greatly among NOM fractions, modeling efforts are made much more difficult by the structural heterogeneity of NOM, which ranges from humic acids to low-molecular-weight organic acids (Tipping et al., 2006). The absence of reliable models for multimetal interactions is a further difficulty. Synergistic or antagonistic effects of cooccurring metals are not taken into consideration by the majority of current frameworks, such as the BLM, which is intended for single-metal scenarios. Organisms are frequently exposed to metal combinations in their natural habitats, which might cause compensatory biological reactions or compete for binding sites. For example, copper and nickel may show additive toxicity, whereas zinc may reduce cadmium toxicity by occupying shared transport routes. Developing predictive models that consider these interactions necessitates a better comprehension of metal-specific transport proteins, cellular feedback mechanisms, and competitive binding dynamics (Santore et al., 2021).

Moreover, redox variations and temporal variability add even more intricacy. Metal speciation and mobility can be altered by redox conditions that are influenced by seasonal variations, microbial activity, and hydrological events. The steady-state assumptions of equilibrium-based models make it challenging to represent these dynamic processes. Incorporating feedback loops and kinetic factors into speciation models remains a top research priority. Standardized procedures and cross-disciplinary integration are also urgently needed. Variability in data interpretation, analytical methods, and experimental design complicates the comparison of studies. Building comprehensive frameworks that accurately represent environmental reality will require bridging the gaps between geochemistry, toxicology, and molecular biology (Leclerc and Wilkinson, 2014).

4.11 Applications and implications

The study of metal bioavailability has broad implications for agriculture, public health, environmental research, and policymaking (Table 4.1). One of its most important functions is in environmental risk assessment, where a better understanding of metal speciation and bioavailability allows for more precise ecological impact projections. To ensure that requirements represent real toxicity

TABLE 4.1 Applications and implications of metal bioavailability in environmental and health sciences.

Domain	Application area	Role of bioavailability	Representative examples/tools	References
Environmental risk assessment	Ecological impact prediction	Differentiates total metal concentrations from biologically active fractions, improving toxicity predictions	Biotic Ligand Model (BLM), site-specific water quality criteria	Di Toro et al. (2001); Campbell (1995)
Regulatory frameworks & policy	Standards and guideline development	Enables adaptive, site-specific regulations that reflect real toxicity	USEPA Copper Criteria, EU Water Framework Directive	United States Environmental Protection Agency (2007); Alloway (2013)
Environmental monitoring	Pollution hotspot identification	Detects labile and bioavailable metal species rather than total metals	DGT, anodic stripping voltammetry, passive samplers	Davison and Zhang (1994); Florence (1986)
Remediation strategies	Soil and water remediation	Guides immobilization or removal of bioavailable metal fractions	Phytore mediation, biochar, and compost amendments; liming	Salt et al. (1998); Alloway (2013)
Engineered treatment systems	Targeted metal removal	Optimizes design based on metal speciation and mobility	Constructed wetlands, permeable reactive barriers (PRBs)	Vymazal (2014); Fu and Wang (2011)
Agriculture & soil management	Crop nutrition and safety	Balances essential micronutrient availability while preventing toxicity	Zn and Cu fertilization, soil pH adjustment	Marschner (2012); McLaughlin et al. (2000)

Continued

Table 4.1 Applications and implications of metal bioavailability in environmental and health sciences—cont'd

Domain	Application area	Role of bioavailability	Representative examples/tools	References
Food Chain safety	Metal transfer to crops	Predicts accumulation in edible plant tissues and food products	Cd uptake in rice, Pb uptake in leafy vegetables	Meharg et al. (2013); Grant et al. (2008)
Public health	Exposure and health risk assessment	Identifies the most toxic and bioaccessible metal species	Pb bioaccessibility, As(III)/As(V) speciation	Ruby et al. (1999); Smedley and Kinniburgh (2002)
Water treatment technologies	Drinking water safety	Improves treatment efficiency by targeting bioavailable metal forms	Coagulation–flocculation, ion exchange, membrane filtration	Fu and Wang (2011); World Health Organization (2017)
Climate Change studies	Altered metal behavior	Evaluates the effects of redox shifts, temperature, and DOC on metals	Fe^{2+}/Fe^{3+} cycling, DOC–metal interactions	Gadd (2010); Wetzel (2001)
Research & modeling	Predictive ecosystem modeling	Improves fate, transport, and toxicity predictions	Visual MINTEQ, WHAM, PHREEQC	Tipping (1994); Parkhurst and Appelo (2013)
Ecosystem management	Biodiversity protection	Supports the protection of sensitive aquatic species	Fish and benthic invertebrate risk mapping	Rainbow (2002); Campbell (1995)

rather than total metal concentrations, regulatory bodies are increasingly relying on models such as the BLM to develop site-specific water quality criteria. This strategy promotes environmental protection without placing an undue financial burden on the environment by avoiding both overregulation and underregulation (Peijnenburg and Jager, 2003).

Assessments based on bioavailability are used in environmental monitoring to identify pollution hotspots and gauge how well rehabilitation initiatives are working. Methods like voltammetry and DGT enable the real-time detection of labile metal species, providing information on dynamic changes in aquatic systems. These instruments are especially useful in polluted areas, where conventional measurements cannot adequately reflect the actual danger caused by metals bonded to biological materials or sediments. Remedial strategy design is also influenced by the idea of bioavailability. For instance, the efficacy of phytoremediation depends on the choice of plant species that can withstand and collect metals in bioavailable forms. Likewise, the selection of amendments, such as compost or charcoal, depends on their capacity to bind metals and decrease their mobility. Speciation data is used to optimize built wetlands and permeable reactive barriers (PRBs) in engineered systems to target particular metal types (McLaughlin et al., 1999).

Adding bioavailability to regulatory frameworks improves the scientific validity of environmental standards from a policy standpoint. It facilitates the creation of adaptive management plans, in which data from monitoring drives iterative enhancements to pollution prevention. In light of new pollutants and climate change, which can change redox conditions and metal behavior in unforeseen ways, this is particularly pertinent. Understanding metal bioavailability aids in crop safety and soil fertility management in agriculture. Essential micronutrients include metals like copper and zinc, but in order to prevent toxicity or deficiencies, their availability needs to be carefully controlled. In regions impacted by mining or industrial activities, bioavailability models help determine the risk of metal uptake in food crops and establish suitable fertilization schedules. Lastly, the health effects of metal bioavailability are not limited to drinking water safety; they also include exposure through the food chain. In order to guide treatment technologies and public health actions, speciation analysis assists in identifying the most dangerous forms of metals, such as lead and arsenic. As studies progress, incorporating bioavailability into interdisciplinary frameworks will be essential to protecting communities and ecosystems.

4.12 Conclusion

Redox dynamics, complexation, and speciation interact intricately to control the bioavailability of metals in environmental systems. These activities are not distinct; rather, they are intricately linked and influenced by a wide range of environmental factors, including microbial activity, ionic strength, organic matter, and pH. A metal's chemical form, which influences its reactivity, mobility, and toxicity, is determined by speciation. Complexation alters the bioavailability and transport pathways of metals by binding them to ligands, thereby modifying speciation. This picture is further complicated by redox dynamics, which change the oxidation states and influence the behavior of metals across different time and spatial scales. Comprehending these mechanisms is crucial for precise risk evaluation, regulatory decision-making, and remediation strategy development. Researchers can now test and simulate metal behavior with greater accuracy thanks to major advancements in analytical methods and modeling tools. However, the measurement of free ion concentrations, the modeling of multimetal interactions, and the capture of dynamic environmental variables remain challenging tasks.

References

Allen, H.E., Fu, G., Deng, B., 1993. Analysis of acid-volatile sulfide (AVS) and simultaneously extracted metals (SEM) for the estimation of potential toxicity in sediments. Environ. Toxicol. Chem. 12 (8), 1441–1453. doi:10.1002/etc.5620120812.

Alloway, B.J., 2013. Heavy Metals in Soils: Trace Metals and Metalloids in Soils and Their Bioavailability, third ed. Springer. doi:10.1007/978-94-007-4470-7.

Amiard, J.-C., Amiard-Triquet, C., Barka, S., Pellerin, J., Morin, B., 2006. Metallothioneins in aquatic invertebrates: their role in metal detoxification and their use as biomarkers. Aquat. Toxicol. 76 (2), 160–202. doi:10.1016/j.aquatox.2005.08.015.

Campbell, P.G.C., 1995. Interactions between trace metals and aquatic organisms: a critique of the free-ion activity model. Environ. Sci. Technol. 29 (3), 695–705. doi:10.1021/es00003a001.

Davison, W., Zhang, H., 1994. In situ speciation measurements of trace components in natural waters using thin-film gels. Nature 367 (6463), 546–548. doi:10.1038/367546a0.

Di Toro, D.M., Allen, H.E., Bergman, H.L., Meyer, J.S., Paquin, P.R., Santore, R.C., 2001. Biotic ligand model of the acute toxicity of metals. Environ. Toxicol. Chem. 20 (10), 2383–2396. doi:10.1002/etc.5620201034.

Domingos, R.F., Gélabert, A., Carreira, S., Cordeiro, A., Sivry, Y., Benedetti, M.F., 2015. Metals in the aquatic environment—interactions and implications for the speciation and bioavailability: a critical overview. Aquat. Geochem. 21, 231–257. doi:10.1007/s10498-015-9251-x.

Erickson, R.J., 2013. The biotic ligand model approach for addressing effects of exposure water chemistry on aquatic toxicity of metals: genesis and challenges. Environ. Toxicol. Chem. 32 (6), 1212–1214. doi:10.1002/etc.2204.

Filella, M., Town, R.M., 2008. Speciation of trace elements in natural waters: a review of electrochemical methods. Environ. Chem. 5 (4), 250–267. doi:10.1071/EN08022.

Florence, T.M., 1986. Electrochemical techniques for trace metal analysis. Anal. Chim. Acta 184, 25–37. doi:10.1016/S0003-2670(00)87067-4.

Fortin, C., 2024. Metal bioavailability in aquatic systems—beyond complexation and competition. Front. Environ. Chem. 5, 1345484. doi:10.3389/fenvc.2024.1345484.

Franklin, N.M., Stauber, J.L., Lim, R.P., Petocz, P., 2000. Toxicity of metal mixtures to a tropical freshwater alga (Chlorella sp.): the effect of interactions between copper, cadmium, and zinc. Environ. Toxicol. Chem. 19 (1), 60–71. doi:10.1002/etc.5620190107.

Fu, F., Wang, Q., 2011. Removal of heavy metal ions from wastewaters: a review. J. Environ. Manag. 92 (3), 407–418. doi:10.1016/j.jenvman.2010.11.011.

Gadd, G.M., 2010. Metals, minerals and microbes: geomicrobiology and bioremediation. Microbiology 156 (3), 609–643. doi:10.1099/mic.0.037143-0.

Gagnon, C., Saulnier, I., 2003. Distribution and fate of metals in the Saguenay Fjord, Canada, following a major flood event. Mar. Pollut. Bull. 46 (6), 806–815. doi:10.1016/S0025-326X(03)00062-6.

Gensemer, R.W., Playle, R.C., 1999. The bioavailability and toxicity of aluminum in aquatic environments. Crit. Rev. Environ. Sci. Technol. 29 (4), 315–450. doi:10.1080/10643389991259209.

Giraldo-Gómez, V.M., Petrizzo, M.R., Bottini, C., Möller, C., Wagner, T., 2021. Bottom water redox dynamics during the Early Cretaceous Weissert Event reconstructed from benthic foraminiferal assemblages. Palaeogeogr. Palaeoclimatol. Palaeoecol. 581, 110795. doi:10.1016/j.palaeo.2021.110795.

Grant, C.A., Clarke, J.M., Duguid, S., Chaney, R.L., 2008. Selection and management of plant species for phytoremediation of soils contaminated with trace elements. Can. J. Plant Sci. 88 (3), 513–522. doi:10.4141/CJPS07060.

Leclerc, S., Wilkinson, K.J., 2014. Bioavailability of lead to freshwater algae: influence of chemical speciation and carbonate complexation. Environ. Chem. 11 (3), 276–284. doi:10.1071/EN13113.

Magalhães, D.P., Marques, M.R.C., Baptista, D.F., Buss, D.F., 2015. Metal bioavailability and toxicity in freshwaters. Environ. Chem. Lett. 13 (1), 69–87. doi:10.1007/s10311-014-0491-9.

Marschner, P. 2012. Mineral Nutrition of Higher Plants, third ed. Academic Press.

McLaughlin, M.J., Parker, D.R., Clarke, J.M., 1999. Metals and micronutrients—food safety issues. Field Crops Res. 60 (1–2), 143–163. doi:10.1016/S0378-4290(98)00137-3.

McLaughlin, M.J., Parker, D.R., Clarke, J.M., 2000. Metals and micronutrients—food safety issues. Field Crops Res. 60 (1–2), 143–163. doi:10.1016/S0378-4290(98)00137-3.

Meharg, A.A., Norton, G., Deacon, C., Williams, P., Adomako, E.E., Price, A., Zhao, F.J., 2013. Variation in rice cadmium related to human exposure. Environ. Sci. Technol. 47 (11), 5613–5618. doi:10.1021/es400521h.

Niyogi, S., Wood, C.M., 2004. Biotic ligand model: a flexible tool for developing site-specific water quality guidelines for metals. Environ. Sci. Technol. 38 (23), 6177–6192. doi:10.1021/es0496524.

Parkhurst, D.L., Appelo, C.A.J., 2013. Description of Input and Examples for PHREEQC Version 3—A Computer Program for Speciation, Batch-reaction, One-dimensional Transport, and Inverse Geochemical Calculations (USGS Techniques and Methods, Book 6, Chap. A43). U.S. Geological Survey.

Peijnenburg, W.J.G.M., Jager, T., 2003. Monitoring approaches to assess bioaccessibility and bioavailability of metals: matrix issues. Ecotoxicol. Environ. Saf. 56 (1), 63–77. doi:10.1016/S0147-6513(03)00051-0.

Rainbow, P.S., 2002. Trace metal concentrations in aquatic invertebrates: why and so what? Environ. Pollut. 120 (3), 497–507. doi:10.1016/S0269-7491(02)00238-5.

Ruby, M.V., Schoof, R., Brattin, W., Goldade, M., Post, G., Harnois, M., Galagan, P., 1999. Advances in evaluating the oral bioavailability of inorganics in soil for use in human health risk assessment. Environ. Sci. Technol. 33 (21), 3697–3705. doi:10.1021/es990479z.

Salt, D.E., Smith, R.D., Raskin, I., 1998. Phytoremediation. Annu. Rev. Plant Physiol. Plant Mol. Biol. 49, 643–668.

Santore, R.C., Croteau, K., Ryan, A.C., Schlekat, C., Middleton, E., 2021. Water quality factors affecting nickel bioavailability to aquatic organisms: refinement of the biotic ligand model. Environ. Toxicol. Chem. 40 (5), 1345–1360. doi:10.1002/etc.4973.

Santore, R.C., Ryan, A.C., Di Toro, D.M., 2001. The effect of dissolved organic carbon on the bioavailability of copper to fathead minnows. Environ. Toxicol. Chem. 20 (3), 493–499. doi:10.1002/etc.5620200303.

Sigg, L., Xue, H., 1994. Metal speciation: concepts, analysis and effects. In: G. Bidoglio, W. Stumm (Eds.), Chemistry of Aquatic Systems: Local and Global Perspectives. Springer, pp. 153–181.

Slaveykova, V.I., Wilkinson, K.J., 2002. Physicochemical aspects of bioavailability and toxicity of metals in aquatic systems. Environ. Sci. Technol. 36 (3), 337–342. doi:10.1021/es010151g.

Slaveykova, V., Wilkinson, K.J., 2005. Predicting the bioavailability of metals and metal complexes: critical review of the biotic ligand model. Environ. Chem. 2 (1), 1–10. doi:10.1071/EN04076.

Smedley, P.L., Kinniburgh, D.G., 2002. A review of the source, behaviour and distribution of arsenic in natural waters. Appl. Geochem. 17 (5), 517–568. doi:10.1016/S0883-2927(02)00018-5.

Tercero Espinoza, L.A., van den Berg, C.M.G., 2006. Absence of gradients and Nernstian equilibrium stripping (AGNES): a new electrochemical technique for measuring free metal ion concentrations. J. Electroanal. Chem. 588 (2), 138–149. doi:10.1016/j.jelechem.2005.12.003.

Tipping, E., 1994. WHAM—a chemical equilibrium model and computer code for waters, sediments, and soils incorporating a discrete site/electrostatic model of ion-binding by humic substances. Comput. Geosci. 20 (6), 973–1023. doi:10.1016/0098-3004(94)90038-8.

Tipping, E., Lofts, S., Lawlor, A.J., 2006. Modelling the chemical speciation of trace metals in surface waters. Sci. Total Environ. 362 (1–3), 167–182. doi:10.1016/j.scitotenv.2005.09.017.

Town, R.M., van Leeuwen, H.P., Blust, R., 2009. Biophysical description of metal ion binding to biotic ligands: a multi-site complexation model. Environ. Sci. Technol. 43 (19), 7397–7402. doi:10.1021/es9010464.

United States Environmental Protection Agency, 2007. Aquatic Life Ambient Freshwater Quality criteria—Copper. USEPA.

Unsworth, E.R., van Leeuwen, H.P., 2005. Metal speciation dynamics and bioavailability: in situ techniques and modeling approaches. Environ. Sci. Technol. 39 (23), 8942–8950. doi:10.1021/es050697f.

VanBriesen, J.M., Small, M., Weber, C., Wilson, J., 2011. Modelling chemical speciation: thermodynamics, kinetics and uncertainty. In: G. Hanrahan (Ed.), Modelling of Pollutants in Complex Environmental Systems, vol. II. ILM Publications, pp. 133–149.

Viarengo, A., Nott, J.A., 1993. Mechanisms of heavy metal cation homeostasis in marine invertebrates. Comp. Biochem. Physiol. C 104 (3), 355–372. doi:10.1016/0742-8413(93)90036-2.

Vymazal, J., 2014. Constructed wetlands for treatment of industrial wastewaters: a review. Ecol. Eng. 73, 724–751.

Wetzel, R.G. 2001. Limnology: Lake and River Ecosystems, third ed. Academic Press.

World Health Organization, 2017. Guidelines for Drinking-water Quality, fourth ed., incorporating the 1st addendum. WHO Press.

Zhang, Z., Furman, A., 2021. Redox dynamics at a dynamic capillary fringe for nitrogen cycling in a sandy column. J. Hydrol. 603, 126899. doi:10.1016/j.jhydrol.2021.126899.

Chapter 5

Metal–radical interactions: Synergistic effects on food chain toxicodynamics

Safeera Akbar[a], Sumira Tyub[a], Farheen Mushtaq[a], Aabroo Fatima[b], Uzma Ali[a], and Syed Nasir Ahmad[a]
[a]*Centre of Research for Development (CORD), University of Kashmir, Srinagar, India*
[b]*Department of Botany, University of Kashmir, Srinagar, India*

5.1 Introduction

The role of the complex interaction of trace metals and reactive species in the regulation of toxic effects in ecological systems has become an increasing focus in environmental toxicology. Pollutants like mercury, cadmium, arsenic, and lead are known contaminants in the terrestrial and aquatic trophic webs, and reactive oxygen species (ROS), reactive nitrogen species (RNS), and lipid-derived radicals act as the main sources of cellular injury. Despite the fact that the disciplines of metal-mediated toxicity and radical biology have conventionally been described as two autonomous fields of study, recent discoveries indicate that their mutual interactions are critical determinants of the dynamics of toxicity in food chains (Khan and Lang, 2023).

Toxicodynamics is defined as the biochemical and physiological impacts of toxicants on living organisms, as compared to toxicokinetics, which is the absorption, distribution, metabolism, and excretion (Timbrell, 2021). The toxicodynamics of trophic systems are especially complex since metals and radicals rarely act independently but rather interact with one another in a process of mutual reinforcement. Radicals can be produced using metals, and metal speciation, migration, and natural toxicity can also be altered by radicals (Valko et al., 2016). These positive feedback loops often contribute to the magnification of negative impacts at several different trophic levels, including primary producers (like plankton and crops), secondary consumers (like fish and livestock), and humans.

The current chapter aims to explain the processes by which metal and radical interactions occur in food chains. It begins with background concepts on

The Metallome in Motion. https://doi.org/10.1016/B978-0-443-44299-5.00003-1

radical chemistry and transition metal toxicology, moves on to analyze environmental transport mechanisms, bioaccumulation mechanisms, and subsequent toxicodynamics, and concludes with an evaluation of the synergistic effects on human health. Case studies, experimental evidence, and mitigation approaches are included to emphasize the global importance of these interactions. Its overall aim is to provide a holistic, human-oriented approach that combines and unites molecular processes with ecological and social outcomes.

5.2 Fundamentals of metal–radical chemistry

Free radicals are atoms or molecules that are distinguished by their unpaired electrons and, therefore, are strongly reactive and capable of damaging biomolecules. In biological systems, the most relevant radicals fall into three broad categories (Halliwell and Gutteridge, 2015).

1. ROS, including hydroxyl radicals, superoxide, and hydrogen peroxide.
2. RNS, such as nitric oxide and peroxynitrite, are important molecules in various biological processes.
3. Lipid-derived radicals, generated during lipid peroxidation.

Transition metals such as iron (Fe), copper (Cu), and manganese (Mn) play physiological roles in enzymes and redox reactions. However, at high concentrations, that is, in nonphysiological forms, they are toxic. Toxic heavy metal elements such as mercury (Hg), cadmium (Cd), arsenic (As), and lead (Pb) do not engage in a classical redox cycle but rather cause the antioxidant systems to be disrupted, indicating that they indirectly promote the generation of radicals (Valko et al., 2005a).

A central mechanism of metal–radical interplay is the Fenton reaction: $\mathbf{Fe^{2+} + H_2O_2 \rightarrow Fe^{3+} + OH^- + \cdot OH}$.

The reaction of ferrous iron with hydrogen peroxide produces hydroxyl radicals, which are among the most reactive species in biological systems (Prousek, 2007). Superoxide and hydrogen peroxide are also involved in radical generation through the associated Haber-Weiss reaction. Consequently, metals can act as radical catalysts in food webs, where organisms accumulate the metal and the radical products.

Radicals are not only generated by metals, but metal speciation is also affected. As an example, the Fenton cycle is maintained as Fe^{3+} is reduced by superoxide to Fe^{2+}. Lipid peroxidation chelates metal products, thus changing their bioavailability (Schaich, 1992). This feedback mechanism is critical to the fact that, as they develop, metal–radical interactions increase in a self-perpetuating way, spreading oxidative stress across tissues and ecosystems (Valko et al., 2005a) as shown in Fig. 5.1.

Part of your document could not be imported, as it contained an unsupported element. For more information about unsupported elements, please visit the Support Center.

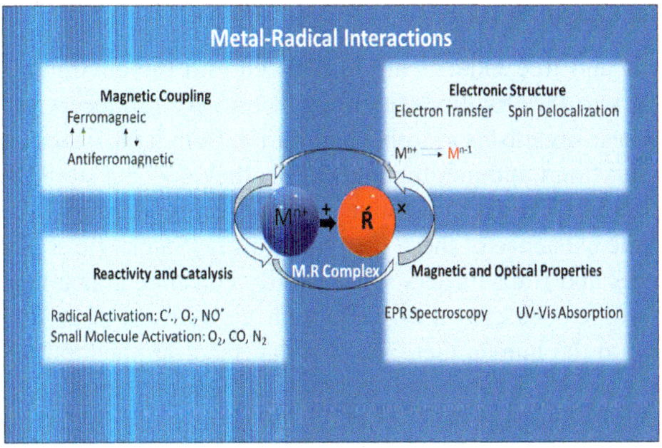

FIG. 5.1 Conceptual diagram of metal–radical interactions.

5.3 Environmental sources and pathways

There are various sources of entry of metals and radicals into ecosystems, both natural and anthropogenic. The determination of these pathways and their description is a prerequisite for the assessment of the bioaccumulation of toxicants and their subsequent interactions throughout trophic networks within food webs (Streit, 1992).

Geogenic processes are the main source of natural inputs; e.g., volcanogenic activity releases arsenic, mercury, and sulfur species into the environment. Lithogenic materials break down (weathering) to release trace elements like manganese, chromium, and iron, which are all deposited in terrestrial soils and aquatic ecosystems (Kar, 2022). Furthermore, biogenic reactions, specifically microbial metabolic processes, produce ROS, such as superoxide and hydrogen peroxide, which are common in natural aqueous reservoirs.

Modern pollution patterns are mainly anthropogenic. The release of heavy metals through industrial discharges, mining activities, smelting processes, and coal burning occurs in large quantities into the atmospheric, terrestrial, and water compartments (Kumar et al., 2023). Cadmium and arsenic find their way into agricultural setups through agricultural inputs such as phosphate fertilizers. Pesticides and herbicides also contribute organometallic residues with the ability to produce oxidative radicals during degradation. The waste discharges in urban areas, especially electronic wastes, produce intricate combinations of metals that, over time, are integrated into the larger biosphere.

Radical generation is often a co-occurring process in these processes. Burning fossil fuels produces both metallic particulates and ROS. Treatment plants might fail at degrading the organic pollutants entirely, leaving behind leftover precursors that produce radicals through photolytic or microbiological degradation (Lindsey, 2018). This is a concomitant intoxication of metals and radicals that preludes synergism before the emergence of bioaccumulation.

5.4 Food chain dynamics

When metals and free radicals are introduced into the environment, they are incorporated into the trophic webs through primary producers such as plants and algae. These organisms absorb the pollution from land, water, and air. Since metals are very inert and non-biodegradable, they become stored in biological tissues, and radicals trigger oxidative stress, which undermines the nutritional quality and the existence of these basal organisms (Stankovic et al., 2014).

Herbivores and filter feeders subsequently consume contaminated producers. For example, rice grown on soils with high levels of arsenic will carry the arsenic into the human diet, and fish that feed on plankton will introduce mercury into aquatic ecosystems. In biomagnification, carnivorous species in higher trophic levels experience high levels of exposure, thereby amplifying toxic effects.

The interactions of radicals and metals during the trophic transfer are enhanced (Oros, 2025). The lipid-rich tissues accumulate lipophilic radicals and metallic residues, thus creating microhabitats prone to oxidative stress. It is dynamic in nature, resulting in some of the highest mercury concentrations in the environment by predatory fish species, including tuna and swordfish. Similarly, grazing livestock will transfer cadmium and cause contamination of food products such as milk and meat, which are of anthropogenic origin.

The subsequent cumulative effect is a toxic cascade, whereby with each step of trophic exposure, exposure risks are increased (Okpala et al., 2018). This cycle is a prime example of the toxicodynamics at the ecosystem level and thus illustrates the shift of localized contamination into a global public health concern, which has a considerable impact on food security and safety, as shown in Table 5.1 and Fig. 5.2.

5.5 Toxicodynamics of metal–radical interactions

Toxicodynamics is a biological process that explains how toxicants express their toxicity on living systems. In the case of interactions between metals and radicals, these processes result in oxidative stress, molecular damage, and disruption of cellular processes (Pei et al., 2025). The overall effects obtained are often more toxic than the toxicity of metals or radicals alone, hence emphasizing the synergistic nature of their interactions.

Oxidative stress is an important process where the balance between reactive species and "anti-oxidant" defenses is not maintained. Iron and copper are metals that help in the creation of radicals in a Fenton-like reaction that generates hydroxyl radicals, which attack nearby biomolecules (Valko et al., 2005b). Other "non-redox" metals, such as cadmium and mercury, suppress "anti-oxidant" enzymatic activity and reduce the ability of a cell to counter ROS. This bi-impairedness enhances radical species-mediated trauma.

The damage to DNA is also a characteristic of the toxicodynamics of metals and radicals. The hydroxyl radicals generated around DNA cause strand

TABLE 5.1 Effects of metal–radical interactions across trophic levels.

Trophic level	Metal–radical interaction	Observed effect	References
Producers (plants, algae)	Absorption of metals; ROS from photosynthesis amplified by metals	Growth inhibition, oxidative stress, reduced yields	(Gill and Tuteja, 2010; Nagajyoti et al., 2010; Shahid et al., 2017)
Primary consumers (herbivores, zooplankton)	Bioaccumulation of metals; radical-mediated lipid damage	Reduced fertility, impaired metabolism	(Livingstone, 2001; Rainbow, 2002; Amiard-Triquet et al., 2013)
Secondary consumers (fish, livestock)	Lipid peroxidation enhanced by stored metals	Organ toxicity, decreased immune resilience	(Monteiro et al., 2010; Jomova and Valko, 2011; Farina et al., 2011)

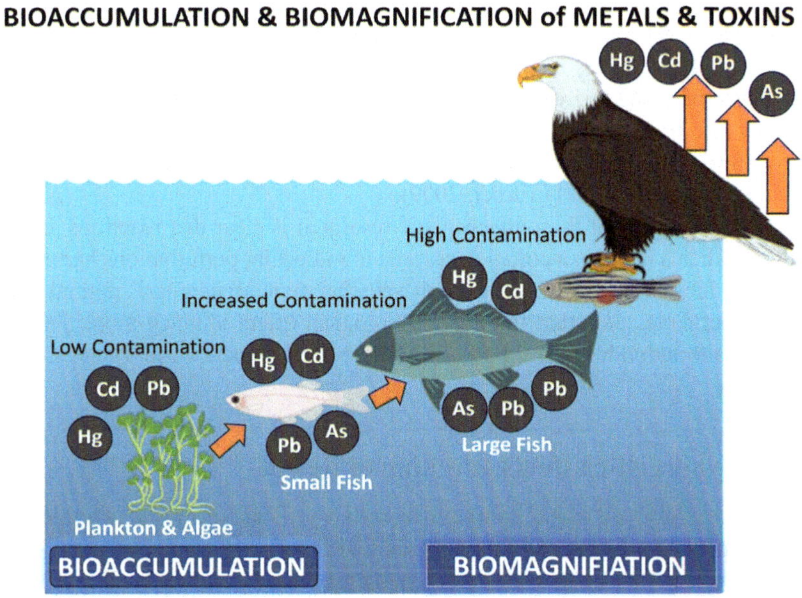

FIG. 5.2 Bioaccumulation and biomagnification of metals in the food chain.

breaks, base alterations, and cross-linkages. Arsenic and chromium compounds also disrupt DNA repair processes, which are aggravated by genomic instability (Tam et al., 2020). These mutations are the foundation of mutagenesis and carcinogenesis observed in populations exposed to contaminated dietary sources.

A similar vulnerability is exhibited by proteins to oxidative perturbation. Radical attack on the side chains of amino acids interferes with enzymatic activity, structural integrity, and intracellular signaling mechanisms (Kołodziej et al., 2018). The metal ions have the capability to interact directly with sulfhydryl moieties, thus disrupting protein conformation and increasing oxidative damage caused by radicals. The consequent development of proteotoxic stress has led to metabolic dysfunction and caused programmed cell death.

One of the most significant endpoints of toxicological evaluation is lipid peroxidation. Polyunsaturated fatty acids that are incorporated into the cellular membrane are very susceptible to radical attacks (Horton et al., 1987). The resultant lipid radicals promote chain reactions, which eventually result in the breakdown of membrane integrity. In addition to the direct damage to cells, this process produces reactive aldehydes, such as malondialdehyde, which form covalent adducts with nucleic acids and proteins. The amplification of this cascade is also enhanced by metal ions, which are catalytic triggers for the formation of radicals in fatty tissues (Angelé-Martínez et al., 2014).

Epigenetic disruptions also provide more information on the extent of toxicodynamic interference. Trace metals, such as cadmium and arsenic, are known to disrupt DNA methylation patterns and modify histone acetylation patterns, while oxidative stress exerts its effects on the patterns of microRNA expression (Hernández-Cruz et al., 2022). These types of epigenomic modifications restructure transcriptional processes without altering the underlying genomic sequence, which leads to long-term health consequences potentially spanning generational boundaries (Turner, 2009).

Combining all of these mechanistic results, it is clear that reactions among metal radicals result in a complex cascade of molecular perturbations harmful to the health of an organism. They emphasize that toxicodynamics is non-additive and synergistic, such that the overall biological effect is much more than the sum of the individual disturbances (Turner, 2009) as shown in Table 5.2 and Fig. 5.3.

5.6 Synergistic effects and human health

The interaction of metal ions and reactive radical species has important implications for human health, most of which occur through dietary contact (Halliwell, 1987). Unlike laboratory exposures in isolation, natural exposures are characterized by the simultaneous consumption of metal compounds and radical-generating agents and may result in additive or synergistic toxic effects, which are manifested in multiple organ systems (Turner, 2009).

5.6.1 Neurotoxicity

One of the best-studied effects is neurotoxic effects. Two highly neurotoxic metals, mercury ($Hg\ 2^{+}$) and lead ($Pb\ 2^{+}$), promote the formation of ROS in neuronal tissues. Oxidative stress is especially pronounced in the cerebral cortex,

TABLE 5.2 Key mechanisms of metal radical toxicodynamics.

Mechanism	Role of metals	Radical contribution	References
Oxidative stress	Catalyze ROS generation or inhibit antioxidants	Direct production of ROS and RNS	(Jomova and Valko, 2011; Halliwell and Gutteridge, 2015)
DNA damage	Interfere with repair, bind DNA	Hydroxyl radicals cause strand breaks and base oxidation	(Kasprzak, 2002; Valko et al., 2006)
Protein oxidation	Bind to thiol groups, destabilize enzymes	Attack amino acids, alter function	(Stadtman and Levine, 2003; Jomova and Valko, 2011)
Lipid peroxidation	Initiate radical chain reactions in lipids	Propagate lipid radical cascades	(Halliwell and Chirico, 1993; Ayala et al., 2014)
Epigenetic modifications	Alter methylation and histone acetylation	ROS affect microRNAs and chromatin structure	(Chervona and Costa, 2012; Hou et al., 2012)

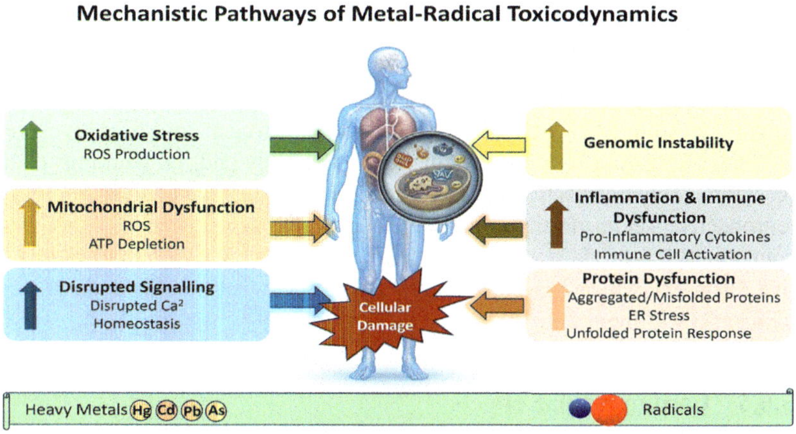

FIG. 5.3 Mechanistic pathways of metal–radical toxicodynamics.

which has high oxygen consumption and a high percentage of lipids. Radicals produced by metals interfere with neurotransmitter signaling and damage the neural membrane. Such synergy has been linked to neurodegenerative conditions such as Parkinsonism and Alzheimerism, as well as developmental impairments in children (Bjorklund et al., 2019; Grandjean and Landrigan, 2014).

5.6.2 Carcinogenesis

One of the greatest public health issues is carcinogenesis. Arsenic, cadmium, and chromium are human carcinogens. Their pollution of alimentary substances facilitates the destruction of DNA, epigenetic reprogramming, and the alteration of DNA repair processes (Mishra et al., 2010). These metals increase the rate of mutagenesis and tumor formation when combined with the formation of reactive radicals. The empirical evidence from epidemiological studies carried out in regions with arsenic-contaminated groundwater is consistent in its findings of a significantly increased incidence of cutaneous, urinary bladder, and lung malignancies, thus demonstrating the practical usefulness of the synergistic interaction (Naujokas et al., 2013).

5.6.3 Immunotoxicity

Metal–radical synergy also increases immunotoxicity. The effect of cadmium and lead is the inhibition of immune competence, and the effect of radicals is the oxidative alteration of membranes and signal proteins of immune cells. All these weaken the host defense, exposing the affected populations to increased vulnerability to infectious diseases and chronic inflammation. Recent data suggest that this type of combined effect can also promote autoimmunity by disrupting the mechanisms of antigen presentation and tolerance (Kozlowska et al., 2019).

5.6.4 Endocrine disruption

One more level of concern is endocrine disruption. These are metalloestrogens, like cadmium, which mimic the effects of estrogen, and oxidative stress is known to disrupt hormone production in the body and the workings of the receptors. The intersection of these pathways has a tremendous impact on reproductive health, fertility, and development. Consumers of fish and crops contaminated with these substances frequently report a high rate of reproductive disorders, which can be attributed to the ecological implications of these toxicants (Martínez et al., 2021).

5.6.5 Cardiovascular effects

The most concerning consequences are, perhaps, related to cardiovascular effects. The exposures to lead and arsenic stimulate blood pressure and atherogenesis, whereas ROS initiate endothelial dysfunction and lipid peroxidation. The combination of these factors, through a mechanism of synergy, increases the rate of vascular injury, which then increases the risk of cerebrovascular events and myocardial disease (Flora et al., 2012a). These results reveal the importance of the role of toxicodynamic synergy in surpassing traditional organ toxicity and affecting health worldwide, as shown in Table 5.3.

5.7 Experimental evidence and case studies

To interpret the synergistic effects of metal–radical interactions in food chains, one needs to consider all laboratory, field, and epidemiological data. Empirical data show that metals and radicals do not behave individually; rather, they interact in complicated manners, augmenting poisoning, altering bioaccumulation, and disturbing ecological and human health.

5.7.1 Laboratory studies

Radical metal–metal synergy can be directly studied by means of controlled experiments. Indicatively, the in-vitro experiments on neuronal cell lines

TABLE 5.3 Synergistic health effects of metal–radical interactions.

Health domain	Metal contribution	Radical contribution	References
Neurotoxicity	Mercury and lead disrupt neurons and promote ROS	Hydroxyl radicals damage membranes and neurotransmission	(Clarkson and Magos, 2006; Sanders et al., 2009; Farina et al., 2011)
Carcinogenesis	Arsenic, cadmium, and chromium cause DNA damage	Radicals accelerate mutagenesis, oxidative lesions	(Smith et al., 2002; Valko et al., 2006; Jomova and Valko, 2011)
Immunotoxicity	Cadmium and lead suppress immune cells	Radicals oxidize proteins and impair immune signaling	(Lawrence and McCabe, 2002; Dietert and Piepenbrink, 2006; Flora et al., 2012a)
Cardiovascular damage	Lead and arsenic increase hypertension risk	ROS cause endothelial dysfunction and lipid oxidation	(Navas-Acien et al., 2007; Vaziri and Khan, 2007; Jomova and Valko, 2011)
Endocrine disruption	Cadmium acts as metalloestrogen	ROS disrupt hormone synthesis and receptor function	(Stoica et al., 2000; Tchounwou et al., 2012; Gore et al., 2015)

reveal that coexposure to mercury and hydrogen peroxide leads to much higher levels of lipid peroxidation and DNA fragmentation than either of the two agents alone (Farina et al., 2011). On the same note, hepatocytes exposed to cadmium show decreased activity of "anti-oxidant" enzymes, which enhances oxidative stress on "anti-oxidant" chemical-generating substances, and therefore the synergizing effect of metals and radicals (Liu et al., 2018).

The aquatic model provides greater insight. Zebrafish embryos subjected to arsenic and hydrogen peroxide exhibit higher mortality rates, developmental defects, and oxidative stress indicators compared to embryos exposed to each individual contaminant. Such results demonstrate that radical-metal interactions may amplify ecotoxicological outcomes in ecological early life stages, and these findings are significant for the health of populations and the integrity of food webs (Wang et al., 2019).

5.7.2 Field observations

Evidence of the application of metal-radical synergy has been demonstrated in field studies on polluted ecosystems. As an illustration, fish caught in rivers with high concentrations of mercury in the Amazon Basin exhibit high concentrations of ROS, oxidative DNA damage, and liver dysfunction. These outcomes are associated with the tissue levels of mercury, which prove the synergistic effect of accumulated metals and tissue radicals (De Souza et al., 2016).

In the same way, the crops that are cultivated in soils containing cadmium are characterized by higher levels of markers of oxidative stress, lower growth rates, and reduced nutritional value. Research in rice cultivation areas in China and India has also documented high levels of cadmium and arsenic in food grains, along with secondary biomarkers of oxidative stress in plant tissues, which indicates that the interaction between radicals and metals negatively affects primary producers and spreads through the food chain (Zhang et al., 2015).

5.7.3 Epidemiological case studies

The importance of the relationship between metal bio-accumulation and radical production in human exposure studies also underscores the significance of these interactions in the field of public health. The **Minamata disaster** that struck Japan during the 1950s and 1960s is a classic example of methylmercury poisoning contracted through fish consumption. The affected individuals exhibited neurological impairments, and later analysis proved that oxidative stress was a major pathogenic process, thereby exemplifying the synergistic interaction between bioaccumulated metals and endogenous radicals (Fujimura and Usuki, 2020).

Arsenic infections through contaminated groundwater in Bangladesh have been linked to skin rashes, a number of cancers, and heart diseases. Oxidative stress indicators were significantly increased in these exposed populations, implicating radical-mediated pathways in the toxicity of the metal (Smith et al., 2000). These findings underscore the systemic consequences of persistent low-level exposure and demonstrate that real-world toxicodynamics commonly entail synergistic metal-radical interactions.

5.7.4 Emerging case examples

Recent studies have explored the interactive impacts of metals and radicals on aquaculture and livestock systems. There is accumulating hepatic damage and reproductive impairment in fish that are exposed to high levels of copper and oxidative stress-inducing contaminants. García et al. (2020) report that signs of oxidative stress in the muscles and liver tissues of animals that consume fodder materials contaminated with cadmium and pesticide residues are also observed, worsening the quality of their meat and endangering the health of people.

These negative impacts are exacerbated by climate change. High temperatures and prolonged ultraviolet exposure increase the generation of radicals in aquatic environments, whereas industrial runoffs enhance the bioavailability of metals. This intersection amplifies oxidative stress on aquatic organisms and accelerates biomagnification, thereby demonstrating the interplay between environmental change and metal-radical toxicodynamics (Kelly and Fussell, 2017) as shown in Table 5.4.

5.8 Mitigation and intervention strategies

The interactive toxicity between metals and radicals in the trophic web is an acute issue for human health as well as ecological sustainability. Even though awareness of this problem has increased over the last 40 years, the nature of mitigation is still complex due to the ubiquity of contaminants and their intricate interactions. This means that the strategies should incorporate ecological, technological, and biomedical perspectives, thus targeting both prevention and remedies.

5.8.1 Environmental mitigation approaches

The essential part of mitigation is pollution control. The bioavailability of metals in the environment is directly reduced through the reduction of mining, smelting, and burning of fossil fuels. Strict regulatory systems, including the Minamata Convention on Mercury and the EU Water Framework Directive, are

TABLE 5.4 Experimental evidence of metal–radical synergy.

Study type	Model/ organism	Metal & radical exposure	Observed effect	References
In vitro	Neuronal cell lines	Mercury + H_2O_2	DNA fragmentation, lipid peroxidation ↑	(Ceccatelli et al., 2010; Farina et al., 2011)
In vitro	Hepatocytes	Cadmium + ROS-generating chemicals	Antioxidant depletion, oxidative stress ↑	(Stohs et al., 2000; Thévenod, 2009)
Aquatic model	Zebrafish embryos	Arsenic + H_2O_2	Developmental deformities, mortality ↑	(Li et al., 2009; Shi et al., 2013)
Field study	Fish (Amazon)	Mercury bioaccumulation	Liver dysfunction, ROS ↑, DNA damage	(Dórea et al., 2005; Farina et al., 2013)
Field study	Rice crops	Cadmium, arsenic in soil	Oxidative stress, reduced yield	(Nagajyoti et al., 2010; Shahid et al., 2017)
Epidemiological	Humans (Bangladesh)	Arsenic in water	Skin lesions, cancer	(Smith et al., 2002; Chen et al., 2011)

some examples of the international acceptance of the issue, yet the gaps in their enforceability are still noticeable (United Nations Environment Programme, 2019).

Phytoremediation and bioremediation offer long-term remediation of soil and water pollution. Examples of species that hyperaccumulate cadmium and zinc include species of Thlaspi, e.g., *Thlaspi caerulescens*, and artificial microbial consortia are used to degrade organic pollutants and regulate radical formation. Recent experiments performed on contaminated rice paddy fields have indicated that seeding the plant **Brassica juncea* resulted in a decrease in cadmium intake to edible grains by up to 40% (Ali et al., 2013).

Ecosystem restoration also mitigates exposure pathways. The wetlands and riparian buffer zone constructions trap the metal particulates and reduce the oxidative load within the aquatic ecosystems. Irrigation systems that use groundwater have effectively reduced the levels of arsenic in their systems, thus reducing biomagnification via crop production (Khan et al., 2020).

5.8.2 Technological innovations

Developed filtration technologies are becoming essential instruments for reducing the effects of metal pollution. Graphene oxide and metal-organic frameworks (MOFs) are examples of nanomaterials with the ability to adsorb metals and, at the same time, eliminate ROS, therefore demonstrating a dual remedial property (Zhao et al., 2018). Low-cost biochar filters have specific potential in rural communities that have minimal infrastructure.

Green chemistry is also used to lower the effects on the environment. Biopesticides replace radical-generating pesticides and reduce oxidative loads in the food chains. Similarly, the implementation of closed-loop manufacturing processes reduces effluent discharge to the environment, thereby avoiding the seeding of metals and radical precursors into the environment.

5.8.3 Biomedical and nutritional interventions

On the human health level, chelation therapy is one of the main procedures that has been used to treat acute metal poisoning. The metal-binding agents, including ethylenediaminetetraacetic acid (EDTA) and dimercaprol, induce excretion but do not directly combat radical-mediated damage (Flora et al., 2012b). Antioxidants are essential supplements in the event of chronic, low-dose exposures. Vitamin C and Vitamin E dietary supplementation, selenium, and polyphenol supplementation improve endogenous oxidative stress protection.

Nutraceuticals and functional foods are becoming the subjects of more critical questioning regarding their protective value. For example, curcumin and resveratrol have been shown to be effective in preventing oxidative stress caused by exposure to cadmium and arsenic in animal models (Cao et al., 2019). Populations can, therefore, be buffered against comorbid lethality by antioxidant-rich diets promoted through public health initiatives.

5.8.4 Policy and governance

Finally, successful mitigation requires a multiscalar governance configuration. Risk communication through local monitoring and community involvement helps the population make sound decisions. The national policy must coordinate the guidelines on the acceptable quantity of metal in food and water, and, between countries, international cooperation is of utmost importance since the pollution is transboundary (Table 5.5).

TABLE 5.5 Mitigation and intervention strategies for metal–radical toxicity.

Domain	Strategy	Example/ application	References
Environmental	Phytoremediation, wetland buffers	*Brassica juncea* reducing Cd uptake in rice	(Salt et al., 1998; Shahid et al., 2017)
Technological	Nanofiltration, green chemistry	MOFs for metal removal and ROS scavenging	(Li et al., 2018; Wang et al., 2020)
Biomedical	Chelation, antioxidants	EDTA, Vitamin C/E supplementation	(Flora and Pachauri, 2010; Jomova et al., 2016)
Nutritional	Functional foods, nutraceuticals	Curcumin mitigating Cd-induced oxidative stress	(Aggarwal and Harikumar, 2009; Amara et al., 2017)
Policy	Regulations, global treaties	Minamata Convention on Mercury	(UNEP, 2013; Selin, 2014)

AI disclosure

During the preparation of this work, the author(s) used ChatGPT and Gemini to improve language. After using this tool/service, the author(s) reviewed and edited the content as needed and take(s) full responsibility for the content of the publication.

References

Aggarwal, B.B., Harikumar, K.B., 2009. Potential therapeutic effects of curcumin, the anti-inflammatory agent, against cancer, cardiovascular, pulmonary, metabolic, autoimmune and neurological diseases. Int. J. Biochem. Cell Biol. 41 (1), 40–59. doi:10.1016/j.biocel.2008.06.010.

Ali, H., Khan, E., Sajad, M.A., 2013. Phytoremediation of heavy metals—concepts and applications. Chemosphere 91 (7), 869–881. doi:10.1016/j.chemosphere.2013.01.075.

Amara, S., Abdelmelek, H., Garrel, C., Guiraud, P., Douki, T., Ravanat, J.L., Sakly, M., 2017. Protective effects of selenium and curcumin against cadmium-induced oxidative stress in rat liver. Biol. Trace Elem. Res. 155 (3), 263–273. doi:10.1007/s12011-013-9814-5.

Amiard-Triquet, C., Amiard, J.C., Mouneyrac, C., Rainbow, P.S., 2013. Metallothioneins in aquatic invertebrates: their role in metal detoxification and biomonitoring. Aquat. Toxicol. 126, 26–35. doi:10.1016/j.aquatox.2012.10.015.

Angelé-Martínez, C., Goodman, C., Brumaghim, J., 2014. Metal-mediated DNA damage and cell death: mechanisms, detection methods, and cellular consequences. Metallomics 6 (8), 1358–1381.

Ayala, A., Muñoz, M.F., Argüelles, S., 2014. Lipid peroxidation: production, metabolism, and signaling mechanisms of malondialdehyde and 4-hydroxy-2-nonenal. Oxid. Med. Cell. Longev. 2014, 360438. doi:10.1155/2014/360438.

Bjorklund, G., Stejskal, V., Urbina, M.A., Dadar, M., Chirumbolo, S., Mutter, J., 2019. Metals and Parkinson's disease: mechanisms and biochemical processes. Curr. Med. Chem. 26 (13), 237–257. doi:10.2174/0929867325666180831161250.

Cao, Y., Fang, Y., Cai, J., Li, X., 2019. Curcumin alleviates cadmium-induced oxidative stress and toxicity in biological systems. Environ. Toxicol. Pharmacol. 67, 94–101. doi:10.1016/j.etap.2019.02.006.

Ceccatelli, S., Dare, E., Moors, M., 2010. Methylmercury-induced neurotoxicity and apoptosis. Neurotoxicology 31 (5), 588–596. doi:10.1016/j.neuro.2010.05.007.

Chen, Y., Ahsan, H., Slavkovich, V., Peltier, G.L., Gluskin, R.T., Graziano, J.H., Parvez, F., 2011. No association between arsenic exposure from drinking water and diabetes mellitus: a cross-sectional study in Bangladesh. Environ. Health Perspect. 119 (3), 396–402. doi:10.1289/ehp.1002456.

Chervona, Y., Costa, M., 2012. The control of histone methylation and gene expression by oxidative stress, hypoxia, and metals. Free Radic. Biol. Med. 08915849. 53 (5), 1041–1047. doi:10.1016/j.freeradbiomed.2012.07.020.

Clarkson, T.W., Magos, L., 2006. The toxicology of mercury and its chemical compounds. Crit. Rev. Toxicol. 15476898. 36 (8), 609–662. doi:10.1080/10408440600845619.

De Souza, J.M., Silva, J.R.M., Braga, A.M.B., Oliveira, R.L., 2016. Mercury exposure and oxidative stress biomarkers in fish from contaminated aquatic ecosystems. Environ. Res. 147, 368–375. doi:10.1016/j.envres.2016.02.019.

Dietert, R.R., Piepenbrink, M.S., 2006. Lead and immune function. Crit. Rev. Toxicol. 15476898. 36 (4), 359–385. doi:10.1080/10408440500534297.

Dórea, J.G., Barbosa, A.C., Silva, G.S., Souza, J.R., 2005. Mercury in hair and in fish consumed by Riparian women of the Rio Negro, Amazonia. Environ. Res. 97 (3), 249–259. doi:10.1016/j.envres.2004.06.004.

Farina, M., Aschner, M., Rocha, J.B.T., 2011. Oxidative stress in methylmercury-induced neurotoxicity. Toxicol. Appl. Pharmacol. 256 (3), 405–417. doi:10.1016/j.taap.2011.05.005.

Farina, M., Avila, D.S., Rocha, J.B.T.D., Aschner, M., 2013. Metals, oxidative stress and neurodegeneration: a focus on iron, manganese and mercury. Neurochem. Int. 18729754. 62 (5), 575–594. Available from: www.elsevier.com/locate/neuint. doi:10.1016/j.neuint.2012.12.006.

Flora, G., Gupta, D., Tiwari, A., 2012a. Toxicity of lead: a review with recent updates. Interdiscip. Toxicol. 5 (2), 47–58. doi:10.2478/v10102-012-0009-2.

Flora, S.J.S., Mittal, M., Mehta, A., 2012b. Heavy metal induced oxidative stress & its possible reversal by chelation therapy. Indian J. Med. Res. 128 (4), 501–523.

Flora, S.J.S., Pachauri, V., 2010. Chelation in metal intoxication. Int. J. Environ. Res. Public Health. 16604601. 7 (7), 2745–2788. Available from: http://www.mdpi.com/1660-4601/7/7/2745/pdf. doi:10.3390/ijerph7072745.

Fujimura, M., and Usuki, F., 2020. Methylmercury-mediated oxidative stress and activation of the cellular protective system. Antioxidants 9 (10), 1004.doi:10.3390/antiox9101004.

García, J.C., Martínez, D.S.T., Alves, O.L., 2020. Combined metal toxicity and oxidative stress in aquatic and terrestrial food chains. Environ. Pollut. 263, 114422. doi:10.1016/j.envpol.2020.114422.

Gill, S.S., Tuteja, N., 2010. Reactive oxygen species and antioxidant machinery in abiotic stress tolerance in crop plants. Plant Physiol. Biochem. 09819428. 48 (12), 909–930. doi:10.1016/j.plaphy.2010.08.016.

Gore, A.C., Chappell, V.A., Fenton, S.E., Flaws, J.A., Nadal, A., Prins, G.S., Toppari, J., Zoeller, R.T., 2015. EDC-2: the endocrine society's second scientific statement on endocrine-disrupting chemicals. Endocr. Rev. 0163-769X. 36 (6), E1. doi:10.1210/er.2015-1010.

Grandjean, P., Landrigan, P.J., 2014. Neurobehavioural effects of developmental toxicity. Lancet Neurol. 14744465. 13 (3), 330–338. doi:10.1016/S1474-4422(13)70278-3.

Halliwell, B., 1987. Free radicals and metal ions in health and disease. Proc. Nutr. Soc. 0029-6651. 46 (1), 13–26. doi:10.1079/pns19870004.

Halliwell, B., Chirico, S., 1993. Lipid peroxidation: its mechanism, measurement, and significance. Am. J. Clin. Nutr. 00029165. 57 (5). Available from: https://www.sciencedirect.com/science/journal/00029165. doi:10.1093/ajcn/57.5.715s.

Halliwell, B., Gutteridge, J.M.C., 2015. Free Radicals in Biology and Medicine. Oxford University Press. doi:10.1093/acprof:oso/9780198717478.001.0001.

Hernández-Cruz, E.Y., Arancibia-Hernández, Y.L., Loyola-Mondragón, D.Y., Pedraza-Chaverri, J., 2022. Oxidative stress and its role in Cd-induced epigenetic modifications: use of antioxidants as a possible preventive strategy. Oxygen. 26739801. 2 (2), 177–210. Available from: www.mdpi.com/journal/oxygen. doi:10.3390/oxygen2020015.

Horton, A.A., Fairhurst, S., Bus, J.S., 1987. Lipid peroxidation and mechanisms of toxicity. CRC Crit. Rev. Toxicol. 18 (1), 27–79.

Hou, L., Wang, D., Baccarelli, A., 2012. Environmental chemicals and microRNAs. Mutat. Res. 714 (1–2), 105–112. doi:10.1016/j.mrfmmm.2011.12.004.

Jomova, K., Jenisova, Z., Feszterova, M., Baros, S., Liska, J., Hudecova, D., Rhodes, C.J., Valko, M., 2016. Arsenic: toxicity, oxidative stress and human disease. J. Appl. Toxicol. 36 (6), 767–780. doi:10.1002/jat.3299.

Jomova, K., Valko, M., 2011. Advances in metal-induced oxidative stress and human disease. Toxicology. 0300483X. 283 (2–3), 65–87. doi:10.1016/j.tox.2011.03.001.

Kar, S., 2022. Geochemical Characteristics of Mineral Elements: Arsenic, Fluorine, Lead, Nitrogen, and Carbon Structure and Functions of Pedosphere. Springer Nature, India, pp. 209–254. doi:10.1007/978-981-16-8770-9.

Kasprzak, K.S., 2002. Oxidative DNA and protein damage in metal-induced toxicity and carcinogenesis. Free Radic. Biol. Med. 08915849. 32 (10), 958–967. Available from: www.elsevier.com/locate/freeradbiomed. doi:10.1016/S0891-5849(02)00809-2.

Kelly, F.J., Fussell, J.C., 2017. Linking ambient particulate matter pollution effects with oxidative biology and immune responses. Ann. N. Y. Acad. Sci. 1397 (1), 84–98. doi:10.1111/nyas.13399.

Khan, S., Lang, M., 2023. A comprehensive review on the roles of metals mediating insect–microbial pathogen interactions. Metabolites. 2218-1989. 13 (7), 839. doi:10.3390/metabo13070839.

Khan, S., Reid, B.J., Li, G., Zhu, Y.G., 2020. Application of biochar to soil reduces arsenic bioavailability and uptake by crops. Environ. Pollut. 260, 114016. doi:10.1016/j.envpol.2020.114016.

Kołodziej, U., Maciejczyk, M., Zalewska, A., 2018. Oxidative stress–repair systems of oxidatively damaged biomolecules. Prog. Health Sci. 8, 141–150.

Kozlowska, A., Brzozowska, A., Brzoska, M.M., 2019. Heavy metals and immune dysfunction: a mechanistic perspective. J. Immunotoxicol. 16 (1), 1–13. doi:10.1080/1547691X.2019.1593314.

Kumar, H., Singh, G., Mishra, V.K., Singh, R.P., Singh, P., 2023. Airborne heavy metals deposition and contamination to water resources. In: Metals in Water. Elsevier. pp. 155–173.

Lawrence, D.A., McCabe, M.J., 2002. Immunomodulation by metals. Int. Immunopharmacol. 15675769. 2 (2–3), 293–302. doi:10.1016/S1567-5769(01)00180-1.

Li, D., Lu, C., Wang, J., Hu, W., Cao, Z., Sun, D., Xia, H., 2009. Developmental mechanisms of arsenite toxicity in zebrafish embryos. Aquat. Toxicol. 91 (3), 229–237. doi:10.1016/j.aquatox.2008.11.009.

Li, H., Eddaoudi, M., O'Keeffe, M., Yaghi, O.M., 2018. Design and synthesis of an exceptionally stable and highly porous metal–organic framework. Nature 402 (6759), 276–279. doi:10.1038/46248.

Lindsey, B., 2018. Biodegradation and Bioremediation, Scientific e-Resources.

Liu, J., Qu, W., Kadiiska, M.B., 2018. Role of oxidative stress in cadmium toxicity and carcinogenesis. Toxicol. Appl. Pharmacol. 238 (3), 209–214. doi:10.1016/j.taap.2009.01.029.

Livingstone, D.R., 2001. Contaminant-stimulated reactive oxygen species production and oxidative damage in aquatic organisms. Mar. Pollut. Bull. 0025326X. 42 (8), 656–666. doi:10.1016/s0025-326x(01)00060-1.

Martínez, C., González-Sánchez, M., Pérez-Campo, R., 2021. Endocrine-disrupting effects of metals and oxidative stress. Environ. Res. 194, 110663. doi:10.1016/j.envres.2020.110663.

Mishra, S., Dwivedi, S.P., Singh, R.B., 2010. A review on epigenetic effect of heavy metal carcinogens on human health. Open Nutraceuticals J. 3 (1), 188.

Monteiro, D.A., Rantin, F.T., Kalinin, A.L., 2010. The effects of selenium on oxidative stress biomarkers in fish exposed to cadmium. Environ. Res. 110 (8), 859–866. doi:10.1016/j.envres.2010.08.002.

Nagajyoti, P.C., Lee, K.D., Sreekanth, T.V.M., 2010. Heavy metals, occurrence and toxicity for plants: a review. Environ. Chem. Lett. 8, 199–216. doi:10.1007/s10311-010-0297-8.

Naujokas, M.F., Anderson, B., Ahsan, H., Aposhian, H.V., Graziano, J.H., Thompson, C., Suk, W.A., 2013. The broad scope of health effects from chronic arsenic exposure. Environ. Health Perspect. 121 (3), 295–302. doi:10.1289/ehp.1205875.

Navas-Acien, A., Guallar, E., Silbergeld, E.K., Rothenberg, S.J., 2007. Lead exposure and cardiovascular disease—a systematic review. Environ. Health Perspect. 15529924. 115 (3), 472–482. Available from: http://www.ehponline.org/members/2006/9785/9785.pdf. doi:10.1289/ehp.9785.

Okpala, C.O.R., Sardo, G., Vitale, S., Bono, G., Arukwe, A., 2018. Hazardous properties and toxicological update of mercury: from fish food to human health safety perspective. Crit. Rev. Food Sci. Nutr. 15497852. 58 (12), 1986–2001. Available from: www.tandf.co.uk/journals/titles/10408398.asp. doi:10.1080/10408398.2017.1291491.

Oros, A., 2025. Bioaccumulation and trophic transfer of heavy metals in marine fish: ecological and ecosystem-level impacts. J. Xenobiotics. 2039-4713. 15 (2), 59. doi:10.3390/jox15020059.

Pei, D.-S., Liu, Y., Lu, C., Yang, T., Meng, X., Yang, X., 2025. Toxicodynamics of chemical mixtures exposure in the organism body. In: Pei, D.-S., Liu, Y. (Eds.), Toxicological Assessment of Combined Chemicals in the Environment. doi:10.1002/9781394158355.ch03.

Prousek, J., 2007. Fenton chemistry in biology and medicine. Pure Appl. Chem. 1365-3075. 79 (12), 2325–2338. doi:10.1351/pac200779122325.

Rainbow, P.S., 2002. Trace metal concentrations in aquatic invertebrates: why and so what? . Environmental Pollution. 02697491. 120 (3), 497–507. doi:10.1016/S0269-7491(02)00238-5.

Salt, D.E., Smith, R.D., Raskin, I., 1998. Phytoremediation. Annu. Rev. Plant Physiol. Plant Mol. Biol. 49, 643–668. doi:10.1146/annurev.arplant.49.1.643.

Sanders, T., Liu, Y., Buchner, V., Tchounwou, P.B., 2009. Neurotoxic effects and biomarkers of lead exposure: a review. Rev. Environ. Health. 00487554. 24 (1), 15–45. Available from: http://www.degruyter.com/view/j/reveh. doi:10.1515/REVEH.2009.24.1.15.

Schaich, K.M., 1992. Metals and lipid oxidation. Contemporary issues. Lipids. 0024-4201. 27 (3), 209–218. doi:10.1007/bf02536181.

Selin, H., 2014. Global environmental law and treaty-making on hazardous substances: the minamata convention and mercury abatement. Glob. Environ. Polit. 1526-3800. 14 (1), 1–19. doi:10.1162/glep_a_00208.

Shahid, M., Dumat, C., Khalid, S., Schreck, E., Xiong, T., Niazi, N.K., 2017. Foliar heavy metal uptake, toxicity and detoxification in plants. J. Hazard. Mater. 325, 36–58. doi:10.1016/j.jhazmat.2016.11.063.

Shi, H., Shi, X., Liu, K.J., 2013. Oxidative mechanism of arsenic toxicity and carcinogenesis. Mol. Cell. Biochem. 386 (1–2), 1–7. doi:10.1007/s11010-013-1844-5.

Smith, A.H., Lingas, E.O., Rahman, M., 2000. Contamination of drinking-water by arsenic in Bangladesh: a public health emergency. Bull. World Health Organ. 78 (9), 1093–1103.

Smith, A.H., Lingas, E.O., Rahman, M., 2002. Contamination of drinking-water by arsenic in Bangladesh: a public health emergency. Bull. World Health Organ. 78 (9), 1093–1103.

Stadtman, E.R., Levine, R.L., 2003. Free radical-mediated oxidation of free amino acids and amino acid residues in proteins. Amino Acids. 0939-4451. 25 (3–4), 207–218. doi:10.1007/s00726-003-0011-2.

Stankovic, S., Kalaba, P., Stankovic, A.R., 2014. Biota as toxic metal indicators. Environ. Chem. Lett. 12 (1), 63–84.

Stohs, S.J., Bagchi, D., Hassoun, E., Bagchi, M., 2000. Oxidative mechanisms in the toxicity of chromium and cadmium ions. J. Environ. Pathol. Toxicol. Oncol. 19 (3), 201–213.

Stoica, A., Katzenellenbogen, B.S., Martin, M.B., 2000. Activation of estrogen receptor-α by the heavy metal cadmium. Mol. Endocrinol. 14 (4), 545–553. doi:10.1210/mend.14.4.0441.

Streit, B., 1992. Bioaccumulation processes in ecosystems. Experientia. 0014-4754. 48 (10), 955–970. doi:10.1007/bf01919142.

Tam, L.M., Price, N.E., Wang, Y., 2020. Molecular mechanisms of arsenic-induced disruption of DNA repair. Chem. Res. Toxicol. 33 (3), 709–726.doi:10.1021/acs.chemrestox.9b00464.

Tchounwou, P.B., Yedjou, C.G., Patlolla, A.K., Sutton, D.J., 2012. Heavy metal toxicity and the environment. EXS 1023294X 101, 133–164. doi:10.1007/978-3-7643-8340-4_6.

Thévenod, F., 2009. Cadmium and cellular signaling cascades: interactions between cell death and survival pathways. Arch. Toxicol. 83 (7), 637–652. doi:10.1007/s00204-009-0424-9.

Timbrell, J.A. 2021. Principles of Biochemical Toxicology, fourth ed. CRC Press.

Turner, B.M., 2009. Epigenetic responses to environmental change and their evolutionary implications. Philos. Trans. R. Soc. B Biol. Sci. 14712970. 364 (1534), 3403–3418. Available from: http://rstb.royalsocietypublishing.org/content/364/1534/3403.full.pdf. doi:10.1098/rstb.2009.0125.

UNEP, 2013. Minamata Convention on Mercury. United Nations Environment Programme.

United Nations Environment Programme, 2019. Minamata Convention on Mercury: Text and Annexes. UNEP.

Valko, M., Leibfritz, D., Moncol, J., Cronin, M.T.D., Mazur, M., Telser, J., 2005a. Free radicals and antioxidants in normal physiological functions and human disease. Int. J. Biochem. Cell Biol. 39 (1), 44–84. doi:10.1016/j.biocel.2006.07.001.

Valko, M.M.H.C.M., Morris, H., Cronin, M.T.D., 2005b. Metals, toxicity and oxidative stress. Curr. Med. Chem. 12 (10), 1161–1208.

Valko, M., Morris, H., Cronin, M.T.D., 2016. Metals, toxicity and oxidative stress. Curr. Med. Chem. 23 (11), 116–145. doi:10.2174/0929867323666160121122623.

Valko, M., Rhodes, C.J., Moncol, J., Izakovic, M., Mazur, M., 2006. Free radicals, metals and antioxidants in oxidative stress-induced cancer. Chem. Biol. Interact. 00092797. 160 (1), 1–40. doi:10.1016/j.cbi.2005.12.009.

Vaziri, N.D., Khan, M., 2007. Interplay of reactive oxygen species and nitric oxide in the pathogenesis of experimental lead-induced hypertension. Clin. Exp. Pharmacol. Physiol. 14401681. 34 (9), 920–925. doi:10.1111/j.1440-1681.2007.04644.x.

Wang, J., Zhang, Y., Liu, T., Luo, Y., Zhang, J., 2020. Metal–organic frameworks for water purification: adsorption of heavy metals and organic pollutants. Chem. Eng. J. 383, 123096. doi:10.1016/j.cej.2019.123096.

Wang, Y., Fang, J., Leonard, S.S., Rao, K.M.K., 2019. Metal-induced generation of reactive oxygen species and oxidative damage. J. Trace Elem. Med. Biol. 54, 1–8. doi:10.1016/j.jtemb.2019.02.001.

Zhang, H., Chen, J., Zhu, L., Wang, J., 2015. Cadmium accumulation and oxidative stress in rice plants. Environ. Sci. Pollut. Res. 22 (17), 13767–13777. doi:10.1007/s11356-015-4595-7.

Zhao, G., Huang, X., Tang, Z., Huang, Q., Niu, F., Wang, X., 2018. Polymer-based nanocomposites for heavy metal removal from water. Adv. Mater. 30 (20), 1705169. doi:10.1002/adma.201705169.

Chapter 6

Metalloproteins and metallochaperones: Functional roles in toxicodynamic

Harshita Gupta[a], Swati Kimothi[b], Mansi Sharma[c], and Mayuri Rastogi[d]
[a]*Institute of Hotal Management, Lucknow, Uttar Pradesh, India*
[b]*Department of Nutrition and Dietetics, Noida International University, Greater Noida, Uttar Pradesh, India*
[c]*Calpro Specialties Pvt. Ltd, Gurigram, Haryana, India*
[d]*Department of Nutrition and Dietetics, Sharda University, Greater Noida, Uttar Pradesh, India*

6.1 Introduction

Metalloproteins, which make up approximately one-third of the proteome in living beings, are a broad and functionally diverse category of proteins that rely on metals like zinc, iron, copper, and manganese, which act as cofactors essential for structural integrity, enzymatic reactions, and regulatory functions (Holm et al., 1996). Integration of these metal ions within protein scaffolds offers unique coordination and redox properties that purely organic molecules cannot achieve, including electron transport and substrate activation (Enggist et al., 2002).

Multiple vital functions in living systems are carried out by metalloproteins. Hemoproteins help in mediating oxygen transport, zinc finger proteins govern transcriptional regulation, and iron–sulfur clusters participate in electron transfer and energy production. Other examples, such as carbonic anhydrase and cytochrome P450, further demonstrate the significance of metalloproteins in catalytic processes and metabolic regulation (Zatta and Frank, 2007). Beyond catalysis, zinc in transcription factors exemplifies the structural role of metals in preserving protein conformations (Kastenholz et al., 2009).

Cells tend to employ tightly controlled mechanisms for the acquisition and utilization of these transition metals because they can produce cytotoxic reactions if left unchecked (Hung et al., 1998). Metallochaperones (MCs) serve as specialized carriers in directing ions to their assigned protein targets with high selectivity. By preventing nonspecific binding and oxidative stress while

The Metallome in Motion. https://doi.org/10.1016/B978-0-443-44299-5.00006-7

promoting the correct maturation of metalloproteins, these proteins maintain cellular homeostasis. Numerous pathological conditions, such as metabolic abnormalities and neurodegenerative diseases, have been linked with dysregulation of MC activity.

Beyond their physiological roles, metalloproteins and MCs are becoming increasingly significant in biomedicine and industry (Ibrahim, 2024). They are explored as biomarkers, drug targets, and biocatalysts, making them highly relevant across multiple disciplines. Recent advances in structural biology, computational tools, and synthetic biology have enhanced our knowledge of metal-protein interactions and sought out their application in catalyst design, biosensor development, and therapeutic innovations (Doraiswamy and Finefrock, 2004).

This chapter outlines the functional diversity of metalloproteins and MCs, with an emphasis on their structural characteristics, regulatory mechanisms, disease associations, and emerging technological applications.

6.2 Metalloproteins—Biology and function

6.2.1 Definition and general characteristics

Proteins that have one or more metal ions as cofactors, which are necessary for their structure or operation, are known as metalloproteins. These metal ions, which include iron, zinc, copper, and manganese, are coordinated with prosthetic groups or amino acid residues inside the protein. Metal ion incorporation into protein structures enables a variety of chemical reactivities that are superior to those of solely organic molecules, facilitating processes such as oxygen transport, electron transfer, and substrate activation.

In the words of Holm et al., "The structural and functional diversity of metal sites in biology is vast, encompassing active sites for electron transfer, substrate binding and activation, and stabilization of protein structure". Depending on their functions, these proteins may have metal cores that are visible on the surface or deeply buried. Their functional specificity is influenced by the great variability of their metal coordination geometries.

6.2.2 Types of metalloproteins

Based on the metal ion and its particular function, metalloproteins can be divided into a number of groups. Hemoproteins, zinc finger proteins, and iron–sulfur proteins are some of the most researched classes (Fig. 6.1).

6.2.2.1 Hemoproteins

An iron ion arranged within a porphyrin ring is part of the heme group found in hemoproteins. Redox processes and oxygen transport are the main functions of these proteins. Two well-known hemoproteins that are involved in oxygen binding and storage are hemoglobin and myoglobin. Furthermore, hemoproteins

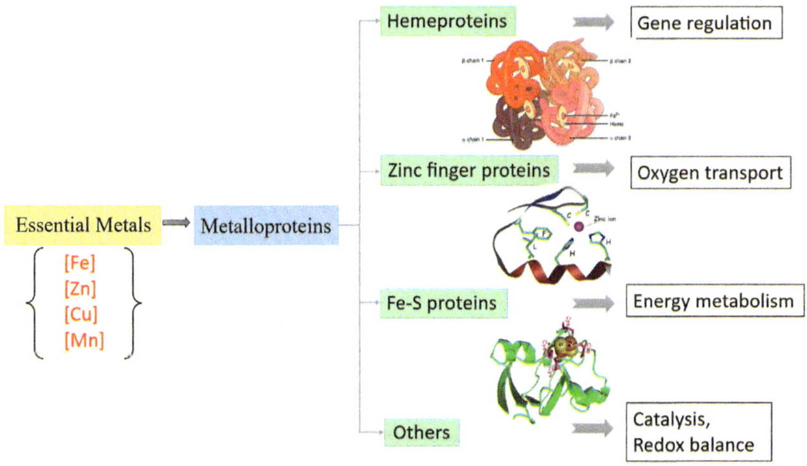

FIG. 6.1 Classes of metalloproteins and their biological roles.

called cytochromes play a role in the transport of electrons during cellular respiration. Zhang et al. point out that "heme-containing proteins are central to biological oxidation-reduction processes, particularly in respiratory and photosynthetic electron transport chains" (Zhang and Zheng, 2020).

6.2.2.2 *Zinc finger proteins*

Zinc finger proteins create stable folds that usually interact with DNA by coordinating one or more zinc ions with conserved cysteine and histidine residues. They are able to control transcription thanks to these structural motifs. Crucially, zinc preserves protein structure but does not take part in redox processes. According to Cassandri et al., "Zinc finger domains are essential modules for DNA recognition in transcription factors and stabilize protein structure" (Cassandri et al., 2017).

6.2.2.3 *Iron–sulfur proteins*

In iron–sulfur proteins, cysteine thiol groups control the arrangement of iron and sulfur atoms in clusters such as [2Fe-2S] or [4Fe-4S]. These proteins are involved in catalysis and electron transfer, particularly in nitrogen fixation and mitochondrial electron transport chains. Iron–sulfur clusters are versatile redox cofactors that mediate single or multiple electron transfers in biological systems (Solomon et al., 2014).

6.2.3 Role in enzymatic activity, transport, and redox reactions

Catalysis, electron transport, molecular stability, and oxygen metabolism all depend on metalloproteins.

6.2.3.1 *Electron transport*

During aerobic respiration, electron flow is facilitated by proteins such as iron–sulfur clusters and cytochromes. Adenosine triphosphate (ATP) production is made possible by the gradual acceptance and donation of electrons by these molecules. Electron-transfer metalloproteins are central components of respiration and photosynthesis (Holm et al., 1996).

6.2.3.2 *Catalysis*

Catalytic activity depends on metals like iron in cytochrome P450 and zinc in carbonic anhydrase. Iron in heme permits the oxidation of substrates, whereas zinc stabilizes hydroxide ions. "Metal ions can act as Lewis acids, redox partners, or stabilize transition states, depending on their chemical environment," according to Solomon et al.

6.2.3.3 *Oxygen transport*

Using their heme-iron centers, hemoglobin and myoglobin reversibly bind oxygen, which is essential for gas exchange and muscle metabolism. "The iron in hemoproteins allows reversible binding of molecular oxygen, essential for aerobic life," Zhang et al. observed.

6.2.3.4 *Structural stability*

Zinc ions are necessary for zinc finger domains to maintain their folded shape. Gene regulation, signal transduction, and protein-DNA interaction all depend on these structures. Cassandri et al. remarked, "Zinc is essential not for catalysis but to preserve the structural folding and integrity of finger-like domains".

6.2.4 Biomedical and industrial relevance

Metalloproteins are becoming more and more significant in industrial biocatalysis, drug development, and medical diagnostics. Neurodegenerative disorders target enzymes that help neutralize reactive oxygen species (ROS), such as superoxide dismutase (with copper/zinc). Engineered hemoproteins for biosensors and artificial catalysts are examples of biotechnological uses. Rational drug design and the creation of biomimetic materials are aided by an understanding of their mechanisms. According to Holm et al., "Design of metalloenzyme mimics with tailored activity has been made possible by insights into metal–protein interactions".

6.3 Metallochaperones—gatekeepers of metal trafficking

MCs, a unique class of proteins that facilitate the integration of metal ion cofactors into metalloenzymes and metalloproteins, are crucial for the correct operation of cells despite being much smaller than cells. MCs, also known as intracellular metal ion carriers, distribute metals within cells and ensure that a particular metalloenzyme acquires the right metal. MCs, a class of soluble metal receptor proteins, bind and shield metal ions and cofactors by aiding in the intracellular trafficking of metal ions to safeguard the cell. Numerous metalloenzymes, or proteins that bind metal ions and employ them as cofactors to carry out vital biological processes, including DNA synthesis and cellular respiration, are target sites for metal/cofactor delivery and antioxidant defense.

Up to one-third of all proteins in cells are metalloproteins, which aid in the proper insertion of metal ions into metalloenzymes. This sector is thought to be one of the fastest-growing. Free metal ions are bound by and moved between different transporters, MCs, and storage proteins in a generic model of intracellular transport, trafficking, and delivery of metal ions like Cu, Fe, and Zn, as published by published (Cammack and Hughes, 2007). The concentration of free, unbound metal ions is often very low, and they may also be held in intracellular organelles. To prevent excessive free metal species from damaging cells, transition metals must be handled carefully inside cells.

For all creatures to survive, transition metal ion equilibrium is, therefore, vital. Each metalloprotein must attach to the right metal ion at the right time, even if many of them have the ability to bind a variety of metals. Metal-specific MC proteins are able to accomplish this metal selectivity in eukaryotes.

6.3.1 Metallochaperones

A number of findings in the late 1990s indicated that the MC, an auxiliary protein, is necessary for the incorporation of the metal. Proteins called MCs carry metals, minerals, and cofactors through interstitial fluid, chaperone them to the appropriate enzymes, and shield them from scavengers. The idea behind metal chaperones is that certain proteins temporarily attach metallic cofactors to convey them to the enzymes where they work; as a result, metal chaperones serve both a transport and a protective purpose (Enggist et al., 2002). A review of the literature indicates that MCs are necessary for the correct operation of cells because they transport metal ions, including copper, iron, nickel, manganese, vanadium, cobalt, zinc, molybdenum, and arsenic, to particular locations within a cell.

Several metalloenzymes, or proteins that bind metal ions, are the target sites for metal delivery. MCs are different from chaperones in that the former help fold proteins, while the latter protect and transport metal ions (Bukau et al., 2000). Copper MCs target copper-transporting ATPases and the Wilson's and Menkes disease proteins in humans (Krupanidhi and Sanjeevi, 2008; Zatta and Frank, 2007).

In addition to preventing neurological conditions, including Alzheimer's disease (AD) and amyotrophic lateral sclerosis, as well as discomfort brought on by metal ion imbalance, MCs aid in restoring metal ion homeostasis (Burdette and Lippard, 2003).

The majority of what is currently known about metal chaperones and metal trafficking pathways has been discovered, and many human diseases have been connected to MCs' improper metal delivery. A potential connection between oxidative stress and metal homeostasis in AD was identified through a copper-binding site in the cytoplasmic domain of BACE1 (Dingwall, 2007).

For research targeted at creating novel and etiological therapeutics for protein-misfolding illnesses, including AD, MCs are a potential class of molecules (Kastenholz et al., 2009). Atx-like MCs are antioxidants with a copper-binding motif (Hung et al., 1998). Through the interaction of electrostatics, hydrogen bonds, and hydrophobic interactions, MCs and their physiological partner ATPases from various phylogenetic kingdoms are able to recognize one another in a way that accurately positions the metal-binding side chains for quick metal transfer between otherwise tightly binding sites (Arnesano et al., 2002).

6.3.2 Specificity of MCs

Every metal in the body has a specific function, and each MC is trained to deal with a particular kind of metal. This guarantees that every protein or enzyme gets the right metal for its job.

6.3.2.1 Copper MCs

Because copper is incorporated into so many proteins in all living things, including humans, it is considered vital. Within cells, copper is constantly linked to metalloproteins rather than existing in a free state. Certain MCs shield cells against the harmful effects of intracellular free copper by escorting copper to a variety of sites within the cell.

1. Through direct contact between the chaperone and the target protein's metal-binding site, CCS provides copper to superoxide dismutase (Bartnikas and Gitlin, 2001).
2. By docking with two P-type ATPases, Atox1 transports copper to the secretory route. Furthermore, Wilson disease is caused by mutations in ATP7B, whereas Menkes disease is caused by a nonfunctional protein called ATP7A. Copper metabolism MURR1 domain) and X-linked inhibitor of apoptosis protein, two more intracellular hepatic copper-binding proteins, might also be necessary for excretion. Amyloid precursor protein and metallothionein may be additional proteins involved in copper homeostasis (Prohaska, 2008).
3. COX17 provides copper to other mitochondrial chaperones so that cytochrome c oxidase can be synthesized.

Understanding disorders like variants of amyotrophic lateral sclerosis, which are linked to copper and oxidative stress, requires research on MCs. Scientists are one step closer to developing treatments and solutions for debilitating disorders involving copper imbalance when they understand the function of copper and the processes by which homeostasis is achieved (Bertini and Cavallaro, 2008).

6.3.2.2 Zinc MCs

Zinc is a transition metal that is only found in biological systems in the + 2-oxidation state. It is crucial for the function of proteins in all living cells. Excess Zn(II) is hazardous to cells, even though it is necessary for the structural and catalytic functions of many cellular proteins. Therefore, the potential toxicity of zinc ions must be weighed against their intracellular availability.

Zinc and chaperones are essential for healthy immunological function. As people age, their immune system, stress response, and zinc status all deteriorate. In the lymphocytes of elderly donors, short-term oral zinc supplementation safely and effectively triggers the stress response, which could be a potential mechanism linking zinc deficiency to aging and immunosenescence. Accordingly, adequate zinc intake in the diet has become known as an immune system antiaging mechanism and chaperone inducer (Putics et al., 2008).

1. Following a reaction with L-homocysteine, metallothionein, a common intracellular zinc-chaperone and superoxide anion radical scavenger, lost its function. This demonstrated that L-homocysteine specifically targeted intracellular metallothionein by forming a mixed-disulfide conjugate and that the loss of function followed homocysteinylation (Barbato et al., 2007).
2. Znt proteins (Znt1–Znt8) → Regulate zinc movement

6.3.2.3 Iron MCs

Iron, a crucial element in heme and iron-sulfur clusters, is necessary for almost all life forms. Iron-sulfur clusters and hemes are both used by proteins to carry out functions like ATP synthesis and O_2 delivery. It has been documented that Isa1p and Isa2p iron MCs are necessary for the transport of iron to cellular active sites (Jensen and Culotta, 2000).

1. Frataxins are tiny, vital proteins that are deficient in a variety of metabolic disorders, such as oxidative stress, iron-sulfur cluster deficiencies, and deficiencies in heme synthesis, energy metabolism, sulfur amino acid metabolism, stress response, and mitochondrial function. Understanding the pathophysiology of Friedreich ataxia requires an understanding of the function of frataxin in mitochondria.
2. Mammals' ability to retain iron in ferritin is crucial to their survival. Iron is delivered to ferritin by the cytosolic iron chaperone known as human poly (rC)-binding protein 1 (PCBP1). When expressed in yeast, PCBP1 enhanced the quantity of iron loaded into ferritin. In vitro, PCBP1-ferritin promoted iron loading into ferritin. In human cells, PCBP1 depletion enhanced cytosolic iron pools and prevented ferritin iron loading (Shi et al., 2008).

6.3.2.4 Manganese MCs

Almost every type of life accumulates and uses manganese, which is a vital trace element. In addition to being a poison, this vital metal is also a nutrient. A Parkinsonian-like condition called "manganism" can result from severe brain damage caused by manganese exposure in humans. Therefore, the uptake and transportation of this ion must be carefully regulated by cells.

Superoxide dismutase (SOD_2), which is found in manganese, is vital for many species to survive and plays a crucial role in protecting against mitochondrial oxidative stress. The inner membrane of the mitochondria contains the protein MTM_1. The Mtm1p protein, which is derived from the MTM_1 gene, is situated in close proximity to the matrix translocation site of SOD_2. This suggests that Mtm1p plays a role in the mitochondrial activation of SOD_2 by specifically facilitating the insertion of the necessary manganese cofactor, indicating that the manganese insertion by Mtm1p into the SOD_2 receptor occurs as the SOD_2 protein enters the mitochondrial matrix (Luk et al., 2003).

Mechanism of metal delivery to the target protein

For metal ions like copper (Cu), zinc (Zn), iron (Fe), and manganese (Mn) to be safely delivered to particular target proteins inside the cell, MCs are essential. This process prevents toxicity from unbound metal ions while ensuring that metals are used appropriately (Rae et al., 1999; Robinson and Winge, 2010).

Step-by-step mechanism

1. **Metal ion uptake**
   Membrane transporters allow metal ions to enter the cytoplasm. To avoid free circulation in the cytosol, which may result in oxidative damage, they are rapidly bound by certain MCs (Lutsenko et al., 2007).
2. **Binding by MC**
   Using coordinating amino acids like cysteine, histidine, or methionine residues, the MC binds the metal ion with remarkable selectivity (Finney and O'Halloran, 2003; Rae et al., 1999). For instance, cysteine motifs are used by the CCH Atox1 to bind Cu^+ ions.
3. **Shielding and transport**
   The chaperone transports the metal ion through the cytoplasm safely, while protecting it from causing harm to the cell. In addition, this prevents metal-induced protein misfolding and nonspecific interactions (Huffman and O'Halloran, 2001; Robinson and Winge, 2010).
4. **Protein–protein interaction**
   A regulated handoff is initiated when the MC binds selectively to the target protein, which is frequently in an apo-form. Structural recognition and binding domains ensure this specificity (Robinson and Winge, 2010).

5. **Metal transfer (ligand exchange)**
By means of a ligand exchange mechanism, the metal ion is moved from the chaperone to the target protein. Both the target and the chaperone frequently undergo conformational changes that facilitate this procedure (Finney and O'Halloran, 2003).
6. **Activation of target protein**
The protein becomes functionally active and capable of carrying out its function, such as signaling, electron transfer, or catalysis, once a metal is inserted (Lutsenko et al., 2007; Rae et al., 1999).
Example:
Atox1 → ATP7A/ATP7B → Ceruloplasmin
Atox1 transports copper ions to the Golgi's copper-transporting ATPases, which then incorporate Cu^{+} into enzymes such as ceruloplasmin (Lutsenko et al., 2007).

6.4 Protective roles of MCs in metal toxicity

MCs are found in both animals and plants, emerging as multifunctional proteins that play significant roles in plant growth, development, and responses to biotic and abiotic stresses (Zhao et al., 2022; Abreu-Neto et al., 2013). These proteins are essential in safeguarding cells against metal toxicity by facilitating the transport, sequestration, and detoxification of metals (Fig. 6.2). They function

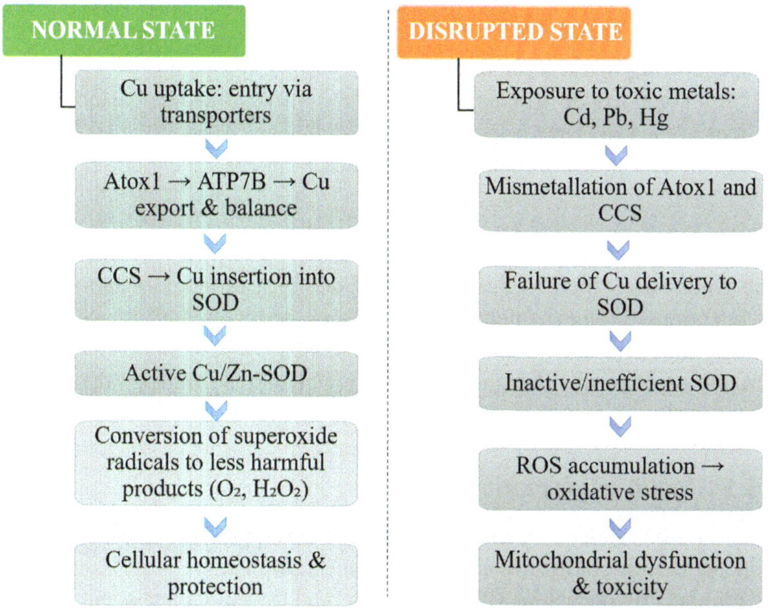

FIG. 6.2 Protective vs. disrupted metallochaperone pathways in copper trafficking.

as delivery proteins, ensuring that vital metals are directed to their appropriate targets while mitigating the detrimental effects of excess or improperly localized metals. This protective role is crucial for sustaining cellular homeostasis and averting damage from both essential and nonessential toxic metals (Bhattacharya, 2022). The different strategies to protect cells from metal toxicity include:

1. **Preventing uncontrolled reactions**
   Free metal ions possess high reactivity and can engage in undesirable chemical reactions, which may lead to the damage of cellular components such as proteins, DNA, and lipids. MCs effectively bind to these ions, thereby inhibiting their involvement in these detrimental reactions.
2. **Facilitating metal delivery**
   MCs transport metal ions to designated cellular locations, including metalloenzymes, which require them for optimal functioning. This precise delivery guarantees that metals are used effectively and avoids their buildup in other regions where they might lead to toxicity.
3. **Assisting in metal detoxification**
   Some MCs are involved in metal detoxification processes by transporting toxic metal ions to proteins or transporters that facilitate their elimination from the cell. For instance, the ArsD protein conveys arsenic to the ArsAB pump for excretion.
4. **Antioxidant properties**
   Some MCs, including metallothioneins (MTs), possess antioxidant properties that help neutralize harmful ROS generated by metal toxicity. This antioxidant role also protects cells from oxidative damage.
5. **Regulating metal homeostasis**
   MCs are essential for maintaining metal homeostasis—the balance of metal ions in the cell. They help prevent both deficiencies and toxicities by managing the transport and availability of metals.

6.5 Metal sequestration and detoxification

The processes of metal sequestration and detoxification are essential biological functions through which organisms, such as plants and microorganisms, handle and neutralize harmful heavy metals. These functions encompass intricate mechanisms designed to avert metal toxicity and maintain cellular homeostasis.

6.5.1 Metal sequestration

Sequestration refers to the process of binding or trapping metal ions, effectively reducing their mobility and bioavailability. **Examples:**

Plants: Phytochelatins (PCs) and MTs bind to heavy metals and are stored in vacuoles.

Microorganisms: Bacteria and fungi have the ability to bind metals to their cell walls or release chelating agents to eliminate them from the environment.

Mechanisms involve in metal sequestration:

1. **Cellular compartmentalization**
   Metals are transported to specific cellular compartments, like vacuoles in plants or intracellular vesicles in microorganisms, where they are stored and isolated from sensitive cellular components.
2. **Complexation with ligands**
   Metals can be bound to organic molecules (ligands) like PCs, MTs, or organic acids, forming stable complexes that reduce their toxicity.
3. **Extracellular sequestration**
   In some cases, metals can be bound to the cell wall or excreted outside the cell, reducing their uptake and impact.

6.5.2 Metal detoxification

Detoxification encompasses the processes that make toxic metals less harmful to living organisms. **Examples:**

- **Plants:** Plants have the ability to detoxify metals by binding them to compounds such as PCs, sequestering them in vacuoles, or converting them into less toxic forms.
- **Microorganisms:** Bacteria can detoxify metals through various mechanisms, including efflux pumps, metal reduction/oxidation, and the synthesis of siderophores.

Mechanisms:

- **Metal reduction:** Certain metals can be transformed into less toxic forms via reduction reactions (for instance, converting Cr(VI) to Cr(III)).
- **Metal oxidation:** In specific instances, metals may be oxidized to forms that are less toxic. Methylation/demethylation: Some metals can undergo methylation or demethylation, which modifies their toxicity and volatility.

Efflux pumps: Specialized proteins that are capable of actively transporting metals out of the cell, thereby preventing their accumulation.

Importance:

Heavy metal toxicity incites various toxicity symptoms, such as inhibition in biomass, germination potential, photosynthesis, alterations in physiological growth parameters, accumulation of excess ROS, and biochemical and metabolic attributes, ultimately culminating in oxidative stress conditions. It is necessary to develop appropriate strategies in order to reduce such potentially toxic metals/metalloids in plant-derived foods. Jasmonates are lesser-known, lipid-derived plant growth regulators that provide protection during heavy metal/metalloid stresses in different plants (Samanta and Roychoudhury, 2025). A study reported that the sequestration occurring at the plant cell wall serves as the primary detoxification mechanism in white birch subjected to acute and chronic metal stress, whereas PCs contribute to alleviating metal toxicity within the cells (Fernández-Fuego et al., 2017). Heavy metals seem to possess various mechanisms through which they exert toxicity, while plants, conversely, implement a range of defense responses to mitigate their effects. Upon exposure to high levels of heavy metals, plants demonstrate unique molecular and biochemical strategies for tolerance. These strategies are mainly focused on inhibiting the buildup of toxic metals within the cells through mechanisms such as apoplastic entrapment, chelation of metals by cytosolic ligands, and sequestration into vacuoles (Agarwal et al., 2025).

Biological techniques, especially those involving bacterial-mediated bioremediation, represent a cost-efficient, practical, and eco-friendly solution for addressing contaminated soil and groundwater, as well as industrial wastewater, effluents, and sludge. Numerous bacterial species, including *Bacillus* spp., serve as effective candidates for bioremediation due to their molecular mechanisms, which indicate the presence of resistance, transport, efflux, and detoxification systems that function in both high and low concentrations of heavy metals, thereby ensuring the maintenance and regulation of metal homeostasis at the cellular level (Alotaibi et al., 2021).

The processes of metal sequestration and detoxification are essential for preserving both cellular and environmental health. These mechanisms enable organisms to withstand elevated metal levels in their surroundings, mitigate metal-induced toxicity, and play a significant role in bioremediation initiatives by decreasing the bioavailability of harmful metals.

Essential trace metals such as zinc (Zn), copper (Cu), and iron (Fe) are crucial for the growth and development of plants (Awasthi et al., 2022). These micronutrients serve as structural and regulatory elements within plant cells, facilitating the functions of numerous enzymes and proteins (Weber et al., 2023). For instance, manganese (Mn) acts as a cofactor for superoxide dismutase and glutamine synthetase, in addition to being a vital component of the photosynthetic machinery (El-Beltagi et al., 2024). Nevertheless, an excess of these elements can be harmful to organisms. Alongside the essential metals, there exists another category of naturally occurring nonessential metals, such as lead (Pb), cadmium (Cd), and mercury (Hg), which are recognized for their nonbiological advantages or toxic effects on living organisms (Rono, 2021). An increase in both categories of metals within plants can interfere with various biological processes, including nutrient absorption, basal metabolism, and physiological responses. Some reactions triggered by toxic metals produce ROS, leading to auto-oxidative damage to lipids, nucleic acids, proteins, and other biomolecules (Fan et al., 2022; Zhao et al., 2022). The accumulation of these toxic metals in plants and crops poses significant risks to human health through the food chain (Sikdar et al., 2022). The negative impacts on human health have been extensively documented, indicating a variety of diseases linked to metal toxicity (Abubakar, 2024). Cadmium is a notably harmful metal whose accumulation can lead to dysfunctions in the skeletal system, liver, and kidneys, as well as provoke a potential carcinogenic immune response characterized by a decrease in white blood cell count (Bhargava, 2024). In addition, several other metals, including chromium (Cr), nickel (Ni), and arsenic (As), are also categorized as Group I carcinogens (Lee et al., 2021).

According to their structural components, MCs can be categorized into two subfamilies: heavy metal-associated plant proteins (HPPs) and heavy metal-associated isoprenylated plant proteins (HIPPs) (Barr et al., 2023). HIPPs have been demonstrated to directly bind metals and engage with other proteins that possess comparable biological functions (Feng et al., 2023). Some types of HIPPs play a role in the allocation of plant mineral nutrients. Arabidopsis CCH is a MC found to mobilize Cu from senescing organs to reproductive tissues, indicating that CCH can redistribute minerals in plants. As industrial and agricultural activities progress, the levels of toxic heavy metals like Cd and Cu in agricultural land and surrounding environments are anticipated to increase steadily. Various methods have been implemented to remediate environments contaminated with heavy metals, including chemical treatment, phytostabilization, sedimentation, excavation and disposal, ion exchange, and filtration (Komárek, 2024).

MCs represent a category of valuable genetic resources that exhibit significant diversity in their biological functions, facilitating plant growth, development, and responses to environmental stress. As of now, many members of the HIPP/HPP family have been discovered in key plant species or crops; however, only a limited number have undergone functional characterization. The extent to which they contribute to metal absorption, allocation, homeostasis, or detoxification in plants remains largely unclear. Furthermore, the recent advancements in research regarding the essential functions of metal-binding proteins in modulating plant responses to various biological processes, including plant growth, development, pathogen stress, and abiotic stresses such as salinity, drought, cold, and light, have already been reviewed.

6.6 Role of MCs in specific stress responses

- **Oxidative stress**
  MCs play a crucial role in safeguarding against oxidative stress by facilitating the optimal functioning of antioxidant enzymes and inhibiting the formation of ROS. For instance, they are instrumental in the maturation of hydrogenases, enzymes that assist in maintaining cellular redox balance.
- **Heavy metal stress**
  In plants, MCs assist in managing heavy metal toxicity by transporting metals to detoxification pathways or facilitating their storage in vacuoles.
- **Bacterial infections**
  In cases of bacterial infections, MCs play a crucial role in the "tug-of-war" between the host and the pathogen for metal ions, assisting bacteria in adapting to the host's environment, which is limited in metal availability.

TABLE 6.1 Metallochaperones and associated detoxification strategies across biological systems in bacteria, plants, and animals.

System/ organism	Representative metallochaperones	Primary functions/detoxification strategies
Bacteria	CopZ, HypA–HypB, ArsD	Copper delivery and homeostasis (CopZ); insertion of Ni into hydrogenases (HypA/HypB); arsenic detoxification (ArsD)
Plants	Mettalothioneies (MTs)	Chelation of toxic metals and sequestration in vacuoles
Humans/ animals	Atox1, CCS, ATP7A, ATP7B, Cu/Zn-SOD, Metallothioneins (MTs)	Copper binding and delivery, transport via ATP7A/ATP7B, metallothionein-mediated sequestration, and SOD activation for oxidative stress defense

- **Stress-activated chaperones**
  Certain MCs are elevated in response to stress conditions, serving as an initial line of defense by rapidly transporting proteins to their active sites, thereby enabling cells to adjust to stress (Table 6.1).

  Examples of MCs:

- **CopZ:** A bacterial MC that plays a role in copper homeostasis and its delivery
- **HypA and HypB:** A complex of bacterial MC and GTPase that is involved in the insertion of nickel into hydrogenases
- **ArsD:** A MC that participates in the detoxification of arsenic in bacteria
- **ATP7A and ATP7B:** Human ATPases that transport copper and exhibit functions similar to MCs

6.7 MCs and different metal toxicity

MCs serve an essential protective function against metal toxicity by facilitating the appropriate distribution and detoxification of both essential and nonessential metals within cellular environments. They function as molecular carriers, guaranteeing that metal ions are transported to the correct metalloenzymes while averting their harmful accumulation or misplacement. This is especially critical for toxic metals such as copper, cadmium, and mercury, as MCs assist in alleviating their adverse impacts.

Copper (Cu): Copper is a vital metal; however, an excess of copper can lead to toxicity. MCs, such as Atox1, play a crucial role in regulating the transport and delivery of copper to enzymes that are essential for cellular respiration and various other processes. In instances of copper toxicity, MCs can mitigate oxidative damage by ensuring that copper is correctly incorporated into proteins rather than remaining free within the cell. **Example:** Atox1 and Copper Homeostasis: Atox1, a MC, plays a vital role in the transport of copper to the ATP7A and ATP7B copper-transporting ATPases. These ATPases are responsible for the export of copper and its delivery to cuproenzymes. Atox1 guarantees the proper delivery of copper to these proteins, thereby preventing its accumulation in the cytoplasm and reducing its potential toxicity.

Cadmium (Cd): Cadmium is a nonessential metal that is extremely toxic. MTs, a category of MCs, are recognized for their ability to bind cadmium ions, thereby diminishing their toxicity. MTs can sequester cadmium, preventing it from engaging with other cellular components and causing harm. Research indicates that organisms with elevated levels of MTs demonstrate increased resistance to cadmium toxicity. **Example:** MTs and Cadmium Detoxification: MTs represent a group of proteins that bind heavy metals, such as cadmium, via cysteine residues. This binding action diminishes the concentration of free cadmium within the cell, thereby preventing its interaction with other proteins and subsequent damage.

Mercury (Hg): Mercury, in its various forms, is also highly toxic. Although specific MCs for mercury are still under investigation, it is believed that proteins such as MTs and others involved in sulfur metabolism contribute to mercury detoxification. These proteins can bind to mercury, potentially averting its interference with enzyme activity or the induction of oxidative stress.

Example: Glutathione and mercury detoxification: Glutathione, a tripeptide, has the ability to bind mercury, resulting in the formation of a glutathione-mercury complex that can either be transported out of the cell or detoxified by various enzymes. This mechanism aids in alleviating the cellular burden of mercury and lessening its toxic effects.

In summary, MCs are crucial for sustaining cellular health by facilitating the correct delivery and use of metal ions, which are vital for a variety of cellular functions and for providing protection against different stress conditions.

6.8 Emerging trends and application

6.8.1 Drug discovery of metalloproteins and chaperones

Metalloproteins, which are proteins that bind metal ions, are being increasingly acknowledged as vital targets in the field of drug discovery and possess considerable therapeutic significance. Their participation in a range of biological processes, such as enzyme catalysis, electron transfer, maintaining structural stability, and the regulation and signaling processes of cells, frequently necessitates specific metal cofactors such as Cu, Fe, Zn, Mn, Ni, and Co, rendering them appealing candidates for therapeutic intervention. The inhibition or modulation of metalloprotein activity has demonstrated potential in the treatment of diseases such as cancer, hypertension, and infections, as well as in processes such as respiration, oxidative stress, photosynthesis, and drug metabolism, making them appealing targets for the development of novel therapies.

Metalloproteins represent promising targets for pharmaceutical development due to their role in a variety of diseases. Inhibiting metalloproteins can interfere with pathways associated with diseases. For instance, targeting metalloproteinases in cancer and creating drugs that disrupt metal-dependent enzymes involved in infections are notable examples. The design and engineering of metalloproteins can result in innovative biocatalysts and biosensors. Examples of a few enzymes include:

A complex enzyme, nitrogenase, is critical for nitrogen fixation in specific bacteria and plants and is heavily dependent on metalloproteins. Another enzyme, carbonic anhydrase, facilitates the hydration of carbon dioxide, playing a vital role in numerous biological processes. The enzyme superoxide dismutase acts as a safeguard for cells against oxidative damage, employing metal ions to catalyze the dismutation of superoxide radicals. Grasping the structure, function, and interactions of metalloproteins is essential for the advancement of new therapies and biotechnological innovations.

Numerous metalloproteins have been established as validated drug targets, while others are under investigation for their therapeutic capabilities. A variety of drugs currently utilized in clinical settings target metalloproteins, including Captopril (an angiotensin-converting enzyme (ACE) inhibitor used for hypertension), Vorinostat (an histone deacetylase (HDAC) inhibitor for cancer treatment), and Raltegravir (an integrase inhibitor for Human Immunodeficiency Virus (HIV)). The metal ions present in metalloproteins, along with the adjacent amino acids, can be targeted by pharmaceuticals to influence their functionality. Fragment-based lead discovery involves screening fragment libraries against metalloproteins, which are proteins that contain a metal ion as a structural or functional component. This approach is particularly useful for targeting metalloenzymes, where the metal ion plays a crucial role in the enzyme's activity.

6.8.2 Therapeutic implications of metalloproteins and chaperones

Metalloenzymes play a vital role in various biological processes, making them key players in the progression of many diseases. This importance positions metalloenzymes as attractive targets for therapeutic development. As awareness of their role in disease increases, there is a growing interest in devising new strategies to develop inhibitors and, ultimately, effective medications (Chen et al., 2018). Metalloproteins make up more than a third of the human proteome and display considerable diversity in their physiological functions and pathological effects, which are influenced by the specific metal or metals involved and the tissue environment. Their functions include catalysis, bioenergetics, redox reactions, DNA repair, cell growth, signaling, transport of vital elements, and immune responses (Ibrahim, 2024).

Metal ions in metalloproteins serve two primary functions: structural and functional. Structural metal ions are crucial for the proper folding of proteins, with zinc finger proteins being a prime example. In these proteins, the Zn^{2+} ion aids in transforming an unstructured polypeptide into a correctly folded domain that can bind to nucleic acids or other proteins. In addition, structural metal ions can regulate protein assembly. Functional metal ions, found at the active sites of metalloenzymes, are involved in various processes such as electron transfer, substrate recognition, and catalysis, contributing to a wide array of biological functions. For example, metalloproteins that utilize well-known Cu centers, Fe–S clusters, or Fe-heme (like cytochrome) cofactors illustrate the role of metal ions in electron transfer (Solomon et al., 2014). In some cases, these redox centers may also act as catalytic sites (Fig. 6.3).

When a functional metal ion aids in catalysis, the metalloprotein is identified as a metalloenzyme. The extensive roles of metalloenzymes in biological systems also link them to the development of various diseases, which can result from overexpression, heightened activation, or mis-regulation of an endogenous metalloenzyme (Fig. 6.4).

Abnormal interactions between copper or iron in the brain and metal-binding proteins (such as amyloid-β peptide or neuromelanin), which result in oxidative stress, have been identified as significant potential mechanisms in brain aging and neurodegenerative diseases. While a controlled study of deferoxamine in AD yielded some encouraging results, concerns regarding toxicity and brain delivery have restricted the trials of conventional chelators. The therapeutic importance of metal dysregulation in neurodegenerative diseases has proven challenging to evaluate (Doraiswamy and Finefrock, 2004).

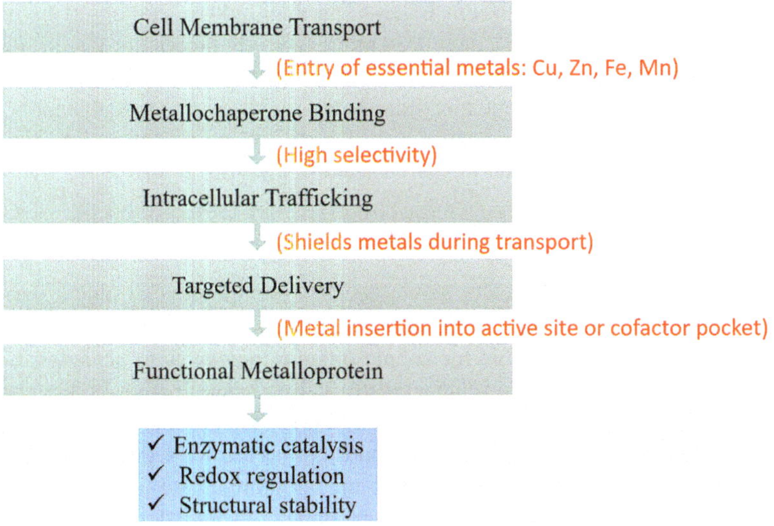

FIG. 6.3 Schematic representing the delivery pathway of metallochaperones.

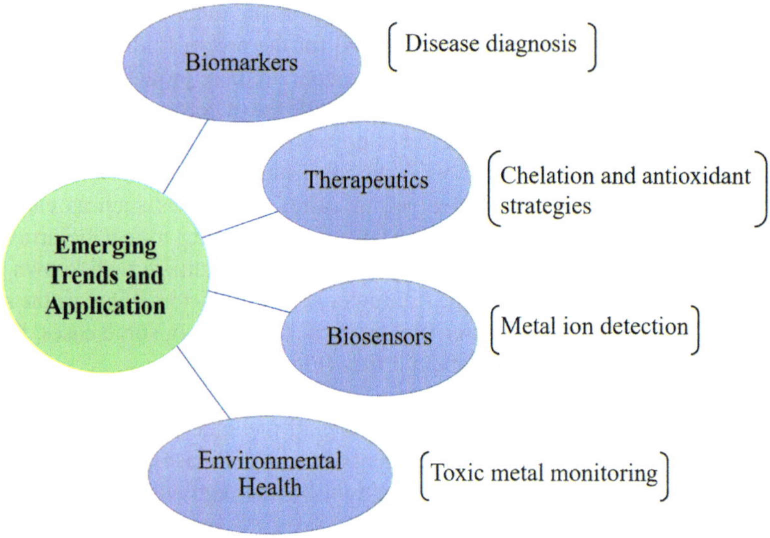

FIG. 6.4 Major application domains of metallochaperones and metalloproteins.

Studies on the human metalloproteome have shown that many families of metalloproteins, as well as individual metalloproteins, are often dysregulated in various clinical conditions. In addition, different types of interactions between redox-active and redox-inert metalloproteins have been identified in both healthy and diseased states. Profiling metalloproteins has revealed specific alterations linked to neurodegenerative diseases, cancer, inflammation, infections, diabetes, and other health issues. This highlights metalloproteins both individually and as groups, thus presenting them as promising targets for a variety of therapeutic approaches. Inhibitors and activators of metalloenzymes, metal chelators, and synthetic metalloproteins could serve as valuable tools for diagnosing and treating numerous diseases, as well as having potential applications in other biomedical and industrial sectors (Ibrahim, 2024).

6.9 Conclusion

A diverse class of biological macromolecules, metalloproteins play a part in catalysis, structural control, and redox processes. They carry out necessary functions that are impossible for simple organic molecules to accomplish by taking advantage of metal ion characteristics. From hemoglobin's oxygen transport to zinc fingers regulating transcription, these proteins are indispensable for cellular function. Their importance in industry and medicine keeps growing as our knowledge of them expands. Novel metalloproteins are being discovered thanks to bioinformatics and other analytical methods, broadening their potential uses in green chemistry, medicine, and diagnostics.

References

Abreu-Neto, B.J., Turchetto-Zolet, A.C., Oliveira, L.F., Zanettini, M.H.B., Margis-Pinheiro, M., 2013. Heavy metal-associated isoprenylated plant protein (HIPP): characterization of a family of proteins exclusive to plants. FEBS J. 280, 1604–1616.

Abubakar, U.S., 2024. Copper and lead as environmental pollutant and their elemental toxicity – a review. Sci. World J. 1597-6343. 19 (2), 342–346. doi:10.4314/swj.v19i2.8.

Agarwal, H., Chaudhary, D., Aggarwal, H., Karala, C., Purkait, N., Sharma, N., Mishra, A., Mishra, V., Kumar, A., Singh, P., Dufossé, L., Joshi, N., 2025. Molecular underpinning of heavy metal sequestration through advanced remediation strategies in higher plants. Plant Stress. 2667064X. 16, 100881. doi:10.1016/j.stress.2025.100881.

Alotaibi, B.S., Khan, M., Shamim, S., 2021. Unraveling the underlying heavy metal detoxification mechanisms of Bacillus species. Microorganisms 9 (8), 1628.

Arnesano, F., Banci, L., Bertini, I., Ciofi-Baffoni, S., Molteni, E., Huffman, D.L., O'Halloran, T.V., 2002. Metallochaperones and metal-transporting atpases: a comparative analysis of sequences and structures. Genome Res. 1088-9051. 12 (2), 255–271. doi:10.1101/gr.196802.

Awasthi, S., Chauhan, R., Srivastava, S., 2022. The importance of beneficial and essential trace and ultratrace elements in plant nutrition, growth, and stress tolerance. In: Plant Nutrition and Food Security in the Era of Climate Change. Academic Press. pp. 27–46.

Barbato, J.C., Catanescu, O., Murray, K., DiBello, P.M., Jacobsen, D.W., 2007. Targeting of metallothionein by L-homocysteine. A novel mechanism for disruption of zinc and redox homeostasis. Arterioscler. Thromb. Vasc. Biol. 27, 49.

Barr, Z.K., Werner, T., Tilsner, J., 2023. Heavy metal-associated isoprenylated plant proteins (HIPPs) at plasmodesmata: exploring the link between localization and function. Plants 12 (16), 3015.

Bartnikas, T.B., Gitlin, J.D., 2001. How to make a metalloprotein. Nat. Struct. Biol. 8 (9), 733–734. doi:10.1038/nsb0901-733.

Bertini, I., Cavallaro, G., 2008. Metals in the "omics" world: copper homeostasis and cytochrome c oxidase assembly in a new light. J. Biol. Inorg. Chem. 09498257. 13 (1), 3–14. doi:10.1007/s00775-007-0316-9.

Bhargava, M., 2024. Evolution of Haematology in India: A Haematologist's Perspective, Cambridge Scholars Publishing.

Bhattacharya, S., 2022. Protective role of the essential trace elements in the obviation of cadmium toxicity: glimpses of mechanisms. Biol. Trace Elem. Res. 0163-4984. 200 (5), 2239–2246. doi:10.1007/s12011-021-02827-7.

Bukau, B., Deuerling, E., Pfund, C., Craig, E.A., 2000. Getting newly synthesized proteins into shape. Cell 00928674. 101 (2), 119–122. Available from: https://www.sciencedirect.com/journal/cell. doi:10.1016/S0092-8674(00)80806-5.

Burdette, S.C., Lippard, S.J., 2003. Meeting of the minds: metalloneurochemistry. Proc. Natl. Acad. Sci. U. S. A. 100 (7), 3605–3610. doi:10.1073/pnas.0637711100.

Cammack, R., Hughes, M.N., 2007. Considerations for the specification of enzyme assays involving metal ions. Proceedings of the Beilstein-Institut Workshop, September 23rd – 26th, 93–107.

Cassandri, M., Smirnov, A., Novelli, F., Pitolli, C., Agostini, M., Malewicz, M., Melino, G., Raschellà, G., 2017. Zinc-finger proteins in health and disease. Cell Death Discov. 2058-7716. 3 (1). doi:10.1038/cddiscovery.2017.71.

Chen, Z., Yoo, S.H., Takahashi, J.S., 2018. Development and therapeutic potential of small-molecule modulators of circadian systems. Annu. Rev. Pharmacol. Toxicol. 58, 231–252.

Dingwall, C., 2007. A copper-binding site in the cytoplasmic domain of BACE1 identifies a possible link to metal homoeostasis and oxidative stress in Alzheimer's disease. Biochem. Soc. Trans. 0300-5127. 35 (3), 571–573. doi:10.1042/bst0350571.

Doraiswamy, P.M., Finefrock, A.E., 2004. Metals in our minds: therapeutic implications for neurodegenerative disorders. Lancet Neurol. 14744422. 3 (7), 431–434. Available from: http://www.journals.elsevier.com/the-lancet-neurology/. doi:10.1016/S1474-4422(04)00809-9.

El-Beltagi, H.S., El-Nady, M.F., Al-Daej, M.I., El-Naqma, K.A., Rezk, A.A., El-Afry, M.M., Shehata, W.F., Ismail, A.M., Eltonoby, W.F., Metwaly, M.M.S., 2024. Exogenous application of manganese and arginine alleviates the adverse effects of salinity stress on pea (Pisum sativum L.). Cogent Food Agric. 23311932. 10 (1). Available from: https://www.tandfonline.com/action/journalInformation?journalCode=oafa20. doi:10.1080/23311932.2024.2389445.

Enggist, E., Thöny-Meyer, L., Güntert, P., Pervushin, K., 2002. NMR structure of the heme chaperone CcmE reveals a novel functional motif. Structure. 09692126. 10 (11), 1551–1557. doi:10.1016/s0969-2126(02)00885-7.

Fan, Y., Chen, X., Chen, Z., Zhou, X., Xin, L., Liu, J., 2022. Pollution characteristics and source analysis of heavy metals in surface sediments of Luoyuan Bay, Fujian. Environ. Res. 00139351. 203, 111911. doi:10.1016/j.envres.2021.111911.

Feng, Y., Jin, C., Shihao, L., Zhang, H., Ren, F., Wang, J., 2023. Molecular mechanisms and applications of polyphenol-protein complexes with antioxidant properties: a review. Antioxidants. 2076-3921. 12 (8), 1577. doi:10.3390/antiox12081577.

Fernández-Fuego, D., Bertrand, A., González, A., 2017. Metal accumulation and detoxification mechanisms in mycorrhizal Betula pubescens. Environ. Pollut. 231 (1), 1153–1162.

Finney, L.A., O'Halloran, T.V., 2003. Transition metal speciation in the cell: insights from the chemistry of metal ion receptors. Science 300 (5621), 931–936. doi:10.1126/science.1085049.

Holm, R.H., Kennepohl, P., Solomon, E.I., 1996. Structural and functional aspects of metal sites in biology. Chem. Rev. 96 (7), 2239–2314. doi:10.1021/cr9500390.

Huffman, D.L., O'Halloran, T.V., 2001. Function, structure, and mechanism of intracellular copper trafficking proteins. Annu. Rev. Biochem. 00664154. 70, 677–701. doi:10.1146/annurev.biochem.70.1.677.

Hung, I.H., Casareno, R.L.B., Labesse, G., Mathews, F.S., Gitlin, J.D., 1998. HAH1 is a copper-binding protein with distinct amino acid residues mediating copper homeostasis and antioxidant defense. J. Biol. Chem. 00219258. 273 (3), 1749–1754. doi:10.1074/jbc.273.3.1749.

Ibrahim, I.H., 2024. Metalloproteins and metalloproteomics in health and disease. Adv. Protein Chem. Struct. Biol. 141, 123–176. Available from: https://www.sciencedirect.com/science/bookseries/18761623. doi:10.1016/bs.apcsb.2023.12.013.

Jensen, L.T., Culotta, V.C., 2000. The delivery of iron to active sites in the cell require Isa1p and Isa2p iron metallochaperones. In Role of Saccharomyces Cerevisiae ISA1 and ISA2 in iron homeostasis. Mol. Cell Biol. 20, 3918–3927.

Kastenholz, B., Garfin, D.E., Horst, J., Nagel, K.A., 2009. Plant metal chaperones: a novel perspective in dementia therapy. Amyloid 16, 81–83.

Komárek, M. (2024). The use of sulfidated nano zero-valent iron for stabilization of soil contaminants-implication on plants [(Doctoral dissertation]. Czech University of Life Sciences, Prague.

Krupanidhi, A.S., Sanjeevi, C.B., 2008. Copper and biological health. Indian J. Med. Res. 128, 448–461.

Lee, K.H., Lee, S., Park, J.H., Lee, S.S., Kim, H.Y., Lee, W.J., Cha, E.S., Kim, K.P., Lee, W., Lee, J.Y., Lee, K.H., 2021. Risk of hematologic malignant neoplasms from abdominopelvic computed tomographic radiation in patients who underwent appendectomy. JAMA Surg. 21686262. 156 (4), 343–351. Available from: http://archsurg.jamanetwork.com/issues.aspx. doi:10.1001/jamasurg.2020.6357.

Luk, E., Carroll, M., Baker, M., Culotta, V.C., 2003. Manganese activation of superoxide dismutase 2 in Saccharomyces cerevisiae requires MTM1, a member of the mitochondrial carrier family. Proc. Natl. Acad. Sci. U. S. A. 100 (18), 10353–10357. doi:10.1073/pnas.1632471100.

Lutsenko, S., Barnes, N.L., Bartee, M.Y., Dmitriev, O.Y., 2007. Function and regulation of human copper-transporting ATPases. Physiol. Rev. 15221210. 87 (3), 1011–1046. Available from: http://physrev.physiology.org/cgi/reprint/87/3/1011. doi:10.1152/physrev.00004.2006.

Prohaska, J.R., 2008. Role of copper transporters in copper homeostasis. Am. J. Clin. Nutr. 00029165. 88 (3), 826S. doi:10.1093/ajcn/88.3.826s.

Putics, A., Vödrös, D., Malavolta, M., Mocchegiani, E., Csermely, P., Soti, C., 2008. Zinc supplementation boosts the stress response in the elderly: hsp70 status is linked to zinc availability in peripheral lymphocytes. Exp. Gerontol. 05315565. 43 (5), 452–461. doi:10.1016/j.exger.2008.01.002.

Rae, T.D., Schmidt, P.J., Pufahl, R.A., Culotta, V.C., O'Halloran, T.V., 1999. Undetectable intracellular free copper: the requirement of a copper chaperone for superoxide dismutase. Science. 0036-8075. 284 (5415), 805–808. doi:10.1126/science.284.5415.805.

Robinson, N.J., Winge, D.R., 2010. Copper metallochaperones. Annu. Rev. Biochem. 00664154. 79, 537–562. doi:10.1146/annurev-biochem-030409-143539.

Rono, D.K., 2021. Health and Environmental Risks of Using Wastewater in Vegetable Production in Urban and Peri-Urban Areas of Nairobi City, Kenya (Doctoral thesis). Masinde Muliro University of Science and Technology.

Samanta, S., Roychoudhury, A., 2025. Unravelling the Protective Role of Jasmonates during Heavy Metal Stress Biotechnological Applications of Jasmonates: A Group of Less Well-Known Plant Growth Regulators. Apple Academic Press, India, 141–167. Available from: https://www.appleacademicpress.com/biotechnological-applications-of-jasmonates-a-group-of-less-well-known-plant-growth-regulators/9781774919569.

Shi, H., Bencze, K.Z., Stemmler, T.L., Philpott, C.C., 2008. A cytosolic iron chaperone that delivers iron to ferritin. Science. 10959203. 320 (5880), 1207–1210. doi:10.1126/science.1157643.

Sikdar, A., Jeyasundar, P.G.S.A., Debnath, B., Hossain, M.S., Islam, M.A., Ahammed, G.J., 2022. Cadmium Contamination in the Soil Environment: Impact on Plant Growth and Human Health Agrochemicals in Soil and Environment: Impacts and Remediation. Springer Nature, Bangladesh, pp. 367–408. Available from: https://doi.org/10.1007/978-981-16-9310-6. doi:10.1007/978-981-16-9310-6_16.

Solomon, E.I., Heppner, D.E., Johnston, E.M., Ginsbach, J.W., Cirera, J., Qayyum, M., Kieber-Emmons, M.T., Kjaergaard, C.H., Hadt, R.G., Tian, L., 2014. Copper active sites in biology. Chem. Rev. 15206890. 114 (7), 3659–3853. Available from: http://pubs.acs.org/journal/chreay. doi:10.1021/cr400327t.

Weber, J.N., Minner-Meinen, R., Behnecke, M., Biedendieck, R., Hänsch, V.G., Hercher, T.W., Hertweck, C., van den Hout, L., Knüppel, L., Sivov, S., Schulze, J., Mendel, R.R., Hänsch, R., Kaufholdt, D., 2023. Moonlighting Arabidopsis molybdate transporter 2 family and GSH-complex formation facilitate molybdenum homeostasis. Commun. Biol. 23993642. 6 (1). Available from: https://www.springer.com/journal/42003. doi:10.1038/s42003-023-05161-x.

Zatta, P., Frank, A., 2007. Copper deficiency and neurological disorders in man and animals. Brain Res. Rev. 01650173. 54 (1), 19–33. doi:10.1016/j.brainresrev.2006.10.001.

Zhang, Y., Zheng, J., 2020. Bioinformatics of metalloproteins and metalloproteomes. Molecules. 1420-3049. 25 (15), 3366. doi:10.3390/molecules25153366.

Zhao, Y.N., Wang, M.Q., Li, C., Cao, H.W., Rono, J.K., Yang, Z.M., 2022. The metallochaperone OsHIPP56 gene is required for cadmium detoxification in rice crops. Environ. Exp. Bot. 00988472. 193. Available from: https://www.elsevier.com/inca/publications/store/2/6/7. doi:10.1016/j.envexpbot.2021.104680.

Chapter 7

Transgenerational effects of metal toxicity in aquatic and terrestrial organisms

Vandana Singh[a], Ankush Verma[b], Amit Pratap Singh Chouhan[b], Pradeep Kumar[c], and Ajay Kumar[c]

[a]*Department of Microbiology, Sharda School of Allied Health Sciences, Sharda University, Greater Noida, Uttar Pradesh, India*

[b]*Department of Radiology, School of Allied Health Sciences, Galgotias University, Greater Noida, Uttar Pradesh, India*

[c]*MRIT, Santosh Medical College, Uttar Pradesh, India*

7.1 Introduction

Environmental metal pollution has been accelerating dramatically since the Industrial Revolution, and anthropogenic inputs vastly exceed natural geochemical contributions for most toxic metals by several orders of magnitude. Global production and use of metals have multiplied exponentially to meet the demands of industrialization, urbanization, technological progress, and agricultural intensification. An estimated 20 million tons of toxic metals are released into the environment each year, posing a serious threat to ecosystems and human health. These metals originate from a range of activities such as mining and smelting, the use of fossil fuels, metal fabrication and processing, the application of metallic pesticides and fertilizers in agriculture, and the dumping of electronic waste materials, among other types of industrial activities. In contrast to organic constituents that can biodegrade through microbial or chemical decay, metals are elements that cannot be destroyed in any way, nor can they be permanently removed from the environment. Instead, they remain indefinitely cycling among various environmental compartments and chemical states, preserving their intrinsic toxicological significance (Anastasiadi and Piferrer, 2023). This legacy has resulted in background levels of these metals in soil, water, air, and biota that have never been higher in many parts of the world due to widespread anthropogenic inputs, accompanied by the persistent reuse and re-release of some metals into the global environment.

The Metallome in Motion. https://doi.org/10.1016/B978-0-443-44299-5.00004-3

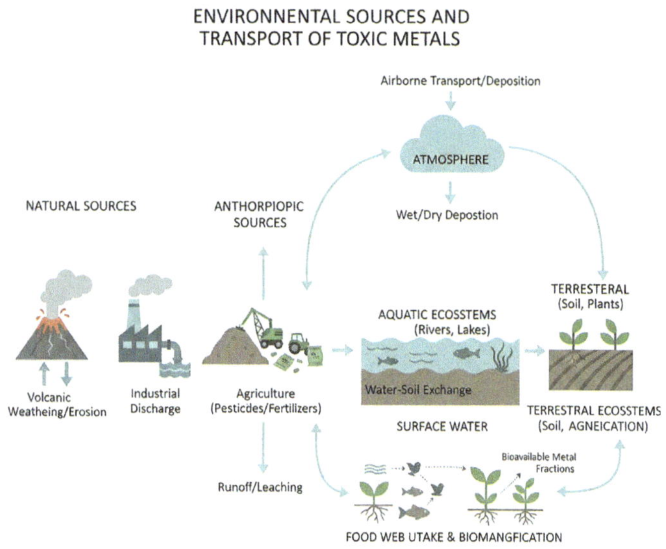

FIG. 7.1 Environmental sources, transport, and bioavailability of toxic metals.

In addition, metals have the ability to be transported over long distances through atmospheric deposition, water, and biotic vectors, given their environmental persistence (Fig. 7.1). Industrial sources tend to release atmospheric emissions over thousands of kilometers, so that deposited contaminants may be found in remote ecosystems far beyond the initial dispersal areas. Waterborne metal pollution may also be transported along river systems, groundwater aquifers, and ocean currents, influencing aquatic ecosystems at the basin to global scales (Bollati and Baccarelli, 2022). This ubiquitous metal pollution has implications for the ecological health of our planet because there are few terrestrial and aquatic ecosystems in which metal exposure is truly absent. Yet, under such conditions, they do not appear to exert a major impact on biodiversity. The "metal time bomb" effect, which refers to continuous deposition and accumulation at a rate greater than rates of natural elimination, has occurred in many ecosystems that are approaching or even exceeding their ability to assimilate these poisonous contaminants (Burggren, 2020). This widespread and long-term global distribution of metal pollution further provides the rationale for examining not only the direct toxicities of exposed organisms but also potential transgenerational consequences and has recently been raised as an important issue in environmental toxicology and risk assessment.

7.1.1 Concept of transgenerational toxicology

Transgenerational toxicology marks a paradigm shift in the way researchers think about the relationship between environmental exposures and human health, moving from a historical focus on direct exposure to including effects that are observed in future generations. A basic principle of transgenerational toxicology is that environmental exposures occurring in parental or ancestral generations can promote biological alterations transmitted to their offspring and beyond, including multiple unexposed generations (Eirin-Lopez and Putnam, 2019). This idea explicitly contradicts the classical view of toxicology, which has traditionally focused on direct exposure-dose relationships and immediate or delayed effects occurring within an exposed individual's lifespan. The expanding realm of transgenerational toxicology is based on the concept that environmental stressors, such as metals, can induce molecular "memories" in exposed organisms that persist beyond exposure and affect the phenotype, physiology, and fitness of their progeny. It is important to note that transgenerational effects are distinct from those of multigenerational effects, which involve ongoing exposures across generations. The transgenerational nature of toxicity has been a growing area of research over the last 20 years, with epigenetic alterations identified as the predominant mechanism by which environmental exposures can be passed between generations.

Epigenetics refers to heritable changes in gene expression through mechanisms that do not involve changes to the underlying DNA sequence, including DNA methylation, histone modifications, and noncoding RNAs (ncRNAs). These epigenetic marks can be induced by environmental cues, such as metal exposure, and maintained through cell divisions, in some cases even across generations. The capacity of metals to cause transgenerational effects has significant implications for understanding how environmental pollutants may impact population dynamics, evolutionary processes, and ecosystem health on scales much longer than the duration of pollution events. The transgenerational perspective also necessitates a re-evaluation of environmental risk assessment guidelines, which have traditionally focused on direct toxicity to the exposed individual rather than considering the potential for effects to cascade across generations.

7.1.2 Significance in environmental and ecological risk assessment

Acknowledgment of transgenerational effects in toxicity studies would have tremendous implications for environmental and ecological risk assessments, which generally rely on short-term tests to assess acute or chronic impacts on directly exposed organisms. Indeed, classical toxicity testing guidelines [e.g., Organization for Economic Co-operation and Development (OECD) and worldwide regulatory agencies] are usually conducted over durations ranging from hours to a few weeks and most often remain within the boundary of a single generation, while sometimes extending to two generations (Fallet et al., 2020). These tests yield important information on direct toxicity and are used to derive regulatory threshold values such as No Observed Effect Concentrations (NOECs) and Lowest Observed Effect Concentrations (LOECs) for use in water quality criteria, soil quality guidelines, and other standards. Nevertheless, these approaches may fail to detect or forecast impacts as generations born after metal exposure ends respond, possibly underestimating the long-term ecological costs of metal pollution. If metals are able to induce transgenerational effects at lower concentrations than those that would elicit acute or chronic toxicity in directly exposed individuals, current risk assessment methods might fail to protect ecosystem functioning and services (Heindel and Vandenberg, 2022).

The ecosystemic relevance of transgenerational metal toxicity extends beyond its traditional emphasis on organismal health to effects at the scale of population biology, community dynamics, and ecosystem function. Transgenerational effects on reproductive success, developmental trajectories, behavior, immune function, and tolerance to stress could modify population growth rates, age structure, and genetic diversity for several generations, in turn affecting the persistence of populations under additional stressors. At the community level, transgenerational shifts in species interactions, competitive abilities, and predator–prey associations might lead to reorganized ecological communities and altered ecosystem functioning through processes such as nutrient cycling, primary production, and decomposition. The additive pattern of transgenerational effects, with each generation being able to exhibit more severe or complex phenotypes than the previous one, can result in delayed population reductions or sudden ecosystem crashes after a tipping point is reached (Ricardo and Hyo, 2011). These longer-term and population- or ecosystem-level outcomes are rarely considered in traditional risk assessments, which focus on protecting the individual organism more than the long-term health and resilience of populations and ecosystems. Integration of transgenerational endpoints in ERA may therefore reflect a paradigmatic shift toward an approach that is more precautionary and ecologically relevant for the protection of the environment and chemical regulation.

7.2 Classification and environmental fate of toxic metals

7.2.1 Essential versus nonessential metals

Biologically, metals can be classified into two categories according to their requirement for organismal functioning: essential and nonessential metals. Essential metals, such as iron (Fe), zinc (Zn), copper (Cu), manganese (Mn), cobalt (Co), and molybdenum (Mo), are crucial for all living organisms to perform normal physiological functions, as they act as structural elements, enzyme cofactors, and signaling molecules (Jeremias et al., 2022). These metals are indispensable for many vital biological processes, such as oxygen delivery, electron transfer, antioxidant function, and gene expression, and they are involved in signal transduction. For instance, iron is an integral part of hemoglobin and cytochromes; zinc is essential for the activity of over 300 enzymes as well as DNA-binding proteins; and copper participates in the enzymatic machinery that fuels energy production, antioxidant defense systems, and connective tissue construction. Living organisms possess complex homeostatic systems for the import, distribution, and storage of essential metals, as well as their export and/or recycling, to maintain ideal levels without risking deficiency or poisoning. These protective mechanisms include membrane transport proteins, intracellular chaperones, metallothioneins, and metal-binding proteins, which together help ensure the availability of essential metals where required while keeping them unavailable at sites where they could be harmful. However, essentiality does not confer immunity to toxicity, as even essential metals can be toxic in excess by disturbing the physiological functions of cells due to competition with other metals, inappropriate binding to metalloproteins, and the generation of oxidative stress.

In contrast, nonessential metals are of no known biological importance and act strictly as toxicants when sequestered in living systems. Such a category comprises elements like lead (Pb), cadmium (Cd), mercury (Hg), arsenic (As), chromium (Cr), nickel (Ni), as well as aluminum (Al) and silver (Ag), which enter the environment essentially through human activities. Organisms have never had particular biological demands for these elements and, therefore, possess no specialized regulatory structures for uptake, distribution, or detoxification regarding them; consequently, they are particularly dangerous when present in the environment. Nonessential metals frequently gain access to cells via transport pathways designed to deliver essential metal ions that possess similar chemical behavior, in a process referred to as the molecular mimicry effect, which bypasses normal cellular defense mechanisms and leads to accumulation in tissues. Once inside cells, nonessential metals exert toxicity via various mechanisms that interfere with metabolism, including displacement of essential metal ions from their binding sites, enzyme inhibition, and membrane disruption, leading to the generation of reactive oxygen species (ROS) (Kandola and Giesy, 2024). The categorization of metals into essential and nonessential is useful conceptually, but it is not always a clear distinction because some "nonessential" metals may exert beneficial effects at very low concentrations or in particular situations, while so-called "essential" metals can also be toxic at levels slightly greater than the optimal range. In addition, the toxic effects of essential and nonessential metals are largely related to their chemical form (speciation), bioavailability, as well as the presence of other cooccurring metals/oxides, whether they interact additively, synergistically, or antagonistically.

7.2.2 Major toxic metals (Cd, Pb, Hg, As, Cr, Ni, Cu, Zn)

Among these metals, those that are most often implicated in environmental toxicity and transgenerational impacts are both nonessential (Cd, Pb, Hg, As) and essential at high doses (Cu, Zn, Cr, Ni). Cadmium is a hazardous nonessential metal, which mostly originates from the mining, smelting, battery production, phosphate fertilizer, and plastics stabilizer industries. Cadmium builds up primarily in the kidneys and liver, causing renal damage, osteomalacia, and carcinogenesis. Its toxicity is associated with its capacity to bind sulfhydryl groups of proteins and create oxidative stress, as well as its long biological half-life (10–30 years in humans), which favors bioaccumulation and chronic exposure. Another nonessential metal, lead, has been widely utilized in paints, gasoline, batteries, and soldering materials, resulting in general environmental pollution (Skinner, 2021). Toxicity produced by lead primarily attacks the nervous system, manifesting as developmental neurotoxicity in children and neurological disorders, cognitive, sensory, and behavioral aberrations even at lower levels of exposure. Lead disrupts not only calcium signaling and neurotransmitter function but can also replace calcium in biological substances, thereby inhibiting normal cellular behavior. The legacy of leaded gasoline has caused global soil contamination, which lasted for several decades after its phase-out and continues to impose transgenerational risks.

There are several forms of mercury, including metallic or elemental mercury, inorganic compounds of mercury, and organic methylmercury, which differ significantly in terms of their toxicological responses and environmental fate. Mercury is emitted through coal-combustion, artisanal gold mining, chlor-alkali industries, and other industrial processes. Methylmercury (MeHg), produced by the methylation of inorganic mercury (Hg) resulting from microbial activity in wetlands, is of greatest concern due to its propensity for biomagnification and neurotoxicological effects (Al-Asadi et al., 2023). Methylmercury biomagnifies in the aquatic food chain, with the highest levels occurring in apex predators, including large predatory fish, marine mammals, and human consumers. Methylmercury exposure during prenatal or early life results in persistent neurological damage, manifested as loss of cognitive function, motor control, and sensation. Although arsenic is not a true metal but a metalloid, it is grouped with the toxic metals on these pages because of its prevalence in the environment and long history of use, coupled with the plethora of adverse health effects that it can cause. Arsenic poisoning arises from natural geological processes as well as industrial sources such as mining, smelting, pesticide application, and wood preservation (Chen et al., 2022). Inorganic arsenic is a powerful human carcinogen and also produces a range of noncancer health effects, such as skin lesions, cardiovascular disease (CVD), and neurotoxicity. Arsenic toxicity is greatly affected by the arsenic species, which exhibit variation in toxic effects; e.g., inorganic arsenic species (arsenite and arsenate) are more toxic than organic forms, while arsenite is generally more toxic than arsenate (Da Silva et al., 2024).

Chromium has two predominant redox states with significantly different toxicities: while trivalent chromium (Cr (III)) is relatively nontoxic and an essential micronutrient in glucose metabolism, hexavalent chromium (Cr (VI)) is highly toxic, carcinogenic, and mobile in the environment. Cr (VI) pollution arises from industrial treatments such as electroplating (1), leather tanning (2), pigment manufacturing, and stainless-steel welding. Cr (VI) can easily penetrate cell membranes via anion transporter channels and is intracellularly reduced to Cr (III), forming reactive oxygen species that lead to DNA damage, lipid peroxidation, and protein oxidation. Nickel, a second transition metal, is emitted by mining, smelting ore both for] nickel and other metals, and preparing battery materials (Gu et al., 2023). Although nickel is necessary for the function of certain microbial and plant enzymes, it is not an essential element for humans or animals, and exposure to nickel compounds, especially insoluble Ni sulfides and oxides, has been linked to respiratory toxicity, allergic contact dermatitis, and carcinogenic potential (Guan and Wang, 2021). Some of the mechanisms by which nickel exerts its toxic effects include disruption of calcium homeostasis, induction of oxidative stress, and epigenetic changes such as DNA hypermethylation and histone modifications. When the environment becomes highly contaminated by mine tailings, industrial discharges, and agricultural regions where metal fungicides or fertilizers are used, metals can reach toxic levels. Copper toxicity to aquatic organisms, particularly fish and invertebrates, occurs through interference with osmoregulation and gill function as well as induction of oxidative stress. Zinc toxicity may inhibit the physiological processes of essential metals, including copper and iron, and result in developmental abnormalities and immune dysfunction in both aquatic and terrestrial species. The bioavailability and toxicity of each of these metals are largely dependent on environmental conditions such as pH, redox potential, organic matter content, or the presence of complexing ligands that condition their geochemical state, and in turn, their interaction with biological membranes and intracellular targets.

7.2.3 Bioavailability, speciation, and environmental transformation

Environmental toxicity and bioaccumulation of metals are controlled by their speciation in the environment and not by total concentrations, which can change dramatically with environmental conditions and chemical reactivity. Metal speciation is described as the various chemical forms in which an element occurs, such as free hydrated ions, inorganic complexes with small molecular-weight anions such as hydroxide, chloride, and carbonate ligands, organic complexes with natural organic matter, or colloidal- or particle-bound states. Chemical reactivity, biological availability, and toxicological behavior vary widely between different metals. The free hydrated metal ion is, in most cases, the most bioavailable and toxic form for many metals, as it can directly interact with biological membranes and transport proteins. However, some metal complexes, especially hydrophobic organic ones, can also be highly bioavailable and, in some cases, more toxic than free ions (Huang et al., 2025). Environmental conditions such as pH, redox potential (Eh), solution temperature, ionic strength, and concentrations of complexing ligands can all significantly influence the speciation of metals and subsequent bioavailability. The bioavailability of cationic metals, including Cu, Zn, Cd, and Pb, is expected to increase as pH declines due to reduced competition between metal and hydrogen ions for binding sites and enhanced solubilization of the metal.

The influence of natural organic compounds, such as humic and fulvic acids derived from the degradation of plant and animal material, is particularly important because they form organometal complexes due to strong interactions with many heavy metals. These organic compounds (OCs) are able to either decrease metal bioavailability and toxicity by complexing metals into nonbioaccessible forms, which cannot directly interact with biological receptors, or, under certain circumstances, increase bioavailability through facilitated transport across biological membranes (Jeong et al., 2022). Likewise, anthropogenic complexing agents, e.g., EDTA [ethylene diamine tetra(methylene phosphonic acid)] and nitrilotriacetic acid (NTA), which are applied as industrial input compounds and in consumer products, may strongly complex metals, thus altering their environmental dynamics and bioavailability. Time-space variant environmental changes, such as acid-base reactions, redox reactions, precipitation-dissolution, adsorption-desorption, and complexation–decomplexation, constantly modify metal speciation and bioavailability. These changes result from abiotic processes, including photodegradation, as well as microbial activity, which can reduce or oxidize metals, convert inorganic mercury to more bioavailable methylmercury, and transform arsenic between various valency states of differing toxicity. Multistep, complex processes, such as those described for the formation of natural $Cu_xPb_{1-x,}$ relate directly to our ability to predict the toxicity and bioavailability of metals. However, estimating genuine metal speciation for risk assessment and bioremediation is hampered by the dynamic nature of metal behavior in the environment (Jiang et al., 2024).

7.2.4 Metal cycling in aquatic and terrestrial ecosystems

Metals move in cycles between various environmental reservoirs in intricate biogeochemical processes, which lead to the distribution of metals among the atmosphere, hydrosphere, lithosphere, and biosphere. Metals penetrate aquatic systems through atmospheric deposition, surface runoff, groundwater recharge, industrial disposal, and natural weathering of rocks and minerals (Liu et al., 2023). In water bodies, the metals remain in solution, associate with suspended particles, or deposit on sediments depending on their species and hydrological conditions. Sediments serve as both a sink and a secondary source of metals, which are retained under stable conditions but can be exchanged with the overlying water when environmental conditions change or through sediment resuspension caused by storms, dredging, or bioturbation. The benthic sediment-water interface is recognized as a highly active area where cosmogenic redox gradients lead to the speciation or transmutation of metals; some become more mobile and bioavailable, while others are immobilized (Li et al., 2022). In aquatic organisms, metals are absorbed directly from water over respiratory surfaces, including gills; through the consumption of contaminated food; and occasionally via dermal exposure. The phenomenon of biomagnification, where metal concentration increases with trophic position, is particularly significant for metals that form lipophilic organic complexes such as methylmercury, which can reach concentrations orders of magnitude higher in top predators than in water or at lower trophic levels (Liu et al., 2023).

Metals in terrestrial ecosystems are mainly introduced through atmospheric deposition, metal-containing fertilizers, pesticides, sewage sludge application, and the discharge of industrial waste. The mobility and bioavailability of metals in the soil are governed by factors such as soil pH, redox potential, organic matter content, clay mineralogy, cation exchange capacity, and the presence of competing ions (Luo et al., 2024). Metal mobility and bioavailability are enhanced by lower soil pH, which leads to higher dissolution from solid phases and reduced competition for binding sites. Soil microorganisms play a role in several metal transformations, including reduction-oxidation, methylation, and complexation, which alter the mobility and toxicity of metals. The uptake of metals from soil occurs via plant roots and varies depending on metal bioavailability, plant species and genotype, physiological status, and mycorrhizal relationships. A subset of plant species can accumulate metals to an extreme extent, hyperaccumulating metals at levels hundreds to thousands of times higher than those found in normal plants—a trait that is useful for phytoremediation. In terrestrial animals, metals are introduced primarily through ingestion of contaminated food and soil, inhalation of dust, and, less frequently, dermal contact. Soil invertebrates, including earthworms and nematodes, serve as an important route of transfer by which metals can move through terrestrial food webs, taking up metals from the soil and providing a source for higher trophic levels (Onsanit et al., 2022). There is also an exchange of metals between aquatic and terrestrial systems via the movement of organisms (e.g., insect emergence from water and migration), runoff from land to water, atmospheric particulate settling, and other processes. Such cross-ecosystem transport can result in geographic regions becoming contaminated even if no direct pollution source exists there, creating challenging exposure scenarios for organisms that move or feed across ecosystem boundaries.

7.3 Mechanisms of metal toxicity across generations

7.3.1 Cellular and molecular toxicity pathways

The cellular and molecular basis of metal toxicity is complex due to a range of chemical properties observed among various metals as well as their interactions with biological macromolecules (Fig. 7.2). At the cellular level, metals can disrupt almost any biological process, such as membrane transport, energy generation, gene expression, and cell division. One of the basic mechanisms of metal toxicity is interference with the homeostasis of essential metals, wherein toxic elements compete with essential metals for binding sites on proteins, transporters, enzymes, etc. Such molecular mimicry can provide toxic metals with access to the transport apparatus intended for the transportation of essential

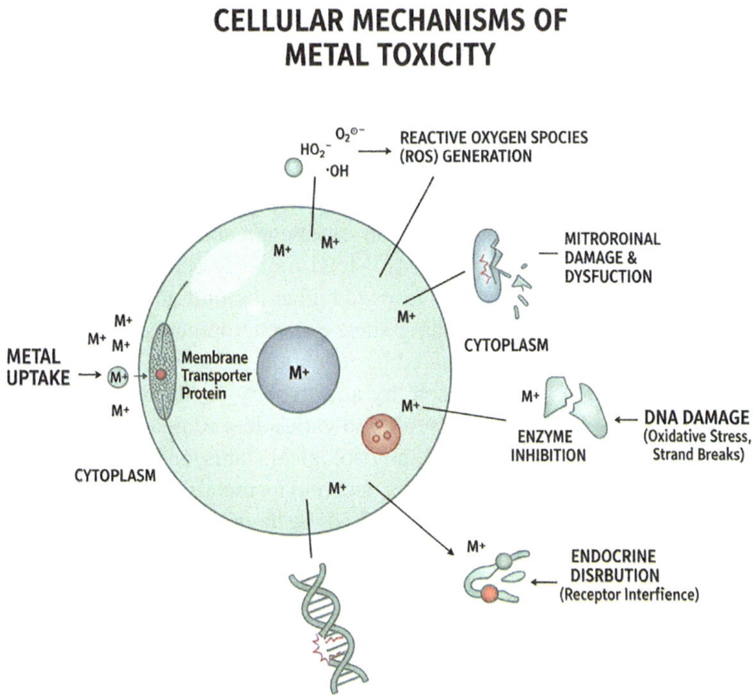

FIG. 7.2 Cellular and molecular mechanisms of metal toxicity.

ones, enabling them to later avoid competition with these metals and subsequently eject them from their physiological sites. Cadmium, for instance, can enter cells via calcium channels and zinc transporters, displacing zinc and specifically calcium from metalloproteins (and calmodulin) while increasing the cytoplasmic concentrations of these cations, thus modulating cellular signaling and enzyme activity. In addition, lead can replace calcium in calcium-dependent events such as neurotransmitter release and second messenger signaling, as well as inhibit enzymes that depend on zinc or other cofactors. Such displacement of functionally necessary metals from their primary binding sites is detrimental to protein and cellular processes and triggers downstream cascades of events that are ultimately responsible for metal toxicity.

Besides directly replacing essential metals, other metals contribute to their toxic action or effect through interactions with -SH groups in proteins or other compounds. SH groups are crucial for the structure and activity of several proteins, serving as ligands for metal-binding sites, participating in disulfide bonds that maintain the tertiary structure of certain proteins, and functioning as nucleophiles in enzymatic actions. Both mercury and methylmercury are metal compounds with a strong affinity for sulfhydryl groups. The methylated product of mercury is not only lipophilic but also binds extensively to reduced sulfur in proteins, which can denature these enzymes, leading to inhibition or interference with cellular functions. For example, mercury has a strong binding capacity to the sulfhydryl moiety of molecules and can bind to cysteine in the sulfur groups found in proteins, resulting in structural malfunction and loss of function. This binding can alter proteins involved in antioxidant defense, membrane transport, signal transduction, and DNA repair, all of which are critical cellular processes. In addition, metals may cause protein misfolding and aggregation by disrupting the normal folding of proteins, potentially leading to proteotoxic stress and activation of unfolded protein responses. These protein-level effects can significantly impact cellular homeostasis and, if they affect germ cells or early embryonic development, may contribute to the production of transgenerational effects.

Alterations in membrane structure and function are also a major causes of metal toxicity. Metals may bind to phospholipid membranes, causing changes in membrane fluidity and permeability, as well as alterations in the activity of plasma membrane proteins. For example, copper may induce lipid peroxidation through the production of ROS, leading to a consequent loss of membrane integrity and increased permeability to ions and molecules that would otherwise be excluded. Mercury can directly bind to membrane proteins, especially those with sulfhydryl groups, thereby interfering with ion transport, signal transduction, and cell-to-cell communication. Lead may influence calcium channels and other membrane transporters, modulating calcium homeostasis and cell signaling (Pereira et al., 2023). Intracellular disruption of lipid metabolism is harmful enough, but the effects on membranes in general disrupt cellular integrity and interfere with nutrient and ion transport, as well as intercellular communications such as Cx-based gap junction communication systems that are crucial for normal development and tissue function. If such effects occur in germ cells or during early stages of embryogenesis, they may result in heritable alterations, driving transgenerational toxicity.

7.3.2 Oxidative DNA damage and stress

The induction of oxidative stress through the formation of ROS and/or the inhibition of antioxidant defense mechanisms represents one of the most widely accepted mechanisms underlying metal toxicity. Several metals, such as redox-active metals like Cu, Fe, Cr, Ni, and V, are able to directly participate in the Fenton/Haber-Weiss reactions that form hydroxyl radicals from hydrogen peroxide and superoxide. Metals, even those that are not directly involved in redox cycling, such as cadmium, lead, and mercury, can also generate oxidative stress indirectly through the reduction of antioxidant species (e.g., glutathione), inhibition of antioxidant enzymes (e.g., superoxide dismutase, catalase, and glutathione peroxidase), or by modulating mitochondrial respiratory chain function, resulting in electron leakage and ROS production within the mitochondrial matrix. The subsequent oxidative stress can affect lipids, proteins, and nucleic acids (DNA), damaging each type of biomolecule through lipid peroxidation, protein oxidation, and DNA damage. Lipid peroxidation leads to the destruction of cellular membranes, compromising their function and integrity, as well as generating reactive aldehydes like malondialdehyde and 4-hydroxynonenal, which form adducts with proteins and DNA that propagate oxidative damage. Protein oxidation is associated with changes in protein conformation and functional properties, thereby resulting in enzyme deactivation, cellular signaling interruption, and dysfunctionality, as well as reduced activity for the clearance of degraded proteins (Riar et al., 2023).

One particularly important sequela of metal-induced oxidative stress is the genotoxic damage to DNA, which may provoke mutations or even be a source of genomic instability and heritable changes that lead to effects in forthcoming generations effects. Metal-induced ROS can lead to different types of DNA damage, such as single-strand breaks, double-strand breaks, base modifications like 8-hydroxy-2'-deoxyguanosine (8-OHdG), and DNA-protein cross-links. For instance, intracellular reduction of chromium (VI) to chromium (III) leads to ROS production, resulting in DNA strand breaks, DNA–protein cross-links, and chromosomal abnormalities. Nickel can suppress DNA repair enzymes as well as induce DNA hypermethylation, which leads to genome instability and carcinogenicity (Sun et al., 2022). Levels of oxidized DNA damage are also increased in response to arsenic exposure, and altered patterns of DNA methylation may contribute to transgenerational epigenetic effects; we refer the reader elsewhere for further discussion. Direct damage to DNA via DNA binding or indirect damage due to ROS production and impaired DNA repair are among the mechanisms of cadmium-induced genotoxicity. Mercury, especially methylmercury, causes oxidative DNA damage and decreases the activity of DNA repair enzymes, which exacerbates genotoxic consequences. Lead exposure is related to elevated oxidative DNA damage and chromosomal damage, which may somehow influence its neurotoxicity and carcinogenicity.

The possibility that metal-induced damage to DNA occurs early enough in the lifecycle to accumulate and express an effect transgenerationally is a function of when the DNA damage occurs and how successfully it is repaired. DNA damage in somatic cells will primarily affect the exposed individual, whereas DNA damage occurring in germ cells might be transmitted to offspring if not repaired before gametogenesis. In addition, oxidative DNA damage in germ cells may evoke subsequent epigenetic changes involved in the genomic defense against genotoxic stress, which might underlie transgenerational epigenetic inheritance. It has been shown that parental exposure to metals can lead to oxidative sperm DNA damage and abnormal DNA methylation in offspring, providing a potential mechanism for the inheritance of metal-induced effects through multiple generations. In addition, maternal metals could induce oxidative damage to the growing oocytes and early embryos during pregnancy, which might even lead to poor long-term health consequences over a number of generations (Wang et al., 2024a). The contribution of metal-induced DNA damage as a direct cause of mutations transferred to the next generations versus inducing epigenetic changes that may alter expression patterns of genes is also an ongoing area of research, with both mechanisms probably playing a role in transgenerational toxicity.

7.3.3 Endocrine disruption and reproductive toxicity

Metals are now considered to be significant environmental endocrine-disrupting chemicals (EDCs) that may inhibit hormone production, metabolism, transport, binding, and action. Endocrine disruption is a major mechanism of action by which metals may influence reproductive development and function, with the potential for transgenerational effects if endocrine-mediated alterations are transmitted through germ plasm or occur during critical developmental windows. The endocrine modulatory effects of metals are varied and metal-specific, based on their distinct chemical characteristics and interactions with components of the endocrine system. Metals may also disrupt the functioning of the hypothalamic-pituitary-gonadal axis (which governs reproduction), leading to alterations in the synthesis and secretion of gonadotropin-releasing hormone, follicle-stimulating hormone, luteinizing hormone, and sex steroids such as estrogen, progesterone, and testosterone. For instance, cadmium can function as a metalloestrogen by attaching to and activating estrogen receptors, thereby exerting an estrogenic-like effect (Wu et al., 2023). Exposure to cadmium has been linked with lower testosterone levels, as well as deficits in spermatogenesis and ovarian follicle development in different animal models. Lead exposure has been associated with reduced fertility, changes in hormones, and altered reproductive development in both men and women. Lead can suppress enzymes involved in steroid hormone synthesis and compromise hypothalamic-pituitary function.

Mercury, especially methylmercury, is a strong reproductive toxicant that interferes with endocrine function. Methylmercury exposure has been linked to a reduction in sperm quality, metabolite levels, and reproductive success in fish and wildlife. In humans, exposure to methylmercury has been associated with menstrual cycle disorders and decreased fertility in women (Zhang et al., 2024). Arsenic exposure can also affect steroidogenesis, leading to changes in sex hormone levels and reproductive dysfunction in males and females. At different levels and in different contexts, arsenic can act as an estrogen receptor agonist or antagonist by interrupting signaling via the glucocorticoid receptor. Exposure to chromium (VI), for example, has been linked to lower sperm counts and motility, changes in hormone levels, and infertility. Nickel compounds may also affect the reproductive system, including changes in sex hormones and spermatogenesis, as well as decreasing the fertility of exposed animals. Elevated concentrations of even essential metals can also cause endocrine disruption, with high copper exposure impacting reproduction in fish and invertebrates and excess zinc lowering steroidogenesis and reproductive hormone levels.

The potential that metal-induced endocrine-disrupting toxicity (ETD) is associated with transgenerational effects is of particular concern because developing organisms, during specific windows of development, are exquisitely sensitive to the modulation of endocrine signals (Zheng et al., 2022). Developmental exposure to endocrine-disrupting metals during embryonic, fetal, or early postnatal growth has the potential to reprogram reproductive and other hormone-sensitive systems for a lifetime, with direct implications for health as well as fertility from cradle to grave. These programming effects might be passed on to future generations via epigenetic mechanisms, which constitute a pathway of transgenerational endocrine disruption. For example, it has been reported that maternal exposure to EDCs such as metals during pregnancy can cause abnormal changes in hormone levels and the reproductive system not only in the directly exposed F1 generation but also in several generations following this one. For instance, previous generational arsenic exposure has been demonstrated to alter the age of pubertal onset and reproductive function within several generations of rats. Likewise, transgenerational impacts on reproduction and behavior can be observed in rodents as a result of lead exposure. Environmental relevance: Together, the findings suggest that metal-induced endocrine disruption occurring at sensitive stages of development may reprogram reproductive and other endocrine functions in subsequent generations, thereby affecting population dynamics and evolutionary responses.

7.3.4 Germline alterations and developmental programming

The germline is the pool of cells from which gametes, and hence progeny, originate, and it constitutes a primary site for metal-induced effects that may be transmitted through generations. Metals may exert influence on germ cells via various pathways, such as direct germ cell toxicity, germline DNA oxidative damage, gametic epigenetic modification, and disruption of processes involved in germ cell development and maturation. The stage responsiveness of germ cells to metal toxicity depends on the stage of germ cell development, as different stages progressing went toward spermatogenesis or oogenesis have distinct turning points in their sensitivities. Spermatogonial stem cells proliferate throughout reproductive life; these cells are sensitive to metal-induced DNA damage and the generation of mutations due to their high rate of proliferation. Metal exposure can cause DNA injury in spermatogonia, which, if not repaired properly before cell division, gets transmitted to sperm cells and subsequent generations. For instance, exposure to cadmium, lead, and mercury has been demonstrated to cause DNA strand breaks and chromosomal aberrations in spermatogonia. Spermatocytes in meiosis are also susceptible to metal toxicants because metals can interfere with meiotic chromosome segregation, leading to sperm aneuploidy (Bi et al., 2023). Although spermatozoa are transcriptionally inactive, they can sequester metals that may be transmitted to the oocyte during fertilization, potentially altering early embryonic development.

Oocytes can also be susceptible to metal toxicity during several stages of their development. Primordial follicles, which store immature oocytes arrested at prophase I, are susceptible to metal-induced damage via oxidative stress and DNA damage that ultimately result in follicular atresia and decreased ovarian reserve. Metal compounds can also interrupt oocyte maturation and ovulation, leading to changes in oocyte quality and fertilization ability. Throughout the growth and maturation of oocytes, remarkable epigenetic reprogramming occurs, such as DNA demethylation/remethylation, changes to histone modifications, and storage of maternal RNA/proteins that support embryonic development in the earliest phases before activation of the embryonic genome. Exposure to metals during these sensitive windows may interfere with these typical epigenetic processes and thus alter the normal epigenetic status of the oocyte, consequently modifying gene expression profiles in the embryo and later (Cao et al., 2024). In fact, maternal exposure to metals can induce changes in the DNA methylation of oocytes, which would subsequently be transmitted to offspring tissues. Moreover, paternal exposure to metals can impact sperm epigenetics, including DNA methylation, histone modifications, and the contents of small ncRNAs that can play a role in offspring development and health.

Developmental programming describes how environmental insults at critical periods of development induce enduring changes in gene expression, physiology, and phenotype, affecting disease risk across the lifespan. The Developmental Origins of Health and Disease hypothesis suggests that prenatal and early postnatal exposure can program individuals for the risk of developing chronic diseases in adulthood, such as metabolic diseases, CVD, neurodevelopmental disorders, and reproductive problems later in life. Metals are known to be developmental toxicants and can induce outcomes of developmental programming that extend later in life and possibly across generations. Lead exposure in utero, for example, is related to cognitive deficits, behavioral problems, and a greater adult risk of hypertension and CVD. Exposure of the fetus to arsenic is linked to a higher risk of respiratory disease, CVD, cancer, and neurodevelopmental disorders. These programming effects are considered to most likely be mediated by epigenetics, which maintain persistent changes in the pattern of gene expression. If these programming effects are transmitted through germ cells or very early embryos, however, they might be transgenerationally inherited as a mechanism of the transgenerational inheritance of developmental programming effects (Diogo et al., 2022). Animal models show that ancestral metal exposure can influence the phenotypic profile of offspring over multiple generations, resulting in changes such as abnormal growth and metabolism, behavioral abnormalities, and impaired reproductive capacity. These transgenerational impacts, in the absence of ongoing exposure, demonstrate that metals can induce heritable epigenetic marks, which endure through generations and affect health and fitness long after the initial contact has ended (Fu et al., 2023).

7.4 Epigenetic basis of transgenerational metal toxicity

7.4.1 DNA methylation and histone modifications

DNA methylation is one of the most commonly studied epigenetic mechanisms associated with the transgenerational transmission of metal toxicity. DNA methylation mainly occurs on cytosines in CpG dinucleotides in mammals and is present not only at CpG but also at CpNpG and CNC sites in plants, usually serving as a gene-silencing mark when located within the promoter region. Metals can cause either global hypomethylation or metal-specific gene hypermethylation or hypomethylation in a dose, time-, and tissue-dependent manner. Such methylation changes can affect gene expression profiles that may participate in the toxicological effects of metals and, when in germ cells, be inherited by offspring. For instance, cadmium exposure has been demonstrated to cause global DNA hypomethylation in different tissues and cell types, possibly through the inhibition of DNMTs and SAM depletion from oxidative stress. The hypermethylation of tumor suppressor gene promoters has also been linked to the carcinogenicity of cadmium. Research in animal models has shown that cadmium exposure can be associated with transgenerational DNA methylation alterations, and abnormal patterns of sperm and offspring tissue Cytosine–phosphate–Guanine site (CpG) methylation have been detected in multiple generations unexposed to the toxicant.

Lead has been shown to be associated with substantial changes in DNA methylation. Epidemiological studies have established that lead exposure is linked to abnormal DNA methylation in blood and other tissues, including genes related to neurological development, immune function, and cellular stress response. It has been reported that lead exposure can alter DNA methylation profiles in brain areas associated with memory and learning processes in animal studies, leading to lead's neurotoxicity and cognitive deficits. Such methylation changes are heritable across generations, as demonstrated in studies that found ancestral lead exposure modifies DNA methylation profiles in sperm and offspring brain tissues (Gao et al., 2022). Arsenic exposure is linked to global hypomethylation, as well as gene-specific hypermethylation, in genes associated with both carcinogenesis and development. Arsenic can disrupt DNA methylation in various ways, such as DNMT inhibition, SAM depletion, and oxidative stress. Ancestral arsenic exposure has been reported to alter the DNA methylation patterns of sperm, oocytes, and offspring tissues transgenerationally, influencing growth, metabolism, and susceptibility to disease.

7.4.2 Noncoding RNAs and gene regulation

Another key group of epigenetic modifiers in transgenerational responses to metal toxicity is ncRNAs [microRNAs (miRNA), long ncRNAs (lncRNAs), and small interfering RNAs (siRNA)]. These RNAs do not encode proteins but are involved in regulating gene expression in a variety of ways, such as through RNA interference and transcription regulation (Grzybowska-Swierkosz et al., 2023). Metals can modulate the presence of ncRNAs in a manner that impacts toxicity and the potential for transmission effects into subsequent generations. miRNAs are approximately 22 nucleotide-long RNAs that posttranscriptionally regulate gene expression by binding to complementary sequences in target mRNAs, causing mRNA turnover or translation repression. Exposure to metals modifies the expression of miRNAs in different tissues and a variety of cell types, targeting genes that mediate oxidative stress response, apoptosis, DNA repair, as well as cell cycle control, among other key networks. For instance, hepatic, renal, and lung miRNA expression is altered by exposure to cadmium, with each organ exhibiting changes in miRNAs that regulate genes corresponding to oxidative stress, metal homeostasis, and apoptosis. There are many studies showing that miRNA expression is dysregulated by lead exposure in brain tissues, especially in those regulating genes associated with neurodevelopment and synaptic function. These miRNA changes are relevant to Pb-induced neurotoxicity and learning disabilities.

Most importantly, miRNAs and other ncRNAs can be carried with the help of extracellular vesicles, such as exosomes and microvesicles, which, when delivered to recipient cells, could reprogram their gene expression. This provides an alternative model for intercellular signaling of metal-associated epigenetic alterations. More relevant for transgenerational inheritance, such small ncRNAs have also been detected in sperm and may be transferred to the oocyte at fertilization, potentially impacting early embryonic development as well as gene expression profiles. Previous studies reported that sperm small RNA content could be affected by paternal exposure to environmental pollutants, such as metals, and the profiled RNAs were linked with offspring phenotypes (Han et al., 2024). For instance, changes in sperm miRNA content due to paternal exposure to lead are accompanied by alterations in the expression of target genes and the behavioral phenotype of offspring. Paternal cadmium exposure also disrupted sperm miRNA profiles, resulting in effects on offspring development and susceptibility to disease.

7.4.3 Epigenetic inheritance and environmental memory

Another significant group of epigenetic regulators, known as ncRNAs, such as miRNAs, siRNAs, and lncRNAs may also contribute to mediating transgenerational effects caused by metal toxicity. While these RNAs do not encode proteins, they exert their effects on gene expression through multiple mechanisms, including posttranscriptional gene silencing, chromatin remodeling, and transcriptional regulation. Metals can alter the expression of ncRNAs, thereby disrupting the balance in their regulatory functions and initiating adverse effects that may be transmitted across generations (Table 7.1). miRNAs are short (~22 nucleotide) RNA molecules that posttranscriptionally regulate gene expression by pairing with the sequence of a target mRNA to promote translational repression or degradation. Metal exposure is known to modify miRNA expression patterns in different tissues and cell types, regulating genes related to oxidative stress response,

TABLE 7.1 Epigenetic inheritance across generations (He et al., 2022).

Epigenetic mechanism	Metal (s) implicated	Biological target	Transgenerational outcome	Representative models	Notes
DNA methylation	Cd, As, Pb	Germline & somatic cells	Altered gene expression, fertility decline	Zebrafish, mouse	Stable inheritance up to F3
Histone modification	Hg, Ni	Chromatin structure	Developmental abnormalities	*Drosophila*, plants	Often reversible but persistent
miRNA dysregulation	Cr, Cd	Posttranscriptional regulation	Growth retardation, stress sensitivity	Fish, mammals	Linked to oxidative stress
Transposon activation	As, Pb	Genome stability	Mutagenesis, phenotypic plasticity	Plants, insects	Adaptive/maladaptive responses

apoptosis, DNA repair, cell-cycle control, and other important processes. For instance, changes in miRNA expression occur in liver, kidney, and lung tissues following cadmium (Cd) exposure, where a group of these miRNAs modulates genes related to oxidative stress response, metal homeostasis, and apoptosis. Lead exposure alters miRNA levels in brain tissues, including those that target neurodevelopment and synaptic genes. Such miRNA alterations are associated with lead-induced neurotoxicity and cognitive dysfunction (He et al., 2022).

7.4.4 Sex-specific epigenetic responses

Sex-differentiated modes of transgenerational inheritance (between maternal and paternal lineages) and responses to metal toxicity are important factors to consider when interpreting the mechanisms underlying transgenerational metal toxicity. Males and females tend to vary in their responses to metal exposure because they differ in physiology, behavior, exposure routes, and hormone regulation. These sex differences also appear to extend to epigenetic responses to metal exposure, as male and female individuals show different patterns of DNA methylation changes, histone modifications, and noncoding RNA expression in response to the same metal exposure. Such sex-specific epigenetic responses could be responsible for observed sex disparities in the effects of metal toxicity and influence sex-specific modes of transgenerational transmission. For instance, it has been evidenced that lead exposure brings about distinct miRNA expression profiles in the male and female brain, which may contribute to sex differences in lead neurotoxicity. Sex-specific epigenetic changes in the reproductive tissues of males and females are also caused by cadmium exposure, which may play a role in their divergent reproductive outcomes.

7.5 Transgenerational effects in aquatic organisms

7.5.1 Fish models: Developmental, behavioral, and reproductive impacts

Changes in behavior are another critical transgenerational effect of metal exposure in fish. This exposure can influence fish behavior, including locomotor activity, predator avoidance, foraging behavior, social behavior, and learning and memory, with some of these behavioral alterations being potentially transgenerational (Table 7.1). For instance, cadmium-treatment causes zebrafish to experience a reduction in their locomotor activity and swimming behaviors that are directly passed on to their progeny, supporting transgenerational inheritance. Exposure to lead in fish is also associated with behavioral changes, such as social behaviors, aggression, and learning dysfunction, some of which can be transmitted across generations via parental exposure. Fish Biology: Mercury exposure, particularly to methylmercury, has been shown to disrupt predator avoidance behaviors, schooling behaviors, and feeding in fish, with documented transgenerational effects existing for a number of fish species. Depending on the context in which these behaviors occur, perturbations may influence feeding efficacy, predator avoidance, and reproductive success, with consequences at both fitness and population levels. The mediators of transgenerational behavioral effects probably include epigenetic changes that target neural developmental and functional genes, especially in brain areas regulating behavior (Hu et al., 2023).

From a population dynamics point of view, reproductive effects are likely the most important transgenerational impact of metal exposure in fish. Metal exposure can interfere with not only with gonad development but also with spawning behavior, gamete production and quality, the success of the fertilization process, and offspring viability in fish. Some of these effects on reproduction can carry over to subsequent generations, with implications for population growth rates and persistence. For instance, when zebrafish were exposed to cadmium, there was a decrease in fecundity and sperm quality alongside altered spawning behavior in the animals, with some of these reproductive deficits observed in nondirectly exposed offspring. Fish exposure to lead is linked to delayed sexual maturation, disturbance of hormone levels, and reduction in reproductive success, while adverse effects on the offspring generation were confirmed in several fish species. Fish reproduction is especially affected by mercury exposure, showing decreased egg production as well as reduced sperm motility, altered hormone levels, and impaired spawning behavior; such effects can be transmitted to several generations. The mechanisms of transgenerational reproductive effects may be associated with epigenetic changes in genes related to steroid synthesis, gonad development, and gametogenesis, as well as potential maternal metal transfer to eggs and impacts on offspring development (Jiang et al., 2025) (Table 7.2).

7.5.2 Invertebrates (Daphnia, mollusks, crustaceans)

Water fleas are promising model organisms for investigating transgenerational metal toxicity because of their ecological relevance, sensitivity to environmental pollutants, and ease of laboratory culturing. Invertebrates, such as Daphnia, mollusks, and crustaceans, are keystone organisms within aquatic ecosystems, serving as primary consumers and prey for higher fauna, and are involved in nutrient cycling and energy transfer. Transgenerational responses to metal exposure have been observed in a number of aquatic invertebrate species, with impacts on reproduction, growth, behavior and stress tolerance, as well as at the population level, extending across several unexposed generations. Such transgenerational effects have important consequences for invertebrate population dynamics, community structure, and ecosystem function, and may provide an overlooked mechanism through which metal pollution influences the health of aquatic ecosystems.

Daphnia are a group of freshwater Cladocerans and, as such, have become model organisms to study transgenerational impacts. They are cyclical parthenogenetic reproducers with relatively short generation times (approximately 1–2 weeks) and are frequently targeted in numerous studies on toxicant exposures due to their sensitivity toward contaminants found within their environment. Ecologically, they are significant as one of the primary consumers within

TABLE 7.2 Transgenerational effects of metal toxicity across aquatic and terrestrial organisms.

Metal	Organism Type	Model Species	Exposure Route	Observed Transgenerational Effects (F1–F3)	Underlying Mechanisms	Key References
Cadmium (Cd)	Aquatic (Fish)	*Danio rerio* (Zebrafish)	Water-borne	Reduced fertility, developmental toxicity, altered behavior in offspring	Oxidative stress, endocrine disruption, altered gene expression and DNA methylation	Wang et al. (2022)
Lead (Pb)	Aquatic (Amphibian)	*Xenopus laevis*	Water/ sediment	Developmental deformities, impaired metamorphosis, neurotoxicity	DNA methylation disruption, histone modification, endocrine interference	Senut et al. (2012)
Mercury (Hg)	Aquatic (Invertebrate)	*Daphnia magna*	Dietary	Reduced survival and fecundity across generations	ROS signaling, mitochondrial dysfunction, epigenetic alterations	Vandegehuchte and Janssen (2014)
Arsenic (As)	Terrestrial (Mammal)	*Mus musculus* (Mouse)	Dietary	Epigenetic reprogramming, metabolic disorders, reproductive toxicity	Germline DNA methylation, ncRNA dysregulation	Skinner and Guerrero-Bosagna (2009)
Chromium (Cr VI)	Terrestrial (Plant)	*Arabidopsis thaliana*	Soil	Growth inhibition, altered stress tolerance across generations	Transgenerational epigenetic memory, DNA methylation changes	Bilichak et al. (2012)
Nickel (Ni)	Terrestrial (Insect)	*Drosophila melanogaster*	Dietary	Reduced lifespan, reproductive impairment	Gene expression modulation, histone modification	Jose et al. (2019)

freshwater systems. Daphnia are capable of both asexual reproduction (producing genetically identical juveniles, or clones) and sexual reproduction. This reproductive variety makes Daphnia a model system for studying transgenerational effects, as clonal reproduction permits the disentanglement of genetic effects from epigenetic effects, while sexual reproduction allows for the study of transgenerational inheritance across sexual generations. Many studies have reported transgenerational effects of metal exposure in Daphnia in terms of reproduction, growth, behavior, and stress tolerance, which persist across multiple unexposed generations (Kim et al., 2023). For instance, Daphnia magna exposed to cadmium exhibit impairments in reproduction, brood size, and growth in the generation directly exposed to the toxicant ($N = 0$), and these effects are also transmitted down two generations of nonexposed descendants. Parallels can be drawn in Daphnia between the effects of other metals and transgenerational inheritance for Cu, Zn, and Ni. The mechanisms underlying these transgenerational effects are likely, in part, due to epigenetic changes, such as DNA methylation, histone modifications, and small RNAs. However, Daphnia have less extensive DNA methylation than vertebrates, suggesting that other epigenetic processes might be more important in this group of organisms.

7.5.3 Metal-induced changes in growth, immunity, and survival

Transgenerational effects of metal exposure on growth, immunity, and survival are key endpoints to evaluate the ecological implications of metal pollution, as these traits directly contribute to fitness and population dynamics. For instance, zebrafish exposed to Cd during early development exhibit smaller body size and growth changes, with such effects being reflected in unexposed progeny, indicative of transgenerational transmission. Similar transgenerational enhancement in growth was previously reported for other metals like lead, mercury, copper, etc., in several fish species.

The immune system is also a candidate target for transgenerational effects of metal exposure in aquatic species. Metals are immunotoxicants that can inhibit or disrupt immune function, leading to increased vulnerability to pathogens and parasites. Transgenerational effects of metal exposure on immunity parameters have also been reported in several aquatic species, where antiinflammatory response, phagocytosis, antibody production, and disease resistance were altered in descendants exposed through parental or ancestral lines. For instance, mussels exposed to cadmium exhibit impaired immune status in the generation directly exposed, and these altered immune parameters are maintained across generations that are not directly exposed, suggestive of transgenerational inheritance (Li et al., 2024). Fish exposed to metals such as copper, zinc, and nickel exhibit transgenerational effects on immune function, encompassing changes in immunogenic gene expression, reductions in disease resistance, and enhanced susceptibility to pathogens in their descendants. These transgenerational immune effects may have important ecological implications by influencing disease dynamics in aquatic populations and potentially even the magnitude of disease outbreaks or population crashes.

7.5.4 Multigenerational and life-cycle exposure studies

Family and life-cycle time exposure studies contribute important insights, as up to now human populations have been perceived from the viewpoint of both long-term and multigenerational metal-exposure reactions, as well as the dynamic processes by which combined effects accumulate or disappear over generations. Genuine multigenerational analyses expose multiple sequential generations—usually F0, F1, F2, F3, and beyond—to metals and observe effects across the generations, with increasing continuous exposures permitting examinations of generational impacts that accrue over time (Fig. 7.3).

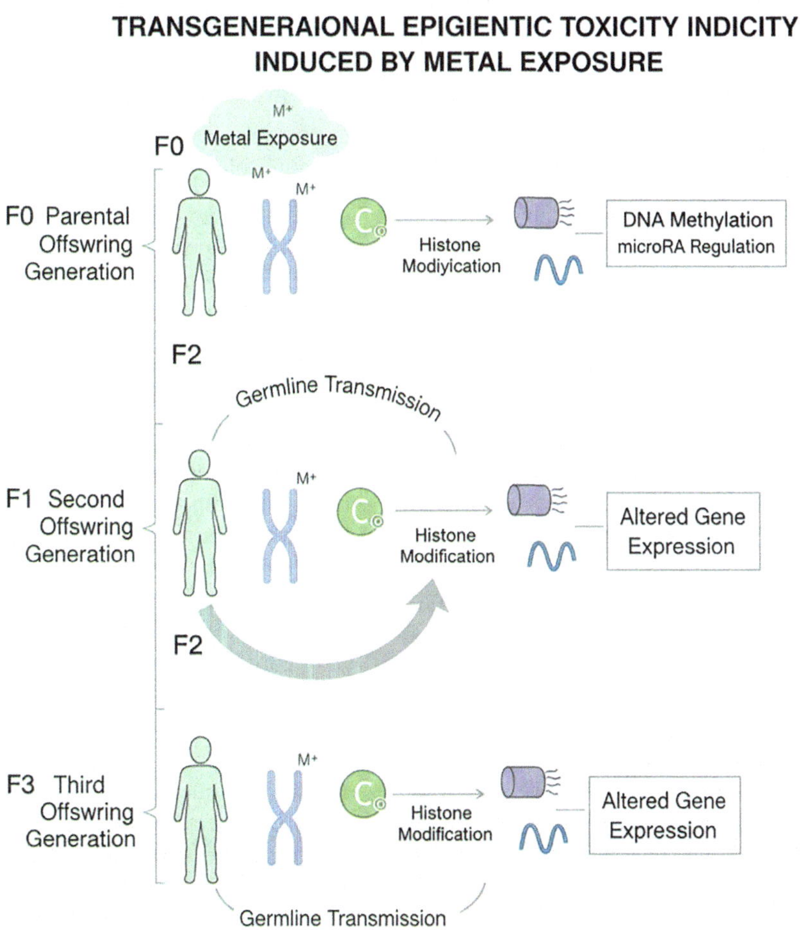

FIG. 7.3 Epigenetic mechanisms driving transgenerational metal toxicity.

7.6 Transgenerational effects in terrestrial organisms

7.6.1 Soil invertebrates (earthworms, nematodes, arthropods)

Soil invertebrates are important constituents of terrestrial systems that contribute to soil formation, the breakdown and decomposition of organic matter, nutrient cycling, as well as food web dynamics (Lavelle et al.) These animals are constantly in contact with metals in the soil by ingestion of soil particles, dermal contact, and also because some nematode species have been experimentally exposed to small quantities of metallic substances bound to the surfaces or adsorbed on solid organic matter; therefore they may be considered bioindicators for metal contamination. Soil invertebrates are also important vectors of transfer for metals through terrestrial food webs, since they can act as metal sinks at their lower trophic levels and make them available to higher trophic levels such as birds, mammals and reptiles (Liu et al., 2022). Transgenerational effects of metals have been observed in several soil invertebrates, including earthworms, nematodes, and arthropods, with consequences for reproduction, growth, behavior, and/or metal uptake patterns that can last over two unexposed generations.

7.6.2 Plants: Metal stress memory and epigenetic priming

As sessile organisms, plants do not have the option of moving to avoid exposure to stressors; hence, they must depend on adaptive responses at cellular and molecular levels in order to avoid death from metal contamination in soil. Plants have developed a range of metal tolerance and detoxification strategies, such as metal exclusion, chelation, sequestration, and antioxidant defense. Strikingly, plants are also capable of exhibiting transgenerational effects of metal exposure, whereby the offspring of exposed parents display modified phenotypes and tolerance to metal stress even when grown in uncontaminated conditions.

The ecological importance of plant transgenerational epigenetic effects (TGEs) lies in their ability to alter plant community composition, succession, and ecosystem function in metal polluted habitats. Inherited metal tolerance can far more quickly enable plant populations to cope with contaminated soils far more quickly than through purely genetic adaptation, contributing to the establishment and/or maintenance of tolerant genotypes at metal-contaminated sites. This can have implications for plant community composition in contaminated areas, where metal-tolerant species may displace sensitive ones (Ma et al., 2023). Transgenerational shifts in metal accumulation patterns may also influence the transfer of metals through terrestrial food webs, as plants with modified metal uptake and distribution traits provide different quantities of metals to herbivores and higher trophic levels. In addition, transgenerational alterations in plant growth and physiology may impact ecosystem processes such as primary production, litter decomposition, and nutrient cycling, potentially modifying the functioning of ecosystems in metal-polluted areas. A better understanding of these transgenerational effects is essential to predict the long-term ecological risks of soil metal contamination and to design efficient phytoremediation strategies that rely on transgenerational metal tolerance.

7.6.3 Mammalian models and wildlife studies

Mammalian models, in particular rodents (mice and rats), are essential for transgenerational analyses of metal toxicity as they closely mimic human physiology and genetics. Their biology is well described, and tools have been developed to examine epigenetic processes. Transgenerational effects of metal exposures are well documented in rodents, where a single exposure affecting reproduction, development, behavior, metabolism, and susceptibility to disease can be transmitted over several unexposed generations (Noguera et al., 2023). These results have potential implications for understanding the likely contribution of metal pollution to wildlife populations and, consequently, to human health through common exposure pathways and mechanisms. Wildlife studies, although more difficult to implement than laboratory studies, enable investigations of the transgenerational effects of metal toxicity in wildlife populations and the ecological relevance of these effects on population dynamics and ecosystem health.

7.6.4 Reproductive fitness and population-level consequences

The transgenerational impact of metal-induced toxicity on reproductive fitness is a major issue influencing long-term ecological and evolutionary trajectories because it is through reproduction, ultimately, that population growth, persistence, and evolution are determined. Metal exposure can have transgenerational impacts on all components of reproductive fitness, including gamete production and quality, mating behaviors, fertilization success, pregnancy outcomes, offspring survival, and overall reproductive output (Pan et al., 2024). These transgenerational impacts on reproduction could lower population growth rates and induce demographic decreases, even if direct exposure ceases, especially under the concurrent effects of stressors. Population-level effects of transgenerational metal toxicity are contingent on the intensity and timing of the initial exposure, as well as which specific reproductive traits are affected, genetic and phenotypic variability within a population, and the mitigating or exacerbating influence of other stressors that can ameliorate or buffer these transgenerational effects.

7.7 Comparative analysis: Aquatic versus terrestrial systems

7.7.1 Exposure routes and bioaccumulation patterns

Metal exposure pathways and bioaccumulation dynamics are fundamentally different in aquatic versus terrestrial systems, resulting in alternative exposure scenarios and likely transgenerational responses. In aquatic environments, organisms are exposed to metals through the water column on respiratory surfaces, including gills in fish and invertebrates, by ingestion of contaminated food and particulate matter, and by dermal absorption. Soil characteristics, such as pH, organic matter content, clay content, cation exchange capacity, and moisture levels, directly affect metal availability in terrestrial environments (Santamaria et al., 2022). Due to contrasting exposure pathways in liquid and solid-phase systems, metal uptake, distribution, and bioaccumulation patterns differ between both systems, which can affect toxicity and transgenerational effects.

7.7.2 Adaptive versus maladaptive transgenerational responses

Transgenerational effects of metal exposure can be adaptive, as they may prepare offspring for a similar environment and increase fitness in this environment, or maladaptive, as reduced fitness may also occur in nonchallenging environments, potentially leading to evolutionary traps. The relative occurrence of adaptive versus maladaptive responses probably depends on the degree of predictability in environmental conditions, the type and severity of the original exposure, the genes and pathways influenced by epigenetic changes, and the genetic and phenotypic diversity within a population. The extent to which these transgenerational effects are adaptive or maladaptive is crucial for predicting long-term population-level responses to metal pollution and for developing effective risk assessment and management strategies (Tao et al., 2024).

The relative contribution of adaptive and maladaptive transgenerational responses could be determined by the dose and duration of the initial exposure; for example, low to moderate doses stimulate adaptive response pathways via hormetic mechanisms, while higher exposures disrupt normal developmental programming, leading to a maladaptive outcome. Selection in response to these patterns may also be influenced by the predictability of environmental conditions, with adaptive responses being more probable when offspring are expected to experience conditions similar to those of their parents.

7.7.3 Ecosystem-specific vulnerabilities

The degree to which ecosystems are vulnerable to transgenerational effects of metal toxicants may depend on the physical, chemical, and biological state of an ecosystem, as well as on the form and patterns of metal contamination in that ecosystem. Aquatic systems, especially freshwater ecosystems, are at high risk of metal pollution because water has high bioavailability for metals, serves as a major dispersing medium, and numerous aquatic organisms are sensitive to metal toxicity. Metal inputs to freshwater ecosystems, of which lakes, rivers, and wetlands are typical examples, derive from point sources such as industrial effluents and mining activities, and nonpoint sources such as agricultural runoffs and atmospheric deposition (Zhang et al., 2023). These inputs may increase metal levels in water and sediment, and aquatic animals can be exposed to metals from more than one pathway, including water, food, and sediment. The high interconnectivity of aquatic systems in terms of metals, with water, sediments, and organisms constantly trading metals amongst themselves, results in an exposure scenario where fish are exposed to metals throughout their lifecycles.

Transgenerational metal toxicity in the soil-plant system varies among terrestrial ecosystems, depending on soil properties, plant species, and land use. Metal contamination of agricultural soils poses a threat to the supply chain of toxic metals in food crops, which may occur due to the use of metal-based agrochemicals and sewage sludge, as well as irrigation with heavy-metal-polluted water. The presence of metals in a fertile soil, which are eventually taken up by crops or soil organisms, can result in transgenerational impacts on plant yields and food quality, as well as on the functioning of soil ecosystems. Urban soils are particularly susceptible to the accumulation of metals from traffic emissions, industrial activities, materials used in construction, and historical pollution. Higher metal concentrations (such as lead, copper, and zinc, among others) present in urban soils can have transgenerational effects on soil organisms, plants, and urban wildlife.

Wetlands are a particularly attractive and vulnerable natural environment for transgenerational metal toxicity to be exhibited, as they exist at the terrestrial-aquatic interface, accumulating metals from both water and sediments (Zhao et al., 2022). Wetlands often serve as sinks for metals by sequestering them from inflowing waters and atmospheric deposition into sediments and wetland biota. This accumulation of metals creates exposure situations for wetland organisms, which can have metal concentrations that are extremely elevated, potentially leading to transgenerational impacts on wetland ecosystem function. Wetlands are also habitats for numerous other species, such as migratory birds and fish that rely on wetlands as breeding or nursery areas, further increasing the possibilities for transgenerational effects to extend beyond a given wetland.

7.8 Methodological approaches for studying transgenerational toxicity

7.8.1 Experimental design and generational exposure models

As a chemical with TMP, bisphenol A (BPA) represents an ideal model for the study of transgenerational toxicity, but such investigation requires meticulous experimental design to differentiate true transgenerational effects from multigenerational effects, in which exposure persists across generations (Fig. 7.4). True transgenerational effects are present in nonexposed future generations, which differ according to the species and its reproductive strategy. In mammals, the F1 generation is exposed in utero as embryos or fetuses through maternal exposure during pregnancy; the F2 generation is exposed to germ cells within the F1—the F3 generation being defined as one unexposed cycle with respect to

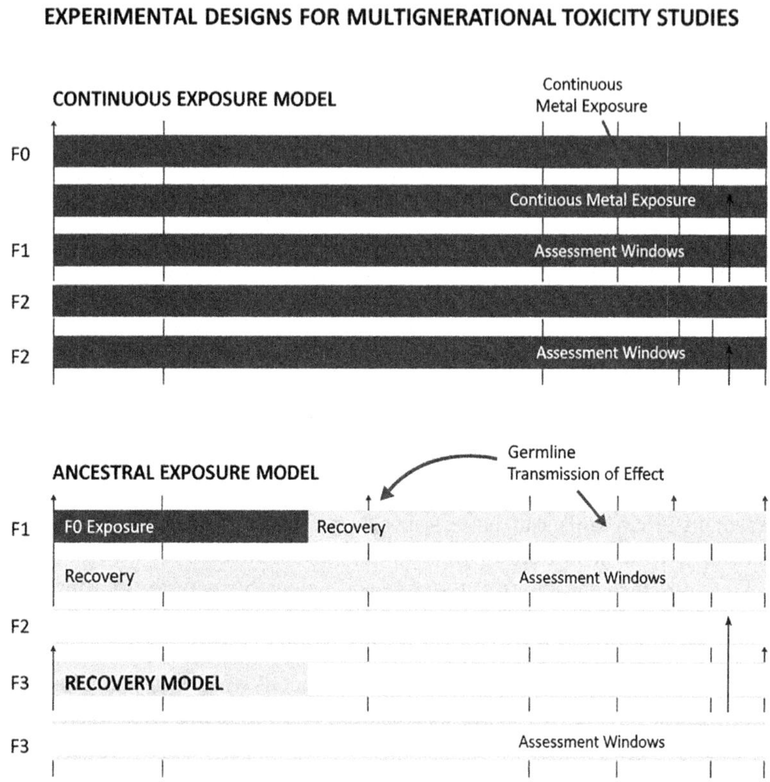

FIG. 7.4 Experimental approaches for multigenerational metal toxicity studies.

any prior exposure, and so on in organisms with external fertilization (Amiard-Triquet and Amiard, 2023). Differentiating multigenerational from transgenerational effects is important for causal inference with respect to mechanisms of inheritance and for risk estimates, since effects that are transgenerationally transmitted beyond the F1, after exposure stops, are more serious than those that only last as long as the exposure.

7.8.2 Molecular, omics, and epigenomic tools

Recent molecular and omics technologies have greatly expanded our tools for studying the transgenerational effects of metal toxicity by observing multiple gene expression patterns, epigenetic changes, and other molecular alterations that are passed between generations. Transcriptomics, especially RNA sequencing (RNA-seq), enables a genome-wide assay of transcriptomic alterations in exposed and nonexposed generations, thereby revealing the pathways and functions targeted by metal exposure and potentially inheritable via an epigenetic route. For instance, transgenerational up and downregulation of gene expression has been identified in metal homeostasis, oxidative stress resistance, DNA repair, and reproduction following metal treatment in fish, rodents, and invertebrates, as demonstrated by RNA-seq studies. Epigenomics tools make it possible to gain a global perspective on epigenetic marks, such as DNA methylation, histone modification, and chromatin accessibility, which could be responsible for TGE. Whole-genome bisulfite sequencing (WGBS) provides nucleotide-level resolution of DNA methylation genome-wide and facilitates the identification of differentially methylated regions that may be transmitted through the germline across generations (Banni et al., 2024). Transgenerational DNA methylome changes after metal exposure have been detected by WGBS in various species, particularly in genes related to development, reproduction, and stress response. Reduced representation bisulfite sequencing (RRBS) offers a high-throughput, low-cost analysis of DNA methylation over CpG-rich regions of the genome, including promoters and CpG islands, which are critical for gene regulation.

7.8.3 Biomarkers of transgenerational stress

Biomarkers are quantitative measures of the state, exposure, or effect on life processes and health conditions in an individual that can potentially serve to assess transgenerational effects of metal toxicity. Classical bioindicators of metal exposure and toxicity, such as metal tissue accumulation, induction of metallothioneins, criteria of oxidative stress, or DNA damage, have been employed for decades to evaluate the assessment of metal exposures and their toxicity in organisms. However, these classical biomarkers are useful measures of current or short-term past exposure rather than transgenerational effects. Biomarkers targeting transgenerational effects are necessary to quantify whether effects persist over generations not directly exposed and to identify those species or populations with transgenerational epigenetic loads derived from earlier exposures (Bonduriansky, 2021). These transgenerational biomarkers can be identified as deviations from this basic roadmap and include epigenetic changes that can be quantified in germ cells or somatic tissues and may translate into a foreseeable phenotypic outcome across two or more generations.

7.8.4 Statistical and computational modeling

Statistical and computational modeling methods are becoming increasingly valuable for characterizing complex transgenerational patterns, relationships between generations, and predicting potential population-level effects of transgenerational metal toxicity. In models for transgenerational data, the hierarchy of the structure of the data cannot be ignored—individuals belong to a family, which belongs to a generation, and there might be correlated effects within families as well as across generations. Such analyses can be conveniently adjusted for fixed effects of treatment and generation by fitting mixed-effects models to the normalized data, while at the same time controlling for random effects of family and all other nested factors. Such models are able to detect within and between-generation effects of treatment, as well as interactions between treatment and generational differences that can differentiate between constant and dynamic re-allocation patterns (Cedergreen et al., 2012). Bayesian methods can provide the flexibility to model complex transgenerational data and to account for a priori knowledge on likely patterns of transgenerational effects. Bayesian hierarchical models explicitly consider uncertainty at multiple layers, and they can be used to estimate parameters of interest in settings where data may be sparse.

7.9 Ecological and evolutionary implications

7.9.1 Population dynamics and biodiversity impacts

The transgenerational effects of metal toxicity may have implications for population dynamics, including differences in effective population growth rates, population age structure, gene housekeeping, and risk of extinction. Metal-induced transgenerational effects on reproduction, survival, or growth rates can depress population growth rates and, hence, may result in a decline of populations even after the cessation of direct exposure. These effects at the population level can be more severe for species with low reproductive rates, long generation times, and small population sizes (Head et al., 2022). Modeling studies that include transgenerational effects have demonstrated that relatively small reductions in reproductive fitness due to a stressor can result in substantial population size decreases over the long-term, especially when interacting with density-dependent and/or temporally variable aspects of the environment. Such models also indicate that long-term effects may have implications for the decline of populations and local extinction in metal-polluted environments, especially for sensitive species with a low ability to adapt.

Age structure can be trans-generationally influenced by metal toxicity through impacts on the timing of development, age at maturity, and longevity. Metal-induced transgenerational shifts in the rate of development could alter the age structure of populations and cause deviations toward younger or older age classes as a consequence of these effects. Changes in age structure can influence the rate of population growth (population elasticity) and the resistance to additional stress sources, because respective cohorts may play different roles in terms of contribution to population change and may respond differently to environmental perturbations. Longevity could also affect population life history and population dynamics (Kille et al., 2024). These changes in age structure may have consequences for population dynamics and ecosystem processes, given that different age classes often perform different ecological functions.

7.9.2 Metal-induced selective pressure and adaptation

Metal contamination generates strong selective pressure capable of promoting evolutionary change in exposed populations. Individuals and genotypes tolerant to metals have a higher fitness in the contaminated environment and may become more frequent in subsequent generations due to natural selection. This selection may drive rapid evolution of tolerance to metals, especially in species with short generation times and a large number of individuals. Several studies have described evolved tolerance to metals in plants, invertebrates, and vertebrates living on metal-polluted sites, such as grasses and other plants growing on mine tailings, soil invertebrates in polluted soils, or fish from contaminated waters. Such evolved tolerances are commonly associated with physiological mechanisms such as increased exclusion of metals, sequestration of metals in a more inert form, elevated synthesis of metallothionein by the plant, and improved antioxidant defense. The development of tolerance to metals can occur over short periods, and several studies have reported marked increases in metal tolerance within a few generations.

7.9.3 Long-term ecosystem resilience

The long-term resilience of an ecosystem, or the ability of an ecosystem to preserve its structure, function, and/or services following a pestiferous disturbance, may be influenced by transgenerational metal toxicity. The resilience of ecosystems is attributed to several different factors, which can include species diversity, functional redundancy, connectivity, and the ability to recover after a disturbance (Lushchak et al., 2023). Transgenerational metal toxicity may impact the resilience of ecosystems by impoverishing species diversity, modifying functional traits, or affecting ecological interactions, as well as a declining potential to recover populations. Such effects are likely to lower the resiliency of ecosystems to metal pollution and other environmental perturbations, possibly driving ecosystems toward alternative stable states or thresholds beyond which recovery is severely compromised.

7.10 Human health and ecological risk considerations

7.10.1 Linkages between transgenerational wildlife and human toxicity

The relationships between wildlife and human transgenerational toxicity may, therefore, add an essential level to the overall view of metal pollution impacts on health and the environment. Humans and wildlife are exposed to metals in the environment, predominantly through contaminated food sources, drinking water, and air, and may be subject to transgenerational effects by similar molecular mechanisms. Wildlife also act as sentinels of human health, alerting us to environmental threats and predicting possible risks to the human population from similar exposures. Biological systems, physiology, and molecular pathways in humans are similar to those of many wild species, and hence the transgenerational effects observed in wildlife models may be applicable to human health, even if routes of exposure, doses, or life histories vary. The investigation of such links is important for the development of holistic hazard assessment frameworks to safeguard wildlife and human health against transgenerational responses to metal toxicity.

7.10.2 Repercussions for food chains and food security

Somatic stress or other related effects of metal toxicity can leave a transgenerational legacy; such inheritance might be especially important in food chains, with implications for food security, because metals are known to biomagnify through the trophic levels and affect food quality, safety, and availability to humans. The transfer of metals into food chains takes place along several pathways, one being root uptake of metal-contaminated soils (soil-plant), body accumulation in aquatic organisms through contaminated waters and sediments, and subsequent action of both terrestrial and aquatic food webs (Parolini et al., 2022). For the long term, at least, it is possible that transgenerational effects modifying growth, survival, reproduction, or metal accumulation in animal taxa occurring at different trophic positions will impact food chain dynamics and ultimately change abundances or access to available food resources. These impacts may have implications for food security, particularly for human populations dependent on contaminated ecosystems for their subsistence (e.g., subsistence fishers, indigenous communities, and residents of contaminated areas).

7.10.3 Lack of regulation and policy issues

Legislation regarding metal toxicities and environmental risk assessment is not adapted to take into account transgenerational effects. Classic testing guidelines for toxicity, such as those developed by the OECD and regulatory agencies around the world, are based on acute or chronic tests that can last from hours to several weeks (and possibly at most a generation or two), with short-term ecological endpoints, i.e., relatively sensitive organisms. These tests provide insight into direct toxicity and support the development of regulatory thresholds, namely NOECs and LOECs, which are used to derive water quality criteria, soil quality guidelines, and other environmental standards. Nevertheless, these tests alone do not directly address potential transgenerational offspring effects that may develop in response to exposure after its cessation, potentially underestimating the long-term impacts of metal pollution.

7.11 Mitigation strategies and sustainable interventions

7.11.1 Bioremediation and phytoremediation approaches

Bioremediation and phytoremediation are being viewed with optimism as potential measures to minimize metal contamination in the environment and its consequent toxicity, including transgenerational risk. The organisms used in these methods are referred to in the context of bioremediation, wherein biological organisms, typically microorganisms, are applied to detoxify or eliminate metals from a contaminated environment. Plants are used to facilitate the process of phytoremediation, which can include phytoextraction, phytoimmobilization, phytostabilization, and/or rhizodegradation for inorganic or organic contaminants. These approaches provide "green" or low-cost alternatives to more traditional remediation technologies (e.g., excavation, soil washing, chemical treatment) that can be applied to large, diffuse areas of contamination or remote locations not readily accessible by conventional methods and where cost would otherwise be prohibitive.

7.11.2 Reducing metal bioavailability

Reducing the availability of metals is also an important strategy to alleviate metal toxicity and transgenerational hazards. Bioavailability refers to the portion of total metal that can be utilized by organisms, and a reduction in bioavailability may lessen exposure and toxicity without altering total metal levels (Szyf, 2023). Strategies to reduce metal bioavailability include amendments (which modify soil or water chemistry toward promote more favorable metal speciation and forms with lower bioavailability), approaches that minimize the mobility and transport potential of metals, and methods that inactivate, immobilize, or stabilize metals into less bioavailable forms.

7.11.3 Preventive environmental management

Preventive environmental management is the most efficient tool for diminishing metal toxicity and transgenerational hazards by hindering the contamination event before it happens. Compiling preventive strategies with transgenerational effects can help to protect against metal poisoning across generations. Pollution prevention measures focus on reducing or eliminating metal releases at the site's source rather than managing releases after they enter the environment. This involves changes to processes, new material technologies, recovery and reuse, recycling, and better operating practices. Process changes can decrease the quantity of metal used and waste produced through increased efficiency (e.g., closed-loop systems) and substitution for other processes. Substitution of materials can help replace harmful metals with less toxic ones, thereby preventing potential environmental pollution and transgenerational effects. Recycling and reuse can capture metals from waste streams, minimizing the need for virgin resources and avoiding releases (Wang et al., 2024b). Better operating practices, best management practices (BMPs), training, and preventive maintenance can help reduce accidental releases as well as increase the overall efficiency of processes. Such pollution prevention strategies would ultimately diminish background metal levels in the environment, possibly decreasing transgenerational risks of exposure.

7.12 Future aspects

7.12.1 Emerging metals and mixed-metal

New heavy metals, such as rare earth elements, PGMs, and other metalloids used in new technologies, pose a major challenge to the field of transgenerational toxicity. As we move toward an increasingly hi-tech society, with novel technologies including electronics, renewable systems, electric vehicles, and advanced materials being developed, some of these newer metals and metal mixtures are being used in larger quantities (with potential environmental releases) and possibly causing transgenerational effects. Rare earth elements like lanthanum, cerium, neodymium, and others are widely used in electronic industries, magnets, batteries, and catalysts, yet their environmental fate and toxicity, including multigenerational toxicity, have not been well studied. Platinum group metals, such as platinum, palladium, and rhodium, are utilized in catalytic converters along with many other industrial processes, and they flow into the environment mainly in urban areas; however, their transgenerational toxicity has not been well understood. Silver and other newly emerging metals from nanotechnology (e.g., engineered metal nanoparticles) pose special challenges for the study of transgenerational effects because they are highly reactive due to their extraordinary properties and behavior in environmental systems. Further studies are required to assess the environmental fate, toxicity, and trans-generational effects of these novel metals.

7.12.2 Climate change interactions

Climate change factors, such as temperature rise, drought, flooding, and ocean acidification, may also potentially interact with metal exposure to influence transgenerational outcomes. When organisms are exposed to more than one stressor, they can sometimes experience synergistic or antagonistic effects that deviate from expectations derived from single-stressor exposure. For instance, high temperatures can promote metal-induced oxidative stress and possibly amplify transgenerational consequences. The effect of ocean acidification on metal speciation and bioaccessibility in the marine environment may have implications for the transgenerational effects of metals in marine species. Drought effects may lead to metal bioaccumulation in water bodies and higher uptake through drinking water, with possible transgenerational effects. The interaction between climate change stressors and metal exposure on transgenerational effects needs more exploration to determine the mechanisms involved, as well as avenues for making predictions of interactive effects. Future research should examine a range of simulated climate change scenarios, metals and exposures, organisms, and ecosystems.

7.12.3 Translational and cross-species studies

Future directions will involve connecting model system discoveries to translational research. Translational research linking model system findings to ecology and human health is an important direction for the future. The majority of transgenerational metal toxicity studies have been carried out in laboratory models, i.e., rodents, zebrafish, *C. elegans,* and Arabidopsis, which offer insights into mechanisms but have uncertain applicability to natural populations or human health. Translational research is required to fill this gap and to link what is known at the cellular and model level with information from wild populations, across-species comparisons, or through comparisons to health-related scenarios in humans. This would include developing biomarkers found in model systems for use in field populations and humans, confirming trans-generational effects seen in models in wild populations and human cohorts, and translating mechanistic findings from models into interventions. Translational research demands cooperation between basic scientists, ecologists, epidemiologists, clinicians, and public health workers.

7.13 Conclusions

Transgenerational effects of metal toxicity are an important and currently underappreciated aspect of environmental contamination, as they compound the consequences of exposure to metals beyond those experienced by directly exposed organisms. Data from a wide-range of aquatic and terrestrial systems indicate that heavy metals, including cadmium, lead, mercury, arsenic, chromium, nickel, copper, and zinc, can cause heritable (transgenerational) toxic effects on the development, reproduction, behavior, metabolism, immune function, or survival of several aquatic animal species. These persistent effects are largely mediated by epigenetic processes, such as DNA methylation, histone modification, and noncoding RNA regulation, which allow environmental modifications of gene expression to be transmitted without changes in DNA sequence. The ecological consequences of these effects are significant, given that the transgenerational toxicity of pollutants can impact population dynamics, lower reproductive output, change species composition, and interfere with ecosystem functions, for example, through nutrient cycling, productivity, and food chain stability, while also interacting with evolutionary processes underpinning adaptation to contamination or improving resistance in such environments. From a human health standpoint, the conservation of these epigenetic mechanisms across species means that experimental and wildlife studies provide insights that apply to human populations, especially considering long-term environmental exposure and food-chain transfer. However, even though these consequences raise new issues for species survival, long-term regulatory and risk assessment approaches do not usually consider trans-generational endpoints, thereby possibly underestimating the long-term risks to ecological and human health. Therefore, identifying and incorporating transgenerational effects into environmental management, risk assessment, and disease prevention is critical in order to achieve eco system health and human well-being benefits for current and future generations.

References

Al-Asadi, M.S., et al., 2023. Multigenerational effects of cadmium on *Daphnia magna*: life history and molecular responses. Chemosphere 315, 137782.

Amiard-Triquet, C., Amiard, J.C., 2023. Ecotoxicology of Metals in Aquatic and Terrestrial Ecosystems: A Generational Perspective, CRC Press.

Anastasiadi, D., Piferrer, F., 2023. Epigenetic inheritance in fish: mechanisms and implications for adaptation to environmental change. Mar. Environ. Res. 189, 106041.

Banni, M., et al., 2024. The role of non-coding RNAs in metal-induced transgenerational toxicity. Trends Genet. 40 (3), 215–228.

Bi, J., et al., 2023. Transgenerational effects of cadmium on the gut microbiota and immunity of the earthworm *Eisenia fetida*. J. Hazard. Mater. 448, 130942.

Bilichak, A., Ilnystkyy, Y., Hollunder, J., Kovalchuk, I., 2012. The progeny of Arabidopsis thaliana plants exposed to salt exhibit changes in DNA methylation, histone modifications and gene expression. PLoS One 7 (1), e30515.

Bollati, V., Baccarelli, A., 2022. Environmental epigenetics: heredity and the environment. Clin. Chem. Lab. Med. 60 (10), 1541–1549.

Bonduriansky, R., 2021. Plasticity across generations. In: Phenotypic Plasticity & Evolution. CRC Press, pp. 327–348.

Burggren, W.W., 2020. Phenotypic switching resulting from developmental plasticity: fixed or reversible? Front. Physiol. 1664-042X. 10. doi:10.3389/fphys.2019.01634.

Cao, Z., et al., 2024. Multigenerational effects of lead on the life-history traits of Drosophila melanogaster. Chemosphere 349, 140812.

Cedergreen, N., Sørensen, H., Svendsen, C., 2012. Can the joint effect of ternary mixtures be predicted from binary mixture toxicity results? Sci. Total Environ. 427, 229–237.

Chen, Q., et al., 2022. Maternal transfer of silver nanoparticles and its transgenerational effects on zebrafish. Environ. Pollut. 292, 118412.

Da Silva, J.C., et al., 2024. Transgenerational impacts of mercury on the physiology and behavior of neotropical fish. Sci. Total Environ. 908, 168345.

Diogo, R., et al., 2022. Transgenerational impact of arsenic on the fitness and DNA methylation of terrestrial isopods. Environ. Sci. Pollut. Res. 29 (15), 22104–22115.

Eirin-Lopez, J.M., Putnam, H.M., 2019. Marine environmental epigenetics. Annu. Rev. Mar. Sci. 19410611. 11, 335–368. Available from: http://www.annualreviews.org/journal/marine. doi:10.1146/annurev-marine-010318-095114.

Fallet, M., Montagnani, C., Pepey, E., Cosseau, C., 2020. Epigenetic inheritance in environmental adaptation: lessons from aquatic organisms. Epigenomes 4 (3), 18.

Fu, X., et al., 2023. Parental exposure to copper nanoparticles induces transgenerational toxicity in *Caenorhabditis elegans*. NanoImpact 29, 100445.
Gao, M., et al., 2022. Transgenerational effects of heavy metal exposure on soil invertebrates: a systematic review. Appl. Soil Ecol. 170, 104289.
Grzybowska-Swierkosz, J., et al., 2023. Physiological and biochemical responses across generations of earthworms exposed to metal-contaminated soil. Soil Biol. Biochem. 178, 108945.
Gu, Y., et al., 2023. Transgenerational effects of arsenic exposure on the development and immune system of zebrafish. J. Hazard. Mater. 442, 130021.
Guan, R., Wang, W.X., 2021. Transgenerational effects of parental exposure to silver nanoparticles in *Daphnia magna*. Environ. Sci. Nano 8 (1), 125–136.
Han, S., et al., 2024. Transgenerational neurotoxicity of manganese in *C. elegans* mediated by histone modification. Cell Biol. Toxicol. 40 (1), 12.
He, X., et al., 2022. Cadmium-induced transgenerational male infertility is associated with sperm DNA methylation in mice. Environ. Pollut. 310, 119865.
Head, J.A., et al., 2022. DNA methylation as a biomarker of environmental exposure in wildlife. Environ. Toxicol. Chem. 41 (1), 35–48.
Heindel, J.J., Vandenberg, L.N., 2022. Developmental origins of health and disease: a paradigm shift in toxicology. Environ. Health Perspect. 130(2), 025001.
Hu, J., et al., 2023. Transgenerational effects of parental lead exposure on the cognitive behavior of mice. Toxicol. Appl. Pharmacol. 462, 116405.
Huang, Y., et al., 2025. Chronic lead exposure induces transgenerational neurotoxicity in Oryzias latipes. Aquat. Toxicol. 266, 106789.
Jeong, C.B., et al., 2022. Transgenerational effects of heavy metals on marine copepods: a multi-omics approach. Mar. Pollut. Bull. 175, 113354.
Jeremias, G., et al., 2022. Epigenetic mechanisms in the transgenerational toxicity of chemicals. Environ. Sci. Technol. 56 (12), 7412–7425.
Jiang, J., et al., 2024. Maternal transfer and transgenerational toxicity of methylmercury in aquatic food webs. Environ. Sci. Technol. 58 (4), 1892–1904.
Jiang, M., et al., 2025. Multigenerational effects of mercury on the growth and antioxidant status of Acheta domesticus. Environ. Entomol. 54 (1), 112–121.
Jose, C.C., Wang, Z., Tanwar, V.S., Zhang, X., Zang, C., Cuddapah, S., 2019. Nickel-induced transcriptional changes persist post exposure through epigenetic reprogramming. Epigenetics Chromatin. 12 (1), 75.
Kandola, S., Giesy, J.P., 2024. Molecular mechanisms of metal-induced epigenetic modifications. J. Hazard. Mater. 461, 132641.
Kille, P., et al., 2024. Genomic and epigenetic signatures of metal adaptation in soil invertebrates. Nat. Ecol. Evol. 8 (2), 290–305.
Kim, J., et al., 2023. Epigenetic transgenerational inheritance of cadmium-induced metabolic syndrome in terrestrial mammals. J. Toxicol. Environ. Health A 86 (4), 145–160.
Li, M., et al., 2022. Transgenerational effects of hexavalent chromium on the growth and reproduction of *Daphnia similis*. Ecotoxicol. Environ. Saf. 231, 113175.
Li, Y., et al., 2024. Transgenerational effects of copper on the fitness and detoxification enzymes of the silkworm, *Bombyx mori*. Insects 15 (2), 104.
Liu, H., et al., 2022. Long-term effects of chromium on the reproductive strategy of the collembolan *Folsomia candida*. Pedobiologia 90, 150785.
Liu, X., et al., 2023. Maternal exposure to zinc oxide nanoparticles causes transgenerational skeletal defects in zebrafish. Sci. Total Environ. 857, 159421.

Luo, J., et al., 2024. Transgenerational impacts of manganese on the antioxidant system of *Carassius auratus*. Fish Shellfish Immunol. 145, 109292.

Lushchak, V.I., et al., 2023. Metal-induced oxidative stress: from molecular mechanisms to transgenerational effects. Arch. Toxicol. 97 (2), 345–372.

Ma, L., et al., 2023. Transgenerational impacts of arsenic on the development of honeybee (*Apis mellifera*) larvae. Environ. Sci. Technol. 57 (11), 4521–4532.

Noguera, J.C., et al., 2023. Early-life lead exposure induces transgenerational effects on bird growth and telomere dynamics. Proc. R. Soc. B 290 (1995), 20222543.

Onsanit, S., et al., 2022. Bioaccumulation and maternal transfer of toxic metals in marine teleosts. Mar. Pollut. Bull. 180, 113791.

Pan, Y., et al., 2024. Epigenetic mechanisms of transgenerational toxicity induced by nickel in mice. Environ. Sci. Pollut. Res. 31 (5), 7890–7902.

Parolini, M., et al., 2022. Transgenerational effects of contaminants of emerging concern on aquatic organisms: a review. Environ. Int. 160, 107057.

Pereira, J.L., et al., 2023. DNA methylation patterns in *Daphnia magna* across generations of metal stress. J. Appl. Toxicol. 43 (5), 712–725.

Riar, M., et al., 2023. Transgenerational epigenetic responses to salinity and metal stress in freshwater invertebrates. Evol. Appl. 16 (4), 882–895.

Ricardo, M.-Z., Hyo, C.H., 2011. Environmental epigenetics in metal exposure. Nat. Rev. Genet. 6 (7) , 820–827. doi:10.4161/epi.6.7.16250.

Santamaria, C.A., et al., 2022. Transgenerational effects of heavy metals in wild rodent populations from mining sites. Ecol. Indic. 136, 108654.

Senut, M.C., et al., 2012. Lead exposure disrupts global DNA methylation in human embryonic stem cells and alters differentiation. Environ. Health Perspect. 120, 1356–1362.

Skinner, M.K., 2021. Environmental epigenetic transgenerational inheritance. Mol. Cell. Endocrinol. 526, 111210.

Skinner, M.K., Guerrero-Bosagna, C., 2009. Environmental signals and transgenerational epigenetics. Epigenomics 1 (1), 111–117.

Sun, H., et al., 2022. Lead-induced transgenerational neurotoxicity is mediated by DNA methylation in zebrafish. Chemosphere 303, 135118.

Szyf, M., 2023. The epigenome as a mediator of environmental challenges across generations. Ann. N. Y. Acad. Sci. 1522 (1), 45–58.

Tao, J., et al., 2024. Transgenerational effects of soil cadmium on the growth of *Arabidopsis thaliana* and its herbivores. Plant Soil 495, 233–248.

Vandegehuchte, M.B., Janssen, C.R., 2014. Epigenetics in an ecotoxicological context. Mutat. Res. 764–765, 36–45.

Wang, T., et al., 2024a. Impacts of parental copper exposure on the microbiome and fitness of F1 offspring in *Mytilus edulis*. Environ. Res. 241, 117562.

Wang, X., et al., 2024b. Global patterns of transgenerational metal toxicity: a meta-analysis. Glob. Change Biol. 30 (1), e17056.

Wang, Y., Weng, Y., Lv, L., Wang, D., Yang, G., Jin, Y., Wang, Q., 2022. Transgenerational effects of co-exposure to cadmium and carbofuran on zebrafish based on biochemical and transcriptomic analyses. J. Hazard. Mater. 439, 129644.

Wu, L., et al., 2023. Transgenerational effects of cadmium on the development of the nervous system in Danio rerio. Toxicology 486, 153441.

Zhang, C., et al., 2023. Maternal transfer of lead and its impact on the development of the lizard *Eremias argus*. J. Hazard. Mater. 452, 131235.

Zhang, Y., et al., 2024. Multigenerational exposure to mercury causes persistent metabolic disorders in tilapia. J. Hazard. Mater. 465, 133120.

Zhao, X., et al., 2022. Multigenerational effects of arsenic on the development and gene expression of the midge *Chironomus riparius*. Environ. Pollut. 306, 119421.

Zheng, G., et al., 2022. Transgenerational effects of nickel exposure on the reproductive success of *Artemia salina*. Ecotoxicology 31 (6), 945–955.

Chapter 8

Hidden metal reservoirs in the food chain: Soil microaggregates as metal sinks

Ananta Shrivastava[a], Kritika Singh[a], Kaushlendra Kumar[a], Hema Kumari[a], and Bushra Shaida[b]

[a]*Department of Biomedical Science, School of Biosciences and Technology, Galgotia University, Greater Noida, India*

[b]*Center for Nutrition and Dietetics, SIST, Jamia Hamdard, New Delhi, India*

8.1 Introduction to soil microaggregates and metal dynamics

Soil plays a vital role in agricultural productivity and is a major storehouse for environmental pollutants. It forms an essential link or interface between geological, biological, and human systems. The condition of terrestrial soil directly affects public health, ecosystem stability, and food security because the soil-based agriculture system supports nearly 95% of the world's food supply. Metal pollution is one of the most enduring and persistent environmental challenges affecting agriculture worldwide. This problem has intensified over the past hundred years due to rapid industrial growth, urbanization, and intensified agricultural practices (Alloway, 2013).

Because heavy metals do not break down naturally, heavy metals like cadmium (Cd), lead (Pb), zinc (Zn), copper (Cu), and nickel (Ni) remain in soil for a long time. As their persistence increases, bioaccumulation poses long-term threats to human health and agricultural productivity (Kabata-Pendias, 2010).

Certain metals are crucial micronutrients at optimal concentrations, but when they accumulate in excess, they can cause phytotoxicity, lower yields, and food chain contamination (Stephan Clemens, 2016). Metals enter soil through a variety of natural geogenic pathways and significant anthropogenic sources, which mostly include phosphate fertilizers, sewage sludge, industrial effluents, mining operations, and urban runoff (Alloway, 2013; Nanthi Bolan, 2014).

Despite persistent and pervasive pollution, very little is known about the mechanisms controlling metal retention and mobilization in soil.

The Metallome in Motion. https://doi.org/10.1016/B978-0-443-44299-5.00005-5

Recent studies indicate that soil microaggregates (<250 μm), which are tiny structural units formed through organo-metallic interactions, act as hidden reservoirs that majorly impact food chain transfer and metal bioavailability (Six and B, 2004). These microaggregates function as shielding domains through complicated physicochemical processes that include soil pH, redox conditions, cation exchange capacity (CEC), organic matter (OM) complexation, and Fe/Mn/Al oxide interactions (Sparks, 2003). It is important to understand the geochemical processes, ecological effects, and long-term stabilization mechanisms governing metal retention in soil microaggregates in order to evaluate contamination risk, direct remediation strategies, and protect ecosystems and human health in metal-affected environments.

8.2 Sources and types of metals in agricultural soils

Soil microaggregates play a crucial yet underexplored role as hidden reservoirs for metals within terrestrial food chains. These micro-scale structures, formed through complex organo-metallic interactions, serve as sinks for metals such as iron, aluminum, and potentially toxic elements introduced via natural processes and human activities. Recent studies reveal that microaggregates not only stabilize OM through the "organo-metallic glue" mechanism but also influence the mobility and bioavailability of metals, thereby affecting their entry into the food web. Industrial pollution, especially from steelworks, enhances metal accumulation and changes the physicochemical environment of microaggregates, leading to acidification, increased redox potential, and the formation of dissipative structures that further impact OM turnover and metal cycling. Heavy metal stress disrupts soil microbial communities, reduces aggregation, and accelerates OM decomposition, ultimately decreasing soil carbon sequestration and raising the risk of metal transfer to crops and higher trophic levels. Understanding the geochemical processes and ecological effects related to metal retention in soil microaggregates is key for assessing food chain contamination risks, guiding soil remediation efforts, and protecting ecosystem and human health in environments affected by metals.

Because it provides the nutrients, water, and microorganisms needed for cultivation, soil is essential to ecosystems. Nearly 95% of global food production relies on soil-based systems, making the quality of agricultural soils intimately related to human health and food security (Nations, 2022). Soil degradation and contamination have become prevalent during the past century due to rapid industrial growth, urbanization, and increased agriculture. Heavy metals are particularly dangerous among other pollutants because of their inability to decompose, their persistent presence in soils, and their propensity to accumulate in crops and subsequently in people (Alloway, 2013). Metals can linger for decades or even centuries, posing long-term dangers in contrast to organic contaminants that gradually break down over time.

Elements with a density greater than 5 g/cm^3 are commonly referred to as heavy metals, and even small concentrations of them can be dangerous. Certain elements, such as zinc (Zn), copper (Cu), and nickel (Ni), are essential for the metabolism of both plants and animals. On the other hand, lead (Pb) and cadmium (Cd) are poisonous to all living things and have no known beneficial function (P. C. Nagajyoti, 2010). The problem is that some metals can be both toxicants and necessary micronutrients, which makes managing them in soils more difficult. For instance, too much zinc can limit nutrient uptake and impede root growth, while too little zinc might reduce crop yields. Through air deposition, volcanic activity, and rock weathering, metals gradually find their way into soils in natural ecosystems. According to Kabata-Pendias (2010), these activities provide a natural baseline concentration that changes depending on soil type, climate, and geology (Kabata-Pendias, 2010). However, metal levels in agricultural soils around the world are currently dominated by human activity. Higher concentrations of Cd, Pb, Cu, Zn, and Ni in cultivated fields are caused by phosphate rock-based fertilizers, sewage sludge containing industrial waste, livestock manure with metal additions, and irrigation with untreated wastewater (Nanthi Bolan, 2014). Large volumes of metals are released into adjacent agricultural regions as a result of industrial activities, particularly mining and smelting, which exacerbate contamination.

Soil pollution by heavy metals has complex impacts. Metals can disturb microbial communities, reduce enzymatic activity, and impede the cycling of nutrients at the soil level (Giller and Witter, 2009). Metal stress can cause stunted growth, inhibit efficient photosynthesis, and lower crop production. Furthermore, when metals are absorbed by plants, contaminated fruits, vegetables, and cereals provide a direct pathway for human exposure. For example, renal impairment, bone loss, and cancer are associated with long-term exposure to Cd (Organization, 2021). Lead exposure in children can result in developmental delays and cognitive problems (Figs. 8.1–8.3).

Globally, approximately 15% of the world's cropland is estimated to be polluted with toxic levels of heavy metals (Campbell, 2025). Regions in South Asia, Sub-Saharan Africa, and Eastern Europe are particularly vulnerable due to intensive agricultural practices coupled with weak regulatory oversight. At the same time, developed regions such as the European Union and North America face legacy contamination issues stemming from decades of industrial activity and the historical use of leaded petrol.

Given the scale of the problem, it is critical to understand the diverse sources and dynamics of metal contamination in soils. This chapter provides a comprehensive examination of natural and anthropogenic sources, the behavior of common metals in soils, and their ecological and health impacts. It further explores monitoring techniques, risk assessment frameworks, and mitigation strategies, with an emphasis on global regulatory perspectives. The ultimate goal is to support sustainable soil management practices that balance agricultural productivity with environmental protection and food safety.

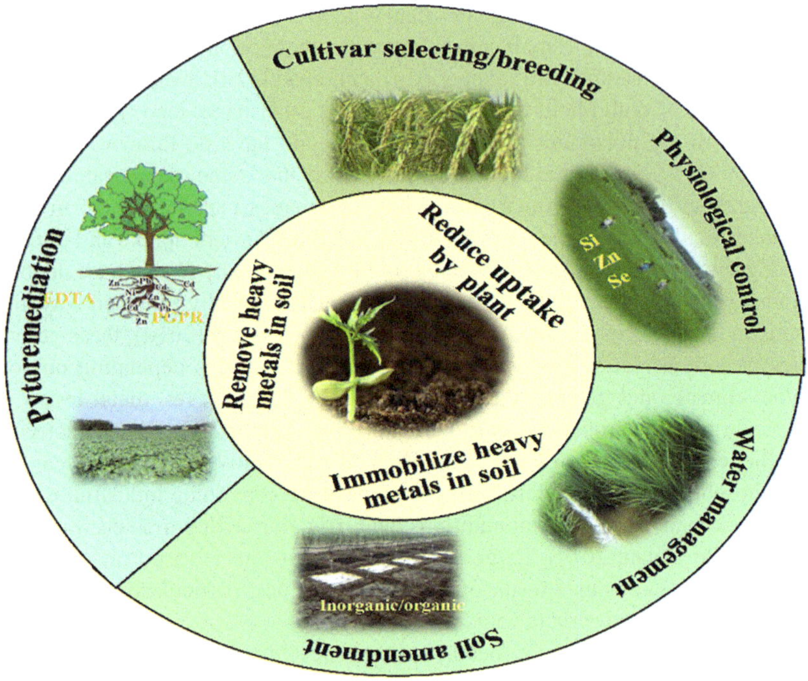

FIG. 8.1 Sustainable strategies for mitigating heavy metal contamination in soils. *(From: Yanan Wan, J.L., 2024. Heavy metals in agricultural soils: sources, influencing factors, and remediation strategies. Impact Heavy Metal Contam. Soil Environ. Adv. Remediat. Strateg. 12 (1), 63.)*

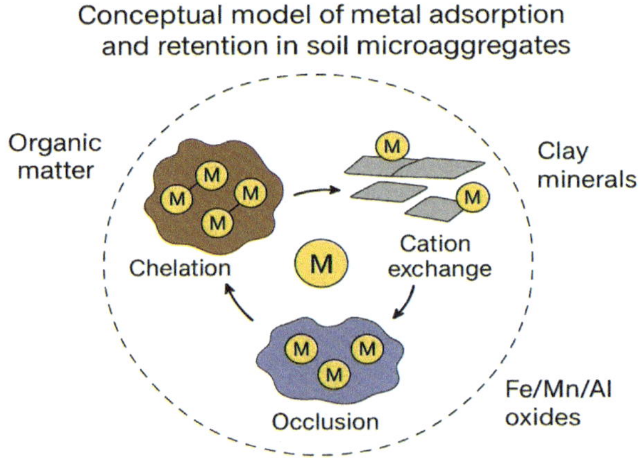

FIG. 8.2 Conceptual model of metal adsorption. *(Source: Alloway, B.J., 2013. Heavy Metals in Soils: Trace Metals and Metalloids in Soils and Their Bioavailability (Third ed.). Springer.)*

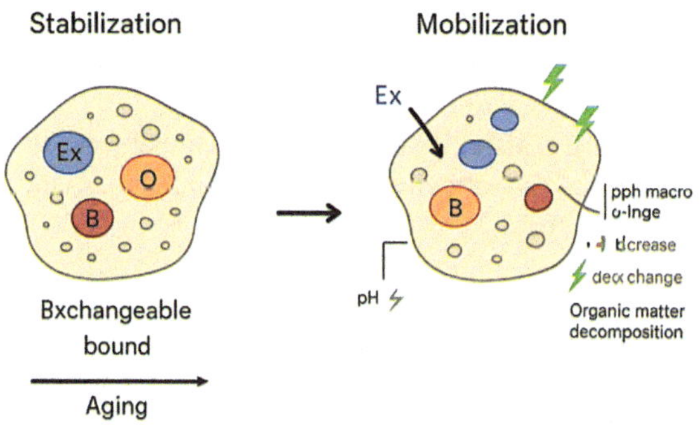

FIG. 8.3 Illustrate Pathways of metal stabilisation an mobilisation in soil microaggregates. *(Adapted from Sparks, D.L. (Ed.), 2003. Environmental soil chemistry: an overview. In: Environmental Soil Chemistry, second ed. Academic Press, pp. 1–42; Alloway, B.J. (Ed.), 2013. Sources of heavy metals and metalloids in soils. In: Heavy Metals in Soils Trace Metals and Metalloids in Soils and Their Bioavailability. Springer Nature, pp. 11–50; Violante, A.U.D.N., Cozzolino, V.U.D.N., Perelomov, L.P.S.U., Caporale, A.G., Pigna, M.U.D.N., 2010. Mobility and bioavailability of heavy metals and metalloids in soil environments. J. Soil Sci. Plant Nutr. 10 (3), 268–292.)*

8.2.1 Natural (geogenic) versus anthropogenic sources

8.2.1.1 Natural (geogenic) sources

- **Parent material/bedrock:** Weathering of rocks releases metals into soils; areas derived from metal-rich lithologies (e.g., ultramafic rocks) show naturally higher Ni and Cr. Soil mineralogy and topography influence baseline concentrations (Zheng Liu, 2023).
- **Atmospheric long-range deposition (natural):** Volcanic ash and wind-blown dust contribute baseline metal inputs in some regions.

8.2.1.2 Anthropogenic sources (dominant in most agricultural areas)

- **Fertilizers and soil amendments:** Certain phosphate fertilizers contain cadmium (Cd) and other trace metals; repeated application over the years increases soil loads (Alengebawy, 2021).
- **Sewage sludge/biosolids and manure:** Sewage biosolids often contain trace metals (Pb, Ni, Cd, Cu, Zn), depending on urban/industrial inputs; land application can be a significant source (Martyna Buta, 2021).
- **Pesticides and agrochemicals:** Historically, some pesticides and their formulations contained metal impurities or metal-based active ingredients (e.g., Cu-based fungicides) (Alengebawy, 2021).
- **Irrigation with contaminated water/wastewater reuse:** Using untreated or partially treated wastewater for irrigation transfers metals to soils and crops (Bibhabasu Mohanty, 2021).

- **Industrial emissions/smelting/mining:** Stack emissions, fugitive dust, and slag deposition from smelters and mines strongly elevate nearby soil metal contents (e.g., Pb, Cu, Zn).
- **Urban runoff and traffic:** Road dust, tire and brake wear, and urban stormwater carry metals (historically Pb, as well as Zn, Cu, and Ni) into peri-urban agricultural soils.

8.2.1.3 Distinguishing natural versus anthropogenic metals

One of the biggest scientific and regulatory challenges is differentiating natural background levels from anthropogenic contamination. For example:

Cadmium may naturally be high in phosphate-rich soils but is also introduced via phosphate fertilizers.

Lead can derive from mineral-rich rocks or urban pollution.

Techniques used to distinguish sources include:

- **Geochemical mapping**—Comparing soils to underlying geology.
- **Isotopic signatures**—Lead isotopes, for instance, can reveal whether Pb comes from petrol, industry, or geology.
- **Enrichment factors (EFs)**—Ratios of trace metals to reference elements (e.g., Al, Fe, Ti) help identify excess contributions above natural levels.

8.2.1.4 Significance of natural metal inputs

Although natural sources generally contribute lower concentrations than anthropogenic inputs, they remain important for several reasons:

- **Baseline assessment**—They set the reference against which pollution is measured.
- **Agricultural productivity**—Many natural metals are micronutrients essential for plant growth.
- **Environmental risk**—In some regions, natural levels of arsenic, cadmium, or nickel already exceed health-based thresholds, making soils inherently risky for agriculture.
- For example, groundwater arsenic contamination in parts of West Bengal and Bangladesh originates from natural geochemical processes rather than industrial discharge, yet it still poses severe health hazards through rice cultivation.

8.2.2 Common metals found in soils (e.g., Cd, Pb, Zn, Cu, Ni)

Heavy metals are naturally present in soils due to geological processes, but their concentrations are increasingly altered by anthropogenic activities such as mining, industrial discharges, fertilizer use, and wastewater irrigation. Among them, cadmium (Cd), lead (Pb), zinc (Zn), copper (Cu), and nickel (Ni) are the most frequently studied because of their widespread occurrence, persistence, and potential risks to agriculture and human health. This section provides a detailed overview of their sources, soil behavior, plant uptake, ecological and health impacts, and regulatory guidelines.

8.2.2.1 Cadmium (Cd)

- **Sources**
- **Natural**: Parent material, phosphate rocks.
- **Anthropogenic**: Phosphate fertilizers (major source), sewage sludge, mining/smelting, electroplating industries, and irrigation with contaminated wastewater (Kabata-Pendias, 2010).
- **Soil behavior**

  Cd is highly **mobile in soils**, especially in acidic and sandy soils.
  Strongly influenced by soil pH and OM; it is more available at low pH.
  It tends to accumulate in the **surface horizon** due to fertilizer inputs.
- **Plant uptake**
  Easily absorbed by cereals, leafy vegetables, and rice.
  Competes with zinc and calcium uptake systems in plants.
  High bioaccumulation factor makes Cd a concern for food safety (Stephan Clemens, 2016).
- **Health and environmental impacts**
  Chronic Cd exposure causes Itai-Itai disease, kidney dysfunction, and bone demineralization.
  Listed as a Group 1 carcinogen by the IARC.
  Adverse effects on soil microbes and enzyme activity, even at low concentrations.
- **Guideline values – EU soil limit**: 1–3 mg/kg.
- **World Health Organization (WHO) food standard**: ≤0.1 mg/kg in cereals.

8.2.2.2 Lead (Pb)

- **Sources**
- **Natural**: Geological mineralization (Galena ore).
- **Anthropogenic**: Leaded petrol (historical legacy), paints, batteries, smelting industries, sewage sludge, and urban dust (Adriano, 2001).
- **Soil behavior**

  Pb is strongly adsorbed onto soil particles, especially clays and OM.
  Immobile under neutral to alkaline conditions but more soluble under acidic conditions.
  Forms stable complexes with phosphates and OM.
- **Plant uptake**
  Low translocation from roots to shoots.
  Most Pb remains in the rhizosphere or root cortex.
  However, leafy vegetables (e.g., spinach, lettuce) can accumulate significant Pb levels when grown in contaminated soils (Sharma and Dubey, 2005).

- **Health and environmental impacts**
  Pb has no biological function and is toxic at all concentrations.
  Causes neurological disorders, cognitive impairment, and developmental delays in children.
  Soil contamination with Pb reduces microbial biomass and alters enzymatic processes.

- **Guideline values—EU soil limit**: 50–300 mg/kg.
- **United States Environmental Protection Agency (US EPA) screening level**: 400 mg/kg for residential soils.

8.2.2.3 Zinc (Zn)

- **Sources**
- **Natural**: Parent rock weathering.
- **Anthropogenic**: Galvanization, mining, Zn-rich fertilizers and pesticides, sewage sludge, and manure (Broadley and J, 2007).
- **Soil behavior**
  Zn is relatively mobile in soils compared to Pb.
  More soluble at acidic pH, while alkaline soils often immobilize zinc (Zn).
  Strongly bound to OM and Fe/Mn oxides.
- **Plant uptake**
  Zn is an essential micronutrient required for enzyme activity, protein synthesis, and plant growth.
  Deficiency is common in calcareous soils, affecting cereals such as wheat and rice.
  Excess Zn, however, causes phytotoxicity: chlorosis, stunted root growth, and nutrient imbalance.
- **Health and environmental impacts**
  Zn is essential for humans, but excessive intake can cause nausea, anemia, and immune dysfunction.
  Soils rich in Zn from industrial wastes can inhibit microbial diversity.

- **Guideline values—EU soil limit**: 150–300 mg/kg.
- **Indian permissible limit in sewage sludge for land application**: 2500 mg/kg (Vasudevan, 2016).

8.2.2.4 Copper (Cu)

- **Sources**
- **Natural**: Parent rocks, volcanic soils.
- **Anthropogenic**: Fungicides (e.g., Bordeaux mixture), mining and smelting, industrial effluents, manure, and sewage sludge.
- **Soil behavior**

Cu is relatively immobile due to strong adsorption to OM and clay minerals.
More readily available in sandy and acidic soils.
Forms stable complexes with humic substances.

- **Plant uptake**
  Essential micronutrient: required for photosynthesis, lignin synthesis, and enzyme activity.
  Deficiency results in chlorosis, reduced reproductive growth, and grain sterility in cereals.
  Toxicity occurs at high concentrations, leading to root necrosis and oxidative stress.
- **Health and environmental impacts**
  Cu is essential for human health (hemoglobin synthesis, enzyme function).
  Excess intake causes liver damage, Wilson's disease, and gastrointestinal problems.
  In soils, excessive Cu reduces microbial activity and earthworm populations.

- **Guideline values— European Union (EU) soil limit**: 50–140 mg/kg.
- **Fppd and Agriculture Organization (FAO) irrigation water guideline**: ≤0.2 mg/L Cu.

8.2.2.5 Nickel (Ni)

- **Sources**
- **Natural**: Ultramafic rocks, serpentine soils (naturally Ni-rich).
- **Anthropogenic**: Electroplating industries, stainless steel production, fertilizers, fossil fuel combustion, and sewage sludge (Cuiyun Chen, 2009).
- **Soil behavior**
  Ni exists mostly in exchangeable and carbonate-bound forms, making it moderately mobile.
  Solubility is strongly influenced by pH: it is more available in acidic soils.
  Often cooccurs with chromium (Cr) and cobalt (Co) in ultramafic soils.
- **Plant uptake**
  Ni is an essential element in small amounts (urease enzyme activation).
  Deficiency is rare, but toxicity occurs when Ni exceeds 50 mg/kg in the soil.
  High accumulation in hyperaccumulator plants (e.g., *Alyssum* spp.) is useful for phytoremediation.
- **Health and environmental impacts**
  Excess Ni in food crops causes allergic dermatitis, respiratory issues, and carcinogenic effects in humans (IARC Group 1 carcinogen).
  Affects nitrogen fixation in legumes and alters the soil microbial community.

- **Guideline values—EU soil limit**: 30–75 mg/kg.
- **Canadian soil quality guideline**: 50 mg/kg for agricultural land.

8.2.3 Agricultural practices that contribute to metal contamination

8.2.3.1 Fertilizer and lime application

Phosphate fertilizers (especially those derived from rock-phosphate) are often the primary agricultural pathway for Cd and other trace metals. Repeated use accumulates metals in cultivated topsoils (Tables 8.1–8.7).

8.2.3.2 Sewage sludge/biosolids and animal manures

Sludge applied as an organic amendment can contain significant metal loads depending on the source; long-term application requires monitoring and adherence to limits. Manure may also concentrate metals (from animal feed additives) (Goss, 2013).

8.2.3.3 Pesticides and copper-based fungicides

Copper-based fungicides are widely used in orchards and vineyards; repeated applications can raise Cu levels in surface soils (Alengebawy, 2021).

TABLE 8.1 Common heavy metals—soil behavior and common anthropogenic sources (Alengebawy, 2021).

Metal	Natural sources	Anthro-pogenic sources	Soil behaviour/ toxicity	Anthropogenic sources
Cadmium (Cd)	Phosphate Rocks	Fertilizers, sewage sludge, mining	Highly mobile in acidic soils and readily taken up by crops. Toxic to humans.	Phosphate fertilizers, sewage sludge, and industrial discharges
Lead (Pb)	Galena Ores	Petrol, batteries, smelting	Strongly adsorbed, low mobility, but high risk via ingestion. Neurotoxic.	Legacy petrol emissions, smelting, and urban runoff.
Zinc (Zn)	Parent Rocks	Fertilizers, sewage sludge	Essential nutrient, toxic at high concentrations.	Fertilizers, manure, sludge, industry
Copper (Cu)	Rocks, volcanic soils	Fungicides, sludge, mining	Micronutrient binds to organic matter; toxic at high levels.	Cu-based fungicides, mining, industrial wastes
Nickel (Ni)	Ultramafic rocks	Industry, fuels, fertilizers	Variable behavior, phytotoxic at high levels.	Mining, metal industry, fertilizers

Table showing cadmium, lead, zinc, copper, and nickel with their soil behavior and anthropogenic sources.

TABLE 8.2 Agricultural practice, primary metals of concern, and pathway.

Agricultural practice	Primary metals of concern	Pathway
Phosphate fertilizers	Cd, Pb	Direct soil addition
Sewage sludge/biosolids	Cd, Cu, Zn, Pb, Ni	Amendment application
Livestock manure	Zn, Cu	Amendment application
Wastewater irrigation	Pb, Cd, Ni, Cr, Zn	Irrigation water deposition
Cu-based pesticides	Cu	Foliar deposition → soil wash-off

TABLE 8.3 Industrial runoff versus urban runoff.

Parameter	Industrial runoff	Urban runoff
Main metals	Cd, Cr, Pb, Ni, Cu, As, Hg	Pb, Zn, Cu, Cd, Cr
Pathways	Direct irrigation, effluent discharge, sludge	Stormwater, wastewater reuse, roadside deposition
Crop contamination	High (Cd, Pb in rice & vegetables)	Moderate to high (Pb, Zn in leafy vegetables).
Soil impact	Severe toxicity, reduced microbial activity	Soil enrichment near cities, peri-urban risk.
Health risks	Kidney, liver, cancer risks	Neurological, cardiovascular, developmental issues

TABLE 8.4 Summary of physicochemical controls.

Factor	Influence on metal adsorption
pH	Low pH increases mobility; high pH promotes precipitation and adsorption
CEC	High CEC soils retain more metals; strongly pH-dependent
Redox potential (Eh)	Reducing conditions release metals; oxidizing conditions immobilize them
Organic matter	Chelation immobilizes metals; soluble complexes enhance mobility
Clay mineralogy	2:1 clays strongly retain metals; kaolinite is less effective
Fe/Mn/Al Oxides	Strong sorbents under oxic conditions dissolve and release metals under reducing conditions

Both soil-specific factors (pH, texture, redox state) and metal-specific characteristics (ionic radius, charge, hydrolysis behavior) affect metal adsorption on soil microaggregates.

TABLE 8.5 Key physicochemical factors influencing metal adsorption in soil microaggregates.

Property	Effect on metal retention	Examples
Soil pH	Higher pH reduces solubility and promotes the precipitation of hydroxides and carbonates	Pb^{2+}, Cd^{2+}, Zn^{2+} immobilized at neutral–alkaline pH
Cation exchange capacity (CEC)	Higher CEC increases adsorption capacity	Soils with smectite clays retain Ni^{2+}, Zn^{2+}
Redox potential (Eh)	Reducing conditions dissolve Fe/Mn oxides, releasing metals; oxidizing conditions promote immobilization	As, Mn, Fe
Surface area	Finer soils adsorb more metals due to their greater reactive surface	Clays > silts > sands
Ionic properties	Smaller ions with higher charges form stronger bonds	$Cr^{3+} > Ni^{2+} > Cd^{2+}$

Sources: (Alloway, 2013) and (Sparks, 2003).

TABLE 8.6 Comparative roles of soil components in metal retention.

Component	Key retention mechanisms	Metals most affected	Environmental sensitivity
Organic matter	Chelation, complexation, physical entrapment	Cu, Pb, Cd, Ni	Decomposition may release metals
Clay minerals	Cation exchange, interlayer fixation, surface adsorption.	Pb, Cd, Zn, Ni	Less effective in sandy soils
Fe/Mn/Al oxides	Adsorption, ligand exchange, coprecipitation, occlusion	Pb, Cu, Zn, As, Co	Dissolve under reducing conditions

Sources: (Stevenson, 1999) and (Violante et al., 2010).

8.2.3.4 *Wastewater irrigation*

Use of contaminated or partially treated wastewater concentrates metals in soils and, ultimately, in crop tissues (riskier for root and leafy crops).

8.2.3.5 *Tillage and soil disturbance*

Resuspension of contaminated dust and redistribution of contaminated topsoil layers; no direct addition, but it alters distribution and exposure risk.

TABLE 8.7 Major binding forms of heavy metals in soil microaggregates (Tessier et al., 1979) and (Sparks, 2003).

Fraction	Description	Mobility/ bioavailability	Examples
Exchangeable	Weakly bound via electrostatic interactions; easily displaced.	High (readily available)	Cd, Zn
Carbonate-bound	Associated with carbonate minerals	Moderate (pH-sensitive)	Pb, Zn
Fe–Mn oxide-bound	Adsorbed or occluded in oxide coatings.	Low unless under reducing conditions	As, Pb, Cr
Organic-bound	Complexed with humic substances or microbial biomass.	Low–moderate (released upon OM decay)	Cu, Pb
Residual	Incorporated into mineral lattices	Very low (stable, immobile)	Ni, Cr

Sources: Tessier, A.P.G.C., Campbell, P.G., Bisson, M.J.A.C., 1979. Sequential extraction procedure for the speciation of particulate trace metals. Anal. Chem. 51 (7), 844–851.

8.2.4 Industrial and urban runoff impacts

Industrialization and urbanization are two of the most significant anthropogenic processes contributing to soil contamination worldwide. Rapid population growth, manufacturing expansion, and urban sprawl generate vast amounts of industrial effluents, stormwater, and urban wastes that act as carriers of heavy metals such as cadmium (Cd), lead (Pb), zinc (Zn), copper (Cu), nickel (Ni), mercury (Hg), and chromium (Cr). When discharged directly into waterways or allowed to flow over impervious surfaces, these pollutants eventually reach agricultural fields through runoff, irrigation with contaminated water, atmospheric deposition, and land application of wastes. Unlike diffuse sources such as fertilizers or manure, industrial and urban runoff are often point sources, delivering concentrated pollutant loads to soils adjacent to factories, highways, and metropolitan regions. Their impacts are long-term because metals are persistent, nonbiodegradable, and tend to accumulate in soil matrices.

8.2.4.1 Industrial runoff and effluents

Sources

Mining and smelting—Release of Pb, Cd, Zn, Ni, and As from ore processing and tailings.

- **Electroplating and metal finishing**—Major contributors of Cr, Ni, and Cu.
- **Textile and tannery industries**—Discharge effluents rich in Cr, Cu, and Zn.
- **Paints, pigments, and battery manufacturing**—Significant Pb and Cd emissions.
- **Chemical and pesticide industries**—Contribute Hg, As, and other trace metals.

Industrial zones often lack adequate effluent treatment facilities in low and middle-income countries. As a result, untreated or partially treated wastewater is released into rivers or irrigation canals, contaminating farmlands downstream (Md Saiful Islam, 2015).

Pathways to agricultural soils

- Direct irrigation with untreated industrial wastewater.
- Flooding of nearby farmlands occurs due to industrial discharge into streams.
- Airborne deposition from smelters and chimneys settling on soils.
- Application of contaminated sewage sludge derived from industrial wastewater treatment plants.

Impacts

- **Soil contamination**: Industrial runoff often elevates Cd, Cr, and Pb levels above permissible limits.
- **Crop contamination**: Rice, leafy greens, and vegetables irrigated with wastewater show high Cd and Pb residues.
- **Soil health**: Metals suppress microbial activity, enzymatic processes, and nutrient cycling (Giller and Witter, 2009).
- **Food safety risks**: Chronic dietary exposure to Cd and Pb is linked to cancer, neurological disorders, and kidney damage (Organization, 2021).
- **Case example**: In Tianjin, China, irrigation with industrial wastewater for over 40 years resulted in cadmium (Cd) concentrations in soils exceeding background values by 6–8 times, with rice grains surpassing national food safety limits (Xiuwu Zhang, 2011).

8.2.4.2 Urban runoff

Sources

Urban runoff refers to stormwater and drainage flows from cities, roads, and residential areas. As rainwater washes across impervious surfaces, it mobilizes pollutants such as:

- **Traffic-related emissions**: Brake linings (Cu, Sb), tire wear (Zn, Cd), fuel combustion (Pb, Ni, V).
- **Construction activities**: Dust carrying Cr, Pb, and As.

- **Domestic sources**: Roof runoff contaminated with zinc (Zn) from galvanized materials.
- **Municipal solid waste leachates**: Cd, Pb, Hg.

Pathways to agricultural soils

- **Stormwater discharges** into rivers used for irrigation.
- **Urban wastewater reuse** in peri-urban agriculture.
- **Flooding and runoff spread** from the city's outskirts into the surrounding farmlands.

Impacts

- **Soil contamination**: Urban runoff often elevates Zn, Pb, and Cu levels in peri-urban soils.
- **Crop uptake**: Vegetables grown near highways show Pb and Cd accumulation exceeding WHO limits (Na Zheng, 2007).
- **Human health**: Populations in peri-urban zones face higher exposure risks through contaminated food chains.
- **Case example**: In Delhi (India), peri-urban vegetable farms irrigated with mixed domestic and industrial wastewater had Pb and Cd levels 3–5 times higher in spinach and okra compared to safe limits (Rajesh Kumar Sharma, 2009).

8.2.5 Mitigation and management

- **Effluent treatment**—Enforcement of zero-liquid discharge (ZLD) technologies in industries.
- **Stormwater management**—Green infrastructure, bioswales, and retention ponds to filter metals.
- **Regulation of sludge use**—Testing sewage sludge before land application.
- **Alternative irrigation sources**—Promoting clean groundwater or treated wastewater.
- **Phytoremediation**—planting hyperaccumulator species (e.g., *Brassica juncea*, *Pteris vittata*) to reduce soil metal loads.

8.2.6 Environmental fate, bioavailability, and plant uptake

- **Soil factors:** pH (lower pH increases mobility for many metals, especially Cd), CEC, clay fraction, and OM content strongly control metal speciation and plant-available fractions (Yanan Wan, 2024).
- **Bioavailability:** Total metal concentration is less predictive of plant uptake than labile fractions (DTPA-extractable, $CaCl_2$-extractable, or pore-water concentrations). Monitoring programs use extractable-fraction measurements and bioassays (Sadee, 2022).

- **Crop differences:** Some crops (rice, leafy vegetables, root crops) accumulate more Cd and other metals; cultivar selection influences uptake.

8.2.7 Soil and human health impacts

Soil metal contamination can reduce microbial diversity, harm soil fauna, and impair nutrient cycling, leading to reduced fertility and crop yield at high levels. Human exposure pathways include the consumption of contaminated produce, ingestion of soil/dust, and groundwater contamination. Chronic exposure to Cd, Pb, and Ni is associated with kidney damage, neurodevelopmental effects (Pb), and carcinogenic risks for some metals.

8.2.8 Monitoring, risk assessment, and thresholds

Monitoring approaches: (1) Total metal analysis (acid digestion + ICP-MS/AES), (2) extractable fractions for bioavailability, (3) plant tissue analysis, and (4) sediment and water monitoring for irrigation sources. Spatial sampling strategies (grid or transect) are used for mapping (Senila, 2024).

Risk indices: EF, geo-accumulation index, contamination factor, and ecological risk index (RI) are commonly used in research for quantifying pollution and identifying sources.

8.2.9 Mitigation and management strategies

8.2.9.1 Preventive measures

Source control: Use low-Cd fertilizers where available; pretreat or limit biosolids with high metal loads; enforce industrial effluent standards (Martyna Buta, 2021).

Good irrigation practices: avoid using wastewater without treatment; monitor the quality of irrigation water.

8.2.9.2 Soil management to reduce bioavailability

- pH **management:** Liming acidic soils reduces Cd and some metal availability.
- **Organic amendments:** The addition of compost or biochar can immobilize metals by binding and reducing bioavailable fractions.
- **Phytoremediation and crop selection:** Growing metal-accumulating plants for removal (phytoextraction) or choosing low-accumulating cultivars for food production.

8.2.9.3 Policy and regulation

Regular monitoring programs, the setting of regional soil quality guidelines, and restrictions on the most contaminated amendments (or requirements for limits) help manage long-term risk. International efforts and national regulations vary; local risk assessments should guide policy.

8.3 Mechanisms of metal retention in soil microaggregates

Small soil aggregates are comprised of fine particles (particles <250 μm) that constitute the majority of soil structure. These small flakes are crucial because they help immobilize heavy metals—keeping them from migrating and ensuring that those bits remain stuck over time. Metals may be adsorbed, complexed, cation-exchanged, or immobilized in the soil within these fine particles or other compounds. These reactions usually take place in the presence of organic matter, clay minerals, and iron and manganese oxides. The extent to which the soil retains metals is determined by its physical and chemical properties, including pH, CEC, the presence of oxygen in the soil, and the types of minerals it contains. How metals are distributed within these microaggregates—such as whether they're exchangeable, associated with carbonates or oxides, combined with OM, or preserved as residues—governs how environmentally risky they are and how readily plants can take them up. It's really important to know how these things work for us to be able to check the quality of soil, predict where contaminants are going, and find good ways to clean up contaminated soils in agricultural areas.

Growing crops, protecting the environment, and keeping the soil in good condition all depend on how much and how heavy metals are stored and present in the soil. Various biological components and geochemical interactions can affect the mobility of metals and bioavailability, controlling soil behavior, which may serve as both sources and long-term reservoirs of hazardous metals (Sparks, 2003). Micro-aggregates, which are very small soil particles <250 μm in size, play a key role in soil structure. These tiny clusters create small spaces where metals can attach themselves to organic material and mineral surfaces. This attachment limits how easily metals can move through the soil (Six and B, 2004).

Due to their toxicity, lengthy residence times, and incapacity to break down naturally, a number of heavy metals, including cadmium (Cd), lead (Pb), zinc (Zn), copper (Cu), and nickel (Ni), represent ongoing risks to the environment and human health (Alloway, 2013). Some of these elements, like zinc, copper, and nickel, are essential for plants in small amounts. However, excessive levels of these metals can cause harm, reduce crop growth, and even contaminate the food chain. Microaggregates help control how these metals are stored and moved in the soil through processes like cation exchange, surface adsorption, attachment to OM, and adherence to iron and manganese oxides (Violante et al., 2010). These processes are influenced by several factors, such as the pH level of the soil, its cation exchange capacity, oxygen conditions, and the availability of sites for metals to adhere.

The environmental risk of microaggregates is also determined by their chemical dispersion. Metals can be found in more stable fractions that are far less accessible for biological uptake, such as those bonded to carbonates, oxides, OM, or locked within mineral crystals, or in exchangeable forms that are readily mobilized (Tessier et al., 1979). Changes such as pH shifts, flooding, or OM breakdown may cause metals to change form within the soil and alter their behavior. Understanding how metals remain workable inside microaggregates is crucial for many different fields, like soil chemistry, environmental assessments, soil science, farm management, and pollution reduction. The physical and chemical processes, the interactions that occur, and how metals are trapped in soil microaggregates in the long-term are discussed in more detail in this chapter.

8.3.1 Physicochemical properties influencing metal adsorption

A number of connected physical and chemical factors influence how much metals move and how stable they are in soil micro-aggregates. These factors determine whether metals remain in the aggregates or move into the soil water, where they might be absorbed by plants or leach into groundwater. The most important factors are the pH of the soil, its cation-exchange capacity, the redox conditions, the amount of OM, the types of minerals, and the quantities of iron, manganese, and aluminum oxides present in the soil.

8.3.1.1 Soil pH

It is commonly known that the primary factor influencing the adsorption and retention of metals is the pH of the soil. The capacity of soils to retain metals like Cd, Zn, and Ni is diminished at lower pH levels because extra protons compete with metal ions for sorption sites on clays and OM (McBride, 1994). Negatively charged surfaces become more accessible when pH rises, improving metal adsorption and encouraging the creation of insoluble hydroxides and carbonates (Sparks, 2003). For instance, when soil pH increases from acidic to almost neutral, lead (Pb^{2+}) exhibits noticeably greater adsorption (Bradl, 2004). As a result, metal mobility and plant availability are typically increased by soil acidification, whether it is brought on by excessive fertilizer use, acid rain, or natural processes.

8.3.1.2 Cation exchange capacity

The total negative charge on clay minerals and organic colloids, which have the ability to draw in and hold on to metal ions, is represented by CEC. Compared to sandy, coarse-textured soils, soils rich in expandable clays or high in OM typically have higher CEC and, hence, a greater capacity to sequester metals (Essington, 2004). Crucially, CEC itself rises with pH because soils have a stronger attraction for metal ions at higher pH levels due to the deprotonation of more variable-charge sites (Sparks, 2003). This indicates that clay-dominated, organic-rich soils are particularly good at immobilizing metals.

8.3.1.3 Redox potential

Another crucial element is redox potential, which regulates metals' solubility and valence state. Under low-oxygen conditions, iron and manganese oxides can decompose and leave behind free metals like arsenic, cobalt, or nickel in the soil (Violante et al., 2010). In contrast, these oxides can also serve as highly effective collectors that retain metals in high-oxygen conditions.

The point is that chromium is a perfect example of this: When it ends up in your body, and the oxygen state changes from Cr(VI) to Cr(III), from hexavalent to trivalent, all of a sudden it becomes immobilized (Alloway, 2013). In wet or waterlogged soils, the redox status often changes quickly, and this influences how metals are stored in and released from micro-aggregates.

8.3.1.4 Organic matter content

The soil OM (SOM) plays two roles in the translocation of metals. It has several active groups—phenolic, carboxyl, and hydroxyl, for example—that can prevent the movement of metals such as copper and lead by creating stable compounds (Tabatabai and S, 2005). However, OM can also create soluble metal-organic compounds that allow those metals to travel more easily through soils (McBride, 1994). What happens to OM in general depends on whether it's lying around loose or mixed into the soil, how much it has already broken down, as well as its composition and interaction with mineral particles.

8.3.1.5 Clay mineralogy

The retention of metals is mediated by clay minerals. Expandable clays (e.g., vermiculite and smectite) have high surface areas as well as high values of negative charge, which enable these materials to adsorb metal ions either through the process of surface complexation or via cation-exchange reactions (Sposito, 2008). Although kaolinite has a low CEC, metals can be firmly attached at its edge positions. Therefore, the extent to which micro-aggregates can retain heavy metals depends largely on the soil's mineral composition.

8.3.1.6 Fe, Mn, and Al oxides

Crystalline and amorphous iron, manganese, and aluminum oxides are excellent for metal-binding by occlusion, complexing at the surface, or adsorption (Violante et al., 2010). Lead and copper attach particularly well to iron oxides, whereas manganese oxides are adept at trapping metals like zinc and cobalt. These oxides can also help metals stay in place by forming complexes with them. However, their effectiveness depends on the redox conditions, as these oxides can dissolve under low-oxygen conditions, which may release the metals back into the soil (Sparks, 2003).

Both soil-specific factors (pH, texture, redox state) and metal-specific characteristics (ionic radius, charge, hydrolysis behavior) affect metal adsorption on soil microaggregates.

8.3.2 Role of OM, clay minerals, and oxides

The main components in soil microaggregates that help retain and stabilize metals are OM, clay minerals, and iron, manganese, and aluminum oxides. These components provide the reactive sites and functional groups that enable complex formations, adsorption, and long-term metal trapping. Together, they influence the movement, persistence, and bioavailability of pollutants in farmland soils.

8.3.2.1 OM

SOM is made up of humic compounds, microbial remains, and broken-down plant matter. It contains many reactive functional groups, such as carboxyl, hydroxyl, phenolic, and carbonyl groups, that can form strong inner-sphere complexes with metal ions (Stevenson, 1994).

- **Chelation and complexation**: Metals like copper and lead bind very tightly to humic and fulvic acids, forming strong complexes that significantly reduce their availability to living things (Nicola Senesi, 2005).
- **Immobilization** versus **mobilization**: The immobilized form discourages metal movement through the soil as compared to suitable soluble organic-metal complexes, i.e., cadmium-humate and nickel-fulvate, in a hypothetical case where it could be leached away (McBride, 1994).
- **Protection within microaggregates**: OM stabilized in microaggregates exposed to metals is less susceptible to remobilization due to reduced solubility (Six and B, 2004).
- **Influence of SOM quality**: Easily degradable organic material (labile SOM) may first dissolve metals when chelate complexes are formed, while OM that is well decomposed typically contributes to keeping the metal stable over a longer period.

Clay minerals

Due to their large surface area, high CEC, and variable electrical charge sites, clay minerals, especially layer silicates, are indispensable for the capturing of metals. Their function is dependent on the type of soil mineral that is present.

- **Expanding clays (smectite, vermiculite):** They interlayer with spaces between them that can be occupied by several metal ions and are adsorbed more strongly. Smectite is particularly effective for Pb and Zn due to the permanent negative charge in the tetrahedral sheets (Sposito, 2008).
- **Nonexpanding clays (kaolinite):** Kaolinite has a low CEC but retains metals through specific adsorption on edge hydroxyl groups, being particularly effective for Al^{3+} and Fe^{3+} (Essington, 2004).
- **Illite:** Provides a permanent negative charge and is efficient at retaining K^+ and other cations, but less so for divalent heavy metals.

- **Mechanisms of retention:** Metals interact with soil through cation exchange, surface adsorption, and inner-sphere complexation at broken edges. For example, Cd^{2+} preferentially binds to smectite interlayers, whereas Pb^{2+} forms inner-sphere complexes at the edges of clays (Bradl, 2004).

Fe, Mn, and Al oxides

Amorphous and crystalline oxides of Fe, Mn, and Al are among the most reactive sorbents for heavy metals. Their high surface area, variable charge properties, and strong affinity for transition metals make them important in immobilizing contaminants.

- **Fe oxides (goethite, hematite, ferrihydrite):** These minerals adsorb Pb^{2+}, Cu^{2+}, and As(V) through surface structure and coprecipitation (Cornell and Schwertmann, 2003).
- **Mn oxides:** Effective in highly oxidizing and adsorbing divalent cations such as Zn^{2+}, Co^{2+} and Ni^{2+}. They can also oxidize As(III) to As(V), reducing toxicity (Violante et al., 2010).
- **Al oxides (gibbsite, boehmite)** Play a role in binding ions such as phosphate and arsenate, but also adsorb metals such as Cu^{2+} and Pb^{2+} via ligand exchange.
- **Redox sensitivity:** Under reducing conditions, the dissolution of Fe and Mn oxides results in the release of previously adsorbed metals into solution (Alloway, 2013). This process is a significant issue for flooded arable soils (e.g., paddy fields).

Microaggregates' synergistic roles

OM, clays, and oxides work together as microaggregates:

- **Organomineral complexes:** The organic materials can coat clay and oxide surfaces to form organomineral complexes, which enhance the stability of composites and provide more adsorption sites.
- **Hierarchical binding:** Organic ligands that are adsorbed on the clay or oxide should first bind to metals in order to be retained inside aggregates.
- **Occlusion:** Metals can be occluded in oxide coatings or pores in the composites, where they lose their ductility and are not biologically active.

While alterations in environmental factors, such as acidification, flooding, or the decomposition of OM, can disturb these interactions, this synergistic relationship endows soils with a significant buffering capacity against metal contamination.

8.3.3 Metal binding forms: Exchangeable, bound, occluded

The retention of metals within soil microaggregates varies among different metals. Rather than being uniform, metals are categorized into distinct binding forms or moieties, which influence their mobility, availability to plants, and long-term stability. These forms are frequently analyzed through sequential extraction methods, such as the one proposed by (for example, (Tessier et al., 1979), which classifies metals into exchangeable, carbonate-bound, oxide-bound, organic-bound, and residual fractions. Within microaggregates, the three forms particularly pertinent to understanding contaminant behavior are exchangeable, bound (to carbonates, OM, and oxides), and occluded (within the mineral lattice or aggregate pores).

8.3.3.1 Exchangeable metals

Exchangeable metals are the most mobile and readily available for plants. They adhere to the negatively charged surfaces of soil colloids (such as soil and OM) through an electrostatic cation exchange mechanism.

- **Characteristics:** These metals are easily displaced by other cations, such as calcium, magnesium, potassium, and hydrogen, and are very sensitive to changes in soil pH and ionic strength (Sparks, 2003).
- **Commonly occurring metals:** Cadmium, zinc, and nickel are often found in the exchangeable pool, especially in acidic soils.
- **Environmental risk:** Because they are soluble and have weak binding, exchangeable metals pose the greatest ecological and health risks due to their ability to be absorbed by plants and to leach into water (Kabata-Pendias, 2010).
- **Influence of microaggregates:** Within microaggregates, exchangeable metals might be physically protected from leaching, but they remain chemically unstable and are available if soil conditions change (Six and B, 2004).

8.3.3.2 Bound metals

Metals that are bound to carbonates, OM, and oxides within microaggregates are more stable than exchangeable metals but can become unstable under certain environmental conditions.

8.3.3.3 Carbonate-bound metals

Metals like lead and cadmium may coprecipitate with or adsorb onto carbonates.

Their stability is strongly affected by soil pH.

In acidic conditions, carbonates dissolve, releasing metals back into the soil solution (McBride, 1994).

8.3.3.4 OM-bound metals

OM provides many functional groups (carboxyl, phenolic, hydroxyl) that form strong complexes with Cu^{2+}, Pb^{2+} and Ni^{2+} (Stevenson, 1994).

While humic complexes immobilize metals, the decomposition of OM (for example, due to microbial activity) can release bound metals, allowing re-mobilization (Tabatabai and S, 2005).

8.3.3.5 *Oxide-bound metals*

Fe and Mn oxides act as powerful sorbents, binding metals through ligand exchange, surface complexation, and coprecipitation (Cornell, 2003).

Metals such as As, Pb, Cu, and Zn are often associated with Fe/Mn oxides.

Under reducing conditions, the dissolution of oxides leads to the sudden release of these bound metals, which is especially important in flooded soils, such as paddy fields (Alloway, 2013).

8.3.3.6 *Occluded metals*

Blocked metals represent the least mobile and most stable fraction in soil microaggregates. They are physically or chemically trapped within mineral structures or aggregate pores.

- **Mechanisms of occlusion:** Metals become incorporated into the crystal lattices of secondary minerals (e.g., silicates, carbonates).
  Metals become encapsulated in oxide coatings or microaggregate interiors during soil formation and pedogenic processes.
- **Examples:** Pb^{2+} and Cr^{3+} often become occluded in Fe/Mn oxides and aluminosilicates over long time scales (Violante et al., 2010).
- **Environmental importance:** Metals are environmentally stable and generally unavailable to plants or microorganisms. However, extreme changes in soil conditions (e.g., acidification, prolonged depletion) can destabilize these pools.
- **Role in long-term stabilization:** Occlusion represents a major mechanism by which soils act as long-term sinks for heavy metals, thereby reducing their ecological risks.

8.3.3.7 *Relative environmental importance of metal forms*

Sequential extraction processes separate metals into operationally defined fractions, which reflect their mobility and stability.

8.3.4 Long-term stability and mobility of metals in microaggregates

Subsequently, processes such as penetration into micropores, occlusion within oxide films, and incorporation in crystalline structures contribute to the metal conversion from a less stable to a more stable state. However, environmental ensembles such as acidification, flooding, and OM decomposition may, as noted in Vol. xxx No. xx Page 176 IJES (www.ijesd.org) cause metals to be released back into the environment (soil–plant–water continuum). The stability and mobility of heavy metals in microaggregates are associated with their binding forms, environmental conditions, and soil formation processes. Even though microaggregates are considered protective structures, some chemical changes and environmental stress may result in the re-mobilization of metals that were previously retained within a fixed soil system. Understanding these processes is important for predicting the behavior of contaminants, determining environmental risk, and testing agroecosystem resilience to pollution.

8.3.4.1 Factors governing long-term stability

Nature of metal binding

Metal phases associated with exchangeable and carbonates are, by nature, unstable and will become even more mobile with acidification or a cation (Kabata-Pendias, 2010). In contrast, oxide-bound and occluded metals are relatively stable over long periods of time and are mobilized only under strongly reducing conditions or very acidic conditions (Violante et al., 2010).

Illustrate Pathways of metal stabilisation an mobilisation in soil microaggregates.

Soil physicochemical properties

- pH: Lead and copper are stabilized by precipitation with carbonates at alkaline pH, while cadmium release is favored under acidic conditions, zinc under neutral to weakly alkaline conditions, and nickel at near-neutral pH (Sparks, 2003).
- **Redox potential (Eh):** In anoxic microniches, reductive dissolution of iron and manganese oxides entails metals bound on to them (Tessier et al., 1979).
- **OM dynamics:** The degradation of humic materials may release previously complexed metals (McBride, 1994).
- **Clay mineralogy:** Smectite and vermiculite also enhance the stabilization of metals over time by a process known as interlayer fixation, with kaolinite showing relatively less retention.

Aggregate protection

Metals are physically entrapped in the SOM-organomineral complex as microaggregates, and the possibility of their leaching process is limited, along with microbial action (Six and B, 2004). Over time, this occlusion is a significant contributor to why metals remain trapped there for long periods.

8.3.4.2 Pathways of metal mobilization

However, a number of environmental processes may further increase the metal release from microaggregates:

Soil acidification

Acid rain, fertilizer inputs (e.g., ammonium-based fertilizers), and organic acids lower soil pH.

This causes the disintegration of carbonates and the displacement of exchangeable metals (Alloway, 2013).

Redox fluctuations

Due to flooding events in wetlands and paddy soils under reduced conditions, Fe/Mn oxides dissolve, and adsorbed Pb, Cu, and As are released (Cornell, 2003).

OM decomposition

Microbial degradation of SOM releases metals bound to humic complexes and increases dissolved organic carbon, thereby enhancing metal mobility through soluble organo-metallic complexes (Stevenson, 1994).

Competitive ion effects

Adding fertilizers (e.g., phosphate, ammonium) and lime materials produces competing ions that can displace metals from colloid surfaces (Bradl, 2004).

Soil erosion and aggregate breakdown

Physical disturbance (tillage, erosion, compaction) breaks up fine aggregates, exposing metals to desorption and transport processes.

8.3.4.3 Long-term sequestration mechanisms (Yin, Yin, J., Zhao, L., Xu, X., Li, D., Qiu, H., & Cao, X.)

Soils also have mechanisms that enhance the long-term immobilization of metals:

Mineral transformation

Metals may be incorporated into newly formed secondary minerals, such as silicates and carbonates.

Aging effect

Over time, labile metals change into less mobile forms through diffusion and recrystallization of oxides in microscopic pores (Sparks, 2003).

Retention within microaggregates

Repeated wet-dry and freeze-thaw cycles increase aggregation, causing metals to become trapped within microstructural domains.

8.3.4.4 Environmental implications

The relationship between stability and mobility in microaggregates carries significant implications:

Soil quality

Long-term separation increases the buffering capacity of the soil and reduces the risk of contamination.

Agricultural productivity

Accumulation of toxic metals (e.g., Cd, Pb) under changing conditions can impair crop growth and threaten food security.

Remediation strategies

Immobilization methods (e.g., liming, organic amendment, biochar application) aim to shift metals to less volatile fractions to ensure long-term stability (Luke Beesley, 2011).

Climate change effects

Increased flooding, acidification, and OM turnover under climate change scenarios could destabilize metal pools, increasing their mobility.

8.3.4.5 Conceptual model

A dynamic equilibrium model can be envisioned, where metals cycle between unstable (exchangeable, carbonate-bound) and stable (oxide-bound, organic-bound, disrupted) forms, with environmental drivers determining the direction of change. For decades, the net trend has been toward stabilization and inhibition, but perturbations can reverse this process, allowing metals to be re-incorporated into the mobile pool.

8.4 Bioavailability and transfer through the food chain

The quality and safety of food are not merely determined by the composition of the nutrients in the food but also by the bioavailability of the nutrients and the transfer of environmental pollutants through the food chain. The portion of an assimilable nutrient or contaminant that is digested, absorbed, and could be used for physiological activities or storage is referred to as bioavailability (Guerrieri, 2024).

Transfer via the food web is the variability and accumulation of environmental nutrients or poisons using autotrophs and, in successive trophic levels, to human beings.

These processes jointly regulate the nutritional adequacy, as well as dietary exposure to toxic substances.

8.4.1 Bioavailability

In Slovakia, a study was carried out, and the results indicated that the concentration of cadmium (Cd) in the soil samples was higher than the acceptable limits during 2017–2019. However, the average concentration of the other metals (Cu, Zn, and Pb) was significantly lower than the acceptable levels, except in the case of Pb, which was higher during the spring seasons. The biological chemical evaluation of heavy metals in the soil revealed that the Cd, Cu, and Zn ratios were lower than the statutory critical values of these elements, which implies that the bioavailability of these elements to plants was low. Nevertheless, there is a high amount of Pb, which indicates an environmental concern that should be addressed.

In the case of winter wheat, the bioaccumulation of Zn and Cu was found to be within safe limits, while Cd and Pb were detected primarily in the roots and other vegetative parts, excluding the grain. These results suggest that the edible portion of the wheat crop remains safe for human consumption, posing no immediate threat to consumer health. Nevertheless, continuous environmental monitoring and the implementation of sustainable soil management practices are recommended to mitigate future heavy metal accumulation, safeguard crop quality, and ensure long-term food safety and agricultural sustainability (Feszterová, 2021).

Environmental pollutants resulting from human activities such as urbanization, mining, and industrialization pose serious threats to humans, animals, and plants. These toxic substances spread across air, water, and soil, where they can directly impact living organisms or accumulate through bioaccumulation and biomagnification (Chormare, 2022).

8.4.1.1 Nutrients

In the case of vital nutrients, bioavailability is a ratio of the amount of consumed material absorbed and used. Chemical form (e.g., heme or nonheme iron), interaction with the food matrix, cooking, and host-related factors (including gut health and microbiome activity) are some of the factors that affect this (Guerrieri, 2024).

8.4.1.2 Contaminants

Bioavailability of toxicants (heavy metals, persistent organic pollutants (POPs), and per- and polyfluoroalkyl substances (PFAS)) is a characteristic of the proportion of the exposure dose that can be absorbed into systemic circulation. The environmental factors that have a significant impact on contaminant uptake in plants are soil pH, redox state, and speciation, whereas the uptake in humans depends on food composition and gastrointestinal conditions (Angon, 2024).

8.4.2 Factors that affect bioavailability in soil-plant systems

In soil-plant interactions, physicochemical characteristics of the soil, such as pH, OM content, CEC, and redox potential, determine the bioavailability of different agrochemicals. The pH of the soil is also a very important factor since it determines the solubility and mobility of minerals and contaminants, which, in turn, affect their absorption by the plant roots. The availability of nutrients and absorption efficiency are further adjusted by the presence of organic ligands, microbial activity, as well as competing ions. In addition, vegetation-specific variables like root structure, transport proteins, and rhizosphere associations play a significant role in dictating how many nutrients or toxic factors are absorbed into edible plant tissues.

8.4.3 Transfer through the food chain

Transference through the food chain can be defined as the transfer of contaminants, toxins, or bioactive compounds among trophic levels via dietary intake. When the primary producers, e.g., plants, absorb heavy metals, pesticides, or other environmentally harmful pollutants found in soil and water, the substances are passed on to the food web and then to the herbivores and further higher consumers. As the trophic level increases, some of the nonbiodegradable substances can be subjected to bioaccumulation and biomagnification, which results in increased concentrations in the highest predators, including humans. The process implicates food safety, the health of people, as well as the sustainability of the ecology.

8.4.3.1 Bioaccumulation and biomagnification

The major environmental processes, which describe how pollutants are sustained and amplified by ecological systems, are the processes of bioaccumulation and biomagnification, which eventually impact the human population. A gradual accumulation of toxic substances, such as pesticides and heavy metals, in organisms is also known as bioaccumulation, whereas the gradual increase in the concentration of these substances as one ascends the food chain is referred to as biomagnification. These processes are particularly concerning for POPs and some heavy metals because the trophic transfer of these substances can result in increased exposure and serious health impacts for the top consumers of the food web, including humans (Awafung, 2025). Heavy metals like cadmium and lead are colonized in soils and crops and spread to animal and human food. Not every metal, however, biomagnifies uniformly at trophic levels (Zhang, 2024).

Trophic transfer can be illustrated by the following.

Mercury

Methylmercury is readily biomagnified in aquatic food webs, and high concentrations are found in predatory fish; therefore, it is a major source of human exposure to mercury through seafood (Huo, 2025). Naturally, heavy metals are released into soils and waters via weathering and volcanic processes; however, human activity, including the disposal of industrial and municipal waste, drastically increases their presence. Aquatic organisms absorb these contaminants via gills and cuticles, among other sensitive tissues. This paper discusses the trophic transfer and biomagnification of heavy metals in water bodies. It states that arsenic tends to decline in freshwater food webs but biomagnifies in marine food webs, particularly in upper-level predator fish. Previously considered to be nonbiomagnifiable, cadmium has been demonstrated to be biomagnifiable in gastropod and epiphyte-based food webs. Mercury exhibits high biomagnification, where it is transferred to higher trophic levels, such as fish, through particulate OM. The paper highlights the importance of safeguarding aquatic environments against pollution in order to conserve biodiversity and prevent environmental destruction.

Persistent organic pollutant and per- and polyfluoroalkyl substance

The invertebrates are also very essential in the movement of nutrients, energy, and pollutants in terrestrial food webs, though there is a limited understanding of how the pollutants move through their trophic chains. The experiment involved the biomagnification and occurrence of POPs in detritivorous, phytophagous, and predatory invertebrates. The highest POP levels were observed in earthworms and dung beetles as detritivorous species. The biomagnification factors (BMFs) and composition patterns differed among species, with negative correlations between BMFs and log K_{ow} in detritivorous and most phytophagous species, and parabolic relationships in snails and predators, which is probably caused by the occurrence of more efficient digestion and absorption. A positive association between basal metabolic rates (BMRs) and BMF is a sign that the greater the metabolic activity, the greater the capacity to biomagnify POPs among animal groups. The general findings indicate that terrestrial predators, particularly those that feed on soil-dwelling invertebrates, are highly exposed to POPs through the food they consume.

The PCBs and dioxins are stored in the fatty tissues, but PFAS vary in their accumulation based on chain length and functional-group.

PFAS are extremely resistant synthetic endocrine disruptors that are retained in fish muscle rich in proteins and are not easily eliminated by cooking. This paper examined 40 PFASs in fish across the trophic levels of the Lake Huron–Lake Erie Corridor to determine bioaccumulation and possible human health impacts. Walleye, yellow perch, and round goby muscle and serum samples collected in 2021 identified 8 PFAS congeners in muscle and 15 in serum, and several new compounds were detected in Great Lakes fish. PFOS was detected in all samples, but the levels were not toxic to fish. Nevertheless, the BMFs of above one across species suggest that PFOS is building up via the food web. The findings reveal the persistent PFAS pollution of water bodies and the relevance of nonlethal sampling in monitoring the exposure to PFAS and the ecological and human health hazards (George, 2023).

Heavy metals

Heavy metals like cadmium and lead are colonized in soils and crops and spread to animal and human food. Not every metal, however, biomagnifies uniformly at trophic levels (Angon, 2024). One of the challenges facing the environment of the world today is heavy metal contamination, which has adverse effects on the food chain and insect natural enemies. Since heavy metals are carried through the soil to the plants and further on to the herbivorous insects and their predators, they become settled and affect the growth, development, and reproduction cycle of these useful insects. These kinds of impairments decrease their effectiveness in managing pests. Though minor exposure can result in a short-term increase in feeding activity as a result of countering detoxification energy requirements, prolonged or excessive exposure causes oxidative stress, production of reactive oxygen species, and disruptions in metabolism. All in all, heavy metal pollution essentially compromises the biological control capacity of insect natural enemies and, as such, threatens the ecological balance and sustainable pest control (Zhang, 2024). Nematodes, constituting >60% of metazoans and approximately 90% of the benthic fauna, are essential components of the marine biosphere and food webs. This paper examined the topic of bioaccumulation of heavy metals in marine nematodes using two independent methods with contaminated sediments. It was found that, although none of the five nematodes are large insects and their life span is relatively short, they can still accumulate heavy metals significantly. It was discovered that the degree of bioaccumulation rose between deposit feeders, microalgal grazers, and microbial and metazoan predators. These findings have shown that nematodes not only help in the accumulation of heavy metals, but they also play a role in biomagnifying the pollutants in marine food webs, thus aiding the movement of the pollutants up the food webs (Danovaro, 2023).

Microplastics

The food plants are the main source of human nutrition, yet, in polluted areas, they are able to absorb contaminants. The impact of the environment and climate change can alter the quality of food; food quality is usually negatively affected and poses a threat to human health. These include heavy metals such as lead, arsenic, cadmium, and chromium, which may occur at different levels in the environment (soil, water, and atmosphere), and these are also widely spread across the world. Moreover, other contaminants may bioaccumulate in food plants, such as new contaminants like POPs, pesticides, and microplastics (MPs). These occur in the roots of food plants and also in the leaves and fruits of food plants, depending on their chemical structure. The literature of recent years was reviewed to determine how contaminants are distributed among food plants. Old agronomical methods, as well as new integrated technologies to clean water, control soil, and monitor crops, have been suggested in the literature to reduce contamination and ensure high food quality as well as a high level of food safety (Guerrieri, 2024).

MP pollution is massive in the sea, and it impacts a variety of species. A metaanalysis of 116 articles investigated the bioaccumulation or biomagnification of MPs and their chemical additives in marine food webs. It was determined that MP bioaccumulation exists at individual trophic levels but does not reflect the presence of biomagnification at higher trophic levels. The bioaccumulation of chemical additives associated with MPs is still unclear, as there is limited and inconsistent information on the issue. Suggestions of trophic transfer from laboratory studies are scant, and field evidence is lacking to support biomagnification. In general, it is clear that as marine species experience an increase in MPs, these particles do not seem to be biomagnified within marine food webs. The research highlights that further studies should be conducted under realistic environmental conditions in the future to gain deeper insight into MP and additive transfer, retention, and depuration across several trophic levels.

8.4.4 Consequences to human health

Dietary guidelines and risk assessment can only be achieved by understanding bioavailability and trophic transfer. Populations with high fish consumption are still under the threat of being exposed to mercury, whereas PFAS and MPs have become new concerns in the sphere of diet. On the other hand, the health outcomes of the population can be improved by enhancing the bioavailability of nutrients (e.g., through fortification or processing). Some of the available policy responses include soil remediation, food advisory, and international regulation of POPs.

Future studies need to incorporate the fields of environmental science, nutrition, and toxicology to offer a comprehensive dietary safety evaluation.

Nutritional and toxicological quality of food is determined through bioavailability and transfer within the food chain. Although nutrients require better methods to increase absorption, contaminants demand strict control and reduction. These two challenges must be addressed as a means of enhancing global food security and human health.

8.4.5 Mechanisms that regulate bioavailability

The chain of interacting factors determines the bioavailability of the nutrients and contaminants:

Source and chemical form: Biological evolution is very vital in the determination of pollutant behavior. The ionic form and type of complex, e.g., methylmercury, as opposed to inorganic mercury, have a significant impact on absorption and toxicity in metals. In the case of organic compounds, distribution in tissues and retention period in the body depend largely on factors such as the size of the molecule and lipophilicity (log Kow).

Polyphenols are secondary metabolites that are very common in plants, and their main bioactive constituents have great health effects. This is because of their structural diversity, which allows them to interact with diverse biomolecules and affect many physiological pathways, making them a significant target in scientific and clinical studies.

8.4.6 Mechanisms controlling bioavailability

Bioavailability of both nutrients and contaminants is determined by a chain of interacting factors.

8.4.6.1 Source and chemical form

Biological evolution plays a critical role in determining pollutant behavior. In metals, the ionic form and type of complex, such as methylmercury compared to inorganic mercury, significantly influence absorption and toxicity. For organic compounds, factors like molecular size and lipophilicity (log Kow) largely dictate how they distribute within tissues and how long they persist in the body. Polyphenols, widely occurring secondary metabolites in plants, are key bioactive compounds with significant health benefits. Their structural diversity enables them to interact with diverse biomolecules and affect many physiological pathways, making them a significant target in scientific and clinical studies (Rudrapal, 2024).

8.4.6.2 Matrix interactions

In foods and soils, the interactions with OM, fibers, phytates, or lipids may alter the way contaminants or nutrients are released in the gut or the bio accessible properties of the environment. Moreover, food processing, like cooking or fermenting, changes the food structure, which can either increase or decrease its availability. The key food matrix effects that affect the bioavailability of the oil-soluble vitamins are underlined: oil content, oil composition, particle size, interfacial properties, and food additives. The human gut droplet size and aggregation condition influence vitamin bioavailability since they alter lipid digestion, vitamin release, and vitamin solubilization. Small and isolated oil droplets generally contain vitamins with a high level of bioactivity compared to those found in large and aggregated droplets. Biological availability may thus be influenced by emulsifiers, stabilizers, or texture modifiers, which may impact droplet size or aggregation (Tan, 2021).

8.4.6.3 Environmental bioaccessibility

In the soil-plant system, the proportion of an intro-relative to the contaminant that is persistently soluble and material to root uptake is one of the major determinants of the integration of that contaminant into plants. The most important factors that determine this bioavailable fraction are the soil pH, redox conditions, and microbial activity. The impact of heavy metals on agricultural soils endangers the productivity of crops, the health of the soil, as well as human health. The toxic metals include Cr, As, Ni, Cd, Pb, Hg, Zn, and Cu, which reduce the growth of plants by interfering with metabolic processes and changing soil characteristics, eventually lowering yields. Eating contaminated crops poses severe health hazards to human beings, damaging major organs such as the kidneys, liver, brain, and lungs (Angon, 2024).

8.4.6.4 *Physiological and dietary factors(host)*

Food plants are the basis of the human diet, but under polluted conditions, they are able to take in a variety of contaminants. Lead, arsenic, cadmium, and chromium are heavy metals that are common in soil, water, and air, and their assimilation varies among plant species. The metals usually accumulate in roots and leaves and can reach fruits and seeds, with As and Cd often being detected. Food plants can also bioaccumulate emerging contaminants such as POPs, pesticides and MPs, depending on their chemical characteristics in addition to metals. The latest literature has been highlighting traditional agronomic processes, as well as advanced integrated technologies applied to agronomic processes, to enhance water quality, soil management, and crop surveillance in order to minimize contamination and improve food safety (Guerrieri, 2024).

8.5 Environmental and agricultural implications

8.5.1 Risks to food safety and security

8.5.1.1 *Accumulation/ bioavailability*

Heavy metals are likely to get concentrated in soil microaggregates (<50–250 μm or <53 μm in most studies) as compared to macro-aggregates. Since they are highly surface-active, have small particle size, and are rich in OM, metal oxides, or binding sites, microaggregates are able to entrap and possibly neutralize metals; however, they may also liberate them over time (Deng, 2018).

8.5.1.2 *The exposure is influenced by land-use changes*

The changes in land use (e.g., forest to agricultural land, urban-road soils) modify the structure and distribution of aggregates, increasing the concentration of microaggregates and the exposure risk through dust, plant uptake, and runoff (Deng, 2018).

8.5.1.3 *Plant uptake and accumulation in food*

Higher levels of heavy metals in soil aggregates are associated with high uptake in the food biomass. Research indicates that an increase in soil heavy metal loads is associated with an increase in plant concentrations, which heightens the risk of dietary exposures (Liu et al., 2022).

8.5.1.4 *Health hazards metals*

Health hazards metals such as cadmium (Cd), lead (Pb), and arsenic (As) are often involved. They may lead to long-term health problems such as kidney damage, neurotoxicity, and developmental failures, and food safety may be compromised. The fact that metals are present in some secret forms in aggregates implies that conventional bulk soil tests can underestimate the risk (Zheng, 2022).

8.5.1.5 *Security and yield effects*

An excessive amount of heavy metals can cause reduced crop yields or lead to the contamination of crops to a level where they cannot be traded or consumed. In addition, the health of the soil (microbial activity, nutrient cycling) can be compromised (Deng, 2018).

8.5.2 Strategies for metal risk assessment and monitoring

8.5.2.1 *Aggregate fractionation*

It is important to separate soil into classes of aggregate sizes (e.g., micro- versus macro-aggregates) when determining the heavy metals content. The research indicates that concentration and risk indices differ profoundly with size classes; the smaller aggregates are more likely to be metal-enriched (Zheng, 2022).

8.5.2.2 *Selection of method (wet and dry sieving, etc.)*

This distribution is sensitive to the method of aggregate separation: wet-sieving usually causes more metals to be concentrated in smaller sizes, while dry sieving typically differs in its distribution. In that way, surveillance requires systematization (Zheng, 2022).

8.5.2.3 *Ecological risk indices*

Assuming aggregates of risk, e.g., potential ecological RI, mass loading, and distribution factor, to measure the risk of different metals (Zheng, 2022).

8.5.2.4 *Plant tissue/food crop monitoring*

It is important to measure the actual uptake in the edible tissue of crops rather than the concentration in the soil alone, in order to determine what gets into the human food chain (Liu, 2022).

8.5.2.5 *Monitoring of soil property*

pH, content of OM, redox potential, and binding phase (clay, OM, metal oxides) determine mobilization and bioavailability. These parameters are to be measured in addition to the metal concentrations (Liu, 2022).

8.5.2.6 *Spatial & temporal monitoring*

Map hotspots (e.g., near roads, industrial areas), and time-monitor to detect alterations caused by erosion, land use variations, climate, etc. (Deng, 2018).

8.5.3 Remediation and soil management practices

8.5.3.1 *Addition of OM*

Adding compost, manure, biochar, and mulch may bind up heavy metals or dilute their bioactivity by creating more binding sites and keeping the metals in less mobile states. As an illustration, the Cr-polluted paddy soil was amended with biochar, which lowered levels of Cr uptake in rice and reduced the levels of bioavailable forms of metals (Jia, 2015).

8.5.3.2 pH modification

Soil pH needs to be brought toward neutral (approximately pH 6–7) to reduce the mobilization of most heavy metals (most metals are more soluble under acidic conditions). Additives such as soil liming are also used, as noted by Hinds (2023).

8.5.3.3 Phytoremediation/phytostabilization

Plants (including hyperaccumulators) are used to absorb metals or retain them in roots or soil to make them less mobile. Combined with microorganisms (mycorrhizae, bacteria), they help increase uptake or stabilization (Wang, 2021).

8.5.3.4 Physical removal/replacement of soil

In highly contaminated areas, topsoil can be removed, or raised beds can be placed with clean soil. These methods are disruptive and costly, however, according to Hinds (2023).

8.5.3.5 Amendments/chemical stabilization

Addition of the following agents to fix metals: phosphates, clay minerals, metal oxides, etc. New emerging technologies too, such as nanomaterials and plant/microbe combinations (Luo, 2024).

8.5.3.6 Agronomic strategies

Selecting crops (those that are less prone to uptake heavy metals), crop rotation, and alternating flooding/draining (in rice) to reduce arsenic/lead uptake. For example, arsenic and lead levels in rice fields decreased when wetting and drying were alternated Islam et al. (2020).

8.5.4 Policy frameworks and sustainable agriculture approaches

8.5.4.1 Regulations and safety standards

Governmental agencies (or international bodies) establish maximum allowed concentrations of metals in soils as well as in food crops. Monitoring and enforcement should be done regularly. Although one may not find the exact citation on microaggregates, soil and food safety standards are highlighted in the literature on policies Surls et al. (2017).

8.5.4.2 Best management practices

Agricultural guidelines: keep soil OM intact, do not excessively use fertilizers or pesticides that might contain heavy metals, maintain a good pH balance, minimize erosion, and ensure clean water is used for irrigation. Such BMPs are found in urban agriculture guidance (Hinds, 2023).

8.5.4.3 Incentives and financing remediation

Remediation programs that are subsidized or encourage testing and soil improvement. For example, urban agriculture programs also involve grants and technical assistance for testing the soil and educating growers Surls et al. (2017).

8.5.4.4 Sustainable agricultural systems/regenerative agriculture

Technologies that enhance the health of the soil in general, including reduced tillage, crop rotations, cover crops, and agroforestry, are thought to contribute to the development of soil structure (including aggregates) and OM, which can slow the movement of metals and increase resilience. The global environmental crisis has been driven by the emergence of diverse businesses, emerging technologies, and rising population levels. The rise of various businesses, emergent technologies, and increased population levels have been catalysts for the global environmental crisis.

8.5.4.5 Precautionary & rights-based approach

It is characterized by ensuring that the communities are safeguarded, have fair access to safe food, and receive clear information regarding the dangers of soil that may be contaminated. Policies can demand the involvement and transparency of the stakeholders. The microaggregate literature often makes these assumptions more implicitly, but they form part of the general policy schemes.

8.5.4.6 The surveillance needs and unified procedures

In policy frameworks, standard procedures are commonly required or advised to use for soil sampling, aggregate fractionation, and food testing. This ensures comparability across time and place.

References

Adriano, D.C., 2001. Trace Elements in Terrestrial Environments: Biogeochemistry, Bioavailability, and Risks of Metals. Springer Nature.

Alengebawy, A.A.-Q., 2021. Heavy Metals and Pesticides Toxicity in Agricultural Soil and Plants: Ecological Risks and Human Health Implications. MDPI.

Alloway, B.J. Ed., 2013. Sources of heavy metals and metalloids in soils. In: Heavy Metals in Soils Trace Metals and Metalloids in Soils and Their Bioavailability. Springer Nature, pp. 11–50.

Angon, P.B., 2024. A. Sources, effects and present perspectives of heavy metals contamination: soil, plants and human food chain. Heliyon 10 (7), eXXXXX.

Awafung, E.A., 2025. The impact of bioaccumulation and biomagnification in humans. On J. Clin. 1.

Bibhabasu Mohanty, A.D., 2021. Heavy Metals in Soils and Vegetation from Wastewater Irrigated Croplands near Ahmedabad. Risk to Human Health. Nature Environment and Pollution Technology, Gujarat, pp. 163–175.

Bradl, H.B., 2004. Adsorption of heavy metal ions on soils and soils constituents. J. Colloid Interface Sci. 277, 1–18.

Broadley, M.R., J, P., 2007. Microbes as Hidden or Prominent Players in Plant Life. New Phytologist Foundation.

Campbell, S., 2025. The guardian.org. Retrieved from he guardian.org: https://www.theguardian.com/environment/2025/apr/17/about-15-world-cropland-polluted-toxic-metals-say-researchers.April 17

Chormare, R., 2022. Environmental health and risk assessment metrics with special mention to biotransfer, bioaccumulation and biomagnification of environmental pollutants. Chemosphere 302, 134836.

Cornell, R.M., Schwertmann, U., 2003. The Iron Oxides: Structure, Properties, Reactions, Occurrences and Uses, Wiley, pp. 1–7.

Cuiyun Chen, D.H., 2009. Functions and Toxicity of Nickel in Plants: Recent Advances and Future Prospects. Wiley, pp. 304–313.

Danovaro, R.C., 2023. Bioaccumulation and biomagnification of heavy metals in marine micropredators. Commun. Biol. 6 (1), 1206.

Deng, A.Z., 2018. Soil aggregate-associated heavy metals subjected to land use changes. Environ. Adv. 1, 100003.

Essington, M.E., 2004. Soil and Water Chemistry: An Integrative Approach. CRC Press.

Feszterová, M.P., 2021. The monitoring of selected heavy metals content and bioavailability in the soil-plant system and its impact on sustainability in agribusiness food chains. Sustainability 13 (13), 7021.

George, S.E., 2023. Nonlethal detection of PFAS bioaccumulation and biomagnification within fishes in an urban-and wastewater-dominant Great Lakes watershed. Environ. Pollut. 321, 121123.

Giller, K.E., Witter, E., 2009. Heavy metals and soil microbes. In: Witter, E., Giller, K.E., Soil Biology and Biochemistry. Elsevier, pp. 2031–2037.

Goss, M.T., 2013. A review of the use of organic amendments and the risk to human health. In: Goss, A.T.M.J., Advances in Agronomy. Elsevier, pp. 275–379.

Guerrieri, N.M., 2024. Food plants and environmental contamination: an update. Toxics 12 (5), 365.

Hinds, J., 2023. Soil Remediation, Soil Health and Nutrient Management. SARE Outreach, Sustainable Agriculture Research and Education. https://www.sare.org/publications/best-practices-for-the-sustainable-urban-farm/soil-remediation-soil-health-and-nutrient-management/.

Huo, M.P., 2025. Trophic transfer of mercury in marine food chains from the offshore waters of Changshan Archipelago. Front. Mar. Sci. 12, 1566875.

Islam, S.F.U., Wei, C., Yang, X., Ahmad, A., Yang, J., 2020. Reducing greenhouse gas emissions and grain arsenic and lead levels without compromising yield in organically produced rice (arXiv:2006.02840).

Jia, X.Z., 2015. Soil respiration in relation to soil temperature and soil water content in a maize field in the Loess Plateau, China. Ecol. Res. 30 (3), 433–445.

Kabata-Pendias, A., 2010. Trace Elements in Soils and Plants. Taylor and Francis.

Liu, Q.C., 2022. Health risk assessment of heavy metals in soils and food crops: a case study. Front. Public Health 10, 947525.

Liu, Q., Li, X., He, L., 2022. Health risk assessment of heavy metals in soils and food crops from a coexist area of heavily industrialized and intensively cropping in the Chengdu Plain, Sichuan, China. Front. Chem. 10, 988587. doi:10.3389/fchem.2022.988587.

Luke Beesley, E.M.-J.-E., 2011. A review of biochars' potential role in the remediation, revegetation and restoration of contaminated soils. Environ. Pollut. 159 (12), 3269–3282.

Luo, N., 2024. Methods for controlling heavy metals in environmental soils based on artificial neural networks. Sci. Rep. 14, 2563.

Martyna Buta, J.H., 2021. Sewage sludge in agriculture—the effects of selected chemical pollutants and emerging genetic resistance determinants on the quality of soil and crops—a review. Ecotoxicol. Environ. Saf. 214, 112070.

McBride, M.B. 1994. Environmental Chemistry of Soils. Oxford University Press, Inc., New York.

Md Saiful Islam, -M.K.-A.-M., 2015. Heavy metal pollution in surface water and sediment: a preliminary assessment of an urban river in a developing country. In: Ecological Indicators. Elsevier. pp. 282–291.

Na Zheng, Q.W., 2007. Population health risk due to dietary intake of heavy metals in the industrial area of Huludao city, China. In: Zheng, Q.W.N. (Ed.), Science of the Total Environment. Elsevier, pp. 96–104.

Nanthi Bolan, A.K., 2014. Remediation of heavy metal(loid)s contaminated soils—to mobilize or to immobilize? J. Hazard. Mater. 266, 141–166.

Nations, F.A., 2022. FAO. https://openknowledge.fao.org/items/ff3cfcc4-e895-4df0-a925-c8ce240004ab.

Nicola Senesi, E.L., 2005. Metal ion complexation by soil humic substances. In: Tabatabai, D.S.M.A. (Ed.), Chemical Processes in Soils, vol. 8. Wiley, pp. 469–489.

Organization, W.H., 2021. Cadmium. Retrieved from World Health Organization: https://www.who.int/news-room/fact-sheets/detail/cadmium.

P. C. Nagajyoti, K.D., 2010. Heavy Metals, Occurrence and Toxicity for Plants: A Review. Springer Nature.

Rajesh Kumar Sharma, M.A., 2009. Heavy metals in vegetables collected from production and market sites of a tropical urban area of India. In: Sharma, M.A.R.K. (Ed.), Food and Chemical Toxicology. Elsevier, pp. 583–591.

Rudrapal, M.R., 2024. Dietary polyphenols: review on chemistry/sources, bioavailability/metabolism, antioxidant effects, and their role in disease management. Antioxidants 13 (4), 429.

Sadee, B.A., 2022. Determination of trace metals in vegetables using ICP-MS. ZANCO J. Pure Appl. Sci. 34, 73–83.

Senila, M., 2024. Recent advances in the determination of major and trace elements in plants using inductively coupled plasma optical emission spectrometry. Molecules 29, 3169.

Sharma, P., Dubey, R.S., 2005. Lead toxicity in plants. Braz. J. Plant Physiol. 17.

Six, J., B, H., 2004. A history of research on the link between (micro)aggregates, soil biota, and soil organic matter dynamics. In: Six, H.B.J. (Ed.), Soil and Tillage Research. Elsevier, pp. 7–31.

Sparks, D.L. (Ed.), 2003. Environmental soil chemistry: an overview. In: Environmental Soil Chemistry, second ed. Academic Press, pp. 1–42.

Sposito, G., 2008. The Chemistry of Soils. Oxford university press.

Stephan Clemens, J.F., 2016. Toxic heavy metal and metalloid accumulation in crop plants and foods. Annu. Rev. 67, 489–512.

Stevenson, F.A., 1999. Cycles of Soil (Carbon, Nitrogen Phosphorus Sulfur, Micronutrients). John Wiley and Sons Publishers.

Stevenson, F.J., 1994. Humus Chemistry: Genesis, Composition, Reactions, second ed. Wiley.

Surls, R., Borel, V., Biscaro, A., 2017. Soils in Urban Agriculture: Testing, Remediation and Best Management Practices for California Community Gardens, School Gardens, and Urban Farms. University of California Agriculture and Natural Resources.

Tabatabai, M.A., S, D., 2005. Metal ion complexation by oil humic substances. In: Chemical Processes in Soils, pp. 119 145.

Tan, Y., 2021. Improving the bioavailability of oil-soluble vitamins by optimizing food matrix effects: a review. Food Chem. 348, 129148.

Tessier, A.P.G.C., Campbell, P.G., Bisson, M.J.A.C., 1979. Sequential extraction procedure for the speciation of particulate trace metals. Anal. Chem. 51 (7), 844–851.

Vasudevan, B.U., 2016. Eco-friendly approach for leaching out heavy metals from sewage sludge. In: A. Francis, T. (Ed.), Chemistry and Ecology. Taylor and Francis, pp. 507–519.

Violante, A.U.D.N., Cozzolino, V.U.D.N., Perelomov, L.P.S.U., Caporale, A.G., Pigna, M.U.D.N., 2010. Mobility and bioavailability of heavy metals and metalloids in soil environments. J. Soil Sci. Plant Nutr. 10 (3), 268–292.

Wang, L.J., 2021. Green remediation strategies for heavy metal contaminated soils: a review. Soil Use Manag. 37 (4), 619–635.

Xiuwu Zhang, L.Y., 2011. Impacts of lead/zinc mining and smelting on the environment and human health in China. In: Zhang, L.Y.X. (Ed.), Environmental Monitoring and Assessment. Springer Nature, pp. 2261–2273.

Yanan Wan, J.L., 2024. Heavy metals in agricultural soils: sources, influencing factors, and remediation strategies. Impact Heavy Metal Contam. Soil Environ. Adv. Remediat. Strateg. 12 (1), 63.

Zhang, Z.W., 2024. Transfer of heavy metals along the food chain: a review on the pest control performance of insect natural enemies under heavy metal stress. J. Hazard. Mater. 478, 135587.

Zheng Liu, Y.B., 2023. Driving factors on accumulation of cadmium, lead, copper, zinc in agricultural soil and products of the North China Plain. Sci. Rep. 13, 7429.

Zheng, N.W., 2022. Effect of soil aggregate separation methods on the occurrence characteristics of typical pollutants. Processes 10 (2), 216.

Chapter 9

Advanced analytical approaches in metallome profiling

Akruti Singh[a], Tej Bhan Singh[b], Piyush Verma[a], and Ravinder Kaushik[a]
[a]*School of Health Sciences and Technology, UPES, Dehradun, India*
[b]*Department of Agriculture, Invertis University, Bareilly, India*

9.1 Introduction

9.1.1 Metallomics and its importance

The new area of omics, known as metallomics, specifically refers to the interaction of metals with biomolecular forms, with a primary focus on biological inorganic chemistry (Olivier et al., 2019). This term, "metallomics", was recently developed to provide a means to measure multiple biometals and metalloprotein levels in cellular and tissue systems based on the technical advances achieved by analytical omics-based methodologies that facilitate the global profiling of metabolites and macromolecules in biological matrix systems (Maret, 2021). The metallomics scientific field focuses on identifying, quantifying, and locating the specific forms of metals in cells and organisms. Metallomics data consist of total concentrations of metals in bulk or at a particular site (i.e., a specific tissue or cellular compartment) (Montes-Bayón et al., 2018). While reviewing elemental bio-distribution in cells, Williams used the term "metallome" to describe this new scientific discipline of metallomics, which would subsequently be defined as the study of metal species in biology (Vogiatzis and Zachariadis, 2014). As a result of the impact of metal concentration on the function of metalloproteins, metallomics is a vital and relatively new discipline. Of great insight are the mechanisms of uptake, storage, and transport of metals in hyperaccumulators. Comparative metallomics provides an understanding of the temporal differences in a metallome based on differing levels of exposure to metals. Comparative metallomics ultimately enables researchers to study the effects of heavy metal stress tolerance, reactive oxygen species homeostasis, and metal transport processes (Ningombam et al., 2024).

The Metallome in Motion. https://doi.org/10.1016/B978-0-443-44299-5.00008-0

An important part of the overall role of metal ions in the body is their physiological and biological functions. Metal ions, such as iron, zinc, and copper, play critical roles in a variety of cellular processes, including electron transfer, development, and enzyme activity (Busser et al., 2018; Tian et al., 2025). In addition to the physiological functions of metals, there is an association with a number of diseases, including neurological diseases such as Parkinson's and Alzheimer's, which exhibit abnormalities in metal metabolism as a result of dysregulation in the homeostasis of metals (Mezzanotte and Stanga, 2024). Thus, understanding the biological roles and dynamics of metals can facilitate the understanding of the causes of disease and life processes in mammals. The metallome encompasses many aspects of metallomics, including metal-dependent characteristics of the proteome and metabolome; however, since metallomes are typically divided into groups based on the type of biomolecule that interacts with the inorganic element or metal, the metallo proteome is the most commonly studied subset. This subset consists of the entire proteome or a portion of the proteome that is modified by or interacts with metal ions (Banci and Bertini, 2012). The field of metallomics has increasingly attracted the attention of researchers in many disciplines, including medicine, food safety, geoscience, and architectural engineering, as well as biomedical research. This includes the development of new analytical approaches to the study of biometals, which has led to substantial advancements in this area (Maret, 2022). Eventually, the development of new methods to determine the lowest concentrations of these metals in chemical and instrumental studies will serve as an important milestone in the story of metallomics.

9.1.2 Role of metals in biological systems

Metallomics, a discipline integrating sciences that address biometals and biometalloids, provides new opportunities for discoveries. As part of a systems biology approach, it draws attention to the importance of many chemical elements in biochemistry (Maret, 2018). Organisms depend on essential metals to grow, survive, and reach maturation stages that serve physiological importance in mammals through their function as necessary cofactors for many enzymes and to support numerous different types of cellular metabolism (Katsarou and Pantopoulos, 2020). Metals are required to create biological structures. Their use in the body's support systems and the skeletal system is only one example of the critical living support provided by metals. Currently, more than 75% of elements are classified as metals, whereas only about 2.5% of the human body's mass contains any form of metal. The essential role of metals in the biochemical functions of organisms can be overlooked or only briefly mentioned, specifically because of the critical role that metals play in supporting electron transport in the respiratory chain within mitochondria. Iron and copper centers within proteins are critical to aerobic cell life (Maret, 2018). Using metallomics as part of medical research has produced important evidence of the mechanisms involved in the circulation, retention, toxicity, and homeostasis of metals within living animals, particularly in studies of the effects of toxicants and medical disorders that affect the eyes (Forma et al., 2025).

Metallomics works in tandem with proteomics and genomics because different metal ions and metalloenzymes are essential for the synthesis and metabolic processes of proteins and genes. Two-thirds of our proteins require a metal to function, creating metalloproteins or metalloenzymes (metallomes) (Sussulini and Hauser-Davis, 2018). Water oxidation and photosynthesis are important processes that metalloproteins catalyze. A subclass of metalloproteins, known as metalloenzymes, carries out specific catalytic tasks and interacts with the substrate, a molecule that undergoes a net chemical transformation. They are necessary for biological processes to maintain life (Scassellati et al., 2020). Omic approaches are now essential analytical tools in many fields of study, including environmental analysis, systems biology, biomedicine, and food analysis. The three main ways that metal elements carry out biological tasks are through metal-binding proteins (MBPs) and enzymes, metal ions, and the regulation of gut microbes (Tian et al., 2025).

Metal elements are involved in the life activities of mammals. The survival and well-being of organisms depend on trace metal elements, which also play a variety of roles in their life processes. As necessary cofactors for several enzymes and proteins, trace elements assist with a range of chemical reactions in living organisms and support processes including nutrition, digestion, nutrient transport, and genetic material creation (Wang et al., 2018). MBPs make up about 30% of all proteins in animals and are closely related to the organism's ability to sustain life (Cheng et al., 2023). Maintaining human health is heavily dependent on the relative amount of metals in the body. Homeostatic balance can be disrupted by many different conditions, resulting in pathological disorders. Malnutrition, diseases, and prescription medications are just a few of the factors that can impact how well we process and absorb different metals (Crichton, 2020). Dysfunction and death of nerve cells may result in neurodegeneration via specific disease processes. For example, the neurodegenerative diseases associated with abnormal collective metal metabolism of iron, copper, and zinc are [Alzheimer's Disease (AD); Parkinson's Disease (PD); Huntington's Disease (HD) and Multiple System Atrophy (MS)] also collectively known as metallic disorders (Tian et al., 2025).

9.1.3 Need for advanced analytical tools

As a new and expanding area of research called "metallomics," studying and understanding how metals function in living organisms requires the use of advanced technology to quantify and identify metal compounds/solutions accurately and precisely. Adding metallomics to all other areas may improve our understanding of how metals affect biological processes (Li et al., 2008). To enhance the research capability of metallomics, a combination of interdisciplinary activity is needed (i.e., the use of highly developed analytical techniques). The identification and quantification of metallomes on a large scale (high-throughput) necessitate the use of analytical instruments such as Inductively Coupled Plasma Mass Spectrometry (ICP-MS) and other instruments like Laser Ablation ICP-MS (LA-ICP-MS) and Energy Dispersive X-Ray Fluorescence Spectrometers (EDXRF) to analyze how metals interact with biological molecules and how they are distributed within an organism (Machado and Gambino, 2024). The ability to identify metalloproteins, understand the structure-function relationship, and study metal-containing nanoparticles (nanomaterials) in the body and their bioavailability increases the need to develop new tools and improve existing technologies (Sun and Chai, 2010) Using nuclear technology to measure the distribution and accumulation of metal-based nanomaterials in living organisms will provide further detail about how metals behave in both healthy and diseased states and aid in developing metallodrugs and other areas to improve public health (Machado and Gambino, 2024).

Only specified levels of certain elements are required for the appropriate physiological functioning of certain organs, while trace amounts of other elements may be present (Forma et al., 2025). The appropriate operation of many biochemical and metabolic processes depends on micro- and macro-elements. Nutrient concentrations in bodily fluids and tissues, however, vary significantly due to their unequal distribution throughout the organism (Moksnes et al., 2024). The mineralization process and the application of sophisticated analytical methods, such as ICP-MS, inductively coupled plasma (ICP)-atomic emission spectroscopy (ICP-AES), atomic absorption spectroscopy (AAS), and LA-ICP-MS, are required to measure the concentrations of elements in biological samples (Mohammed, 2021). These are techniques of superior sensitivity for multielement analysis (Scalese et al., 2022). The advancement of certain analytical techniques has shown that combined mass spectrometric instruments remain a desirable substitute. Consequently, numerous metallomics experiments employ hyphenated techniques that integrate high-resolution separation via chromatography or electrophoresis (to prevent the coelution of multiple species of the same heteroelement) with ICP-MS detection or electrospray ionization mass spectrometry (ESI-MS) for structural analysis (Montes-Bayón et al., 2018). The primary benefits of ICP-MS, which is frequently employed in metallomics, are its excellent sensitivity and selectivity. The primary detection method used in analyses is often ICP-MS. As a substitute option for quantifying proteins and peptides, it plays an important role in proteomics (Vogiatzis and Zachariadis, 2014).

The use of X-ray absorption spectroscopy (XAS) and synchrotron X-ray spectroscopy as measuring techniques is emerging, according to recent articles on metallomics. Detection sensitivity from synchrotron radiation-stimulated X-ray fluorescence (XRF) can actually match that of LA-ICP-MS. The emergence of new technology has facilitated significant progress, leading to the integration of genomics, proteomics, metabolomics, and metallomics (Sussulini and Hauser-Davis, 2018). The investigation of novel biological metal species necessitates the development of new analytical instruments (bioanalysis) that replace conventional photon-based atomic detectors (AAS), ICP-AES, and atomic fluorescence spectroscopy with ion-characterizing mass detectors [mass spectrometry (MS) and ICP-MS]. The use of ICP-MS allows for multielemental determinations (García-Barrera et al., 2012) and the absolute quantification of the metallo-biomolecule using species-specific isotopic dilution or species-unspecific isotopic dilution analysis, which overcome matrix effects and problems derived from instrumental drift and avoid the need for correction with dilution or preconcentration factors (Ramirez-Acosta et al., 2021). The spectrum of applications for metallomics has expanded due to the notable advancements in metal detection techniques in recent years. The detection of metal distribution in tissues and the comprehension of the actions of metal elements in biological systems are particularly common applications of MS techniques and new imaging technologies (Tian et al., 2025). The detection of metal elements and metal isotope determination in samples using MS and spectroscopy (Jim et al., 2017) and the structural determination of metal complexes using spectroscopy, crystallography, and cryo-electron microscopy (Zeng et al., 2024) are examples of the growing number of metallomics technologies.

9.2 Sample preparation strategies for metallomics

There are a number of ways that metallomic samples are prepared to allow for the study of metal-based elements in the biological sciences. The microwave-assisted preparation of metallomic samples allows for enhanced extraction and breakdown, which, in turn, makes the study of trace metals and metalloproteins that play essential roles in biological functions significantly easier (Mataveli et al., 2014). The use of LA-ICP-MS in combination with polyacrylamide gel electrophoresis (PAGE) allows for the accurate measurement of MBPs and their interactions in biological systems (Sussulini and Becker, 2011). Currently, sample preparation for the analysis of heavy metals, as well as the sampling, cleaning, and preservation of samples, is critical to obtaining accurate results (Chirila et al., 2010). Therefore, ICP-MS and LA-ICP-MS techniques are preferred for metallomic analyses due to their high sensitivity and capability of quantifying a vast number of elements (Feng, 2024). The combination of these techniques provides valuable information about the roles of metals in living systems and their impacts on human health and the health of the ecosystems where they occur.

9.3 Sample types

9.3.1 Biological (blood, tissues, cells, plants)

Metallomics refers to the study of metal and metalloid species in biological tissues (e.g., blood, tissue, and plant) to gain an understanding of their function and role in health and disease; thus, metallomics is an evolving science encompassing both the study of metal/metalloid species and their function in a variety of complex biological environments. The use of sophisticated analytical methods, such as synchrotron-based XRF (SR-XRF) and ICP-MS, is employed to assess metallomes, which are dynamic and impacted by both environmental and genetic factors (Grabrucker, 2020). By profiling the metal ion concentrations in human biological specimens, cancer research has identified key metal species, specifically copper, as contributing factors with respect to the development of malignancies (Zhang et al., 2022). The qualitative and quantitative investigation of the distribution of metals in animal tissues is facilitated through bioimaging techniques, which increase our understanding of the biological processes associated with metal metabolism (Dressler et al., 2018). Overall, metallomics provides critical insight into the molecular mechanisms by which metals interact with biological systems and their relevance for diagnosis and therapy.

9.3.2 Food and environmental samples

This field of study, known as metallomics, is crucial for understanding how metals interact with living organisms. Studying the way metals and metalloids (the latter being a classification that includes selenium, for example) are present in food and environmental samples allows researchers to determine the point at which these elements become toxic or effective for both human health and environmental remediation (Mo et al., 2007). Recent advances in analytical techniques (e.g., MS and chromatography) have enabled scientists to examine metallobiomolecules in their natural environments, gaining insight into metal toxicity and homeostasis in the environment (Rodríguez-Moro et al., 2018). Using these same technologies to investigate the structural and functional aspects of metalloproteins in many different species or tissues has further advanced the application of metallomics for environmental monitoring (Silva and Silva, 2020). Combining metallomics and metabolomics as applied to plants provides a unique opportunity to evaluate the effects of metal stresses as well as the mechanisms of pollution remediation, including exploring hyperaccumulators and producing food enriched with important elements (Gómez Ariza et al., 2013). In addition, by combining metallomics and metabolomics in model organisms, such as mice and clams, researchers are able to identify biomarkers of environmental pollution and thus provide real-world applications for these findings (Blasco et al., 2020). As such, this holistic approach provides a more comprehensive understanding of the ways organisms respond biologically to exposure to metals while also aiding in the development of techniques for protecting both food safety and the environment.

9.3.3 Digestion and extraction methods

In the context of metallomics, there are many types of digestion/extraction techniques, all of which have their pros and cons. There is evidence to support that the use of chemical acids (particularly nitric acid (HNO3)) to digest plant tissues for the extraction of trace metallic elements (TMEs) is effective. For TMEs, including Cu, Zn, and Fe, the most effective recovery method is typically known as "cold extraction," whereas for TMEs, including Cr and Ba, "hot extraction" methods are more effective (Sleimi et al., 2022). Microwaves (MW) assist digestion is most favorable for extracting certain metals, including cadmium (Cd) and lead (Pb), from MSW (MW produce faster and higher extraction efficiencies) (Ramanathan and Ting, 2015). The use of enzyme-based digestion methods offers a gentler approach that preserves the integrity of sensitive species (such as arsenic (As)) when extracting from biological matrices; however, enzyme methods may yield lower extraction efficiencies compared to other methods when operated under intermediate conditions (Lu et al., 2012). The need to choose the appropriate digestion/extraction technique based on the sample matrix and analytical requirements is illustrated by the use of ultrasonic-assisted digestion techniques, as well as by the differences between open and closed system methods used for the analysis of various sample matrices (Dugo et al., 2012).

9.4 Techniques for measuring total metal content

9.4.1 Inductively coupled plasma-mass spectrometry

Because of its wide dynamic range, high sensitivity, and ability to resolve isotopes, ICP-MS is considered the benchmark method for total metal quantification in metallome-type research. In ICP-MS, an aerosol of the sample is ionized inside an argon (inductively coupled) plasma (6000–10,000 K) (Clases and Gonzalez de Vega, 2022). The ions produced in the ionization process are then separated based on their mass-to-charge ratio (m/z) using one of three primary types of analyzers [quadrupole, sector-field, and time-of-flight (TOF)]. By using collision/reaction cell technology (with He, H_2, and NH_3), polyatomic and isobaric interferences are diminished substantially, and at that point, detection limits can be determined in the ppt to sub-ppt range. Desolvating nebulizers and microflow nebulizers, in addition to modern sample introduction systems, help to enhance the stability of the signal from these metals and lower the tendency to form oxides, thereby increasing accuracy in measuring metallic ions in a complex biological matrix (Michalke, 2022; Retzmann et al., 2023). The features of ICP-MS make it a critical tool for mapping trace-metal isotope ratios and low-abundance trace metals in metallomics workflows. Recently published high-impact review papers summarize the major advancements that have occurred to improve instrument stability, the robustness of the plasma, and expanded isotopic applications (Resano et al., 2023; Chang et al., 2022).

Over the years, there have been transformative developments in ICP-MS, especially with regard to time-resolved and single-entity analysis. These new approaches allow the quantification of elemental content at the single-particle, organelle, or cellular levels, which represent emerging frontiers in cellular metallomics (Resano et al., 2023; He et al., 2024; Gregar et al., 2025). In addition, hyphenated applications such as LC-ICP-MS, CE-ICP-MS, and GC-ICP-MS have become instrumental tools in differentiating between protein-bound, free ion, and nanoparticulate metal species, further facilitating mechanistic insights into metal trafficking (Michalke, 2022). While ICP-MS offers great advantages, strict contamination controls, consistent digestion protocols, and matrix-matched calibration or isotope dilution techniques are necessary to avoid suppression or enhancement effects. Therefore, although operating expenses are high and sensitivity to matrix-induced interferences remains an existing issue, progress in the development of collision/reaction cells, autosamplers, and high-resolution platforms is enabling ICP-MS to remain the preferred method for achieving high-resolution metallome profiling (Diez-Fernández et al., 2020; Dressler et al., 2020).

9.4.2 Inductively coupled plasma-optical emission spectrometry

The high-temperature-initiated ICP allows the measurement of characteristic atomic/ionic emission lines generated in the ICP, which provide robust multi-element detection capability in the form of precise measurements of major and trace elements (Donati et al., 2017; Li et al., 2021). This technique is generally noted for its ability to produce very low levels of detectability in the parts-per-billion (ppb) range. Recent improvements in echelle spectrometry, charge-coupled devices, and the development of improved algorithms for correcting background contributions from the interference of other emission lines have enhanced spectral separation, allowing for fewer errors caused by overlapping spectral emissions (Khan et al., 2022). In addition, ICP-optical emission spectrometry (ICP-OES) has a relatively high tolerance for elevated levels of total dissolved solids compared to MS and is thus an excellent choice for routine utilization in high-throughput screening of digested biological, food, and environmental samples. The expanding use of the ICP-OES technique for systematic multielement surveys and as a routine component of metallomic workflows has been discussed in several recent reviews (Clough et al., 2023).

Plasma stability, optical design, and detector technology have undergone major advancements over the past five years. These advancements have resulted in improved sensitivity, matrix tolerance, and usability of ICP-OES for the analysis of complex biological samples such as plants, animals, and plastic micro-particulates (Sharma, 2020). Relative to the cost-effectiveness of operating an ICP-OES compared to an IC-MC, the lower cost-to-analyst ratio makes ICP-OES well-positioned for larger-scale and longitudinal studies that require the analysis of many elements in thousands of samples (Borowska and Jankowski, 2023). Nonetheless, due to the higher detection limits associated with ICP-OES as opposed to IC-MC and the inherent limitations of ICP-OES caused by signal interference and/or signal overlap, there are restrictions on emission-line selection, calibration against matrix standards, and the utilization of approved internal standards. On the other hand, while ICP-OES cannot provide isotope-specific results or quantification of ultra-trace concentrations, the use of modern ICP-OES is critical to metallomic workflows for determining concentrations of relatively abundant to moderately concentrated metals, as well as corroborating findings from the ICP-MC system. Recent work highlights the importance of ICP history and how ICP-OES can be used as a mechanism for identifying metallomic constituents effectively, cost-effectively, and as a means of achieving a complete characterization of all metallomic constituents (Carter et al., 2016; Patriarca et al., 2022a; Brunnbauer et al., 2024).

9.4.3 Atomic absorption spectroscopy

AAS measures the concentration of metals present in a solution by quantifying the amount of light absorbed during a flame or graphite furnace process (Patriarca et al., 2022b). Flame AAS (FAAS) is the preferred analytical technique for determining metals at mg/L to high μg/L levels and is widely used across the globe for these types of analyses. Graphite Furnace AAS (GFAAS) offers significantly higher sensitivity compared to FAAS (low μg/L to ng/L) due to the combination of electrothermal atomization and extended residence times of the analytes in the optical path (Butcher, 2024). Elements can be detected with greater accuracy using AAS than with other methods because AAS employs either element-specific hollow cathode lamps or electrodeless discharge lamps to produce distinct emission lines, enabling individual detection even in moderately complex matrices. AAS measures one element at a time and is less susceptible to spectral interferences compared to ICP-OES, making it a reliable and cost-efficient method for quantifying specific metals. Recent reviews have emphasized the continued importance of AAS for trace metal analysis in food, clinical, environmental, and biological samples, particularly when sample volume and regulatory testing demand highly accurate results (Momen, 2023).

AAS has a number of advantages for use as a single-element detection tool; however, it has limitations, such as being restricted to one element at a time and having a much narrower dynamic range compared to other techniques that can measure multiple elements on a plasma/MSS (multispecies spectroscopic) basis. Nevertheless, many recent advancements in the design and technology related to thermospray laser atomic absorption spectrometry (TL-AAS), such as high-temperature platform design, improvements in matrix-extraction modifiers (increased sensitivity of matrix extraction), and enhanced atomizer coatings, are making AAS applicable to a wider variety of more complex biological matrices, as well as providing more reproducible and precise limits of detection or limit of quantification (LOD or LOQ) for AAS (Resano et al., 2023; Clough et al., 2023). Through improvements in high-resolution continuum source AAS, fast scanning has been made possible by using multiple lines of detection with an increased signal-to-noise ratio (improved detection). In comparison to the most frequently used multielement analytical techniques (MS and ICP), while AAS does not provide the ultra-trace sensitivity of the modern generation of ICP/MS, it is still a very cost-effective and accurate analysis method for certain key elements, such as Fe, Cu, Zn, Pb, and Cd (Acar, 2024). As an alternative to validated approaches for measuring metal concentrations in metallome studies, AAS has a number of advantages over existing validated approaches for large-scale metallomic profiling. These advantages include the high reproducibility and precision with which it can generate the results necessary for using multiple validated and/or transitional assays that are utilized in metallomics (Gómez-Nieto et al., 2022; Yang et al., 2024).

9.4.4 X-ray fluorescence spectroscopy

XRF determines elemental composition by measuring the characteristic secondary (fluorescent) X-rays emitted when atoms are excited by a primary X-ray beam. It is a fundamentally nondestructive technique that requires little to no sample preparation and enables rapid, multielement screening from ppm to percentage levels. Modern XRF techniques are often called EDXRF and Wavelength Dispersive XRF (WDXRF), which provide broad elemental coverage (Na-U), with WDXRF offering higher spectral resolution and accuracy, particularly for analyses of overlapping lines (Sindhu et al., 2022). XRF is increasingly being used in metallomic studies of biological and environmental materials because it can be applied to samples in solid, tissue, powder, or surface form without requiring sample dissolution, making it possible to preserve the spatial and chemical variability in a sample while also reducing the risk of contamination (Vanhoof et al., 2023; Dhara and Mishra, 2025).

Recent reviews have discussed how laboratory-scale micro-XRF and benchtop EDXRF systems are increasingly being used for high-throughput metallome screening and quality control and assurance workflows (Carter et al., 2021; Revenko and Pashkova, 2023). The development of new technologies, particularly over the last five years, has led to the rapid advancement of XRF technology, including the growth of micro-XRF, SR-XRF, and XRF imaging technologies, which enable the study of cellular and sub-cellular spatially resolved metallomics (Carter et al., 2021). Micro-XRF now achieves spot sizes of 10–20 μm with improved detectors (silicon drift detector (SDDs)), providing semiquantitative maps of metal distribution in tissues, seeds, and biomaterials critical for studying metal localization, trafficking, and toxicity. SR-XRFfurther pushes detection limits to ppm-ppb levels with nanometric spatial resolution, supporting high-impact studies of metalloproteins and metal-dependent cellular processes (Wang et al., 2022). Limitations of XRF include relatively higher detection limits than ICP-MS, challenges in quantifying very light elements (e.g., Li, Be), and the matrix-dependency of calibration. However, ongoing advancements in detector sensitivity, fundamental-parameter quantification algorithms, and portable XRF instrumentation continue to position XRF as a powerful complementary technique for nondestructive metallome characterization (Li et al., 2021; Specht et al., 2024). The techniques, pros, cons, and applications are summarized in Table 9.1.

TABLE 9.1 Attributes and applications of main techniques for total metal analysis.

Technique	Advantages	Limitation	Applications
ICP-MS	• Ultra-trace sensitivity (ppt-sub-ppt) • Wide dynamic range; multielement detection • Isotopic ratio capability • Compatible with hyphenated systems (LC-ICP-MS, CE-ICP-MS) • High throughput	• High cost (instrument + maintenance) • Susceptible to polyatomic/isobaric interferences • Sensitive to contamination; strict sample prep needed • Matrix suppression/enhancement issues	• Advanced metallomics and biomonitoring • Single-cell and nanoparticle elemental analysis • Isotope fingerprinting and environmental forensics • Trace metal profiling in biological, food, and clinical matrices
ICP-OES	• Good sensitivity (low-ppb) • Robust, stable, multielement capability • Tolerates high dissolved solids • Lower operational cost than ICP-MS	• Higher LODs than ICP-MS (not suitable for ultra-trace metals) • Spectral overlaps require careful wavelength selection • No isotopic information	• Routine metal monitoring in environmental, food. and agricultural samples • Large-scale surveys requiring rapid screening • QC/QA laboratories • Profiling moderately abundant metals in biological digests
AAS (FAAS/ GFAAS)	• Highly selective with minimal spectral interference • Low cost; suitable for smaller labs • GFAAS provides good sensitivity ($ng \cdot L^{-1}$) • Excellent accuracy for targeted elements	• Single-element technique • low throughput • Narrow dynamic range • Requires matrix modifiers for complex samples (GFAAS) • Not ideal for broad metallome profiling	• Targeted quantification (Fe, Zn, Cu, Pb, Cd) • Food safety and water quality testing • Pharmaceutical and environmental QC • Validation of ICP-based measurements
XRF (EDXRF/ WDXRF/ Micro-XRF)	• Nondestructive; minimal sample prep • Rapid multielement detection (ppm–%) • Suitable for solids, powders, tissues • Portable XRF enables field analysis • Micro-XRF provides spatial mapping	• Higher LODs than ICPS techniques • Poor sensitivity for light elements (e.g., Li, Be) • Matrix effects influence quantification • Less accurate for trace metals in biological samples	• Spatially resolved metallomics (micro-XRF, synchrotron XRF) • Nondestructive testing in food, archeology, and geology • Rapid field screening using handheld XRF • Semiquantitative screening before ICP analysis

9.5 Speciation and metalloprotein analysis

9.5.1 Why metal speciation matters

Using total metal concentrations on their own often results in misrepresenting the biological role, toxicity, and metabolic activity. A critical step in demonstrating the relationship of metals to biological activity is to first identify and measure the individual forms in which a metal occurs. This step is referred to as speciation or measuring the metal species. Each of the individual metal species has very different chemistry, which influences its reactivity, bioavailability, mode of transport, and toxicity (Capdevila et al., 2024). For example, Cr(III) is a nutrient, while Cr(VI) is a carcinogen; inorganic As(III–V) is much more toxic than the methylated arsenicals, and the biological activity of Cu, Fe, and Zn is highly dependent on whether they are present in solution as free ions or bound to metalloproteins. There is an increasing emphasis by researchers on interpreting data on total metal content in ways that identify biologically relevant mechanistic pathways, particularly those related to oxidative stress, neurodegeneration, microbial resistance to metals, and nutrient transport (Genchi et al., 2021; Lim et al., 2023; Zhou et al., 2024) (Table 9.2).

Most of the biologically active forms of metals in biological systems are metalloproteins, metalloenzymes, or transient metal-ligand complexes. Determining these species is vital for understanding metal homeostasis, signaling networks, and pathological metal imbalances observed in conditions such as Alzheimer's disease, cancer, Parkinson's disease, and metabolic disorders (Du et al., 2024). Speciation also reveals how processing, storage, or environmental exposure alters metal forms, influencing safety and health outcomes. Over the last five years, advances in metalloproteomics and single-cell metal imaging have shown that speciation profiling can uncover early biomarkers of disease, clarify metal-protein interactions, and support precision nutrition strategies. Thus, speciation is now considered a core requirement for any advanced metallomic investigation (Patriarca et al., 2022a; Resano et al., 2023).

9.5.2 Hyphenated techniques for metal speciation (HPLC-ICP-MS, GC-ICP-MS, CE-ICP-MS)

Hyphenated techniques combine a separation method high-performance liquid chromatography (HPLC), gas chromatography (GC), or capillary electrophoresis (CE) with the element-specific, highly sensitive detection of ICP-MS, enabling the characterization of metal species without losing elemental information. HPLC-ICP-MS is the most widely used and is capable of separating ionic species, metal-ligand complexes, and intact metallodrugs with excellent reproducibility (Michalke, 2022). GC-ICP-MS is used for volatile or derivatized organometallic compounds, such as mercury or tin species (Suárez-Criado et al., 2022). CE-ICP-MS provides high-efficiency separation for charged and small-volume biological samples, often outperforming HPLC in resolving

TABLE 9.2 Comprehensive comparison of imaging techniques used in metallome studies.

Technique	Spatial resolution	Detection limits	Type of information	Strengths	Limitations	Applications in metallomics	References
Synchrotron X-ray fluorescence (XRF/XFM)	~30–100 nm (nano-XRF), 1–5 μm (micro-XRF)	ppm to ppb	Elemental distribution, semiquantitative metal concentration	Nondestructive, multielemental, deep penetration, high sensitivity	Requires synchrotron access, limited chemical speciation	Mapping metal distribution in cells/tissues, metal accumulation in diseases, plant metal uptake	(Gorman et al., 2024b; Lovett and Harris, 2021)
X-ray absorption spectroscopy (XAS: XANES/EXAFS)	~1–5 μm (micro-XAS)	ppm	Oxidation state, coordination environment, speciation	Provides chemical bonding info, works in complex matrices	Needs synchrotron, no high-res spatial maps without microprobe	Metal oxidation states, speciation in proteins, toxic metal forms	(Newton et al., 2023)
X-ray diffraction (XRD)	N/A (requires crystals)	N/A	Atomic structure, lattice spacing	High structural accuracy, useful for metalloproteins	Requires crystals; not suitable for intact cells	Metalloprotein structure, biomineral analysis	(Lovett and Harris, 2021)
Nano secondary ion mass spectrometry (Nano-SIMS)	30–50 nm	ppm	Elemental/isotopic mapping, quantitative analysis	Highest spatial resolution, isotopic imaging	Destructive, limited field of view, matrix effects	Subcellular metal imaging, isotopic tracing, metal–metabolite interactions	(Li et al., 2021)
Laser ablation ICP-MS (LA-ICP-MS)	1–5 μm	ppb–ppt	Elemental quantification, 2D mapping	Highly sensitive, quantitative, multielemental	Destructive, lower spatial resolution than XRF	Tissue metal quantification, metallodrug distribution	(Li et al., 2021)

Continued

TABLE 9.2 Comprehensive comparison of imaging techniques used in metallome studies—cont'd

Technique	Spatial resolution	Detection limits	Type of information	Strengths	Limitations	Applications in metallomics	References
Inductively coupled plasma mass spectrometry (ICP-MS) imaging (Laser or Direct Nebulization)	5–20 μm	ppt	Multielemental quantitative maps	Ultra-sensitive, good for trace metals	Requires ablation or sample introduction; destructive	Trace metal profiling, metal exposure studies	(Li et al., 2021)
Magnetic resonance imaging (MRI) for metals	~100–500 μm	μM	Metal ion presence (Fe, Mn), tissue-level mapping	Noninvasive, in vivo imaging	Poor sensitivity, limited to paramagnetic metals	Iron metabolism, ferritin imaging, brain metal dysregulation	(Akdogan and Istanbullu, 2022)
Electron microscopy (TEM/SEM) with EDS	TEM: 1–2 nm; SEM: 5–10 nm	ppm	Ultrastructure + elemental identity	Very high-resolution structural imaging	Limited quantification, small area, sample prep needed	Metal nanoparticles, subcellular metal localization	(Pereira et al., 2025)
Fluorescent metal probes (chemical imaging)	~200–300 nm	μM–nM	Dynamic metal pools, redox-active metals	Live-cell imaging, high speed	Requires specific probes; not all metals detectable	Zn^{2+}, Cu^{+} pools, oxidative stress metals, signalling studies	(Carter et al., 2014)
Infrared (IR) and Raman microscopy	~1–10 μm	μM	Chemical bonding, metal–ligand interactions	Nondestructive, label-free	Poor metal specificity, weak signals	Metal–biomolecule complexes, metallodrug tracking	(Cebi et al., 2023; Saputra et al., 2024)

metalprotein isoforms, labile complexes, and redox-sensitive species (Duroux and Hagège, 2022). Together, these hyphenated techniques offer unmatched capabilities for distinguishing species that differ only slightly in charge, polarity, oxidation state, or molecular mass (He et al., 2024).

In recent years, hyphenated ICP-MS platforms have undergone major improvements in interface design, nebulization efficiency, and low-flow plasma operation, enabling the analysis of labile, transient, and low-abundance metal species with minimal artifact formation. HPLC-ICP-MS plays an integral role in profiling arsenic, selenium, chromium, cobalt, and copper species in foodstuffs, biological fluids, and environmental matrices (Duroux and Hagège, 2022). Additionally, CE-ICP-MS has emerged as a key tool for metalloprotein characterization due to its ability to operate under native conditions, thereby retaining the noncovalent intermolecular metal-protein interactions. Significant advances in GC-ICP-MS methodology have now enabled the sensitive detection of volatile organometallic toxicants (mercury, tin, and lead species) at trace levels. These "hyphenated" methods are rapidly being combined with orthogonal platforms such as ESI-MS/MS, synchrotron-based XAS, and size-exclusion chromatography to create next-generation multidimensional metalloproteomic workflows that will map the metal content and oxidation state of proteins, as well as their binding and posttranslational metalation mechanisms (Michalke, 2022; Yan et al., 2024; Coverdale et al., 2024).

9.5.3 Separation of metalloproteins

Metalloproteins are responsible for between 13% and 75% of total cellular proteins (depending on the organism). The role of the metal cofactor in metalloproteins directly impacts fundamental biochemical processes: catalysis, electron transfer, signaling, and structural preservation (Helmann, 2025). Since the metal-protein interaction is usually weak and redox-sensitive, the ability to separate and characterize metalloproteins without affecting the native metalation state is critical in metalloproteomics. Conventional separation techniques used to characterize proteins (e.g., SDS-PAGE and extreme chromatographic buffer conditions) strip the metals from the proteins during the separation process, causing an artifactually altered metalloprotein background (Tang et al., 2022). The use of nondenaturing, metal-stabilizing separation techniques [based on size exclusion chromatography (SEC), ion exchange chromatography (IEX), native-PAGE, affinity chromatography, and fast protein liquid chromatography (FPLC)] under precisely controlled conditions for pH, ionic strength, and absence of chelating agents preserves the native metal-protein complex while providing the separation of complex mixtures, thus maintaining the integrity of the separated metalloprotein for further downstream analyses (Resano et al., 2023).

Over the past years, there has been significant interest in advanced separation workflows that combine the use of high-resolution chromatography directly with elemental and molecular detection systems. SEC-ICP-MS continues to be a key resource for mapping the distribution of metals found in protein fractions; among its advantages is the ability to rapidly identify metalloprotein peaks based on metal-specific signals (Michalke et al., 2021; Tang et al., 2022; Resano et al., 2023). Affinity-based methods, such as IMAC, metal-chelating resins, and engineered metalloprotein tags, allow targeted purification of Zn, Cu, Ni, and Fe-binding metalloproteins while preserving their native conformation. Native MS, ion mobility spectrometry (IMS), and microfluidic separation techniques provide higher resolution of the isoform, oligomeric state, and redox variants of metalloproteins with reduced sample usage. Collectively, these techniques assist in preserving the native metal stoichiometry and enable accurate identification of biologically relevant metalloproteins within complex samples (Peris-Díaz et al., 2024; Uyeda, 2025).

9.5.4 Basic steps in identifying metal-binding proteins

A systematic approach is typically used to identify MBPs . It starts with preparing biological extracts under conditions designed to preserve metals' ability to bind to proteins (i.e., preventing metal cofactor loss or exchange). Once the extract is prepared, the next step is to separate the extracts into individual candidate metalloproteins. The separation can be done by SEC, IEX, native PAGE, or FPLC (Michalke, 2022). Each fraction obtained from the separation is analyzed for metal content using ICP-MS or SEC-ICP-MS to detect the locations of the metals and the amount of metal present in each sample. Fractions that yield high amounts of enriched metal signal are collected; subsequently, the proteins in these fractions are identified by proteomics (LC-MS/MS), peptide sequencing, or intact protein MS under native conditions. The combination of these methods (i.e., elemental analysis and molecular analysis) ensures that the protein identified corresponds to the specific metal signals detected in each fraction sample (Zhou et al., 2024).

Initial identification of a metalloprotein is followed by confirmation of its authenticity through several additional and independent methods. Examples of these orthogonal methods include UV-Vis spectroscopy, XAS, electron paramagnetic resonance, and native MS. Each of these methods confirms the oxidation state of the metal, the coordination geometry of the ligand, and the stoichiometric ratio of metal to protein as reported (Shafaat et al., 2023). The functional importance or role of the metal in the metalloprotein can be established through mutagenesis, testing for competitive interactions between metals, and in vitro reconstitution. More recent workflows for studying the characterization of ferrous iron metalloproteins include cross-linking MS, hydrogen-deuterium exchange, and computational docking of metals onto proteins. In summary, through the above-mentioned approaches and technologies, metalloproteins can be identified and characterized to their fullest extent in terms of their mechanisms of action and their involvement in the physiology, nutrition, toxicology, and disease biology of metalloproteins (Stofella et al., 2024).

9.6 Advanced imaging and high-resolution techniques

9.6.1 Laser ablation ICP-MS

Laser ablation is one of the finest techniques utilized for the compositional analysis of solid materials (analytes) due to its sensitivity and conceptual simplicity. It is commonly employed in quadrupole, sector field, or TOF mass analyzers to measure laser-generated aerosols with high elemental sensitivity. The small particles, which range from <0.15 μm, are fully evaporated and ionized under plasma, which can limit the accuracy of quantification for larger particles. In addition, matrix effects, data and graphs, and spectral interferences present significant challenges, requiring careful calibration, optimization of plasma conditions, and the use of standardized methods. An important advantage of ICP-MS over solution-based analysis is the absence of solvent-related interferences, enabling cleaner spectra and improved detection quality as well as quantity with multielement analysis at a single time. Various metals, such as Al, Ag, As, Au, Be, Ca, Cd, Co, Cr, Cu, Fe, Ga, Hg, lanthanides, Mg, Mn, Na, Ni, Pb, Se, and Zn, among others, are the focus of metallomics studies on viral infections. For example, arsenic was detected by ICP-MS from a coal sample with *Cyanobacterium glutamicum* ArsC1-C2, suggesting that it can also be used for screening purposes in aqueous samples (Villadangos et al., 2010). Zn is vital for memory, and its loss contributes to cognitive decline. Sophisticated instruments like XRF, LA-ICP-MS, SIMS, and particle-induced X-ray emission (PIXE)are utilized to detect and map Zn restoration in brain regions. In Alzheimer's disease, caused by the accumulation of Zn in amyloid-β plaques, this accumulation was identified by mapping through such techniques (Ellison et al., 2022).

9.6.2 Secondary ion mass spectrometry

Secondary Ion MS (SIMS) is a specific analytical technique where a focused ion beam sputters the sample surface, generating secondary ions that are analyzed by a mass spectrometer. It involves emitting high-energy primary ions (Cs^+, O_2^+, Ga^+) under vacuum over the surface of a sample. After bombarding the surface with energy rays, secondary ions (mass-to-charge ratio) are ejected and then detected. SIMS provides a comprehensive profile of the molecular content of the tissue under investigation, including drugs, proteins, lipids, N-glycans, and other biomolecules (Zhang et al., 2025). A study (Gorman et al., 2024a) reported that matrix-assisted laser desorption/ionization mass spectrometry imaging (MALDI-MSI) was used for imaging intact biomolecules like lipids, and MSI was used to detect metals like Fe (Fig. 9.1).

Nano-SIMS is a high-resolution technique that enables detection at up to 50 nm. After tremendous research in the field of biomedical sciences, Nano-SIMS has advanced in spatial resolution, sensitivity, multiplexity, and the breadth of analytes (Zhou et al., 2024). It analyzes images and quantifies elements and isotopes by sputtering secondary ions with a focused primary ion

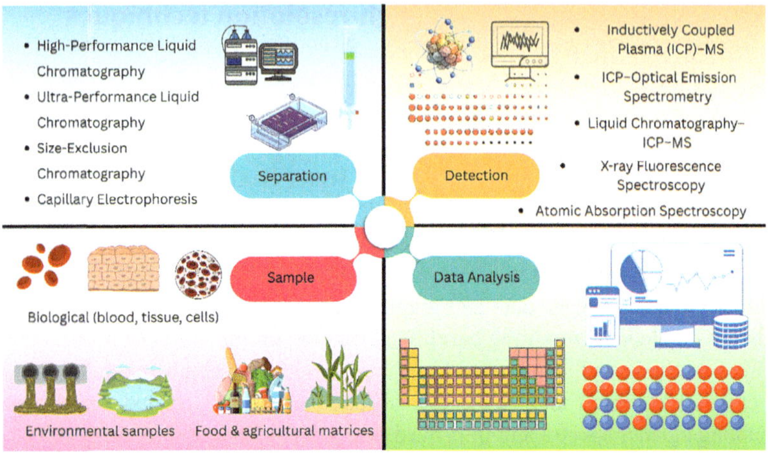

FIG. 9.1 Basic workflow of metallome profiling.

beam. It operates using either Cs^+ or O^- ion sources, enabling precise elemental and isotopic analysis. It is used in several applications, such as studying endogenous elements, drugs, pharmaceuticals, and metallodrugs, including platinum and ruthenium-based anticancer drugs. Elements such as Cu, Zn, N, S, and P are also analyzed (Legin et al., 2014). SIMS provides important information about the distribution, localization, interaction, and mechanisms of elements at the nano scale (Neuditschko et al., 2021).

9.6.3 XRF imaging

XRF spectrometry is based on the principle that individual atoms emit characteristic X-ray photons upon excitation by an external energy source. When X-ray beams strike the sample, they eject electrons from the primary inner-shell, and shortly afterward, the sample undergoes relaxation as higher-energy electrons fill the vacancies. Each electron transition produces specific fluorescence. A detector then records these X-rays, generating high-resolution images that signify the position, concentration, and area of presence of elements (Staufer and Grüner, 2023). The main advantage of XRF imaging is that it is nondestructive, operates under air pressure, and is suitable for liquid samples. Recent studies have shown that SR-XRF can detect multielement; for example, copper (Cu) was found in astrocytes and ependymal cells of the brain's lateral ventricles, as well as in the corpus callosum white matter of mice, rats, and human tissues (Hackett et al., 2019; Lins et al., 2016; Sullivan et al., 2017). Similarly, it has been utilized to identify zinc (Zn) depletion, particularly in specific tissue regions (Fimognari et al., 2018). One of the best examples was reported by Manohar et al. (2016), where XRF was found to be more sensitive than computed tomography (CT). While CT was able to identify a gold-sputtering-marked tumor in a tumor mouse, XRF easily detected the tumor with greater sensitivity (Staufer and Grüner, 2023).

Synchrotron-based methods in metallomics utilize intense, tunable X-ray beams generated by accelerating electrons through magnetic fields to study metals in biological systems. Key techniques include XRF microscopy, which maps elemental distributions by detecting characteristic fluorescent X-rays emitted upon atomic excitation; XAS, including X-ray absorption near edge structure (XANES) and EXAFS, which determine metal oxidation states, coordination geometry, and local atomic environments; and X-ray Diffraction, used for structural determination of metal-containing biomolecules, including metalloproteins, when crystallized. Owing to the exceptional brightness, nanoscale spatial resolution, and multielement detection capability of synchrotron radiation, these methods comprehensively characterize the metallome, identifying which metals are present, their concentrations, spatial localization, and chemical speciation, thus providing critical insights into metal homeostasis, metalloprotein function, and metal dysregulation in diseases such as Alzheimer's and cancer (Fig. 9.2).

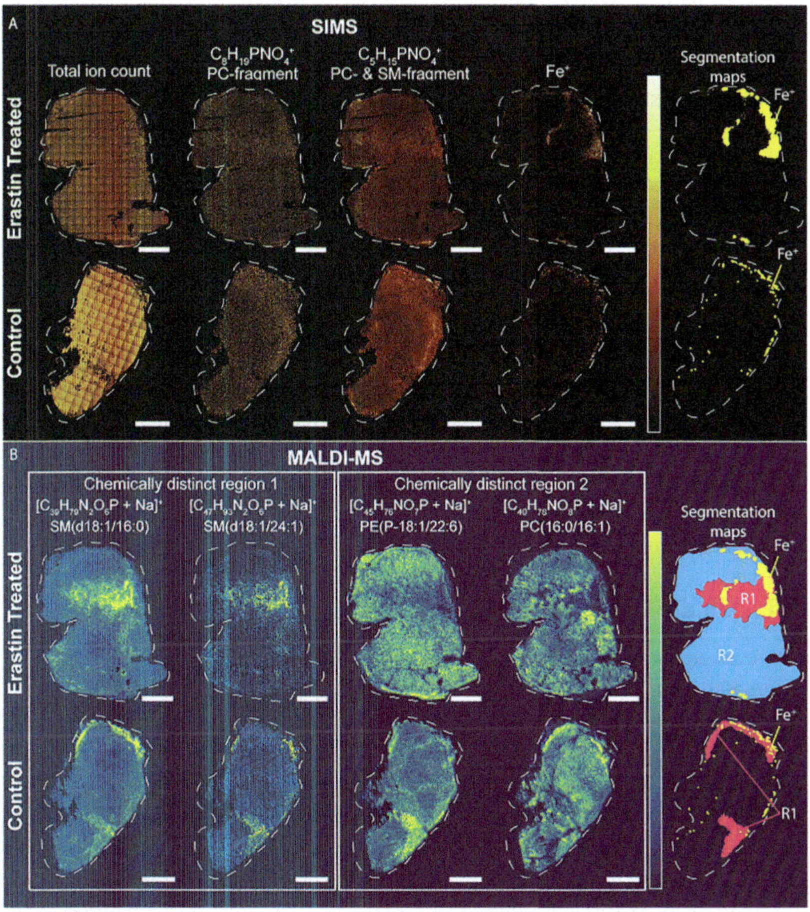

FIG. 9.2 SIMS ion images show the accumulation of Fe in the erastin-treated tumor. *(J. Am. Soc. Mass Spectrom. 2024, 35(1), 5–12).*

9.7 Data analysis and future directions

The quality of data analysis plays a crucial role in accurately interpreting metallome profiling results. Techniques such as ICP-MS, XRF, SIMS, and other hyphenated methods generate complex raw signals that cannot be directly used without proper processing. Raw data typically undergo several correction steps, including background subtraction, instrumental drift correction, normalization using internal standards, and calibration with certified reference materials. These processes are essential for ensuring that the results are accurate, reproducible, and comparable across different instruments and samples, ultimately enabling a reliable understanding of the underlying biological or chemical mechanisms.

The use of advanced data analysis and visualization software greatly enhances the interpretability of complex metallomic datasets. Tools such as Excel, GraphPad Prism, SPSS, and multivariate techniques like Principal Component Analysis help reveal hidden trends, group similarities, and identify associations between metals and biomolecules. Statistical approaches, including hierarchical clustering, k-means, partial least squares regression, and analysis of variance (ANOVA), are commonly applied to classify samples, detect outliers, and establish correlations with biological or environmental factors. By integrating these analytical methods, researchers can efficiently manage multivariate datasets generated from imaging, speciation studies, or multielement quantification. Overall, these tools play a crucial role in extracting, visualizing, and interpreting meaningful information that defines the metallome of a sample.

A growing trend in the field is the integration of metallomics with other omics platforms, including genomics, proteomics, metabolomics, and lipidomics. Such multiomics strategies allow deeper biological interpretation by linking metal distributions to gene expression, metabolic pathways, or protein function. This systems-level perspective enhances our understanding of metal homeostasis, disease mechanisms, and the impacts of environmental exposure. Looking forward, advances such as single-cell metallomics, miniaturized sensors, high-throughput workflows, machine learning, and AI-driven predictive modeling are expected to transform metallome profiling, making it more sensitive, spatially resolved, and biologically informative.

9.8 Challenges, limitations, and future perspective

There are many different types of challenges preventing researchers from advancing metallomic profiling, which is the analysis of ions and their relationships with biological systems. This involves understanding how they relate to and interact with the body's biological functions through the detection of metabolites and other biological substances associated with these molecules. The analytical validity of their data is one type of analytical challenge, and a second major analytical issue is ion suppression resulting from the presence of multiple ion types in complex matrices. Therefore, metallomics researchers must perform thorough analyses of all the metabolites of an organism. The creation and implementation of standardized methods for the analysis of all metabolites is another major challenge. These two major challenges contribute to the validity of metallomics data and, therefore, to the reliability of their results. Metallomics also faces methodological barriers; one example is the preparation of samples, which requires sophisticated techniques to prevent the introduction of contaminants into the sample and to quantify the amount of metal species accurately. Another major methodological barrier is the difficult separation of metalloproteins from their metal cofactors due to the noncovalent nature of the interaction between most proteins and their metal ions. Regarding analytical technology, researchers have found that most current analytical methods are inadequate for detecting low-abundance metal species within complex biological matrices. There is also considerable variation between studies due to differing techniques used to perform metallomic analyses. Researchers continue to have difficulty interpreting the effects of the many ways metals interact with biological systems because metal homeostasis is a constantly changing phenomenon. Therefore, it will be difficult for metallomics to contribute to a better understanding of health or the basic functions of life. As such, continued innovation in methods is required, along with ongoing collaborative efforts between laboratories in multiple disciplines.

With advancements in single-cell analytical technologies, such as real-time measurement in combination with multiomic platforms like proteomics and genomics, we can expect much more from metallomic analysis than was previously possible. Single-cell analysis allows for a thorough investigation into metal distribution within individual cells, providing many new insights into how metals affect cellular function and/or contribute to the pathogenesis of disease. Integration of the metallome with other omics technologies, especially through isotope-labeled metallomics, will open many new avenues for the diagnostics of diseases related to metal exposure. Future metallomic analysis will be enhanced by the use of portable and compact devices, enabling more individualized management of patients on a case-by-case basis.

9.9 Conclusion

Imaging techniques have proven invaluable in the field of metallomics, allowing researchers to obtain important information on the spatial localization, amount, and chemical speciation of trace elements in complex biological samples. While SR-XRF and XAS techniques are highly useful for nondestructive, high-resolution elemental localization and speciation analysis of trace elements, MS-based imaging techniques are highly sensitive and quantitatively precise. Other complementary techniques, such as transmission and scanning electron microscopy, MRI, nuclear imaging techniques, and fluorescent probes targeted at trace elements, further augment the potential scope of metallome analysis by allowing ultrastructural localization analysis, real-time tracking studies, and monitoring of bioavailable trace elements. While each technique has inherent limitations in terms of resolution, sensitivity, sample preparation requirements, and ease of availability, their combined use ensures a comprehensive understanding of metal biology. Advancements in correlative light and electron microscopy, improved spatial resolution, better quantification, and new modalities are expected to further augment studies in metallomics.

References

Acar, O., 2024. The use of chemical modifiers in electrothermal atomic absorption spectrometry. Appl. Spectrosc. Rev. 59 (3), 340–354. doi:10.1080/05704928.2022.2147537.

Akdogan, G., Istanbullu, O.B., 2022. Analysing the effects of metallic biomaterial design and imaging sequences on MRI interpretation challenges due to image artefacts. Phys. Eng. Sci. Med. 45 (4), 1163–1174. doi:10.1007/s13246-022-01183-7.

Banci, L., Bertini, I., 2012. Metallomics and the Cell: Some Definitions and General Comments, vol. 12. Springer Science and Business Media LLC, pp. 1–13. doi:10.1007/978-94-007-5561-1_1.

Blasco, J., Rodríguez-Moro, G., Callejón-Leblic, B., Ramírez-Acosta, S., Arellano-Beltrán, F., Arias-Borrego, A., García-Barrera, T., Luis Gómez-Ariza, J., 2020. Environmental Metallomics and Metabolomics in Free-Living and Model Organisms. Elsevier BV, pp. 91–119. doi:10.1016/b978-0-12-818196-6.00004-2.

Borowska, M., Jankowski, K., 2023. Basic and advanced spectrometric methods for complete nanoparticles characterization in bio/eco systems: current status and future prospects. Anal. Bioanal. Chem. 415 (18), 4023–4038. doi:10.1007/s00216-023-04641-7.

Brunnbauer, L., Jirku, M., Quarles Jr., C.D., Limbeck, A., 2024. Capabilities of simultaneous 193 nm-LIBS/LA-ICP-MS imaging for microplastics characterization. Talanta 269, 125500. doi:10.1016/j.talanta.2023.125500.

Busser, B., Moncayo, S., Coll, J.-L., Sancey, L., Motto-Ros, V., 2018. Elemental imaging using laser-induced breakdown spectroscopy: a new and promising approach for biological and medical applications. Coord. Chem. Rev. 00108545. 358, 70–79. doi:10.1016/j.ccr.2017.12.006.

Butcher, D.J., 2024. Recent advances in graphite furnace atomic absorption spectrometry: a review of fundamentals and applications. Appl. Spectrosc. Rev. 59 (2), 247–275. doi:10.1080/05704928.2023.2192268.

Capdevila, D.A., Rondón, J.J., Edmonds, K.A., Rocchio, J.S., Dujovne, M.V., Giedroc, D.P., 2024. Bacterial metallostasis: metal sensing, metalloproteome remodeling, and metal trafficking. Chem. Rev. 124 (24), 13574–13659. doi:10.1021/acs.chemrev.4c00264.

Carter, K.P., Young, A.M., Palmer, A.E., 2014. Fluorescent sensors for measuring metal ions in living systems. Chem. Rev. 114 (8), 4564–4601. doi:10.1021/cr400546e.

Carter, S., Clough, R., Fisher, A., Gibson, B., Russell, B., 2021. Atomic spectrometry update: review of advances in the analysis of metals, chemicals and materials. J. Anal. At. Spectrom. 36 (11), 2241–2305. doi:10.1039/D1JA90049H.

Carter, S., Fisher, A., Garcia, R., Gibson, B., Marshall, J., Whiteside, I., 2016. Atomic spectrometry update: review of advances in the analysis of metals, chemicals and functional materials. J. Anal. At. Spectrom. 31 (11), 2114–2164. doi:10.1039/C6JA90044E.

Cebi, N., Bekiroglu, H., Erarslan, A., 2023. Nondestructive metabolomic fingerprinting: FTIR, NIR and Raman spectroscopy in food screening. Molecules 28 (23), 7933.

Chang, P.P., Zheng, L.N., Wang, B., Chen, M.L., Wang, M., Wang, J.H., Feng, W.Y., 2022. ICP-MS-based methodology in metallomics: towards single particle analysis, single cell analysis, and spatial metallomics. At. Spectrosc. 10. doi:10.46770/AS.2022.108.

Cheng, Y., Wang, H., Xu, H., Liu, Y., Ma, B., Chen, X., Zeng, X., Wang, X., Wang, B., Shiau, C., Ovchinnikov, S., Xiao-Dong, S., Wang, C., 2023. Co-evolution-based prediction of metal-binding sites in proteomes by machine learning. Nat. Chem. Biol. 1552-4450. 19 (5), 548–555. doi:10.1038/s41589-022-01223-z.

Chirila, Elisabeta, Draghici, C., 2010. Analytical approaches for sampling and sample preparation for heavy metals analysis in biological materials. In: Environmental Heavy Metal Pollution and Effects on Child Mental Development: Risk Assessment and Prevention Strategies. Springer. pp. 129–143.

Clases, D., Gonzalez de Vega, R., 2022. Facets of ICP-MS and their potential in the medical sciences—Part 1: fundamentals, stand-alone and hyphenated techniques. Anal. Bioanal. Chem. 414 (25), 7337–7361. doi:10.1007/s00216-022-04259-1.

Clough, R., Fisher, A., Gibson, B., Russell, B., 2023. Atomic spectrometry update: review of advances in the analysis of metals, chemicals and materials. J. Anal. At. Spectrom. 38 (11), 2215–2279. doi:10.1039/D3JA90038J.

Coverdale, J.P., Polepalli, S., Arruda, M.A., Da Silva, A.B.S., Stewart, A.J., Blindauer, C.A., 2024. Recent advances in metalloproteomics. Biomolecules 14 (1), 104. doi:10.3390/biom14010104.

Crichton, R.R., 2020. An overview of the role of metals in biology. In: Practical Approaches to Biological Inorganic Chemistry, second ed , pp. 1–16.

Dhara, S., Mishra, N.L., 2025. Recent developments in total reflection X-ray fluorescence and applications. X-Ray Fluoresc. Spectrosc. Chemometr. Instrum. Tech. Appl., 113–137. doi:10.1007/978-3-031-98375-7_5.

Diez-Fernández, S., Isnard, H., Nonell, A., Bresson, C., Chartier, F., 2020. Radionuclide analysis using collision–reaction cell ICP-MS technology: a review. J. Anal. At. Spectrom. 35 (12), 2793–2819. doi:10.1039/D0JA00211A.

Donati, G.L., Amais, R.S., Williams, C.B., 2017. Recent advances in inductively coupled plasma optical emission spectrometry. J. Anal. At. Spectrom. 32 (7), 1283–1296. doi:10.1039/C7JA00103G.

Dressler, V.L., Hiedrich, G.M., Neves, V.M., Müller, E.I., Pozebon, D., 2020. Metallomics imaging. In: Metabolomics. Springer US, New York, NY, pp. 267–304. doi:10.1007/978-1-0716-0864-7_21.

Dressler, V.L., Müller, E.I., Pozebon, D., 2018. Bioimaging metallomics. Metallomics 1055, 139–181.

Du, X., Li, X., Liu, Q., 2024. Pathometallomics: taking neurodegenerative disease as an example. Appl. Metallomics 311–347. doi:10.1002/9783527840397.ch10.

Dugo, G., Di Bella, G., Rando, R., Saitta, M., 2012. Sample preparation for the determination of metals in food samples. Compr. Sampl. Sample Prep. 4, 495–519. Available from: http://www.sciencedirect.com/science/referenceworks/9780123813749. doi:10.1016/B978-0-12-381373-2.00146-0.

Duroux, C., Hagège, A., 2022. Interactions between copper (II) and β-amyloid peptide using capillary electrophoresis–ICP–MS: kd measurements at the nanogram scale. Anal. Bioanal. Chem. 414 (18), 5347–5355. doi:10.1039/D1JA90007B.

Ellison, G., Hollings, A.L., Hackett, M.J., 2022. A review of the "metallome" within neurons and glia, as revealed by elemental mapping of brain tissue. BBA Adv. 2, 100038. doi:10.1016/j.bbadva.2021.100038.

Feng, L., 2024. Metrometallomics☆. Appl. Metallomics 1055, 153–191.

Fimognari, N., Hollings, A., Lam, V., Tidy, R.J., Kewish, C.M., Albrecht, M.A., Takechi, R., Mamo, J.C.L., Hackett, M.J., 2018. Biospectroscopic imaging provides evidence of hippocampal Zn deficiency and decreased lipid unsaturation in an accelerated aging mouse model. ACS Chem. Neurosci. 9 (11), 2774–2785.

Forma, A., Torbicz, A., Teresiński, G., Maciejewski, R., Baj, J., 2025. Metallomic profiling of the human eye and its relevance to ophthalmic diseases. Appl. Sci. 2076-3417. 15 (16), 8934. doi:10.3390/app15168934.

García-Barrera, T., Gómez-Ariza, J.L., González-Fernández, M., Moreno, F., García-Sevillano, M.A., Gómez-Jacinto, V., 2012. Biological responses related to agonistic, antagonistic and synergistic interactions of chemical species. Anal. Bioanal. Chem. 1618-2642. 403 (8), 2237–2253. doi:10.1007/s00216-012-5776-2.

Genchi, G., Lauria, G., Catalano, A., Carocci, A., Sinicropi, M.S., 2021. The double face of metals: the intriguing case of chromium. Appl. Sci. 11 (2), 638. doi:10.3390/app11020638.

Gómez Ariza, J.L., García-Barrera, T., García-Sevillano, M.A., González-Fernández, M., Gómez-Jacinto, V., 2013. Metallomics and Metabolomics of Plants under Environmental Stress Caused by Metals Heavy Metal Stress in Plants. Springer-Verlag Berlin Heidelberg, Spain, pp. 173–201. doi:10.1007/978-3-642-38469-1.

Gómez-Nieto, B., Gismera, M.J., Sevilla, M.T., Procopio, J.R., 2022. Direct solid sampling of biological species for the rapid determination of selenium by high-resolution continuum source graphite furnace atomic absorption spectrometry. Anal. Chim. Acta 1202, 339637. doi:10.1016/j.aca.2022.339637.

Gorman, B.L., Taylor, M.J., Tesfay, L., Lukowski, J.K., Hegde, P., Eder, J.G., Bloodsworth, K.J., Kyle, J.E., Torti, S., Anderton, C.R., 2024a. Applying multimodal mass spectrometry to image tumors undergoing ferroptosis following in vivo treatment with a ferroptosis inducer. J. Am. Soc. Mass Spectrom. 35 (1), 5–12. doi:10.1021/jasms.3c00193.

Gorman, B.L., Torti, S.V., Torti, F.M., Anderton, C.R., 2024b. Mass spectrometry imaging of metals in tissues and cells: methods and biological applications. Biochim. Biophys. Acta Gen. Subj. 1868 (2), 130329. doi:10.1016/j.bbagen.2023.130329.

Grabrucker, A.M., 2020. Biometals in Autism Spectrum Disorders Biometals in Autism Spectrum Disorders. Elsevier, Ireland, pp. 1–205. Available from: https://www.elsevier.com/books/biometals-in-autism-spectrum-disorders/grabrucker/978-0-12-821132-8. doi:10.1016/B978-0-12-821132-8.01001-6.

Gregar, F., Baron, D., Pluháček, T., 2025. Advances in ICP-MS-based nanoparticle characterization: techniques and challenges in biological sample analysis. J. Sep. Sci. 48 (9), e70259. doi:10.1002/jssc.70259.

Hackett, M.J., Hollings, A., Caine, S., Bewer, B.E., Alaverdashvili, M., Takechi, R., Mamo, J.C.L., Jones, M.W.M., De Jonge, M.D., Paterson, P.G., 2019. Elemental characterisation of the pyramidal neuron layer within the rat and mouse hippocampus. Metallomics 11 (1), 151–165.

He, M., Chen, B., Hu, B., 2024. ICP-MS for single-cell analysis in metallomics. Appl. Metallomics 391–427. doi:10.1002/9783527840397.ch14.

Helmann, J.D., 2025. Microbial metal physiology: ions to ecosystems. Nat. Rev. Microbiol. 23 (12), 805–819. doi:10.1038/s41579-025-01213-7.

Jim, V., LaViolette, C., Briehl, M.M., Ingram, J.C., 2017. Spatial distribution of uranium in mice kidneys detected by laser ablation inductively coupled plasma mass spectrometry. J. Appl. Bioanal. 2405710X. 3 (3), 43–48. doi:10.17145/jab.17.007.

Katsarou, A., Pantopoulos, K., 2020. Basics and principles of cellular and systemic iron homeostasis. Mol. Aspects Med. 00982997. 75, 100866. doi:10.1016/j.mam.2020.100866.

Khan, S.R., Sharma, B., Chawla, P.A., Bhatia, R., 2022. Inductively coupled plasma optical emission spectrometry (ICP-OES): a powerful analytical technique for elemental analysis. Food Anal. Methods 15 (3), 666–688. doi:10.1007/s12161-021-02148-4.

Legin, A.A., Schintlmeister, A., Jakupec, M.A., Galanski, M.S., Lichtscheidl, I., Wagner, M., Keppler, B.K., 2014. NanoSIMS combined with fluorescence microscopy as a tool for subcellular imaging of isotopically labeled platinum-based anticancer drugs. Chem. Sci. 5 (8), 3135–3143.

Li, X., Liu, T., Chang, C., Lei, Y., Mao, X., 2021. Analytical methodologies for agrometallomics: a critical review. J. Agric. Food Chem. 69 (22), 6100–6118. doi:10.1021/acs.jafc.1c00275.

Li, Y.-F., Chen, C., Qu, Y., Gao, Y., Bai, L., Zhao, Y., Chai, Z., 2008. Metallomics, elementomics, and analytical techniques. Pure Appl. Chem. 1365-3075. 80 (12), 2577–2594. doi:10.1351/pac200880122577.

Lim, S.Y., Dayal, H., Seah, S.J., Tan, R.P.W., Low, Z.E., Laserna, A.K.C., Li, S.F.Y., 2023. Plasma metallomics reveals potential biomarkers and insights into the ambivalent associations of elements with acute myocardial infarction. J. Trace Elem. Med. Biol. 77, 127148. doi:10.1016/j.jtemb.2023.127148.

Lins, B.R., Pushie, J.M., Jones, M., Howard, D.L., Howland, J.G., Hackett, M.J., 2016. Mapping alterations to the endogenous elemental distribution within the lateral ventricles and choroid plexus in brain disorders using x-ray fluorescence imaging. PLoS One 11 (6), e0158152.

Lovett, J.H., Harris, H.H., 2021. Application of X-ray absorption and X-ray fluorescence techniques to the study of metallodrug action. Curr. Opin. Chem. Biol. 61, 135–142. doi:10.1016/j.cbpa.2020.12.004.

Lu, M., Wang, H., Geisel, J., Le, X.C., 2012. Enzyme Digestion for Speciation of Arsenic, vol. 3. Elsevier BV, 421–433. doi:10.1016/b978-0-12-381373-2.00150-2.

Machado, I., Gambino, D., 2024. Metallomics: an essential tool for the study of potential antiparasitic metallodrugs. ACS Omega. 2470-1343. 9 (14), 15744–15752. doi:10.1021/acsomega.3c10200.

Manohar, N., Reynoso, F.J., Diagaradjane, P., Krishnan, S., Cho, S.H., 2016. Quantitative imaging of gold nanoparticle distribution in a tumor-bearing mouse using benchtop x-ray fluorescence computed tomography. Sci. Rep. 6 (1), 22079.

Maret, W., 2018. Metallomics: the science of biometals and biometalloids. Metallomics 1055, 1–20. doi:10.1007/978-3-319-90143-5_1.

Maret, W., 2021. An appraisal of the field of metallomics and the roles of metal ions in biochemistry and cell signaling. Appl. Sci. 2076-3417. 11 (22), 10846. doi:10.3390/app112210846.

Maret, W., 2022. The quintessence of metallomics: a harbinger of a different life science based on the periodic table of the bioelements. Metallomics. 1756-591X. 14 (8). doi:10.1093/mtomcs/mfac051.

Mataveli, L.R.V., Barbosa, H.S., Arruda, M.A.Z., 2014. Microwave-assisted sample preparation focusing on 'omics' areas. In: Microwave-Assisted Sample Preparation for Trace Element Analysis. Elsevier, pp. 313–343.

Mezzanotte, M., Stanga, S., 2024. Brain iron dyshomeostasis and ferroptosis in Alzheimer's disease pathophysiology: two faces of the same coin. Aging Dis. 16 (5), 2615–2640. doi:10.14336/AD.2024.0094 .

Michalke, B., 2022. Review about powerful combinations of advanced and hyphenated sample introduction techniques with inductively coupled plasma-mass spectrometry (ICP-MS) for elucidating trace element species in pathologic conditions on a molecular level. Int. J. Mol. Sci. 23 (11), 6109. doi:10.3390/ijms23116109.

Michalke, B., Berthele, A., Venkataramani, V., 2021. Simultaneous quantification and speciation of trace metals in paired serum and CSF samples by size exclusion chromatography–inductively coupled plasma–dynamic reaction cell–mass spectrometry (SEC-DRC-ICP-MS). Int. J. Mol. Sci. 22 (16), 8892. doi:10.3390/ijms22168892.

Mo, S., Liang, L.N., Cai, Y., Mou, S., 2007. Speciation analysis of selenium in biological and environmental samples. J. Instrum. Anal. 26 (3), 438.

Mohammed, A.M., 2021. Elemental analysis using atomic absorption spectroscopy. Eur. J. Eng. Technol. Res. 2736-576X. 6 (7), 48–51. doi:10.24018/ej-eng.2021.6.7.2639.

Moksnes, M.R., Hansen, A.F., Wolford, B.N., Thomas, L.F., Rasheed, H., Simić, A., Bhatta, L., Brantsæter, A.L., Surakka, I., Zhou, W., Magnus, P., Njølstad, P.R., Andreassen, O.A., Syversen, T., Zheng, J., Fritsche, L.G., Evans, D.M., Warrington, N.M., Nøst, T.H., Olav Åsvold, B., Flaten, T.P., Willer, C.J., Hveem, K., Brumpton, B.M., 2024. A genome-wide association study provides insights into the genetic etiology of 57 essential and non-essential trace elements in humans. Commun. Biol. 2399-3642. 7 (1). doi:10.1038/s42003-024-06101-z.

Momen, A.A., 2023. Evaluation of some spectroscopic techniques for trace elements assessment in human biological samples during 2000–2022: a review. Orient. J. Chem. 39 (3), 635. doi:10.13005/ojc/390314.

Montes-Bayón, M., Sharar, M., Corte-Rodriguez, M., 2018. Trends on (elemental and molecular) mass spectrometry based strategies for speciation and metallomics. TrAC Trends Anal. Chem. 104, 4–10.

Neuditschko, B., Legin, A.A., Baier, D., Schintlmeister, A., Reipert, S., Wagner, M., Keppler, B.K., Berger, W., Meier-Menches, S.M., Gerner, C., 2021. Interaction with ribosomal proteins accompanies stress induction of the anticancer metallodrug BOLD-100/KP1339 in the endoplasmic reticulum. Angew. Chem. Int. Ed. 60 (10), 5063–5068. doi:10.1002/anie.202015962.

Newton, M.A., Zimmermann, P., van Bokhoven, J.A., 2023. X-ray absorption spectroscopy (XAS): XANES and EXAFS. In: Springer Handbook of Advanced Catalyst Characterization. Springer, pp. 565–600.

Ningombam, L., Hazarika, B.N., Yumkhaibam, T., Heisnam, P., Singh, Y.D., 2024. Heavy metal priming plant stress tolerance deciphering through physiological, biochemical, molecular and omics mechanism. S. Afr. J. Bot. 02546299. 168, 16–25. doi:10.1016/j.sajb.2024.02.032.

Olivier, M., Asmis, R., Hawkins, G.A., Howard, T.D., Cox, L.A., 2019. The need for multi-omics biomarker signatures in precision medicine. Int. J. Mol. Sci. 1422-0067. 20 (19), 4781. doi:10.3390/ijms20194781.

Patriarca, M., Barlow, N., Cross, A., Hill, S., Robson, A., Taylor, A., Tyson, J., 2022a. Atomic spectrometry update: review of advances in the analysis of clinical and biological materials, foods and beverages. J. Anal. At. Spectrom. 37 (3), 410–473. doi:10.1021/acs.jafc.1c00275.

Patriarca, M., Barlow, N., Cross, A., Hill, S., Robson, A., Taylor, A., Tyson, J., 2022b. Atomic spectrometry update: review of advances in the analysis of clinical and biological materials, foods and beverages. J. Anal. At. Spectrom. 37 (3), 410–473. doi:10.1039/D2JA90005J.

Pereira, J.S., Fornazaro Moraes, B., Leutz, A.C.N., Nicolau, H.C.D.S., Santos, R.C., Tartari, T., Gomes, B.P.F.D.A., de Jesus Soares, A., Janini, A.C.P., Pelepenko, L.E., 2025. Metallomic characterization of induced periapical lesions—in vivo study. Int. Endod. J. 58, 1584–1615.

Peris-Díaz, M.D., Orzeł, A., Wu, S., Mosna, K., Barran, P.E., Krezel, A., 2024. Combining native mass spectrometry and proteomics to differentiate and map the metalloform landscape in metallothioneins. J. Proteome Res. 23 (8), 3626–3637. doi:10.1021/acs.jproteome.4c00271.

Ramanathan, T., Ting, Y.-P., 2015. Selection of wet digestion methods for metal quantification in hazardous solid wastes. J. Environ. Chem. Eng. 22133437. 3 (3), 1459–1467. doi:10.1016/j.jece.2015.05.006.

Ramirez-Acosta, S., Arias-Borrego, A., Navarro-Roldan, F., Selma-Royo, M., Calatayud, M., Collado, M.C., Huertas-Abril, P.V., Abril, N., García Barrera, T., 2021. Omic methodologies for assessing metal (-Loid) s-host-microbiota interplay: a review. Anal. Chim. Acta 1176, 338620.

Resano, M., Aramendía, M., García-Ruiz, E., Bazo, A., Bolea-Fernandez, E., Vanhaecke, F., 2023. Living in a transient world: ICP-MS reinvented via time-resolved analysis for monitoring single events. Chem. Sci. 13 (16), 4436–4473. doi:10.1039/D1SC05452J.

Retzmann, A., Faßbender, S., Rosner, M., von der Au, M., Vogl, J., 2023. Performance of second generation ICP-TOFMS for (multi-) isotope ratio analysis: a case study on B, Sr and Pb and their isotope fractionation behavior during the measurements. J. Anal. At. Spectrom. 38 (10), 2144–2158. doi:10.1039/d3ja00084b.

Revenko, A.G., Pashkova, G.V., 2023. X-ray fluorescence spectrometry: current status and prospects of development. J. Anal. Chem. 78 (11), 1452–1468. doi:10.1134/S1061934823110072.

Rodríguez-Moro, G., Ramírez-Acosta, S., Arias-Borrego, A., García-Barrera, T., Luis Gómez-Ariza, J., 2018. Environmental Metallomics, vol. 1055. Springer Science and Business Media LLC, pp. 39–66. doi:10.1007/978-3-319-90143-5_3.

Saputra, R.R., Ariefin, M., Kumalasari, M.R., Dongoran, J., Tampubolon, M.J.L., Sulistiawati, P., Simangunsong, S.Y., Ariska, R., Paksi, P.G.R., Siska, A., 2024. Advancements in NMR and IR spectroscopy: enhancing metabolomics and disease diagnostics in the health sector: a comprehensive review. Indones. J. Chem. Anal. 7 (2), 77–88.

Scalese, G., Kostenkova, K., Crans, D.C., Gambino, D., 2022. Metallomics and other omics approaches in antiparasitic metal-based drug research. Curr. Opin. Chem. Biol. 13675931. 67, 102127. doi:10.1016/j.cbpa.2022.102127.

Scassellati, C., Bonvicini, C., Benussi, L., Ghidoni, R., Squitti, R., 2020. Neurodevelopmental disorders: metallomics studies for the identification of potential biomarkers associated to diagnosis and treatment. J. Trace Elem. Med. Biol. 0946672X. 60, 126499. doi:10.1016/j.jtemb.2020.126499.

Shafaat, H.S., Manesis, A.C., Yerbulekova, A., 2023. How to build a metalloenzyme: lessons from a protein based model of acetyl coenzyme a synthase. Acc. Chem. Res. 56 (9), 984–993. doi:10.1021/acs.accounts.2c00824.

Sharma, I., 2020. ICP-OES: an advance tool in biological research. Open J. Environ. Biol. 5 (1), 027–033. doi:10.17352/ojeb.

Silva, B.M.S., Silva, C.R., 2020. Metalômica: metodologias e Aplicações Em Estudos Ambientais. http://rvq.sbq.org.br/.

Sindhu, R.K., Yadav, S.K., Kaur, A., Kumar, M., Kumar, P., 2022. X-Ray Fluorescence in Biological Sciences. John Wiley & Sons. doi:10.1002/9781119645719.

Sleimi, N., Bankaji, I., Kouki, R., Dridi, N., Duarte, B., Caçador, I., 2022. Assessment of extraction methods of trace metallic elements in plants: approval of a common method. Sustainability. 2071-1050. 14 (3), 1428. doi:10.3390/su14031428.

Specht, A.J., Adesina, K.E., Read, D.E., Weisskopf, M.G., 2024. Benchtop x-ray fluorescence to quantify elemental content in nails non-destructively. Sci. Total Environ. 918, 170601. doi:10.1016/j.scitotenv.2024.170601.

Staufer, T., Grüner, F., 2023. Review of development and recent advances in biomedical X-ray fluorescence imaging. Int. J. Mol. Sci. 24 (13), 10990. doi:10.3390/ijms241310990.

Stofella, M., Grimaldi, A., Smit, J.H., Claesen, J., Paci, E., Sobott, F., 2024. Computational tools for hydrogen–deuterium exchange mass spectrometry data analysis. Chem. Rev. 124 (21), 12242–12263. doi:10.1021/acs.chemrev.4c00438.

Suárez-Criado, L., Queipo-Abad, S., Rodriguez-Cea, A., Rodriguez-Gonzalez, P., Alonso, J.I.G., 2022. Comparison of GC-ICP-MS, GC-EI-MS and GC-EI-MS/MS for the determination of methylmercury, ethylmercury and inorganic mercury in biological samples by triple spike species-specific isotope dilution mass spectrometry. J. Anal. At. Spectrom. 37 (7), 1462–1470. doi:10.1039/D2JA00086E.

Sullivan, B., Robison, G., Pushkar, Y., Young, J.K., Manaye, K.F., 2017. Copper accumulation in rodent brain astrocytes: a species difference. J. Trace Elem. Med. Biol. 39, 6–13.

Sun, H., Chai, Z.-F., 2010. Metallomics: an integrated science for metals in biology and medicine. Annu. Rep. Sect A (Inorg. Chem.) 0260-1818. 106, 20. doi:10.1039/b920672h.

Sussulini, A., Becker, J.S., 2011. Combination of PAGE and LA-ICP-MS as an analytical workflow in metallomics: state of the art, new quantification strategies, advantages and limitations. Metallomics 3 (12), 1271–1279.

Sussulini, A., Hauser-Davis, R.A., 2018. Metallomics Applied to the Study of Neurodegenerative and Mental Diseases, vol. 1055. Springer Science and Business Media LLC, pp. 21–37. doi:10.1007/978-3-319-90143-5_2.

Tang, Y., Liu, L., Nong, Q., Guo, H., Zhou, Q., Wang, D., Jiang, G., 2022. Sensitive determination of metalloprotein in salt-rich matrices by size exclusion chromatography coupled with inductively coupled plasma-mass spectrometry. J. Chromatogr. A 1677, 463303. doi:10.1016/j.chroma.2022.463303.

Tian, X., Teng, Y., Deng, Y., Zhang, Q., Caihong, H., Feng, J., 2025. Advances in mammalian metallomics: new insights into metal dynamics and biological significance. Int. J. Mol. Sci. 1422-0067. 26 (19), 9729. doi:10.3390/ijms26199729.

Uyeda, K.S., 2025. Roles of Transition Metal Ions in Biological Oxidations: Mechanistic Insights into Metalloenzymes and Microbial Metabolism (Doctoral dissertation, University of California, Irvine).

Vanhoof, C., Bacon, J.R., Fittschen, U.E., Vincze, L., 2023. 2023 atomic spectrometry update–a review of advances in X-ray fluorescence spectrometry and its special applications. J. Anal. At. Spectrom. 38 (9), 1730–1743. doi:10.1039/D3JA90026F.

Villadangos, A.F., Ordóñez, E., Muñoz, M.I., Pastrana, I.M., Fiuza, M., Gil, J.A., Mateos, L.M., Aller, A.J., 2010. Retention of arsenate using genetically modified coryneform bacteria and determination of arsenic in solid samples by ICP-MS. Talanta 80 (3), 1421–1427. doi:10.1016/j.talanta.2009.09.046.

Vogiatzis, C.G., Zachariadis, G.A., 2014. Tandem mass spectrometry in metallomics and the involving role of ICP-MS detection: a review. Anal. Chim. Acta. 00032670. 819, 1–14. doi:10.1016/j.aca.2014.01.029.

Wang, C., Guan, Y., Lv, M., Zhang, R., Guo, Z., Wei, X., Xiaoxia, D., Yang, J., Tong, L., Wan, Y., Xiaodong, S., Huang, X., Jiang, Z., 2018. Manganese increases the sensitivity of the cGAS-STING pathway for double-stranded DNA and is required for the host defense against DNA viruses. Immunity. 10747613. 48 (4), 675. doi:10.1016/j.immuni.2018.03.017.

Wang, M., Gu, Y., Lu, H., Ge, L., Zhang, Q., Zeng, G., 2022. Matrix effect correction method based on the main spectral parameters for rock samples in an in situ energy dispersive X-ray fluorescence analysis. Spectrochim. Acta B 193, 106438. doi:10.1016/j.sab.2022.106438.

Yan, X., Xu, M., Wang, Q., 2024. Methodology and Tools for Metallomics. Applied Metallomics: From Life Sciences to Environmental Sciences. Wiley-VCH, pp. 377–390. doi:10.1002/9783527840397.ch13.

Yang, Q., Zhao, Y., Yu, H., Xiong, X., Huang, K., 2024. Recent advances of sample separation and preconcentration techniques for analytical atomic spectrometry. Appl. Spectrosc. Rev. 59 (5), 652–677. doi:10.1080/05704928.2023.2231537.

Zeng, X., Wei, T., Wang, X., Liu, Y., Tan, Z., Zhang, Y., Feng, T., Cheng, Y., Wang, F., Bin, M., Qin, W., Gao, C., Xiao, J., Wang, C., 2024. Discovery of metal-binding proteins by thermal proteome profiling. Nat. Chem. Biol. 1552-4450. 20 (6), 770–778. doi:10.1038/s41589-024-01563-y.

Zhang, D., Zhang, H., Yang, Y., Jin, Y., Chen, Y., Wu, C., 2025. Advancing tissue analysis: integrating mass tags with mass spectrometry imaging and immunohistochemistry. J. Proteomics 316, 105436. doi:10.1016/j.jprot.2025.105436.

Zhang, Y., He, J., Jin, J., Ren, C., 2022. Recent advances in the application of metallomics in diagnosis and prognosis of human cancer. Metallomics. 1756-591X. 14 (7). doi:10.1093/mtomcs/mfac037.

Zhou, Y., Li, H., Tse, E., Sun, H., 2024. Metal-detection based techniques and their applications in metallobiology. Chem. Sci. 15 (27), 10264–10280. doi:10.1039/D4SC00108G.

Chapter 10

Toxicometallomics: Linking metal exposure to biomarkers in humans

Pratibha Singh and Aneesha
Department of Nutrition and Dietetics, Manav Rachna International Institute of Research and Studies, Faridabad, Haryana, India

10.1 Introduction

Metals occur naturally in our surroundings and serve important functions in the human body. While some metals are necessary in small, trace amounts to support vital biological functions, many can become harmful—or even deadly—when their levels exceed the safe threshold (Hollenberg, 2010).

Humans have been exposed to metals for thousands of years. Historical records show that early civilizations, like the Greeks and Romans, recognized both the harmful and healing effects of metals. For instance, ancient physicians documented symptoms of metal poisoning among miners and metalworkers (Boateng et al., 2019). Throughout history, metals have been widely used for tools, jewelry, and machines. Activities like mining and smelting have significantly increased metal levels in our environment. Today, its heavy use in the medical field, industries, and agriculture has increased exposure among occupational workers and the common man through polluted air, water, food, and soil (Jaishankar et al., 2014).

Out of over 80 metallic elements, about 30 have been found to be toxic to humans. As technology advances, new metals may emerge as health risks due to their growing use in electronics, nanotechnology, and pharmaceuticals. The harmful effects of metal exposure depend on several factors, such as the exposure mechanism (inhalation, ingestion, skin contact), the form of the metal (solid, vapor, salt, or compound), and its strength (Long et al., 2021). They can interfere with the body's normal functions in many ways. To affect the body, a metal must enter cells, where it can disrupt essential biochemical processes. Common mechanisms of toxicity include Blocking or damaging enzymes, damaging DNA or cell membranes, replacing essential metals in proteins, producing

The Metallome in Motion. https://doi.org/10.1016/B978-0-443-44299-5.00011-0

harmful free radicals, and affecting gene expression. These effects can harm multiple organs, including the brain, kidneys, lungs, and reproductive system. Several variables affect how harmful a metal can be. These include the metal's half-life (how long it stays in the body), the age of the individual (children and the elderly are more vulnerable), immune system function (especially for metals that trigger allergic reactions), and the fact that metals cannot be broken down like organic toxins (Singh (Sankhla et al., 2016). However, they can bind to proteins in the body to reduce their harmful effects. For example, metallothioneins are proteins that can neutralize certain toxic metals.

Metal toxicity is a major concern in occupational and environmental risks, with specific fields such as metallotoxicology driving its study. Metals can cause reprotoxicity, developmental birth defects, and growth impairment (Tchounwou et al., 2012). The type of manifestation is determined by the exposure stage and toxicokinetics (Jaishankar et al., 2014). Preclinical investigations have demonstrated that a variety of metals, including Al, As, Cd, Co, Cr, Cu, Ga, Hg, Li, Mn, Pb, and Zn, can cause embryonic mortality and deformities. Understanding metal toxicity is complex (Iavicoli et al., 2009). Many factors—such as how much metal someone is exposed to, for how long, and the person's age or health—play a role (WHO, 2017). Continued research is needed to better understand how metals affect the body, how to detect exposure early, and how to reduce health risks, especially as new technologies introduce us to more metal-based materials (Cai et al., 2005).

Every toxic metal possesses a unique toxicity profile. Lead raises blood pressure and damages the kidneys in adults, disrupts heme-synthesis, and affects neurological growth in children (Bellinger, 2011). Mercury is neurotoxic, especially methylmercury, which impairs motor, cognitive, and sensory abilities. Long-term exposure can cause cognitive deterioration, eye issues, and tremors (Clarkson and Magos, 2006). According to Nordberg et al. (2011), cadmium builds up mostly in the kidneys and bones, where it can cause osteomalacia, proteinuria, and an elevated risk of lung cancer over time. Arsenic has been linked to lesions of the skin, heart diseases, and cancers such as skin, bladder, and lung (Rahaman et al., 2022).

Toxicometallomics is an emerging field that seeks to explore toxic metal exposure leading to molecular changes in the body. Metabolomics aids in the investigation of physiological responses to hazardous metal exposure and physiological changes. It merges the study of all metals, metabolic science, and toxicology in the body. It provides a mechanism for understanding metabolic shifts that lead to molecular damage. This improves our ability to trace exposures to adverse outcomes and supports more accurate risk assessment. While many studies report on the exposure to environmental heavy metals such as arsenic, cadmium, lead, and mercury and their adverse effects on the body, there is still a lack of molecular-level monitoring of their effects.

These enter the body through various routes, such as inhaling industrial emissions, consuming contaminated food, occupational contact, and drinking polluted water. These metals remain in the body for years due to their long biological half-lives. For example, cadmium continues to accumulate in the kidneys, while lead preferentially deposits in bone. Over time, such bioaccumulation raises the risk of chronic illnesses such as kidney disease, neurodevelopmental effects, and cancer (Rajkumar et al., 2023).

Earlier, total metal content alone was considered for assessing the risk, but now there are many toxicometallomics biomarkers, such as exposure markers, like metal levels in blood or urine; effect markers, such as signs of oxidative stress or enzyme disruption caused by metals; and susceptibility markers, including genetic differences that influence individual responses to metals. The importance of this field has expanded due to rising metal exposure from human activities. Widespread industrial growth and modern farming practices, even in isolated regions, have increased people's contact with harmful metals. Health risks, like mercury in seafood, arsenic in drinking water, and cadmium in soil, continue to threaten communities (Rajkumar et al., 2023). Without effective detection methods, harmful health impacts may remain undetected until they cause permanent harm. Toxicometallomics also includes the branch of exposomics, the study of a person's lifetime environmental exposures. By integrating metal-related data into broader exposure analysis, scientists can more accurately determine how metals interact with other factors to influence disease development.

Toxicometallomics remains in its initial phase, still in the early stages of development. Researchers are currently working to establish consistent methods for sample handling, analyzing multiple metal forms, and linking findings to broader biological processes. Despite these challenges, cutting-edge technologies—such as advanced mass spectrometry, which can identify specific metal compounds—are improving our ability to track how various metal types interact with and impact the human body.

Metallomics, metabolomics, and exposomics are interconnected fields. Metallomic studies show how metals interact with proteins, emphasizing their role in enzymatic reactions, maintaining molecular structures, and cellular networks. Metabolomics includes the pathways of metabolic changes due to metal exposure. It identifies the indicators and cellular responses to metal toxicity. Exposomics shows the complete individual exposure to toxic metals throughout the life cycle and their effects on health. When all three fields are considered collectively, they provide a detailed mechanism of exposure to molecular changes leading to detrimental biological effects. This integrated concept helps to identify early signs of metal toxicity and supports the planning and execution of appropriate health interventions.

10.2 Pathways of human metal exposure

The presence of hazardous metals in the environment has increased, raising community health risks across the globe. There are diverse sources of toxic metals, such as industrial air releases, industrial wastewater, agricultural farming activities that include the excessive use of chemicals for crop productivity and quality, traffic due to vehicle overload, common household activities, incineration activities, etc. (Rajkumar et al., 2023). These metals enter the human body through multiple routes, such as contaminated air, food/water, or skin absorption.

Heavy metals exist naturally in our surroundings and play crucial roles in biological processes, yet they can turn dangerous when they build up in living systems. Common environmental contaminants among these metals include mercury, cadmium, arsenic, chromium, nickel, copper, and lead—elements that pose significant health risks when their concentrations exceed safe levels (Mitra et al., 2022).

Metalloids enter the environment through both geogenic (natural) and anthropogenic (human-made) activities (Mandal and Suzuki, 2002). Geogenic sources include weathering of metal-rich rocks, volcanic eruptions, etc. These processes release metalloids into soil, water, and the atmosphere. Anthropogenic sources include industrial processes such as mining, smelting, metal plating, and paper production (Nordberg et al., 2011); agricultural practices such as the use of phosphate fertilizers and pesticides (Alengebawy et al., 2021); fossil fuel emissions from burning coal and oil (Vouk and Piver, 1983); and waste disposal practices such as landfill leachates, industrial wastewater, and sewage (Rani Saha et al., 2022). These activities release toxic metalloids (e.g., arsenic, antimony) into the environment, where they persist due to their nonbiodegradable nature (Nordberg et al., 2011; Rani Saha et al., 2022). Contamination of soil, water, and food by metalloids poses serious risks to human health (e.g., cancer, neurological disorders) and ecosystems (e.g., bioaccumulation in aquatic life) (Hughes et al., 2011).

Industrial occupational exposure to heavy metals, such as in mining, smelting, battery manufacturing, welding, and waste recycling, is of major concern today. Workers in these fields inhale hazardous dust and fumes containing cadmium, lead, nickel, chromium, and arsenic, leading to both acute and chronic health effects. Other routine sources, like lead-based paints, contaminated cosmetics, and certain cookware, further increase exposure risks. Adulteration of foods, such as the use of lead chromate in turmeric, has led to cases of poisoning (Witkowska et al., 2021). Tobacco plants absorb cadmium from the soil, which then transfers to smokers through cigarette use (Vacchi-Suzzi et al., 2016). Since the lungs absorb cadmium more efficiently than the digestive system, smokers face significantly higher exposure compared to dietary intake alone (Vacchi-Suzzi et al., 2016).

10.3 Metalloids

Metalloids are a group of elements characterized by their high molecular weight and density. Even in small amounts, these elements are recognized as major environmental pollutants. Some metalloids, including cadmium (Cd), nickel

(Ni), mercury (Hg), arsenic (As), chromium (Cr), thorium (Th), zinc (Zn), antimony (Sb), copper (Cu), and lead (Pb), have relatively high densities ranging from 3.5 to 7 g/cm^3. Pollution caused by metalloids presents a serious threat to ecosystems and living organisms (Kumar et al., 2022). According to the United States Environmental Protection Agency (EPA), the eight most common metalloid contaminants are lead, chromium, arsenic, zinc, copper, cadmium, nickel, and mercury (Kumar et al., 2022).

These metalloids have a tendency to accumulate in the environment; hence, their concentrations are higher than permitted limits. The concentrations can lead to a number of issues, including Parkinson's disease, Alzheimer's disease, and cancer, if they exceed permissible limits. In order to keep pollution levels below the allowed limit, a number of researchers have developed remediation approaches in response to the issue of metalloid contamination. The earth's shell is full of these metalloids, which are indestructible. The human body absorbs these metals through food, water, and air. At trace levels, certain metalloids play a vital role in human metabolism, but at greater quantities, they can be hazardous. Mining and industrial operations can release them into the atmosphere, where they may end up in soils and bodies of water (Kumar et al., 2022).

A study shows that over 90% of human metal intake occurs via contaminated vegetables, rice, and other plant foods (Mitra et al., 2022). Heavy metals enter ecosystems through both natural processes and human activities, presenting significant environmental and health challenges. Cadmium exposure occurs through atmospheric deposition, industrial discharge, and agricultural runoff, contaminating water systems and accumulating in sediments. Humans primarily encounter cadmium through contaminated food, water, and air. Unlike some micronutrients, cadmium offers no known benefits to plant physiology (Hayat et al., 2018).

Mercury exists naturally but has become increasingly prevalent in the environment due to anthropogenic activities. In aquatic environments, it transforms into methylmercury—a potent neurotoxin that bioaccumulates in fish and seafood. Upon consumption, this organic mercury compound enters the bloodstream and can cause severe neurological impairments (Mitra et al., 2022; Rice et al., 2014).

Lead persists indefinitely in the environment as a nondegradable element. Industrial operations, mining activities, and combustion processes have substantially increased atmospheric lead concentrations. While naturally occurring levels are minimal, elevated exposure poses serious health risks, particularly to children who may ingest lead-contaminated dust (Loh et al., 2016; Mitra et al., 2022).

Manganese occurs in multiple oxidation states and serves essential biological functions. However, the combustion of MMT gasoline additives releases manganese oxides into the air. Excessive exposure to these compounds can override manganese's beneficial effects, leading to toxicity (Loranger and Zayed, 1995; Mitra et al., 2022; O'Neal and Zheng, 2015).

Chromium exists primarily in two forms with differing toxicities. While chromium(III) is relatively benign, industrial processes often produce the more dangerous chromium(VI). The ferrochrome industry represents a major emission source, significantly impacting local environments (Kimbrough et al., 1999; Mitra et al., 2022; Coetzee et al., 2020).

Cobalt occurs widely in nature and has industrial applications, particularly in alloy production. Although environmental release rates are typically low, concentrated exposure can be lethal despite cobalt's role in certain biological processes (Domingo, 1989; Mitra et al., 2022).

Nickel's natural abundance and industrial utility make it a common environmental contaminant. Inhalation of nickel particles has been linked to respiratory cancers, allergic reactions, and organ damage (Genchi et al., 2020; Mitra et al., 2022).

Copper serves as a crucial micronutrient in human health. Both deficiency and excess can disrupt biological systems (Mitra et al., 2022). Copper enters the human system through several exposure pathways. Contaminated drinking water, due to corroded copper pipes or plumbing systems, primarily contains inorganic Cu(II) ions in soluble forms (WHO, 2017). Dietary supplements frequently deliver copper as Cu(II) salts, such as copper gluconate or copper sulfate, which are more bioavailable than inorganic forms (Turnlund et al., 2004). Industrial activities, including mining, smelting, and welding operations, generate exposure to particulate forms of copper, including airborne dust and fumes containing metallic copper or copper oxides (Poland et al., 2022). Additionally, genetic conditions like Wilson's disease represent an endogenous exposure pathway, where copper accumulates abnormally in tissues due to defects in the copper transporter protein (Brewer, 2000; Schilsky et al., 2022). These varied sources demonstrate how copper's chemical speciation—whether as dissolved ions, salt complexes, metallic particles, or biologically incorporated forms—fundamentally influences its bioavailability and subsequent metabolic handling in the human body (Schilsky et al., 2022).

Zinc participates in numerous enzymatic reactions as a cofactor. Mining and smelting operations represent primary emission sources, with excessive environmental zinc affecting entire ecosystems (Mitra et al., 2022; Zhang et al., 2012).

Antimony exposure occurs through natural phenomena and industrial activities. Workers in affected industries may develop respiratory conditions, organ damage, and an increased cancer risk from inhalation exposure (He et al., 2019; Mitra et al., 2022).

Thallium ranks among the most toxic heavy metals, entering the environment through both natural water systems and industrial emissions. Even minimal exposure can cause severe health consequences (Mitra et al., 2022).

10.4 Toxicokinetics of metals

Metalloids can exist in inorganic or organic forms, with varying toxicity levels. Their mobility and transformation depend on pH and temperature, the presence of living organisms (e.g., microbial methylation), cation exchange capacity, evaporation, and adsorption processes (Wang and Mulligan, 2006) (Figs. 10.1–10.3).

The human body absorbs toxic metals through various pathways depending on the type of exposure. If the human body inhales fine metal particles (such as cadmium and lead), they reach deeper into lung tissues (Satarug et al., 2010). Exposure through food ingestion leads to absorption via the digestive system (Abadin et al., 2007). Topical applications of cosmetics can cause skin absorption (Al-Ashban et al., 2004). Once inside the body, metals distribute differently based on their chemical properties. Lead binds to erythrocytes initially and later starts accumulating in bones (Barry, 1975; Bergdahl and Skerfving, 2008). Elimination rates vary substantially among metals. The body retains cadmium for decades, as cadmium hinders its ability to excrete through the kidneys (Järup and Åkesson, 2009; Nordberg et al., 2007). Methylmercury can easily cross the blood-brain barrier and cause damage to the brain (Clarkson and Magos, 2006). Biological processes transform these metals into different

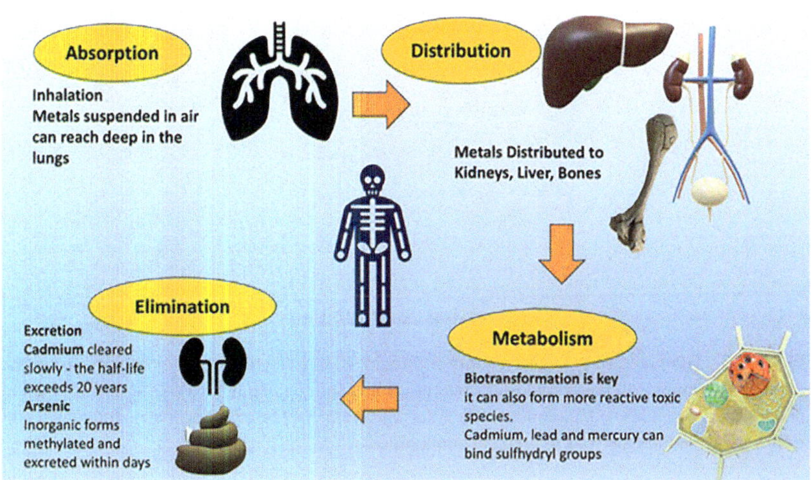

FIG. 10.1 Absorption, distribution, metabolism, and excretion (ADME) of toxic metals in humans. *Note:* Pathways and organ targets vary by metal speciation and dose.

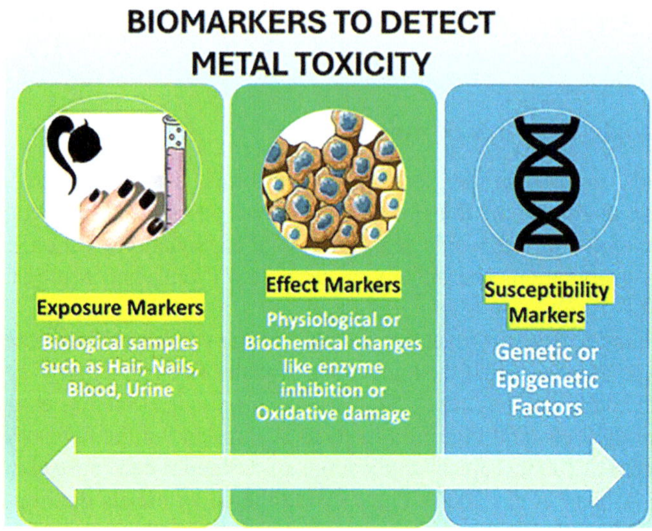

FIG. 10.2 Biomarker classification matrix for metal exposure, effect, and susceptibility. *Note:* Rows group biomarker purposes (exposure, effect, susceptibility); columns show matrices (blood, urine, hair/nails, teeth/bone, exhaled breath condensate). Icons indicate the typical timeframe captured (recent vs. cumulative).

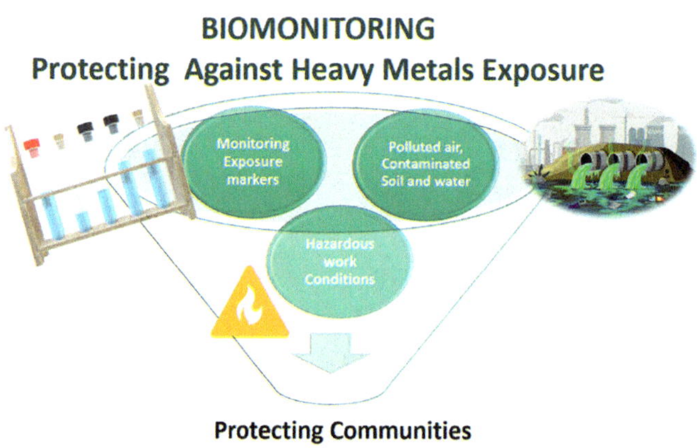

FIG. 10.3 Biomonitoring pathway: From environmental metal sources to community protection. *Note.* Icons summarize major exposure sources (polluted air; contaminated soil and water, hazardous workplace conditions), common biomonitoring specimens (blood, urine, hair), and how results inform targeted interventions to protect communities.

chemical states; for example, arsenic undergoes methylation (Thomas and Bradham, 2016). Certain aquatic microorganisms convert inorganic mercury into its more dangerous organic form, methylmercury, which contaminates seafood. When consumed, it accumulates in the body and causes toxicity (Ullrich et al., 2001) (Tables 10.1–10.5).

10.5 Biomarkers of metal exposure in humans

Monitoring exposure requires the use of detection techniques. Metal levels in biological tissues, including blood, urine, hair, and nails, are measured using techniques such as atomic absorption spectrometry (AAS), inductively coupled plasma mass spectrometry (ICP-MS), and X-ray fluorescence (Magos, 1976; Jaishankar et al., 2014). Due to their sensitivity and specificity, these methods enable early detection and the avoidance of chronic poisoning.

Biomarkers occasionally overlap and serve as indications of exposure, impact, or susceptibility. Biomarkers can be categorized into three types, such as exposure biomarkers, effect biomarkers, and susceptibility biomarkers (Mussali-Galante et al., 2013).

Exposure markers are external substances, their derivatives, or products resulting from interactions between xenobiotic agents and target molecules or cells, which can be measured in biological compartments (Committee on Biological Markers of the National Research Council, 1987; Mussali-Galante et al., 2013; Polkowska et al., 2006). These markers, also known as "*biological dosimeters* or *biomarkers of internal dose*", are classified as "*biomarkers of biological effective dose*" when they assess the consequences of interactions with target molecules. Such biomarkers can be detected in various biological samples, including cells, tissues, blood, nails, hair, and body fluids (Mussali-Galante et al., 2013; WHO, 1993).

Biomarkers of effect refer to measurable biochemical, genetic, physiological, or behavioral alterations within an organism that may indicate an existing or developing health impairment or disease (Mussali-Galante et al., 2013; WHO, 1993). Effect biomarkers indicate that metal exposure can cause physiological or biochemical changes, including enzyme inhibition or oxidative damage. Examples of such biomarkers include DNA breaks, chromosomal abnormalities, micronucleus formation, and enzyme inhibition. Additionally, biomarkers of biochemical effect may reflect changes in enzyme activity, such as alterations in metal-binding proteins, DNA repair enzymes, and oxidative damage to proteins and DNA (Balali-Mood et al., 2021; Hughes, 2006; Ryu et al., 2015).

Susceptibility biomarkers are genetic or epigenetic factors that increase vulnerability to metal poisoning (Smith and Steinmaus, 2009). Research has identified several enzymes associated with disease susceptibility, including glutathione S-transferase, N-acetyltransferase, and cytochrome P-450 (CYP) isoforms, which exhibit significant interindividual variability in activity

TABLE 10.1 Human absorption routes, biological half-lives, elimination pathways, and primary storage sites for selected metals.

Metal	Main absorption route(s)	Biological half-life	Main elimination route(s)	Primary storage site(s)	References
Cadmium (Cd)	Inhalation (efficient); ingestion (poor); dermal (minimal)	≈10–30 y	Urine (slow), feces	Kidneys, liver, lungs, bone	(Rafati Rahimzadeh et al., 2017)
Nickel (Ni)	Inhalation, ingestion, dermal (soluble salts)	11–39 h (water-soluble); 30–54 h (poorly soluble)	Urine (main), feces, sweat	Kidneys, liver	(Dudek-Adamska et al., 2020; Min et al., 2024)
Mercury (Hg)	Inhalation (elemental); ingestion (organic); dermal (methylmercury)	≈30–60 d (species-dependent)	Inorganic → urine; organic → feces; elemental → breath	Brain (organic), kidneys (inorganic)	(Park and Zheng, 2012)
Arsenic (As)	Ingestion (main), inhalation; dermal (minor)	≈2–4 d (inorganic)	Urine (major), feces, sweat	Hair, nails, skin, liver	(Ro et al., 2022)
Chromium (Cr) [Cr(VI)]	Inhalation (highly absorbed); ingestion (low); dermal	≈15–41 h (Cr(VI))	Urine (main), feces	Blood, kidneys, lungs (inhaled), bones	(National Center for Biotechnology Information, 2025)
Thorium (Th) [Th-232]	Inhalation (main); ingestion (low); dermal (negligible)	≈200–400 y	Feces (major), urine (minor)	Reticuloendothelial system (spleen, liver, lymph nodes, bone marrow)	(Rubesin, 2010; National Center for Biotechnology Information, 2025)
Zinc (Zn)	Ingestion (efficient); inhalation (occupational); dermal (minimal)	Whole body ≈ 280 d; plasma ≈ 12 h	Feces (major), urine (minor), sweat	Muscle, bone, liver	(Maret and Sandstead, 2006)
Antimony (Sb)	Inhalation (occupational), ingestion (low), dermal	≈76 h (pentavalent); longer for trivalent	Urine (main), feces	Liver, lungs, spleen	(National Center for Biotechnology Information, 2025)
Copper (Cu)	Ingestion (main); inhalation (industrial); dermal (minor)	Liver: 3.9–21 d; kidney: 5–35 d; heart: 23–662 d; brain: ≈ 457 d; whole body: 13–33 d	Bile/feces (primary), urine (minor)	Liver, brain, muscle, bone	(Agency for Toxic Substances and Disease Registry (ATSDR), 2020)
Lead (Pb)	Inhalation (fine particles); ingestion (notably in children); dermal (organic forms)	Blood ≈ 25 d; soft tissue ≈ 40 d; bone ≈ 25 y	Urine, feces, sweat, hair, breast milk	Bone (~90%), teeth, liver, kidneys, brain	(Klein and Snodgrass, 2003; Wani et al., 2015)

Note: Units: h = hours; d = days; y = years; RES = reticuloendothelial system.

TABLE 10.2 Effect biomarkers and mechanisms of action for selected metals.

Metal	Key effect biomarkers	Mechanism of action
Lead (Pb)	ZPP; δ-ALA; cognitive tests	Heme synthesis inhibition; neurotoxicity
Mercury (Hg)	Urinary porphyrins; sensory dysfunction	Mitochondrial and neuronal damage
Cadmium (Cd)	β2-microglobulin; NAG; proteinuria	Renal tubular toxicity
Arsenic (As)	8-oxo-dG; suppression of DNA-repair proteins	Oxidative and genotoxic stress
Chromium (VI) [Cr(VI)]	DNA adducts; micronucleus assay	Genotoxicity; immune alteration
Copper (Cu)	ALT; AST; bilirubin; oxidative markers	Hepatic overload; redox imbalance
Nickel (Ni)	Cytokines; allergen-specific T-cell responses	Immunotoxicity; dermal hypersensitivity
Aluminium (Al)	ALT; AST (liver); β-amyloid (neuro markers)	Neuronal interference
Cobalt (Co)	Polycythemia; cardiomyopathy biomarkers; ROS	Erythropoietin stimulation; ROS generation
Uranium (U)	NAG; proteinuria; GFR markers	Nephrotoxicity; oxidative DNA damage
Thallium (Tl)	Nerve conduction; alopecia	Neurotoxicity; mitochondrial inhibition

Note: Table summarizing effect biomarkers and mechanisms for 11 metals (Pb, Hg, Cd, As, Cr(VI), Cu, Ni, Al, Co, U, Tl); ZPP = zinc protoporphyrin; δ-ALA = delta-aminolevulinic acid; NAG = N-acetyl-β-D-glucosaminidase; 8-oxo-dG = 8-oxo-2′-deoxyguanosine; ALT = alanine aminotransferase; AST = aspartate aminotransferase; ROS = reactive oxygen species; GFR = glomerular filtration rate. Biomarkers listed are illustrative and context-dependent; confirm clinical cut-points with current guidelines.

(Mussali-Galante et al., 2013). Certain trace metals, such as lead (Pb) and mercury (Hg), have been found to modulate CYP expression. These enzymes play roles in either activating or detoxifying chemical exposures. Advances in genetic research have enabled the identification of polymorphisms and phenotypic variations in metabolic enzymes, making single nucleotide polymorphism analysis essential in studying responses to metal exposures (Xu, 2024). Heavy metal toxicity is a significant global health concern, with genetic susceptibility affecting metabolism, detoxification, and overall toxicity risk. Key

TABLE 10.3 Genetic determinants influencing metal toxicity and effects.

Gene	Affected metal	Effect
ALAD	Lead (Pb)	Alters lead binding and distribution
AS3MT	Arsenic (As)	Determines methylation efficiency
GSTM1/ GSTT1	Mercury (Hg); Cadmium (Cd); Chromium (Cr)	Detoxification of oxidative intermediates
ATP7B	Copper (Cu)	Copper transport; mutation = Wilson's disease
XRCC1/ OGG1	Chromium (Cr); Arsenic (As)	DNA repair pathways

Note: Pb = lead; As = arsenic; Hg = mercury; Cd = cadmium; Cr = chromium; Cu = copper; DNA = deoxyribonucleic acid. Gene effects are summarized; confirm variant-specific impacts in primary sources.

TABLE 10.4 Biological matrices for metal biomonitoring: Common targets and key practical/analytical considerations.

Biological matrix	Metals commonly measured	Practical and analytical considerations
Whole blood	Arsenic, cadmium, lead, mercury, tin	Reflects current or recent systemic levels; sensitive for detecting acute exposure; some metals (e.g., Cd, Pb) also capture mid-term accumulation. Requires strict sample handling to avoid contamination.
Plasma/ serum	Nickel	Sensitive to soluble metal compounds; useful in occupational health contexts; may require rapid processing to prevent redistribution.
Red blood cells	Cadmium, mercury	Captures metals that bind to hemoglobin; suitable for assessing intermediate exposure duration; analytical methods must differentiate between organic and inorganic forms.
Urine	Arsenic, barium, cadmium, lead, mercury, nickel, tin, uranium	Noninvasive and widely accepted; ideal for soluble metals and those cleared renally; timing of collection can influence results; speciation is essential for some metals (e.g., As, Sn).

Biological matrix	Metals commonly measured	Practical and analytical considerations
Hair	Arsenic, cadmium, lead, mercury, uranium	Reflects exposure during hair growth; useful for metals with keratin binding (e.g., Hg, As); requires standardized washing protocols to avoid surface contamination.
Toenails/ fingernails	Arsenic, cadmium, lead, mercury, uranium	Capture longer-term accumulation; growth rate variability can affect interpretation; processing protocols are critical to reducing external contamination.
Teeth	Lead	Different tooth types represent different developmental periods, which are valuable for reconstructing childhood exposure history.
Bone	Lead, tin, uranium	Reflects long-term cumulative storage; noninvasive X-ray fluorescence is possible for Pb, while invasive sampling is needed for others.
Cumulative blood lead index	Lead	Provides an integrated estimate of long-term exposure based on serial blood-lead measurements.
Feces	Barium, cadmium	Reflects recent dietary intake or excretion; rarely used outside of research settings.
Placenta	Arsenic, cadmium, lead, mercury	Can reflect maternal–fetal transfer; variability between maternal and cord blood correlations; limited large-scale validation.
Liver/kidney tissue	Cadmium	Indicates organ burden; usually available only in occupational or postmortem contexts.
Soft tissue	Uranium	Mainly postmortem analysis; used in forensic or occupational exposure cases.
Chelatable urine	Lead	Used with a chelation challenge to estimate mobilizable lead burden; requires medical supervision.

Note: Matrices differ in the exposure timeframe they represent and susceptibility to external contamination. Hair and nails require standardized decontamination; urine often needs speciation (e.g., inorganic vs. methylated arsenic). Bone and teeth reflect cumulative exposure; the cumulative blood lead index integrates serial blood measures.

Source: Adapted from Martinez-Morata, I., Sobel, M., Tellez-Plaza, M., Navas-Acien, A., Howe, C.G., Sanchez, T.R., 2023. A state-of-the-science review on metal biomarkers. Curr. Environ. Health Rep. 10 (3), 215. https://doi.org/10.1007/S40572-023-00402-X.

TABLE 10.5 Primary biomarkers and exposure windows for selected metals.

Metal	Primary biomarker(s)	Exposure window
Lead (Pb)	Blood lead (µg/dL); bone lead (K-shell XRF); urinary lead (postchelation); hair/nails	Blood: Recent; bone/hair/nails: chronic; urinary (postchelation): mobilizable stores
Mercury (Hg)	Blood mercury (speciation for methylmercury/inorganic), hair mercury, and urinary mercury	Blood: Recent; hair: chronic methylmercury; urine: inorganic/elemental exposure
Cadmium (Cd)	Blood cadmium; urinary cadmium; β2-microglobulin; N-acetyl-β-D-glucosaminidase (NAG)	Blood: recent; urine: chronic; β2-mg & nag: early kidney damage
Arsenic (As)	Urinary arsenic speciation (inorganic, MMA, DMA); hair; toenails; blood arsenic	Urine: recent (speciation needed if seafood intake); hair/toenails: chronic
Chromium (Cr(VI))	Urinary chromium; red blood cell chromium; hair; nails	Urine & RBC: recent/occupational; hair/nails: chronic
Copper (Cu)	Serum/plasma copper (ceruloplasmin-bound); urinary copper	Serum/plasma: current status; urine: overload/Wilson's disease
Nickel (Ni)	Urinary nickel; hair; nails	Urine: recent; hair/nails: chronic
Aluminum (Al)	Serum aluminum; urinary aluminum; hair; nails	Serum/urine: acute; hair/nails: chronic
Cobalt (Co)	Blood cobalt; urinary cobalt	Blood/urine: recent
Uranium (U)	Urinary uranium; hair; nails; (research) kidney biopsy	Urine: recent; hair/nails: chronic
Thallium (Tl)	Blood thallium; urinary thallium	Blood/urine: recent

Note: Interpretation of exposure windows depends on chemical speciation, dose, and timing. For arsenic, urinary speciation (inorganic, MMA = monomethylarsonic acid; DMA = dimethylarsinic acid) is essential. For lead, K-shell XRF provides cumulative bone burden; postchelation urinary lead reflects mobilizable stores. Abbreviations: β2-MG = β2-microglobulin; NAG = N-acetyl-β-D-glucosaminidase; RBC = red blood cells; XRF = X-ray fluorescence.

genes, DNA repair mechanisms, antioxidant defense genes, and immune-related differences impact inflammatory responses. Genetic biomarkers can help identify susceptible populations, enabling targeted prevention and treatment strategies. Understanding genetic susceptibility can lead to better preventive measures to reduce heavy metal exposure and its health impacts (Xu, 2024).

10.6 The need for biomonitoring in metal exposure

Metal exposure is a silent public health risk; it remains hidden until it is too late, until clinical symptoms appear. Many metals cause harm gradually when they accumulate and become toxic. They work quietly within the body for years before symptoms appear. Cadmium can slowly damage kidney function, with signs of disease appearing only at advanced stages (Jacquillet et al., 2007).

A key issue is how metals accumulate in human tissues: lead and cadmium are sequestered in bone and kidney, where they can persist for decades and progressively raise the internal toxic burden (Goyer, 1989; Branca et al., 2018). Even small, repeated exposures can have lasting health consequences. Some groups are especially vulnerable, like infants, unborn children, and pregnant women. These vulnerable groups face increased risks because of their growth and developmental physiological changes. Likewise, people with certain genetic traits may be more sensitive to harmful effects, even at exposure levels others might tolerate. The problem is compounded by the fact that exposure sources are widespread—arising from polluted air, contaminated soil and water, unsafe food, or hazardous workplace conditions. The history of the Flint water crisis in the United States illustrates this clearly. When lead leached from aging pipes into the municipal water supply, thousands of residents, including children, were exposed to dangerously high levels. The consequences—cognitive impairment, developmental delays, and chronic health issues—continue to affect the community years later (Kennedy et al., 2019).

Biomonitoring can help us safeguard against such disasters. By measuring biomarkers in blood, urine, hair, or other tissues, scientists and public health authorities can identify exposures early, determine who is most at risk, and act before damage becomes irreversible. Thus, by monitoring, one can plan targeted interventions that protect entire communities. In today's world, where industrial activities and environmental contamination continue to expand, biomonitoring is more than a scientific method—it is an essential public health strategy for preventing silent but devastating harm.

10.7 Approach for monitoring biomarkers

A comprehensive biomonitoring approach must include understanding the toxicokinetics of heavy metals, matrix selection, time frame of exposure, and validated analytical techniques. Understanding how metals are absorbed, distributed, metabolized, and excreted is critical to choosing appropriate biomarkers and matrices. For matrix selection, blood samples are suitable for recent exposure (e.g., Pb, Hg); urinary analysis reflects renal excretion and cumulative exposure (e.g., Cd, As); hair/nails are useful for long-term and retrospective exposure (e.g., methylmercury, arsenic); bone and dental tissues indicate lifetime exposure (e.g., Pb via X-ray fluorescence). Time frame is important as acute and chronic exposure biomarkers differ. For example, methylmercury in hair reflects the past 3–6 months, while urinary arsenic reflects the recent 1–2 days. Analytical techniques include ICP-MS, AAS, and advanced omics approaches.

10.7.1 Metal-specific biomarkers

Lead (Pb) has the standard indicator of exposure as blood lead levels (BLLs). BLLs and δ- Aminolevulinic acid dehydratase (ALA-D) activity have an inverse correlation (Goyer, 1997). It remains one of the most studied environmental toxins, with blood lead concentration (μg/dL) serving as the principal measure of recent exposure. In contrast, bone lead—determined via K-shell X-ray fluorescence—offers a more accurate estimate of cumulative body burden. In certain clinical scenarios, urinary lead, collected postchelation, helps quantify mobilizable stores, while hair and nail analysis may provide retrospective evidence of exposure, though results can be influenced by surface contamination. Lead inhibits δ-ALA-D and ferrochelatase, elevating δ-ALA and zinc protoporphyrin, changes that contribute to anemia and red blood cell abnormalities. Neurological consequences, particularly severe in children, include slowed nerve conduction, learning difficulties, behavioral changes, and intelligence quotient (IQ) decline. Genetic polymorphisms in *ALAD* and micronutrient deficiencies—particularly calcium, zinc, and iron—heighten absorption and toxicity, with fetuses and children being the most vulnerable due to immature neural systems and higher gastrointestinal uptake.

Hair mercury levels are a good indicator of methylmercury exposure. The molar ratio of selenium to mercury in tissues may influence toxicity (Ralston et al., 2008). Mercury (Hg) exposure assessment depends on the chemical form. Total mercury in blood reflects recent contact, with speciation distinguishing methylmercury from inorganic forms. Hair mercury analysis is well-suited for chronic dietary intake evaluation, while urinary mercury is more indicative of elemental or inorganic exposure, such as from dental amalgams or industrial work. Mercury toxicity arises from glutathione depletion, altered porphyrin metabolism, and neurosensory impairments affecting coordination, hearing, and vision. Renal effects are also prominent, manifesting as proteinuria or tubular dysfunction. Variability in genes regulating glutathione synthesis and metallothionein expression influences individual risk. Selenium may counteract some toxic effects, while age and sex also shape susceptibility.

Cadmium: β2-microglobulin screening in industrial settings aids in the detection of cadmium nephrotoxicity. For environmental and occupational health risk assessment and supervision, these biomarkers are essential. The sensitive indicator of renal tubular failure is urinary β2-microglobulin. The body's attempt to store and detoxify cadmium is indicated by the levels of metallothionein (Nordberg et al., 2011). Cadmium (Cd) biomarkers differ according to the exposure window of interest. Blood cadmium reflects short-term exposure, whereas urinary cadmium better represents cumulative accumulation in renal tissues. Early kidney injury may be detected through elevated β2-microglobulin or N-acetyl-β-D-glucosaminidase (NAG), often before overt symptoms. Long-term exposure damages the proximal tubules, leading to proteinuria and glucosuria, and can reduce the glomerular filtration rate. Chronic accumulation also contributes to skeletal fragility, osteomalacia, and osteoporosis. Iron deficiency markedly increases cadmium absorption, a relationship exemplified in the *itai-itai* disease outbreak. Genetic differences in metallothionein expression and metal transport proteins further explain interindividual variability in response.

The detection of heavy metals in the body is guided by biological reference values (indicating typical exposure levels) and toxic limits (thresholds associated with health risks). These standards vary depending on the metal, the type of biological sample (blood, urine, or hair), and guidelines from organizations such as the Centers for Disease Control and Prevention (CDC), the World Health Organization (WHO), the Occupational Safety and Health Administration, and the EPA. For instance, lead levels in blood are considered elevated at ≥5 μg/dL (CDC's action level for children), with severe poisoning requiring treatment at ≥40 μg/dL. Mercury toxicity is indicated at >10 μg/L in blood or >1.5 ppm in hair, while arsenic in urine exceeding 100 μg/L (inorganic form) suggests harmful exposure. Cadmium becomes toxic at >5 μg/L in blood or >2 μg/g creatinine in urine, posing risks to kidney function.

Urinary arsenic speciation allows for the differentiation of inorganic and organic forms. The methylation index [monomethylarsonic acid (MMA)/dimethylarsinic acid (DMA)] ratio indicates both metabolic efficiency and vulnerability to the toxic effects of arsenic (Vahter, 2002). Arsenic (As) is best assessed through urinary speciation, which distinguishes inorganic, monomethyl-, and dimethyl-arsenic species while also revealing methylation efficiency. Hair and toenail arsenic concentrations provide evidence of long-term exposure, whereas blood levels capture recent intake. Clinical manifestations include hyperkeratotic skin lesions, impaired glucose regulation, cardiovascular effects, and genotoxic damage such as oxidative DNA lesions (8-oxo-dG). Arsenic exposure is also linked to compromised DNA repair pathways involving *ERCC1*, *XRCC1*, and *OGG1*. Polymorphisms in *AS3MT* affect methylation capacity, thereby modifying susceptibility.

Chromium (Cr(VI)) exposure, especially in occupational contexts, is commonly monitored through urinary chromium and red blood cell chromium levels. Hair and nail analysis may also reveal prolonged exposure. Once inside the body, hexavalent chromium generates oxidative DNA damage, induces protein carbonylation, forms DNA adducts, and causes chromosomal abnormalities such as micronuclei. It can also promote inflammation and impair immune responses. Susceptibility is influenced by genetic differences in antioxidant and DNA repair mechanisms, while dietary antioxidant intake and preexisting respiratory conditions may alter the severity of toxic outcomes.

Copper (Cu) status is routinely determined from plasma or serum levels, with attention to the ceruloplasmin-bound fraction. Urinary copper excretion is valuable in diagnosing Wilson's disease and assessing overload. Toxicity from excess copper manifests as liver injury—reflected in elevated ALT, AST, and bilirubin—oxidative stress, and lipid peroxidation, with chronic exposure contributing to neurological and hematological complications. Mutations in *ATP7B* impair copper regulation, and differences in antioxidant enzyme activity further shape the toxicological profile.

Among the emerging metals of concern, several have gained attention for their increasing industrial and environmental presence. Nickel (Ni) exposure is measured through urine, hair, and nails. Its toxic profile includes oxidative stress, DNA damage, and respiratory irritation, with risk influenced by iron status and genetic predisposition to hypersensitivity. Aluminum (Al) shows acute exposure in serum and urine, while hair and nail content reflects chronic accumulation. Effects include hepatic injury and possible contribution to β-amyloid–mediated neurodegeneration, particularly in individuals with renal impairment or advanced age. Cobalt (Co), monitored via blood and urine, can affect cardiac rhythm, thyroid function, and oxidative stress balance. Risk is greater in those with preexisting endocrine or cardiovascular disorders and in individuals with genetic variants affecting cobalt metabolism. Uranium (U) exposure is evaluated primarily through urinary measurements, while kidney biopsies—used in research—confirm tissue deposition. Uranium damages proximal tubules, elevating NAG and β2-microglobulin, and increases oxidative stress. Dehydration and renal dysfunction enhance vulnerability. Thallium (Tl) levels in blood and urine indicate exposure, with clinical signs including alopecia, slowed nerve conduction, and peripheral neuropathy. Susceptibility is influenced by the body's detoxification capacity and nutritional status.

In a study by Saravanabhavan et al. (2017), the researchers compared 95th-percentile "upper reference" concentrations (RV95) for multiple metals measured in whole blood from large population surveys conducted in different countries and years. It shows how background levels vary by age group, sex (for manganese), and national context, and it flags when studies applied exclusion criteria (e.g., excluding smokers or recent fish consumption) to make results more comparable. Several patterns stand out. Total arsenic in blood is lower in Italy (about 5.3 μg/L) than in Brazil (about 9.9 μg/L), consistent with dietary and regional differences. Cadmium in blood spans from very low values in German children (<0.3 μg/L) to higher values in Korean adults (~2.9 μg/L); studies that exclude smokers (a major cadmium source) generally report lower RV95s. Cobalt RV95 reported for Italian adults is ~0.44 μg/L. Lead shows the expected historical and geographic spread: late-1990s German adults had higher RV95s (around 70–90 μg/L by sex), while 2000s values are lower in children (Germany ~35 μg/L) and mid-range in contemporary adults (Italy ~51.7 μg/L; Korea ~42.3 μg/L; Spain ~56.8 μg/L). Manganese exhibits sex differences and country variation—Brazilian adult RV95s are around 29–31 μg/L, whereas Italian adults are ~14–15 μg/L, with women slightly higher than men in both settings. Total mercury in blood varies sharply with fish intake: very low in

German children (~0.8 μg/L) when high fish consumers are excluded, but much higher in Korean adults (~9.4 μg/L) even with a 96-hour seafood abstinence rule, reflecting differences in baseline seafood consumption. RV95 values are population descriptors; exceeding them suggests exposure, not necessarily toxicity. They are best used to screen and prioritize follow-up (Saravanabhavan et al., 2017).

They also compared international reference values (RV_{95}) for metals in urine (Saravanabhavan et al., 2017). Notable contrasts include total urinary arsenic, which is ~15 μg/L in Germany (with fish-related exclusions), ~49 μg/L in Belgium, and ~106 μg/L in Korea—differences that largely track seafood intake and speciation. Urinary cadmium—a marker of long-term body burden—ranges from ~0.7–0.8 μg/L in several European adult surveys (Belgium, Spain, Germany) to ~3.1 μg/L in Korea; children's RV95s are lower (e.g., Germany ~0.2 μg/L) but can be higher in some cohorts (Czech children ~1.0 μg/L), with smoking prevalence and age structure influencing adult values. Inorganic mercury in urine shows a wide spread: Czech adults ~9 μg/L vs. Germany ~1 μg/L and Belgium ~1.9 μg/L—differences that tighten when studies exclude subjects with amalgam fillings. Other elements sit at low single-digit RV95s (e.g., antimony ~0.24–0.30 μg/L; nickel ~3–4.7 μg/L; thallium ~0.5–0.6 μg/L). Nutritionally relevant elements can be higher: molybdenum ~116 μg/L and selenium ~61.6 μg/L in Belgian adults, and zinc shows large variability (~1048 μg/L), illustrating that urinary levels reflect both exposure and physiology. The study indicates that urinary RV95s are matrix-, diet-, and method-dependent. They serve as upper-background benchmarks: results above these cut-points warrant checking recent diet, potential sources (e.g., workplace, water), and—where applicable—speciation (especially for arsenic), rather than implying toxicity (Saravanabhavan et al., 2017).

10.8 Recent advances in biomarkers identification for toxic metal exposure

Recent advancements in toxicometallomics and systems biology have broadened the scope of biomarker identification, moving beyond simple metal detection in biological samples.

10.8.1 Omics technologies in biomarker discovery

Modern toxicology leverages high-throughput omics technologies—including transcriptomics, proteomics, metabolomics, and epigenomics—to identify molecular signatures of metal toxicity. These approaches provide a systems-level understanding of how metals like lead, cadmium, and arsenic disrupt biological pathways. For example, transcriptomics can reveal gene expression changes in response to metal exposure, while metabolomics detects altered metabolic profiles associated with toxicity (Mortimer et al., 2022).

10.8.2 Nanomaterial-based biosensors for enhanced detection

Advances in nanotechnology have improved biosensor sensitivity for detecting trace metal levels. Nanotechnology is applied by incorporating nanomaterials into biosensor systems, which strengthens their ability to detect heavy metals through improved sensitivity, selectivity, and signal transmission, using electrochemical, optical, or mass-based methods combined with precise biorecognition components (Maghsoudi et al., 2021).

10.8.3 Epigenetic modifications as early warning signs

Epigenetic biomarkers, particularly DNA methylation changes, are emerging as sensitive indicators of metal-induced toxicity. Arsenic exposure, for instance, is linked to hypermethylation of tumor suppressor genes, increasing cancer risk (Islam et al., 2022; Saintilnord and Fondufe-Mittendorf, 2021; Smeester et al., 2011). Similarly, nickel exposure alters histone modifications, affecting gene regulation. These epigenetic changes often occur before clinical symptoms, making them valuable for early detection (Martinez-Zamudio and Ha, 2011).

10.8.4 Early-warning biomarkers for preventive medicine

Research now prioritizes preclinical biomarkers that detect toxicity before irreversible damage. Mitochondrial DNA mutations have been observed in lead-exposed individuals (Mani et al., 2019). Exosomal miRNAs are identified as early signs of cadmium-induced liver injury (Wen et al., 2025).

10.8.5 Inflammation and oxidative stress biomarkers

Chronic exposure to toxic metals triggers oxidative stress and chronic inflammation, leading to cellular damage. Key biomarkers include C-reactive protein, which is elevated in lead and cadmium exposure (Liu et al., 2022; Welch et al., 2022). 8-oxo-2′-deoxyguanosine (8-oxo-dG) is a marker of oxidative DNA damage (Valavanidis et al., 2009). Malondialdehyde indicates lipid peroxidation due to arsenic or mercury toxicity (Rana et al., 2018). These biomarkers help assess subclinical toxicity before organ damage occurs.

10.8.6 Machine learning for predictive toxicology

Artificial intelligence (AI) and machine learning are transforming biomarker analysis by identifying hidden patterns in large datasets (e.g., linking cadmium exposure to kidney dysfunction), predicting individual susceptibility to metal toxicity based on genetic and environmental factors, and enhancing risk assessment models for occupational and environmental exposures (Nabavi et al., 2025). Predictive models can estimate future disease risk based on biomarker profiles and exposure history. In a study, a simple risk-prediction tool (nomogram) was developed to identify people at high risk of kidney damage from cadmium exposure, using factors like age, sex, and cadmium levels in blood. The tool was about 76%–78% accurate, working slightly better for women than men (Wang et al., 2020). Another study developed a model forecasting renal decline using urinary cadmium and metallothionein levels combined with demographic data (Chen et al., 2006). ICP-MS is one of the multiple-element analysis techniques used to quantify multiple metals simultaneously, and advanced statistical methods like Bayesian Kernel Machine Regression can be applied to analyze these complex datasets (Martinez-Morata et al., 2023).

10.8.7 Wearable devices

Emerging sensor technologies are being researched to detect the presence of metallic substances in biofluids, allowing for near-real-time monitoring via wearable patches or portable devices. These devices attempt to assess urine metals and oxidative stress indicators, possibly allowing for continuous and individualized health monitoring (Backiyalakshmi et al., 2024).

10.9 Linking biomarkers to health outcomes

The relationship between biomarkers and illness risk is supported by numerous studies. For instance, even at levels below 5 μg/dL, the National Health and Nutrition Examination Survey (NHANES) data showed a strong correlation between BLLs and worse IQ in children (Bellinger, 2011). Urinary arsenic levels have been associated with skin lesions and an elevated risk of cancer in Bangladesh (Argos et al., 2010). The dose-response relationship is a crucial component of toxicology. This is frequently nonlinear for metals. Particularly in young and vulnerable groups, even trace levels of lead and arsenic can result in noticeable adverse health effects. To direct public health initiatives, agencies such as the CDC and WHO have set minimum standards (e.g., BLL$<$ 5 μg/dL in children) (Betts, 2012). Increased ALA-D inhibition in lead-exposed workers may lead to workplace changes prior to the onset of clinical symptoms. Biomarkers make it possible to identify subclinical effects early and take prompt action. For environmental and occupational health risk assessment and supervision, these biomarkers are essential.

Heavy metals harm the body through several intertwined routes. A major one is oxidative stress: metals such as cadmium (Cd), lead (Pb), mercury (Hg), and arsenic (As) spur the formation of reactive oxygen species (ROS) that outstrip our antioxidant defenses. Those ROS then batter lipids, proteins, and DNA. Cadmium is responsible for derailing mitochondria and triggering apoptosis via ROS. Lead worsens the redox imbalance by knocking out key antioxidant enzymes like glutathione peroxidase. Mercury binds tightly to thiol (–SH) groups across tissues, disrupting redox control, while arsenic both generates ROS and interferes with thioredoxin systems, amplifying stress signals inside cells. Chromium (especially Cr(VI)), cadmium, and arsenic cause DNA damage such as strand breaks and base oxidation—and can hinder DNA repair. Lead and mercury readily cross the blood–brain barrier, where they spark neuroinflammation and epigenetic changes. In the developing brain, lead disrupts astrocyte support and myelination, while mercury directly injures neurons through oxidative stress, inflammatory signaling, and interference with tubulin and microtubules. Different organs are affected by different metals. Cadmium targets the kidneys, damaging proximal tubules and driving nephrotoxicity. Arsenic is a well-established carcinogen for skin, lung, and bladder, promoting cancer through genomic instability. Taken together—oxidative stress, protein disruption, genotoxicity, and organ-specific damage—these mechanisms explain why heavy metals are hazardous even at relatively low exposures: they tamper with core cellular processes that keep multiple body systems running.

10.10 Public health and regulatory implications

Agencies such as the WHO and the United States EPA increasingly build protective values—reference doses and tolerable weekly intakes—around biomarker evidence because these measurements tie exposure to health consequences with unusual precision. In practice, risk assessment now revolves around biomarkers: hazard identification relies on biomonitoring to verify that toxic metals are present in defined populations; dose–response assessment links specific concentrations (for example, blood lead or urinary cadmium) to clinical and subclinical outcomes in epidemiologic cohorts; exposure assessment tracks temporal and geographic trends using repeated measurements in blood and urine; and risk characterization integrates hazard and exposure results to estimate both the likelihood and magnitude of harm for individuals and communities.

WHO-coordinated efforts that aggregate standardized biomarker datasets enable cross-country comparisons and support harmonized policy responses over time. Similar goals drive national surveys such as Canada's Canadian Health Measures Survey (CHMS) and Germany's Herman Environmental Survey (GerES), which deploy multimetal panels to establish population baselines and pinpoint demographic groups at greater risk. In the United States, NHANES provides metals data from nationally representative samples and informs benchmarks like the CDC childhood lead reference value, creating a long-running empirical spine for trend analysis and intervention planning.

Guidelines and legal thresholds increasingly mirror what biomarkers reveal about real-world exposure. The WHO drinking-water limit for arsenic (10 μg/L) is based on cancer risk evidence underpinned by biomarker-linked epidemiology, while tolerable intake values for methylmercury (about 1.6 μg/kg body weight per week) rely on blood and hair measurements to evaluate dietary exposure in vulnerable groups. For lead, the CDC uses 3.5 μg/dL as the pediatric blood-lead reference value to trigger follow-up and prevention, and U.S. occupational rules set an action level near 30 μg/dL, with medical removal typically at or above 50 μg/dL. Cadmium policy similarly reflects biomarker interpretation: urinary cadmium above roughly 2 μg/g creatinine is considered elevated in the EU, whereas about 5 μg/g is used as an occupational benchmark in China.

Maternal and child health programs incorporate early-life screening for lead and, where diet or environment suggests higher risk, targeted testing for cadmium and mercury during pregnancy. In high-risk industries such as battery manufacturing and metal fabrication, routine monitoring—blood lead, urinary cadmium—anchors removal and return-to-work decisions using clear thresholds. Community-based initiatives in arsenic-affected regions, including parts of Bangladesh, use periodic urine arsenic speciation to guide well switching, remediation choices, and risk communication, pairing local action with continuous measurement.

Fish-consumption advisories issued by the FDA/EPA draw directly on hair and blood mercury data from coastal communities, balancing nutritional benefits against neurodevelopmental risks for pregnant people and children. Biomonitoring evidence of elevated pediatric blood-lead levels has underwritten national and subnational restrictions on lead-based paint and related products, and the historical "Itai-Itai" cadmium-in-rice crisis in Japan led to stricter soil standards, remediation, and sustained surveillance—examples of how measurements translate into enforceable protections and measurable outcomes.

10.11 Research and technical challenges

Although science has advanced quickly, biomarker-driven toxicometallomics still wrestles with ethical, technical, and translational hurdles. Privacy, consent, and the potential for stigma or discrimination sit uneasily beside the promise of finely resolved risk prediction; any framework that uses personal biomarker data must shield individuals from misuse by employers or insurers while minimizing anxiety and ensuring fair access to mitigation. Against this backdrop, validation remains a moving target: panels discovered in one setting—such as miRNA signatures or extracellular vesicle cargo—often underperform when transported to populations with different genetic backgrounds, dietary patterns, coexposures, or disease burdens. Even when signals replicate, inconsistent preanalytical handling can erase reproducibility; without harmonized procedures for specimen collection, storage, processing, and assay interpretation, laboratories and field teams will continue to produce results that are difficult to compare. A further scientific gap is conceptual rather than logistical: a unified multiomic architecture that links metal body burden to coordinated molecular, metabolic, proteomic, and epigenomic responses is still incomplete, which limits mechanistic inference and the precision of risk models.

In practical terms, four issues keep resurfacing. First, candidate biomarker panels require testing across diverse ancestries and exposure contexts before they can be treated as generalizable tools. Second, standardized protocols—covering everything from tube type and temperature control to bioinformatic thresholds—are essential if accuracy and reproducibility are to be trusted outside the discovery lab. Third, integration across omic layers is needed to convert fragmented signals into causal pathways that connect exposure with cellular injury and clinical endpoints. Fourth, ethical governance must keep pace: clear guidance on privacy, informed consent, secondary use, and equitable distribution of exposure-reduction resources is necessary to maintain public trust.

10.12 Translational implications

Looking forward, progress will hinge on well-powered, longitudinal cohorts that track multimodal biomarkers in step with exposure metrics and health outcomes; these studies can anchor temporal inference and sharpen dose–response estimation. Equally important are cross-sector consortia—universities working with public health agencies, community organizations, and industry—to validate assays in real-world settings. Investment in enabling technologies should continue, from portable diagnostics and wearable biosensors to AI-assisted analytic platforms that can handle high-dimensional data streams. Finally, policy architectures must translate science into action by defining guardrails for ethical data use, prioritizing protections for vulnerable groups, and creating pathways that carry validated biomarkers into surveillance, regulation, and clinical decision support.

Adoption will look different across end users, but the throughline is early detection that leads to timely prevention. National public health systems can fold advanced biomarkers into existing biomonitoring models (for example, NHANES-style designs), improving horizon scanning for emerging metal risks and enabling rapid course corrections. The next wave of prevention depends on integrating biomarker streams with source data, clinical outcomes, socioeconomic indicators, and geospatial context to target policies more precisely and evaluate them faster. Personalization of action thresholds—moving beyond population averages toward risk-based triggers for individuals, such as tailored targets for blood lead or urinary cadmium—will make interventions more responsive. Access must also improve: point-of-care and wearable sensing can reduce dependence on centralized laboratories and speed decisions in the field. Finally, expanding high-quality biomonitoring in low- and middle-income settings, where environmental burdens are often highest, will close critical data gaps and extend the benefits of toxicometallomics to the populations that need them most.

Clinicians, particularly those serving high-risk populations, can incorporate metal biomarker profiles into routine screening to individualize counseling, chelation decisions, nutritional support, and environmental referrals. Policymakers can draw on population-level biomarker distributions to set evidence-based thresholds, prioritize remediation, and evaluate program impact with measurable before-and-after changes. At the community level, transparent communication of biomonitoring results, paired with education and locally led interventions, empowers residents to modify behaviors, advocate for safer infrastructure, and ultimately lower exposure burdens.

10.13 Conclusion

The widespread distribution and capacity for bioaccumulation of metals, including lead, mercury, cadmium, and arsenic, make them poisonous and present a continuous threat to global health. How these metals are absorbed, dispersed, and cause their harmful effects at the molecular and cellular levels can be understood by comprehending their toxicokinetics and toxicodynamics. Biomarkers serve as the basis for public health interventions by offering strong instruments to assess exposure and forecast health effects. Future biomarker discovery is predicted to improve the accuracy and predictive power of toxicological evaluations, thereby enhancing protection for at-risk groups, owing to advances in omics technologies and personalized therapy. In the coming years, toxicometallomics could be used as a precision monitoring method along with personalized medicine. Real-time exposure tracking, early detection diagnostics, and data-analyzed interventions could transform metal toxicity from reactive treatment to proactive prevention.

References

Abadin, H., Ashizawa, A., Stevens, Y.W., et al., 2007. Toxicological Profile for Lead. Agency for Toxic Substances and Disease Registry (US), Atlanta (GA). Available from: https://www.ncbi.nlm.nih.gov/books/NBK158766/.

Agency for Toxic Substances and Disease Registry (ATSDR), 2020. Toxicological Profile for Lead. U.S. Department of Health and Human Services, Public Health Service, Atlanta, GA. doi:10.15620/CDC:95222.

Al-Ashban, R.M., Aslam, M., Shah, A.H., 2004. Kohl (surma): a toxic traditional eye cosmetic study in Saudi Arabia. Public Health 118 (4), 292–298. doi:10.1016/j.puhe.2003.05.001.

Alengebawy, A., Abdelkhalek, S.T., Qureshi, S.R., Wang, M.Q., 2021. Heavy metals and pesticides toxicity in agricultural soil and plants: ecological risks and human health implications. Toxics. 23056304. 9 (3), 1–34. Available from: https://www.mdpi.com/2305-6304/9/3/42/pdf. doi:10.3390/toxics9030042.

Argos, M., Kalra, T., Rathouz, P.J., Chen, Y., Pierce, B., Parvez, F., Islam, T., Ahmed, A., Rakibuz-Zaman, M., Hasan, R., Sarwar, G., Slavkovich, V., Van Geen, A., Graziano, J., Ahsan, H., 2010. Arsenic exposure from drinking water, and all-cause and chronic-disease mortalities in Bangladesh (HEALS): a prospective cohort study. Lancet. 01406736. 376 (9737), 252–258. Available from: http://www.journals.elsevier.com/the-lancet/. doi:10.1016/S0140-6736(10)60481-3.

Backiyalakshmi, G., Snekhalatha, U., Salvador, A.L., 2024. Recent advancements in non-invasive wearable electrochemical biosensors for biomarker analysis—a review. Anal. Biochem. 692, 115578. doi:10.1016/J.AB.2024.115578.

Balali-Mood, M., Naseri, K., Tahergorabi, Z., Khazdair, M.R., Sadeghi, M., 2021. Toxic mechanisms of five heavy metals: mercury, lead, chromium, cadmium, and arsenic. Front. Pharmacol. 16639812. 12. Available from: http://www.frontiersin.org/Pharmacology. doi:10.3389/fphar.2021.643972.

Barry, P.S.I., 1975. A comparison of concentrations of lead in human tissues. Br. J. Ind. Med. 00071072. 32 (2), 119–139. doi:10.1136/oem.32.2.119.

Bellinger, D.C., 2011. The protean toxicities of lead: new chapters in a familiar story. Int. J. Environ. Res. Public Health. 16604601. 8 (7), 2593–2628. Available from: http://www.mdpi.com/1660-4601/8/7/2593/pdf. doi:10.3390/ijerph8072593.

Bergdahl, I.A., Skerfving, S., 2008. Biomonitoring of lead exposure—alternatives to blood. J. Toxicol. Environ. Health A. 10872620. 71 (18), 1235–1243. doi:10.1080/15287390802209525.

Betts, K.S., 2012. CDC updates guidelines for children's lead exposure. Environ. Health Perspect. 15529924. 120 (7), a268. doi:10.1289/ehp.120-a268.

Boateng, T.K., Opoku, F., Akoto, O., 2019. Heavy metal contamination assessment of groundwater quality: a case study of Oti landfill site, Kumasi. Appl. Water Sci. 9 (2). doi:10.1007/S13201-019-0915-Y.

Branca, J.J.V., Morucci, G., Pacini, A., 2018. Cadmium-induced neurotoxicity: still much ado. Neural Regen. Res. 13 (11), 1879–1882. doi:10.4103/1673-5374.239434.

Brewer, G.J., 2000. Recognition, diagnosis, and management of Wilson's disease. Proc. Soc. Exp. Biol. Med. 00379727. 223 (1), 39–46. Available from: www.blackwellscience.com/journals/experiment/index.html. doi:10.1046/j.1525-1373.2000.22305.x.

Cai, L., Li, X.K., Song, Y., Cherian, M.G., 2005. Essentiality, toxicology and chelation therapy of zinc and copper. Curr. Med. Chem. 09298673. 12 (23), 2753–2763. doi:10.2174/092986705774462950.

Chen, L., Lei, L., Jin, T., Nordberg, M., Nordberg, G.F., 2006. Plasma metallothionein antibody, urinary cadmium, and renal dysfunction in a Chinese type 2 diabetic population. Diabetes Care. 01495992. 29 (12), 2682–2687. Available from: http://care.diabetesjournals.org/cgi/reprint/29/12/2682.pdf. doi:10.2337/dc06-1003China.

Clarkson, T.W., Magos, L., 2006. The toxicology of mercury and its chemical compounds. Crit. Rev. Toxicol. 15476898. 36 (8), 609–662. doi:10.1080/10408440600845619.

Coetzee, J.J., Bansal, N., Chirwa, E.M.N., 2020. Chromium in environment, its toxic effect from chromite-mining and ferrochrome industries, and its possible bioremediation. Expo. Health 12 (1), 51–62. doi:10.1007/S12403-018-0284-Z.

Committee on Biological Markers of the National Research Council, 1987. Biological markers in environmental health research. Environ. Health Perspect. 74, 3–9. doi:10.1289/EHP.74-1474499

Domingo, J.L., 1989. Cobalt in the environment and its toxicological implications. Rev. Environ. Contam. Toxicol. 01795953. 108, 105–132. doi:10.1007/978-1-4613-8850-0_3.

Dudek-Adamska, D., Lech, T., Konopka, T., Kościelniak, P., 2020. Nickel content in human internal organs. Biol. Trace Elem. Res. 199 (6), 2138–2144. doi:10.1007/s12011-020-02347-w.

Genchi, G., Carocci, A., Lauria, G., Sinicropi, M.S., Catalano, A., 2020. Nickel: human health and environmental toxicology. Int. J. Environ. Res. Public Health. 16604601. 17 (3). Available from: https://www.mdpi.com/1660-4601/17/3/679/pdf. doi:10.3390/ijerph17030679.

Goyer, R.A., 1989. Mechanisms of lead and cadmium nephrotoxicity. Toxicol. Lett. 03784274. 46 (1–3), 153–162. doi:10.1016/0378-4274(89)90124-0.

Goyer, R.A., 1997. Toxic and essential metal interactions. Annu. Rev. Nutr. 01999885. 17, 37–50. doi:10.1146/annurev.nutr.17.1.37.

Hayat, M.T., Nauman, M., Nazir, N., Ali, S., Bangash, N., 2018. Environmental hazards of cadmium: past, present, and future. In: Cadmium Toxicity and Tolerance in Plants: From Physiology to Remediation, pp. 163–183. doi:10.1016/B978-0-12-814864-8.00007-3.

He, M., Wang, N., Long, X., Zhang, C., Ma, C., Zhong, Q., Wang, A., Wang, Y., Pervaiz, A., Shan, J., 2019. Antimony speciation in the environment: recent advances in understanding the biogeochemical processes and ecological effects. J. Environ. Sci. (China). 18787320. 75, 14–39. Available from: http://www.journals.elsevier.com/journal-of-environmental-sciences/. doi:10.1016/j.jes.2018.05.023.

Hollenberg, P.F., 2010. Introduction: mechanisms of metal toxicity special issue. Chem. Res. Toxicol. 15205010. 23 (2), 292–293. doi:10.1021/tx900456p.

Hughes, M.F., 2006. Biomarkers of exposure: a case study with inorganic arsenic. Environ. Health Perspect. 114 (11), 1790–1796. doi:10.1289/EHP.9058/ASSET/E68766F9-13BB-455E-9BBC-57EC9A6038DE/ASSETS/GRAPHIC/EHP0114-001790E1.JPG.

Hughes, M.F., Beck, B.D., Chen, Y., Lewis, A.S., Thomas, D.J., 2011. Arsenic exposure and toxicology: a historical perspective. Toxicol. Sci. 10960929. 123 (2), 305–332. doi:10.1093/toxsci/kfr184.

Iavicoli, I., Fontana, L., Bergamaschi, A., 2009. The effects of metals as endocrine disruptors. J. Toxicol. Environ. Health B. 12 (3), 206–223. doi:10.1080/10937400902902062. WGROUP:STRING:PUBLICATION.

Islam, R., Zhao, L., Wang, Y., Lu-Yao, G., Liu, L.-Z., 2022. Epigenetic dysregulations in arsenic-induced carcinogenesis. Cancers. 2072-6694. 14 (18), 4502. doi:10.3390/cancers14184502.

Jacquillet, G., Barbier, O., Rubera, I., Tauc, M., Borderie, A., Namorado, M.C., Martin, D., Sierra, G., Reyes, J.L., Poujeol, P., Cougnon, M., 2007. Cadmium causes delayed effects on renal function in the offspring of cadmium-contaminated pregnant female rats. Am. J. Physiol. Renal Physiol. 1931-857X. 293 (5), F1450. doi:10.1152/ajprenal.00223.2007.

Jaishankar, M., Tseten, T., Anbalagan, N., Mathew, B.B., Beeregowda, K.N., 2014. Toxicity, mechanism and health effects of some heavy metals. Interdiscip. Toxicol. 13379569. 7 (2), 60–72. Available from: http://versita.com/science/medicine/it/. doi:10.2478/intox-2014-0009.

Järup, L., Åkesson, A., 2009. Current status of cadmium as an environmental health problem. Toxicol. Appl. Pharmacol. 0041008X. 238 (3), 201–208. doi:10.1016/j.taap.2009.04.020.

Kennedy, C., Yard, E., Dignam, T., Buchanan, S., Condon, S., Brown, M.J., Raymond, J., Rogers, H.S., Sarisky, J., de Castro, R., Arias, I., Breysse, P., 2019. Blood lead levels among children aged <6 years—Flint, Michigan, 2013–2016. MMWR Morb. Mortal. Wkly. Rep. 65 (25), 650–654. doi:10.15585/MMWR.MM6525E1.

Kimbrough, D.E., Cohen, Y., Winer, A.M., Creelman, L., Mabuni, C., 1999. A critical assessment of chromium in the environment. Crit. Rev. Environ. Sci. Technol. 10643389. 29 (1), 1–46. doi:10.1080/10643389991259164.

Klein, G.L., Snodgrass, W.R., 2003. Heavy metal toxicology. In: Encyclopedia of Food Sciences and Nutrition, pp. 3050–3057. doi:10.1016/B0-12-227055-X/00588-5.

Kumar, P., Gacem, A., Ahmad, M.T., Yadav, V.K., Singh, S., Yadav, K.K., Alam, M.M., Dawane, V., Piplode, S., Maurya, P., Ahn, Y., Jeon, B.H., Cabral-Pinto, M.M.S., 2022. Environmental and human health implications of metal(loid)s: source identification, contamination, toxicity, and sustainable clean-up technologies. Front. Environ. Sci. 2296665X. 10. Available from: https://journal.frontiersin.org/journal/environmental-science. doi:10.3389/fenvs.2022.949581.

Liu, Y., Yang, D., Shi, F., Wang, F., Liu, X., Wen, H., Mubarik, S., Chuanhua, Y., 2022. Association of serum 25(OH)D, cadmium, CRP with all-cause, cause-specific mortality: a prospective cohort study. Front. Nutr. 2296-861X. 9. doi:10.3389/fnut.2022.803985.

Loh, N., Loh, H.-P., Wang, L.K., Wang, M.-H.S., 2016. Health effects and control of toxic lead in the environment. Nat. Resour. Control Process. 233–284. doi:10.1007/978-3-319-26800-2_5.

Long, Z., Huang, Y., Zhang, W., Shi, Z., Daming, Y., Chen, Y., Liu, C., Wang, R., 2021. Effect of different industrial activities on soil heavy metal pollution, ecological risk, and health risk. Environ. Monit. Assess. 0167-6369. 193 (1), doi:10.1007/s10661-020-08807-z.

Loranger, S., Zayed, J., 1995. Environmental and occupational exposure to manganese: a multimedia assessment. Int. Arch. Occup. Environ. Health. 0340-0131. 67 (2), 101–110. doi:10.1007/bf00572233.

Maghsoudi, A.S., Hassani, S., Mirnia, K., Abdollahi, M., 2021. Recent advances in nanotechnology-based biosensors development for detection of arsenic, lead, mercury, and cadmium. Int. J. Nanomed. 11782013. 16, 803–832. Available from: https://www.dovepress.com/getfile.php?fileID=66251. doi:10.2147/IJN.S294417.

Magos, L., 1976. Toxicology: the basic science of poisons. Occup. Environ. Med. 1351-0711. 33 (4), 282–283. doi:10.1136/oem.33.4.282-b.

Mandal, B.K., Suzuki, K.T., 2002. Arsenic round the world: a review. Talanta. 00399140. 58 (1), 201–235. doi:10.1016/S0039-9140(02)00268-0.

Mani, M.S., Chakrabarty, S., Mallya, S.P., Kabekkodu, S.P., Jayaram, P., Varghese, V.K., Dsouza, H.S., Satyamoorthy, K., 2019. Whole mitochondria genome mutational spectrum in occupationally exposed lead subjects. Mitochondrion. 18728278. 48, 60–66. Available from: https://www.journals.elsevier.com/mitochondrion. doi:10.1016/j.mito.2019.04.009.

Maret, W., Sandstead, H.H., 2006. Zinc requirements and the risks and benefits of zinc supplementation. J. Trace Elem. Med. Biol. 20 (1), 3–18. doi:10.1016/J.JTEMB.2006.01.006.

Martinez-Morata, I., Sobel, M., Tellez-Plaza, M., Navas-Acien, A., Howe, C.G., Sanchez, T.R., 2023. A state-of-the-science review on metal biomarkers. Curr. Environ. Health Rep. 10 (3), 215. doi:10.1007/S40572-023-00402-X.

Martinez-Zamudio, R., Ha, H.C., 2011. Environmental epigenetics in metal exposure. Epigenetics. 15592308. 6 (7), 820–827. Available from: http://www.landesbioscience.com/journals/epigenetics/ZamudioEPI6-7.pdf. doi:10.4161/epi.6.7.16250.

Min, J.H., Lee, S., Lim, H.J., Kang, M.K., Son, H., Kim, B.G., Hong, Y.S., 2024. Characterization of nickel levels considering seasonal and intra-individual variation using three biological matrices. Environ. Sci. Pollut. Res. Int. 31 (2), 2546–2554. doi:10.1007/S11356-023-31252-7/TABLES/3.

Mitra, S., Chakraborty, A.J., Tareq, A.M., Emran, T.B., Nainu, F., Khusro, A., Idris, A.M., Khandaker, M.U., Osman, H., Alhumaydhi, F.A., Simal-Gandara, J., 2022. Impact of heavy metals on the environment and human health: novel therapeutic insights to counter the toxicity. J. King Saud Univ. Sci. 10183647. 34 (3). Available from: http://www.sciencedirect.com/science/journal/10183647. doi:10.1016/j.jksus.2022.101865.

Mortimer, M., Fang, W., Zhou, X., Vodovnik, M., Guo, L.H., 2022. Omics Approaches in Toxicological Studies Advances in Toxicology and Risk Assessment of Nanomaterials and Emerging Contaminants. Springer Nature, China, pp. 61–94. Available from: doi:10.1007/978-981-16-9116-4.

Mussali-Galante, P., Tovar-Sánchez, E., Valverde, M., Castillo, E.R.D., 2013. Biomarkers of exposure for assessing environmental metal pollution: from molecules to ecosystems. Centro de Ciencias de la Atmosfera, Revista Internacional de Contaminacion Ambiental 01884999. 29 (1), 117–140. Available from: http://www.journals.unam.mx/index.php/rica/article/download/30580/32434.

Nabavi, A., Kashkooli, M., Nabavizadeh, S.S., Safari, F., 2025. Heavy metal biomarkers and their impact on hearing loss risk: a machine learning framework analysis. Front. Public Health. 22962565. 13. Available from: http://journal.frontiersin.org/journal/public-health/section/public-health-education-and-promotion#archive. doi:10.3389/fpubh.2025.1471490.

National Center for Biotechnology Information, 2025. PubChem compound summary for CID 23976, chromium.

Nordberg, G.F., Nogawa, K., Nordberg, M., Friberg, L.T., 2007. Cadmium Handbook on the Toxicology of Metals, third ed. Elsevier, Sweden, pp. 445–486. Available from: https://www.sciencedirect.com/book/9780123694133. doi:10.1016/B978-012369413-3/50078-1.

Nordberg, G.F., Nordberg, M., Fowler, B.A., Friberg, L., 2011. Handbook on the Toxicology of Metals, pp. 1024. https://books.google.com/books/about/Handbook_on_the_Toxicology_of_Metals.html?id=nKulgztuzL8C.

Nordberg, G.F., Nordberg, M., Fowler, B.A., Friberg, L., 2011. Handbook on the Toxicology of Metals, third ed. https://books.google.com/books/about/Handbook_on_the_Toxicology_of_Metals.html?id=nKulgztuzL8C.

O'Neal, S.L., Zheng, W., 2015. Manganese toxicity upon overexposure: a decade in review. Curr. Environ. Health Rep. 21965412. 2 (3), 315–328. Available from: http://link.springer.com/journal/40572. doi:10.1007/s40572-015-0056-x.

Park, J.D., Zheng, W., 2012. Human exposure and health effects of inorganic and elemental mercury. J. Prev. Med. Public Health 45 (6), 344. doi:10.3961/JPMPH.2012.45.6.344.

Poland, C.A., Hubbard, S.A., Levy, L., Mackie, C., 2022. Occupational Exposure—International Copper Association. https://internationalcopper.org/. doi:10.1016/j.tox.2022.153221. 474.

Polkowska, Ż., Kozłowska, K., Mazerska, Z., Górecki, T., Namieśnik, J., 2006. Volatile organohalogen compounds in human urine: the effect of environmental exposure. Chemosphere. 00456535. 62 (4), 626 640. doi:10.1016/j.chemosphere.2005.05.036.

Rafati Rahimzadeh, M., Rafati Rahimzadeh, M., Kazemi, S., Moghadamnia, A., 2017. Cadmium toxicity and treatment: an update. Caspian J. Intern. Med. 8 (3), 135–145. doi:10.22088/cjim.8.3.135.

Rahaman, M.S., Mise, N., Ichihara, S., 2022. Arsenic contamination in food chain in Bangladesh: a review on health hazards, socioeconomic impacts and implications. Hygiene Environ. Health Adv. 2, 100004. doi:10.1016/J.HEHA.2022.100004.

Rajkumar, V., Lee, V.R., Gupta, V., 2023. Heavy metal toxicity. Pakistan J. Med. Health Sci. 10 (2), 324. doi:10.1201/9781003637073-6.

Ralston, N.V.C., Ralston, C.R., Blackwell, J.L., Raymond, L.J., 2008. Dietary and tissue selenium in relation to methylmercury toxicity. NeuroToxicology. 0161813X. 29 (5), 802–811. doi:10.1016/j.neuro.2008.07.007.

Rana, M.N., Tangpong, J., Rahman, M.M., 2018. Toxicodynamics of lead, cadmium, mercury and arsenic-induced kidney toxicity and treatment strategy: a mini review. Toxicol. Rep. 5, 704. doi:10.1016/J.TOXREP.2018.05.012.

Rani Saha, T., Khan, M.A.R., Kundu, R., Naime, J., Karim, K.M.R., Ara, M.H., 2022. Heavy metal contaminations of soil in waste dumping and non-dumping sites in Khulna: human health risk assessment. Results Chem. 22117156. 4, 100434. doi:10.1016/j.rechem.2022.100434.

Rice, K.M., Walker, E.M., Wu, M., Gillette, C., Blough, E.R., 2014. Environmental mercury and its toxic effects. J. Prev. Med. Public Health. 19758375. 47 (2), 74–83. Available from: http://synapse.koreamed.org/Synapse/Data/PDFData/0056JPMPH/jpmph-47-74.pdf. doi:10.3961/jpmph.2014.47.2.74.

Ro, S.H., Bae, J., Jang, Y., Myers, J.F., Chung, S., Yu, J., Natarajan, S.K., Franco, R., Song, H.S., 2022. Arsenic toxicity on metabolism and autophagy in adipose and muscle tissues. Antioxidants 11 (4), 689. doi:10.3390/ANTIOX11040689.

Rubesin, S.E., 2010. Case 308. Teaching Files Gastrointest. 654–655. doi:10.1016/B978-1-4160-5944-8.00308-0.

Ryu, H.W., Lee, D.H., Won, H.R., Kim, K.H., Seong, Y.J., Kwon, S.H., 2015. Influence of toxicologically relevant metals on human epigenetic regulation. Toxicol. Res. 22342753. 31 (1), 1–9. Available from: http://ocean.kisti.re.kr/downfile/volume/ksot/DSHHBQ/2015/v31n1/DSHHBQ_2015_v31n1_1.pdf. doi:10.5487/TR.2015.31.1.001.

Saintilnord, W.N., Fondufe-Mittendorf, Y., 2021. Arsenic-induced epigenetic changes in cancer development. Semin. Cancer Biol. 10963650. 76, 195–205. Available from: http://www.elsevier.com/inca/publications/store/6/2/2/9/4/3/index.htt. doi:10.1016/j.semcancer.2021.03.019.

Sankhla, M.S., Kumari, M., Nandan, M., Kumar, R., Agrawal, P., 2016. Heavy metals contamination in water and their hazardous effect on human health—a review. Int. J. Curr. Microbiol. Appl. Sci. 23197692. 5 (10), 759–766. doi:10.20546/ijcmas.2016.510.082.

Saravanabhavan, G., Werry, K., Walker, M., Haines, D., Malowany, M., Khoury, C., 2017. Human biomonitoring reference values for metals and trace elements in blood and urine derived from the Canadian Health Measures Survey 2007–2013. Int. J. Hyg. Environ. Health. 14384639. 220 (2), 189–200. doi:10.1016/j.ijheh.2016.10.006.

Satarug, S., Garrett, S.H., Sens, M.A., Sens, D.A., 2010. Cadmium, environmental exposure, and health outcomes. Environ. Health Perspect. 15529924. 118 (2), 182–190. Available from: http://ehp03.niehs.nih.gov/article/fetchObjectAttachment.action?uri=info%3Adoi%2F10.1289%2Fehp.0901234&representation=PDF. doi:10.1289/ehp.0901234.

Schilsky, M.L., Roberts, E.A., Bronstein, J.M., Dhawan, A., Hamilton, J.P., Rivard, A.M., Washington, M.K., Weiss, K.H., Zimbrean, P.C., 2022. A multidisciplinary approach to the diagnosis and management of wilson disease: 2022 practice guidance on Wilson disease from the American Association for the Study of Liver Diseases. Hepatology. doi:10.1002/HEP.32801.

Smeester, L., Rager, J.E., Bailey, K.A., Guan, X., Smith, N., García-Vargas, G., Razo, L.M.D., Drobná, Z., Kelkar, H., Stýblo, M., Fry, R.C., 2011. Epigenetic changes in individuals with arsenicosis. Chem. Res. Toxicol. 15205010. 24 (2), 165–167. doi:10.1021/tx1004419.

Smith, A.H., Steinmaus, C.M., 2009. Health effects of arsenic and chromium in drinking water: recent human findings. Annu. Rev. Public Health. 01637525. 30, 107–122. Available from: http://arjournals.annualreviews.org/doi/pdf/10.1146/annurev.publhealth.031308.100143. doi:10.1146/annurev.publhealth.031308.100143.

Tchounwou, P.B., Yedjou, C.G., Patlolla, A.K., Sutton, D.J., 2012. Heavy metal toxicity and the environment. EXS. 1023294X. 101, 133–164. doi:10.1007/978-3-7643-8340-4_6.

Thomas, D.J., Bradham, K., 2016. Role of complex organic arsenicals in food in aggregate exposure to arsenic. J. Environ. Sci. (China). 18787320. 49, 86–96. Available from: http://www.journals.elsevier.com/journal-of-environmental-sciences/. doi:10.1016/j.jes.2016.06.005.

Turnlund, J.R., Jacob, R.A., Keen, C.L., Strain, J.J., Kelley, D.S., Domek, J.M., Keyes, W.R., Ensunsa, J.L., Lykkesfeldt, J., Coulter, J., 2004. Long-term high copper intake: effects on indexes of copper status, antioxidant status, and immune function in young men. Am. J. Clin. Nutr. 00029165. 79 (6), 1037–1044. Available from: http://www.ajcn.org/contents-by-date.2005.shtml. doi:10.1093/ajcn/79.6.1037.

Ullrich, S.M., Tanton, T.W., Abdrashitova, S.A., 2001. Mercury in the aquatic environment: a review of factors affecting methylation. Crit. Rev. Environ. Sci. Technol. 31 (3), 241–293. doi:10.1080/20016491089226.

Vacchi-Suzzi, C., Kruse, D., Harrington, J., Levine, K., Meliker, J.R., 2016. Is urinary cadmium a biomarker of long-term exposure in humans? A review. Curr. Environ. Health Rep. 21965412. 3 (4), 450–458. Available from: http://link.springer.com/journal/40572. doi:10.1007/s40572-016-0107-y.

Vahter, M., 2002. Mechanisms of arsenic biotransformation. Toxicology. 0300483X. 181-182, 211–217. doi:10.1016/s0300-483x(02)00285-8.

Valavanidis, A., Vlachogianni, T., Fiotakis, C., 2009. 8-Hydroxy-2′-deoxyguanosine (8-OHdG): a critical biomarker of oxidative stress and carcinogenesis. J. Environ. Sci. Health C Environ. Carcinog. Ecotoxicol. Rev. 27 (2), 120–139. doi:10.1080/10590500902885684.

Vouk, V.B., Piver, W.T., 1983. Metallic elements in fossil fuel combustion products: amounts and form of emissions and evaluation of carcinogenicity and mutagenicity. Environ. Health Perspect. 0091-6765. 47, 201–225. doi:10.1289/ehp.8347201.

Wang, S., Mulligan, C.N., 2006. Natural attenuation processes for remediation of arsenic contaminated soils and groundwater. J. Hazard. Mater. 03043894. 138 (3), 459–470. doi:10.1016/j.jhazmat.2006.09.048.

Wang, X., Chen, X., He, W., Zhu, G., Jin, T., Chen, X., 2020. A nomogram to predict cadmium-induced renal tubular dysfunction. Sci. Rep. 10 (1), 1–7. doi:10.1038/S41598-020-67124-0. SUBJMETA=4111,499,692,704;KWRD=NATURAL+HAZARDS,RISK+FACTORS.

Wani, A.L., Ara, A., Usmani, J.A., 2015. Lead toxicity: a review. Interdiscip. Toxicol. 8 (2), 55. doi:10.1515/INTOX-2015-0009.

Welch, B.M., McNell, E.E., Edin, M.L., Ferguson, K.K., 2022. Inflammation and oxidative stress as mediators of the impacts of environmental exposures on human pregnancy: evidence from oxylipins. Pharmacol. Ther. 01637258. 239, 108181. doi:10.1016/j.pharmthera.2022.108181.

Wen, Q., Qi, M., Wu, Y., Ji, W., Zhan, L., 2025. Exosomal miR-2137 from cadmium-treated hepatocytes drives renal ferroptosis via GPX4 suppression and is alleviated by selenium. Front. Cell Dev. Biol. 2296-634X. 13. doi:10.3389/fcell.2025.1585106.

WHO, 1993. Biomarkers and risk assessment: concepts and principles. Environ. Health Criteria 155, 82. http://www.inchem.org/documents/ehc/ehc/ehc155.htm#SectionNumber:1.1.

WHO, 2017. Guidelines for Drinking-water Quality, fourth edition, incorporating the 1st addendum. World Health Organization, Geneva. https://www.who.int/publications/i/item/9789241549950.

Witkowska, D., Słowik, J., Chilicka, K., 2021. Heavy metals and human health: possible exposure pathways and the competition for protein binding sites. Molecules 26 (19), 6060. doi:10.3390/MOLECULES26196060.

Xu, Q., 2024. Understanding genetic susceptibility to heavy metal toxicity: implications for health and risk assessment. J. Heavy Met. Toxicol. Dis. 9 (1), 15. doi:10.21767/2473-6457.24.1.09.

Zhang, X., Yang, L., Li, Y., Li, H., Wang, W., Ye, B., 2012. Impacts of lead/zinc mining and smelting on the environment and human health in China. Environ. Monit. Assess. 0167-6369. 184 (4), 2261–2273. doi:10.1007/s10661-011-2115-6.

Chapter 11

Metal-mediated disruption of cellular homeostasis in the food chain

Jyoti Kumari[a], Mohammad Shadab[b,*], Tenzin Palden[b], Zeba Parveen[b], Shirsha Chakrabarty[b], Gaurav Kaushik[c], Ankur Vashishtha[d], Rohit Kumar Tiwari[b], and Ratnakar Shukla[b]

[a]*Department of Pharmacology, Sharda School of Allied Health Sciences, Sharda University, Gautam Buddha Nagar, Uttar Pradesh, India*

[b]*Department of Clinical Research, Sharda School of Allied Health Sciences, Sharda University, Gautam Buddha Nagar, Uttar Pradesh, India*

[c]*Sharda School of Allied Health Sciences, Sharda University, Gautam Buddha Nagar, Uttar Pradesh, India*

[d]*Department of Medical Laboratory Technology, Sharda School of Allied Health Sciences, Sharda University, Gautam Buddha Nagar, Uttar Pradesh, India*

11.1 Introduction

Heavy metals, such as lead (Pb), cadmium (Cd), mercury (Hg), arsenic (As), and chromium (Cr), are recognized as significant pollutants with widespread toxicity to plants, animals, and humans (Tchounwou et al., 2012; Balali-Mood et al., 2021). Industrialization, urbanization, improper waste disposal, and the burning of fossil fuels have led to severe ecological contamination, increasing the risk of chronic human exposure to these hazardous substances (Järup, 2003). Unlike organic pollutants, heavy metals are nonbiodegradable, persisting indefinitely in ecosystems and bioaccumulating through food chains, thereby posing long-term threats to human health (Nagajyoti et al., 2010). **Metal-induced oxidative stress** refers to a pathological cellular condition that emerges when exposure to certain metals impairs the balance between **reactive oxygen species (ROS)** production and antioxidant **defense capacity** (Valko et al., 2005). This imbalance results in excessive ROS accumulation, leading to oxidative damage of vital biomolecules such as lipids, proteins, and DNA. Consequently, this damage extends from subcellular dysfunction to systemic organ failure,

---

* Shares first equal authorship.

The Metallome in Motion. https://doi.org/10.1016/B978-0-443-44299-5.00009-2

contributing to cardiovascular disease, neurodegeneration, nephrotoxicity, hepatotoxicity, and carcinogenesis (Rehman et al., 2018). Heavy metals contribute to oxidative stress through two main mechanisms, classified by their redox properties. Firstly, redox-active metals like iron (Fe), copper (Cu), and chromium (Cr) directly participate in electron transfer reactions and generate ROS through Fenton or Fenton-like reactions. These reactions produce highly reactive hydroxyl radicals (·OH) that nonselectively attack various cellular components such as lipids, proteins, nucleic acids, and carbohydrates (Jomova and Valko, 2011).

Secondly, the redox-inactive metals, such as cadmium (Cd), mercury (Hg), and lead (Pb), do not undergo redox cycling themselves but instead **weaken antioxidant defense** mechanisms, particularly by binding to thiol groups present in various key cellular enzymes and proteins, resulting in the depletion of cellular **glutathione (GSH) levels** or the inhibition of key antioxidant enzymes like **superoxide dismutase (SOD), catalase, and GSH peroxidase (GPx)**. These metals disrupt mitochondrial electron transport chain function and impede the DNA repair mechanism (Valko et al., 2006). When ROS levels surpass the neutralizing capacity of antioxidants, oxidative stress develops, leading to mitochondrial dysfunction, cellular signaling disturbances, and potentially apoptosis or necrosis (Tchounwou et al., 2012).

National and regional surveys document widespread heavy metal contamination across many states. One national review and monitoring report indicates hundreds of districts with groundwater contamination by arsenic (As), Cd, Cr and Pb (Contamination of heavy metals in (TERI) https://www.teriin.org/sites/default/files/2021-11/heavy-metals-report.pdf?utm_source=chatgpt.com; available from: 2019; least accesses: 6 Dec 2025). Such contamination increases chronic exposure risks for rural populations dependent on groundwater (Gousalya et al., 2023). Agricultural soils in industrial and mining regions show elevated metal concentrations, such as Cd, Pb, As, and Cr, facilitating crop uptake and dietary exposure (Babu et al., 2024). Assessments of polluted sites in India have shown high proportions of contamination with heavy metals such as Cd, Pb, As, and Cr (Kumari and Yadav, 2023) For example, Pure Earth's India fact sheet highlights that 80% of nearly 500 assessed toxic sites had heavy metal contamination, with many linked to battery recycling and improper e-waste recycling processes (Chatham-Stephens et al., 2013). National and subnational studies estimate very large impacts of Pb exposure in India. Recently, it has been reported that approximately 232,500 deaths and 7 million disability-adjusted life years due to Pb exposure are reported annually in India, indicating that India harbors a substantial proportion of the global Pb burden (Brown et al., 2022). Recent biomonitoring and exposure studies from Indian cities and states also report elevated blood lead or other metal levels in children and adult populations in hotspots (Kumar et al., 2025).

11.2 Entry routes of heavy metals in cellular environment

The principal environmental sources of heavy metal contamination include mining activities, the use of contaminated water for irrigation and drinking, industrial discharge, pesticides and fertilizers, automobile emissions, improper electronic waste recycling, and contaminated food supplies (Laoye et al., 2025). Once released, heavy metals persist for longer durations in air, water, and soil due to their nonbiodegradable nature. Subsequently, they enter the food chain through crops and animals. Their biological entry can occur via inhalation, ingestion, or dermal contact (Briffa et al., 2020). Human intestinal absorption, especially among populations dependent on contaminated groundwater and/or agricultural produce, poses a significant risk, particularly for vulnerable populations like children, pregnant women, and industrial workers. The biological entry of most heavy metals into a cell occurs through various mechanisms as stated below.

11.2.1 Specific membrane transporters

Specific membrane transporters refer to a wide array of proteins that facilitate the movement of particular solutes, such as amino acids, sugars, drugs, and ions, across cellular membranes. Based on their functions and substrates, these membrane transporters are categorized as ion transporters, amino acid transporters—including solute carriers (SLC family)—and sugar transporters such as glucose transporters (GLUTs) family (Yuan et al., 2024). These transporters use various mechanisms, such as ion channels that utilize facilitated diffusion, whereas various pumps and carriers use active transport, all of which are indispensable for their role in maintaining cellular homeostasis. Indeed, many heavy metal cations gain cellular entry through transporters that normally carry essential metal ions, such as Fe, Zn, Cu, and Mn.

Fe is indeed a crucial metal required for maintaining vital cellular functions, including oxygen transport, particularly through hemoglobin/myoglobin, energy production during the electron transport chain, Krebs cycle enzymes like aconitase, DNA synthesis/repair, and supporting immune function by acting as a vital cofactor for numerous enzymes (Abbaspour et al., 2014; Obeagu, 2025). Divalent metal transporter 1 (DMT1), encoded by SLC11A2 gene, is primarily involved in transporting Fe^{2+} but is also responsible for transporting Cd^{2++}, Pb^{2+}, and Mn^{2+} in the intestinal epithelium (Menon et al., 2016). Furthermore, it has been reported that increased DMT1 expression influences the uptake of Cd and Pb in the gut and kidney (Menon et al., 2016).

The Zrt/Irt-like protein (ZIP) family represents a diverse group of membrane transport proteins involved in facilitating the cellular movement of Zn, Fe, Mn, and Cd (Martinka et al., 2014) and plays a vital role in nutrient uptake, distribution, and maintaining cellular homeostasis. Structurally, these transporters are characterized by the presence of eight transmembrane domains with a peculiar histidine-rich loop. Intriguingly, members of the ZIP family are localized on different cell membranes and are thus important in facilitating the bidirectional movement of divalent cations, albeit in a coupled manner, such as in exchange with HCO_{3^-} (bicarbonate/s) (Ajeesh Krishna et al., 2020). Within this family, ZIP8 is involved in transporting essential metals like Zn, Fe, and Mn and is also associated with the cytotoxic Cd^{2+} uptake into renal, hepatic, and neuronal cells (Lin et al., 2017). Indeed, experimental knockdown models of ZIP8 have reported reduced Cd^{2+} uptake in in vitro models (Fujishiro and Himeno, 2019).

Similarly, Copper Transporter 1, or CTR1ia is an integral mammalian protein involved in transporting the crucial trace element Cu with high affinity. CTR1 plays key roles in development, Cu homeostasis, and brain function" is presently correct for its meaning (Sharp, 2003; Kim et al., 2008). Recently, it was shown that CTR1 is involved in the uptake and associated cytotoxicity of Cd^{2+} in human cells (Kwok et al., 2020). Intriguingly, cytotoxic platinum-based chemotherapeutics, such as platinum-based drugs, are also reported to mimic the effect of Cu, initiating CTR1 endocytosis and proteolytic cleavage. This process is further associated with the development of acquired resistance toward this class of chemotherapeutics in cancer cells (Peleg et al., 2025).

Moreover, Hg in humans is transported largely through thiol-binding proteins and amino acid transporters. It is reported that mercury strongly binds to the cysteine (–SH) group, which in turn forms complexes that are easily transported through amino acid transporters, such as the sodium-dependent amino acid transporter System B and the L-type amino acid transporter LAT1 which is a sodium-independent, pH-independent obligatory exchange transporter. ATP-binding cassette transporters, particularly multidrug resistance-associated protein 2 and breast cancer resistance protein transporters, are also involved in transporting Hg across human cells (Bernhoft, 2012).

11.2.2 Passive diffusion

Passive diffusion represents an energy-independent cellular process facilitating the movement of metal ions and/or lipophilic or neutral metal complexes across biological membranes through a concentration gradient. However, it is reported that the ability of a metal to diffuse across biological membranes depends on multiple factors, including the electrical charge on the metal, its molecular size, and its lipid solubility (Wu et al., 2005). Indeed, it was recently reported that the absorption of Al in most biological systems commonly takes place through passive diffusion of neutral complexes with low molecular weight, such as $[Al(OH_3)]^\circ$ (Briffa et al., 2020). Some lipophilic metal or organometallic complexes are reported to cross biological membranes by passive diffusion, but this is less prominent in the case of inorganic heavy metals unless they are attached to hydrophobic ligands. Methylated Hg (CH_3Hg) is reported to be more permeable to biological membranes compared to its inorganic ion counterparts and is thus transported through both mechanisms, such as diffusion and transporter-mediated cellular entry.

Brown, M.J., Patel, P., Nash, E., Dikid, T., Blanton, C., Forsyth, J.E., Fontaine, R., Sharma, P., Keith, J., Babu, B., Vaisakh, T.P., Azarudeen, M.J., Riram, B., Shrivastava, A., Pant, P., 2022. Prevalence of elevated blood lead levels and risk factors among children living in Patna, Bihar, India 2020. PLOS Glob. Public Health. 2767-3375. 2 (10), e0000743. doi:10.1371/journal.pgph.0000743.

Chatham-Stephens, K., Caravanos, J., Ericson, B., Sunga-Amparo, J., Susilorini, B., Sharma, P., Landrigan, P.J., Fuller, R., 2013. Burden of disease from toxic waste sites in India, Indonesia, and the Philippines in 2010. Environ. Health Perspect. 15529924. 121 (7), 791–796. Available from: http://ehp.niehs.nih.gov/wp-content/uploads/121/7/ehp.1206127.pdf. doi:10.1289/ehp.1206127.

Che, R., Yuan, Y., Huang, S., Zhang, A., 2014. Mitochondrial dysfunction in the pathophysiology of renal diseases. Am. J. Physiol. Renal Physiol. 1931-857X. 306 (4), F367. doi:10.1152/ajprenal.00571.2013.

Chowdhury, R., Ramond, A., O'Keeffe, L.M., Shahzad, S., Kunutsor, S.K., Muka, T., Gregson, J., Willeit, P., Warnakula, S., Khan, H., Chowdhury, S., Gobin, R., Franco, O.H., Di Angelantonio, E., 2018. Environmental toxic metal contaminants and risk of cardiovascular disease: systematic review and meta-analysis. BMJ. 17561833. 362. Available from: http://www.bmj.com/. doi:10.1136/bmj.k3310.

Clemente-Suárez, V.J., Redondo-Flórez, L., Beltrán-Velasco, A.I., Ramos-Campo, D.J., Belinchón-deMiguel, P., Martinez-Guardado, I., Dalamitros, A.A., Yáñez-Sepúlveda, R., Martín-Rodríguez, A., Tornero-Aguilera, J.F., 2023. Mitochondria and brain disease: a comprehensive review of pathological mechanisms and therapeutic opportunities. Biomedicines. 22279059. 11 (9). Available from: www.mdpi.com/journal/biomedicines. doi:10.3390/biomedicines11092488.

Diawara, M., 2024. Pharmacogenetics of lead toxicity. Med. Res. Arch. 23751916. 13 (1). doi:10.18103/mra.v13i1.6268.

Ferraro, P.M., Costanzi, S., Naticchia, A., Sturniolo, A., Gambaro, G., 2010. Low level exposure to cadmium increases the risk of chronic kidney disease: analysis of the NHANES 1999-2006. BMC Public Health. 14712458. 10. doi:10.1186/1471-2458-10-304.

Flora, G., Gupta, D., Tiwari, A., 2012. Toxicity of lead: a review with recent updates. Interdiscip. Toxicol. 5 (2), 47–58. doi:10.2478/v10102-012-0009-2.

Flora, S.J.S., Mittal, M., Mehta, A., 2008. Heavy metal induced oxidative stress & its possible reversal by chelation therapy. Indian J. Med. Res. 128 (4), 501–523.

Fujishiro, H., Himeno, S., 2019. New insights into the roles of ZIP8, a cadmium and manganese transporter, and its relation to human diseases. Biol. Pharm. Bull. 0918-6158. 42 (7), 1076–1082. doi:10.1248/bpb.b18-00637.

Galvan, D.L., Green, N.H., Danesh, F.R., 2017. The hallmarks of mitochondrial dysfunction in chronic kidney disease. Kidney Int. 92 (5), 1051–1057. doi:10.1016/j.kint.2017.05.034.

Ganz, T., Nemeth, E., 2012. Hepcidin and iron homeostasis. Biochim. Biophys. Acta Mol. Cell Res. 01674889. 1823 (9), 1434–1443. doi:10.1016/j.bbamcr.2012.01.014.

Gousalya, V., Prabu, D., Raj Mohan, M., Dhamodhar, D., Bharathwaj, V.V., Sindhu, R., Sathiyapriya, S., 2023. Effect of fluoride on oral health status among general population residing in high- and low-level fluoride blocks in Erode District, Tamil Nadu, India: a cross-sectional study. J. Pharm. Bioallied Sci. 0976-4879. 15 (Suppl 1), S752. doi:10.4103/jpbs.jpbs_581_22.

Guo, C.Y., Sun, L., Chen, X.P., Zhang, D.S., 2013. Oxidative stress, mitochondrial damage and neurodegenerative diseases. Neural Regen. Res. 18767958. 8 (21), 2003–2014. Available from: http://www.nrronline.org/temp/NeuralRegenRes8212003-2739579_073635.pdf. doi:10.3969/j.issn.1673-5374.2013.21.009.

Hassan, W., Noreen, H., Rehman, S., Kamal, M.A., da Rocha, J.B.T., 2022. Association of oxidative stress with neurological disorders. Curr. Neuropharmacol. 18756190. 20 (6), 1046–1072. Available from: http://www.eurekaselect.com/603/journal/current-neuropharmacology. doi:10.2174/1570159X19666211111141246.

Heidari, S., Mostafaei, S., Razazian, N., Rajati, M., Saeedi, A., Rajati, F., 2022. The effect of lead exposure on IQ test scores in children under 12 years: a systematic review and meta-analysis of case-control studies. Syst. Rev. 11 (1), 1–8. doi:10.1186/s13643-022-01963-y.

Jaeschke, H., Gores, G.J., Cederbaum, A.I., Hinson, J.A., Pessayre, D., Lemasters, J.J., 2002. Mechanisms of hepatotoxicity. Toxicol. Sci. 10966080. 65 (2), 166–176. doi:10.1093/toxsci/65.2.166.

Järup, L., 2003. Hazards of heavy metal contamination. Br. Med. Bull. 1471-8391. 68 (1), 167–182. doi:10.1093/bmb/ldg032.

John, W.A., Lückel, B., Matschiavelli, N., Hübner, R., Matschi, S., Hoehenwarter, W., Sachs, S., 2022. Endocytosis is a significant contributor to uranium(VI) uptake in tobacco (Nicotiana tabacum) BY-2 cells in phosphate-deficient culture. Sci. Total Environ. 00489697. 823, 153700. doi:10.1016/j.scitotenv.2022.153700.

Jomova, K., Alomar, S.Y., Nepovimova, E., Kuca, K., Valko, M., 2025. Heavy metals: toxicity and human health effects. Arch. Toxicol. 14320738. 99 (1), 153–209. Available from: https://www.springer.com/journal/204. doi:10.1007/s00204-024-03903-2.

Jomova, K., Valko, M., 2011. Advances in metal-induced oxidative stress and human disease. Toxicology. 0300483X. 283 (2–3), 65–87. doi:10.1016/j.tox.2011.03.001.

Kalas, M.A., Chavez, L., Leon, M., Taweesedt, P.T., Surani, S., 2021. Abnormal liver enzymes: a review for clinicians. World J. Hepatol. 19485182. 13 (11), 1688–1698. Available from: http://www.wjgnet.com/1948-5182/index.htm. doi:10.4254/wjh.v13.i11.1688.

Kim, B.-E., Nevitt, T., Thiele, D.J., 2008. Mechanisms for copper acquisition, distribution and regulation. Nat. Chem. Biol. 4 (3), 176–185. doi:10.1038/nchembio.72.

Kumar, D., Awasthi, S., Mahdi, A.A., Singh, S., Pandey, A.K., Agarwal, G.G., Anish, T.S., A.R, S., Kar, S., Nair, S., Mathew, J.L., Bhat, M.A., Mahanta, B.N., Singh, K., Singh, C.M., 2025. Assessment of blood lead level of school children in 10 cities of India: a cross-sectional study. Indian J. Pediatr. 09737693. 92 (2), 131–137. Available from: https://www.springer.com/journal/12098. doi:10.1007/s12098-023-04864-7.

Kumari, H., Yadav, S., 2023. A comparative study on metal pollution from surface dust of informal and formal e-waste recycling sectors in national capital region of New Delhi and associated risk assessment. Sci. Total Environ. 00489697. 904, 166791. doi:10.1016/j.scitotenv.2023.166791.

Kwok, M.L., Li, Z.P., Law, T.Y.S., Chan, K.M., 2020. Promotion of cadmium uptake and cadmium-induced toxicity by the copper transporter CTR1 in HepG2 and ZFL cells. Toxicol. Rep. 22147500. 7, 1564–1570. Available from: http://www.journals.elsevier.com/toxicology-reports/. doi:10.1016/j.toxrep.2020.11.005.

Laoye, B., Olagbemide, P., Ogunnusi, T., Akpor, O., 2025. Heavy metal contamination: sources, health impacts, and sustainable mitigation strategies with insights from Nigerian case studies. F1000Research. 2046-1402. 14, 134. doi:10.12688/f1000research.160148.4.

Lin, W., Vann, D.R., Doulias, P.T., Wang, T., Landesberg, G., Li, X., Ricciotti, E., Scalia, R., He, M., Hand, N.J., Rader, D.J., 2017. Hepatic metal ion transporter ZIP8 regulates manganese homeostasis and manganese-dependent enzyme activity. J. Clin. Invest. 15588238. 127 (6), 2407–2417. Available from: http://www.jci.org/articles/view/90896/version/2/pdf/render. doi:10.1172/JCI90896.

Liu, Y., 2011. Cellular and molecular mechanisms of renal fibrosis. Nat. Rev. Nephrol. 1759-5061. 7 (12), 684–696. doi:10.1038/nrneph.2011.149.

Martinka, M., Vaculík, M., Lux, A., 2014. Plant cell responses to cadmium and zinc. In: Nick, P., Opatrny, Z. (Eds.), Applied Plant Cell Biology: Cellular Tools and Approaches for Plant Biotechnology. Springer, pp. 209–246. doi:10.1007/978-3-642-41787-0_7.

Menon, A.V., Chang, J., Kim, J., 2016. Mechanisms of divalent metal toxicity in affective disorders. Toxicology 339, 58–72. doi:10.1016/j.tox.2015.11.001.

Nagajyoti, P.C., Lee, K.D., Sreekanth, T.V.M., 2010. Heavy metals, occurrence and toxicity for plants: a review. Environ. Chem. Lett. 8 (3), 199–216. doi:10.1007/s10311-010-0297-8.

Nemeth, E., Ganz, T., 2021. Hepcidin-ferroportin interaction controls systemic iron homeostasis. Int. J. Mol. Sci. 1422-0067. 22 (12), 6493. doi:10.3390/ijms22126493.

Nordberg, M., Nordberg, G.F., 2022. Metallothionein and cadmium toxicology—historical review and commentary. Biomolecules. 2218-273X. 12 (3), 360. doi:10.3390/biom12030360.

Obeagu, E.I., 2025. Iron homeostasis and health: understanding its role beyond blood health—a narrative review. Ann. Med. Surg. 2049-0801. 87 (6), 3362–3371. doi:10.1097/ms9.0000000000003100.

Pamphlett, R., Doble, P.A., Bishop, D.P., 2021. The prevalence of inorganic mercury in human kidneys suggests a role for toxic metals in essential hypertension. Toxics 9 (3), 67. doi:10.3390/toxics9030067.

Pan, Z., Gong, T., Liang, P., 2024. Heavy metal exposure and cardiovascular disease. Circ. Res. 134 (9), 1160–1178. doi:10.1161/CIRCRESAHA.123.323617.

Peleg, S., Hofmann, L., Ruthstein, S., 2025. Human CTR1 through the ages: milestones and emerging roles in disease and therapy. Biomolecules 15 (12), 1739. doi:10.3390/biom15121739.

Rehman, K., Fatima, F., Waheed, I., Akash, M.S.H., 2018. Prevalence of exposure of heavy metals and their impact on health consequences. J. Cell. Biochem. 10974644. 119 (1), 157–184. Available from: http://onlinelibrary.wiley.com/journal/10.1002/(ISSN)1097-4644. doi:10.1002/jcb.26234.

Sharp, P.A., 2003. Ctr1 and its role in body copper homeostasis. Int. J. Biochem. Cell Biol. 13572725. 35 (3), 288–291. Available from: http://www.elsevier.com/locate/biocel. doi:10.1016/S1357-2725(02)00134-6.

Simpson, P.G., Hopkins, T.E., Haque, R., 1973. Binding of methylmercury chloride to the model peptide, N-acetyl-L-cysteine. A proton magnetic resonance study. J. Phys. Chem. 77 (19), 2282–2285. doi:10.1021/j100638a005.

Soderland, P., Lovekar, S., Weiner, D.E., Brooks, D.R., Kaufman, J.S., 2010. Chronic kidney disease associated with environmental toxins and exposures. Adv. Chronic Kidney Dis. 15485595. 17 (3), 254–264. doi:10.1053/j.ackd.2010.03.011.

Tchounwou, P.B., Yedjou, C.G., Patlolla, A.K., Sutton, D.J., 2012. Heavy metal toxicity and the environment. EXS. 1023294X. 101, 133–164. doi:10.1007/978-3-7643-8340-4_6.

Valko, M., Morris, H., Cronin, M.T.D., 2005. Metals, toxicity and oxidative stress. Curr. Med. Chem. 12 (10), 1161–1208. doi:10.2174/0929867053764635.

Valko, M., Rhodes, C.J., Moncol, J., Izakovic, M., Mazur, M., 2006. Free radicals, metals and antioxidants in oxidative stress-induced cancer. Chem. Biol. Interact. 00092797. 160 (1), 1–40. doi:10.1016/j.cbi.2005.12.009.

Vaziri, N.D., 2008. Mechanisms of lead-induced hypertension and cardiovascular disease. Am. J. Physiol. Heart Circ. Physiol. 15221539. 295 (2), H454. Available from: http://ajpheart.physiology.org/cgi/reprint/295/2/H454. doi:10.1152/ajpheart.00158.2008.

Wei, Z., Su, W., Lou, H., Duan, S., Chen, G., Yao, X., 2018. Trafficking pathway between plasma membrane and mitochondria via clathrin-mediated endocytosis. J. Mol. Cell Biol. 1759-4685. 10 (6), 539–548. doi:10.1093/jmcb/mjy060.

Wu, H., Yang, Y., Jiang, S.J., Chen, L.L., Gao, H.X., Fu, Q.S., Li, F., Ma, B.G., Zhang, H.Y., 2005. DCCP and DICP: construction and analyses of databases for copper- and iron-chelating proteins. Genomics Proteomics Bioinformatics. 16720229. 3 (1), 52–57. Available from: http://www.elsevier.com/wps/find/journaldescription.cws_home/707637/description#description. doi:10.1016/S1672-0229(05)03008-1.

Wu, W.L., Gong, X.X., Qin, Z.H., Wang, Y., 2025. Molecular mechanisms of excitotoxicity and their relevance to the pathogenesis of neurodegenerative diseases—an update. Acta Pharmacol. Sin. 17457254. 46 (12), 3129–3142. Available from: https://www.nature.com/aps/. doi:10.1038/s41401-025-01576-w.

Xie, J., Ouyang, L., Li, J., Yang, S., Li, Q., Li, Y., Yan, L., Fu, Y., Li, Q., Xia, Y., Chen, X., Ziyang, F., Sun, W., Guihua, D., Zhou, F., Feng, C., Fan, G., 2025. Chronic low-level exposure to Pb, Hg, and Cd mixture triggers brain premature aging in rat. Toxicology. 0300483X. 516, 154196. doi:10.1016/j.tox.2025.154196.

Yan, L.J., Allen, D.C., 2021. Cadmium-induced kidney injury: oxidative damage as a unifying mechanism. Biomolecules. 2218273X. 11 (11). Available from: https://www.mdpi.com/2218-273X/11/11/1575/pdf. doi:10.3390/biom11111575.

Yin, Z., Jiang, H., Syversen, T., Rocha, J.B.T., Farina, M., Aschner, M., 2008. The methylmercury-L-cysteine conjugate is a substrate for the L-type large neutral amino acid transporter. J. Neurochem. 14714159. 107 (4), 1083–1090. Available from: www.blackwellpublishing.com/journals/JNC. doi:10.1111/j.1471-4159.2008.05683.x.

Yuan, D., Wu, X., Jiang, X., Gong, B., Gao, H., 2024. Types of membrane transporters and the mechanisms of interaction between them and reactive oxygen species in plants. Antioxidants. 2076-3921. 13 (2), 221. doi:10.3390/antiox13020221.

Zahoor, S.M., Ishaq, S., Ahmed, T., 2024. Neurotoxic effects of metals on blood brain barrier impairment and possible therapeutic approaches. Vitam. Horm. 126, 1–24. doi:10.1016/bs.vh.2024.04.003.

Zorov, D.B., Juhaszova, M., Sollott, S.J., 2014. Mitochondrial reactive oxygen species (ROS) and ROS-induced ROS release. Physiol. Rev. 94 (3), 909–950. doi:10.1152/physrev.00026.2013.

Chapter 12

Metals in agricultural systems: Uptake, translocation, and accumulation

Tamer Ibrahim Abdel-Wahab[a], **Sherif Ibrahim Abdel-Wahab**[a], **and Eman Ibrahim Abdel-Wahab**[b]
[a]*Crop Intensification Research Department, Field Crops Research Institute, Agricultural Research Center (ARC), Giza, Egypt*
[b]*Food Legumes Research Department, Field Crops Research Institute, Agricultural Research Center (ARC), Giza, Egypt*

12.1 Introduction

The main factors contributing to heavy metal pollution are typically attributed to the fast pace of urbanization, changes in land use, and industrialization, particularly in developing nations (Wu et al., 2011). In agricultural systems, plants can absorb metals through their roots and transport them to other parts of the plant, including edible parts. Excessive metal accumulation in crops can pose a health risk if consumed in large quantities (Rai et al., 2019). The percentages of nickel (Ni) and cadmium (Cd) in Egyptian clay soil varied from 0.02% to 0.05% and 0.05% to 0.1%, respectively (Williams, 2019). This emphasizes how crucial it is to take heavy element content into account when assessing the effectiveness of land use in various locations. Consuming crops with high levels of metal accumulation poses a serious risk to human health (Angon et al., 2024). It can lead to neurological conditions like delayed brain development and decreased IQ, especially in children (Heng et al., 2022). In addition, it can cause cardiovascular disorders, cancer, renal failure, and weaken the immune system (Alissa and Ferns, 2011). Intercropping can help reduce heavy metal levels in soil by utilizing plants that can absorb and accumulate these metals, a process known as phytoremediation (Wang et al., 2024). Phytoremediation, as described by Berti and Cunningham (2000), is a plant-based technique that involves using plants to extract and eliminate elemental pollutants from soil or reduce their bioavailability. This practice enhances soil quality and reduces the risk of heavy

The Metallome in Motion. https://doi.org/10.1016/B978-0-443-44299-5.00010-9

metal contamination in crops grown in the same area (Liu et al., 2025). These metals are absorbed and accumulated in the roots and shoots of soybeans (*Glycine max* (L.) Merrill), which can aid in phytoremediation efforts (Yan et al., 2020). Rhizobia, soil bacteria that fix nitrogen (N), can form a symbiotic relationship with legumes. The host plant and its microsymbiont communicate to start the legume-rhizobial symbiosis (Oldroyd, 2013). By binding to heavy metals and preventing their absorption by the plant, rhizobia lower heavy metal levels (Aryal, 2024). However, some soybean cultivars have the potential to decrease the risk of heavy metal contamination by absorbing and storing metals in their roots, stems, and leaves (Zhi et al., 2020). On the other hand, the ability of maize (*Zea mays* L.) to absorb and store metals in its roots, stems, and leaves may help reduce the risk of heavy metal contamination (Elik and Gül, 2025). Furthermore, nematodes can concentrate heavy metals in their tissues at levels significantly higher than those in their surroundings because of a process known as bioaccumulation (Danovaro et al., 2023). Nematodes have been utilized as bioindicators of soil quality for over 20 years years. They have demonstrated strong potential for evaluating the effects of heavy metal pollution on soil (Chauvin et al., 2020).

Research on intercropping soybean with maize has demonstrated positive outcomes, including higher yields and improved resource utilization efficiency (Galal and Abd El-Rasool, 1962; Galal et al., 1979, 1983; Shafshak et al., 1997; Metwally et al., 2009, 2012; Abdel-Galil et al., 2014a, 2014b, 2014c; El-Shamy et al., 2015; Abdel-Wahab and Abdel-Rahman, 2016; Metwally et al., 2018; Abdel-Wahab et al., 2019a, 2019b, 2019c; Metwally et al., 2019a, 2019b; Abdel-Wahab and Abdel-Wahab, 2020a, 2020b; Metwally et al., 2021a, 2021b; Abdel-Wahab et al., 2024a; Taha and Abdel-Wahab, 2024; Metwally et al., 2024; Abdel-Galil et al., 2025a, 2025b; Abdel-Wahab et al., 2025a, 2025b, 2025c, 2025d). By recognizing a synergistic effect on crop production, Land Equivalent Ratio (LER) synergy can serve as a new tool for sustainable farming, even if LER is defined as the ratio of the area needed for sole cropping to that for intercropping at the same management level to achieve an identical yield. This collaboration has the potential to enhance overall agricultural productivity and efficiency, ultimately leading to more environmentally friendly and sustainable farming practices. By understanding and applying LER synergy, farmers can optimize their resources and land use to increase yields while minimizing negative environmental impacts.

Several studies were conducted at different Agricultural Research Stations in various governorates under the Agricultural Research Center (ARC), Egypt. The soil texture was determined to be clay. Furrow irrigation was the predominant irrigation system used in the region. The studies included three soybean varieties (Giza 22, Giza 35, and Giza 111) in different intercropping systems with maize, as well as sole plantings of both crops. The white maize variety T.W.C. 321 was used in the investigation. Figures 12.1–12.9 show schematic diagrams of different intercropping systems of soybean with maize and sole plantings of both crops.

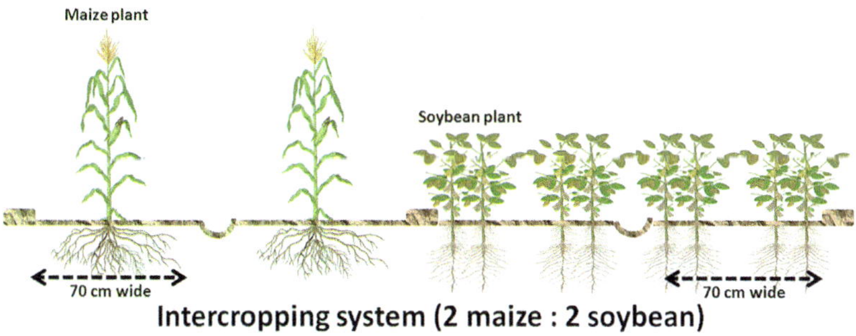

FIG. 12.1 Schematic diagram of intercropping system: 2 maize: 2 soybean.

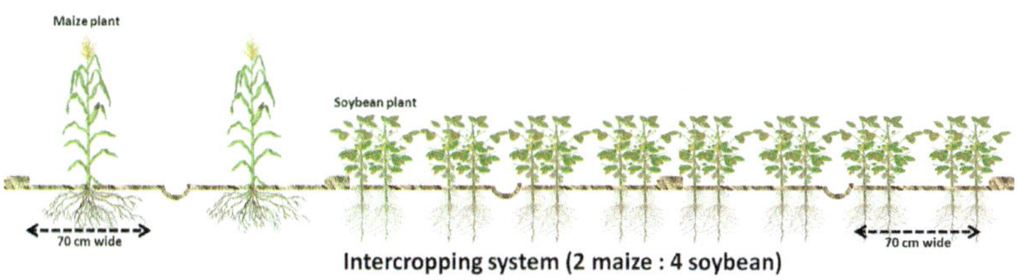

FIG. 12.2 Schematic diagram of intercropping system: 2 maize: 4 soybean.

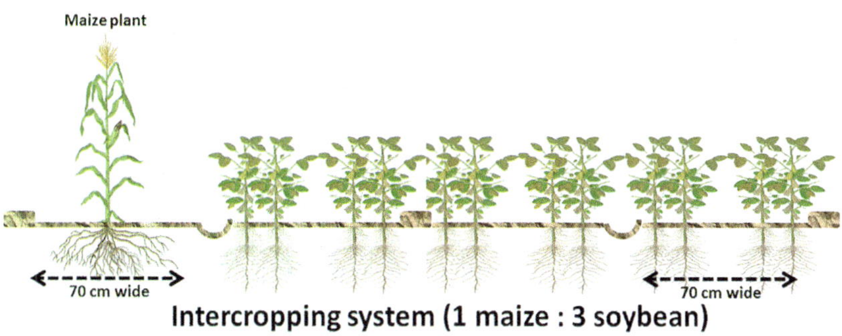

FIG. 12.3 Schematic diagram of intercropping system: 1 maize: 3 soybean.

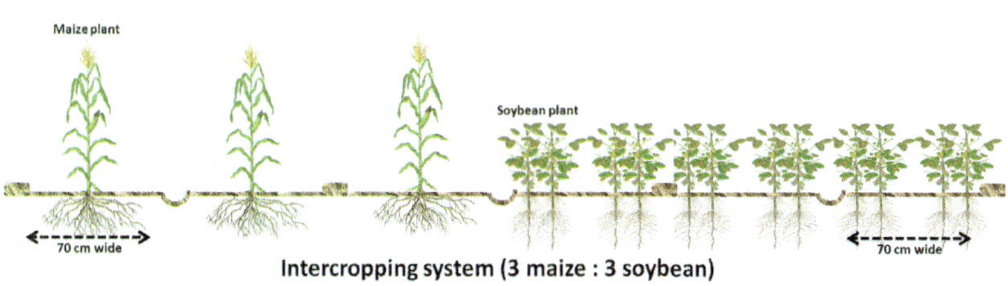

FIG. 12.4 Schematic diagram of intercropping system: 3 maize: 3 soybean.

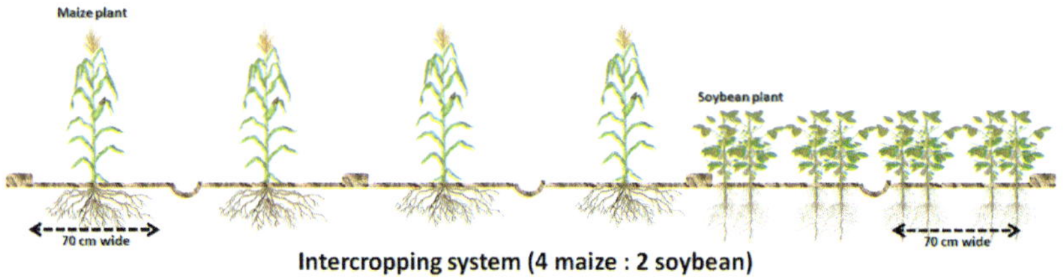

FIG. 12.5 Schematic diagram of intercropping system: 4 maize: 2 soybean.

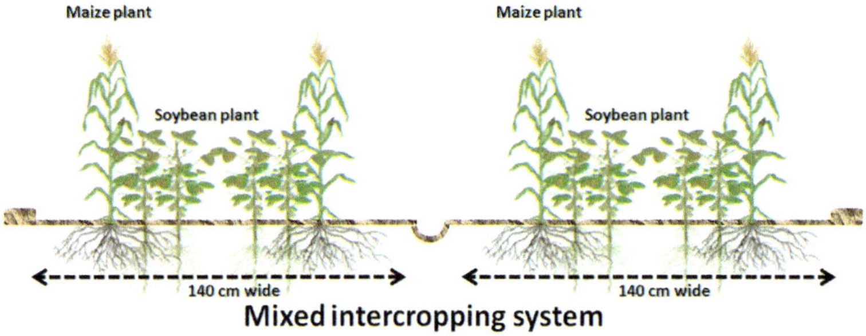

FIG. 12.6 Schematic diagram of mixed intercropping: soybean with maize.

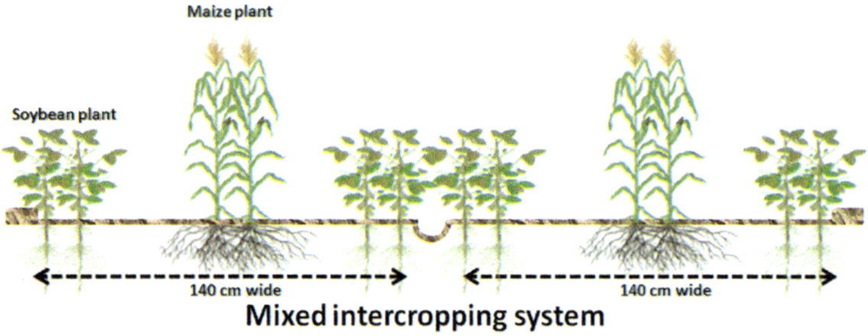

FIG. 12.7 Schematic diagram of mixed intercropping: soybean with maize.

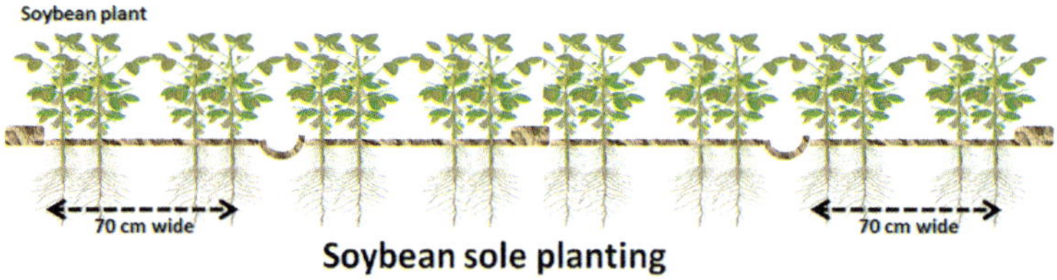

FIG. 12.8 Schematic diagram of soybean sole planting.

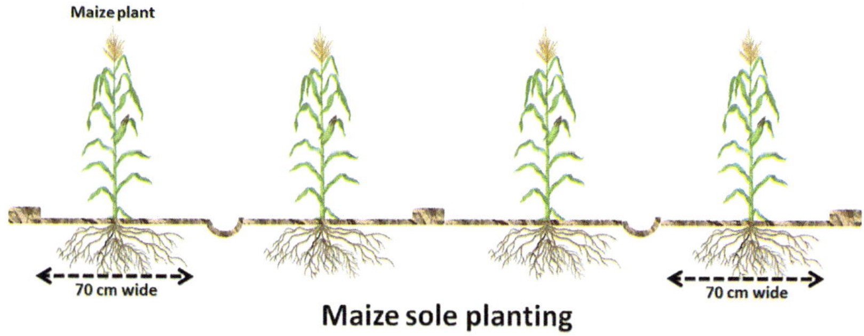

FIG. 12.9 Schematic diagram of maize sole planting.

TABLE 12.1 Origin, pedigree, and maturity group of the tested soybean cultivars.

Cultivar	Origin	Pedigree	Maturity group
Giza 22	Egypt	Giza 21 × 186 k—73	IV
Giza 35	Egypt	Crawford x Celest (early)	III
Giza 111	Egypt	Crawford x Celest (late)	IV

Table 12.1 provides information on the origin, pedigree, and maturity group of the soybean cultivars examined. In both seasons, wheat was the preceding winter crop.

During the two summer seasons, calcium super phosphate (15.5% P_2O_5) was added at a rate of 357 kg per hectare during the soil preparation process. *Bradyrhizobium japonicum* was used to inoculate the soybean seeds, and Arabic gum was used as a sticky substance. Soybean seeds were sown in May, while the maize variety T.W.C. 321 was sown 15 days later. Mineral N fertilizer was provided to maize at a rate of 285.6 kg per hectare as ammonium nitrate (33.5% N) in two equal doses administered before the first and second irrigations, respectively, under intercropping and sole plantings. Additionally, before the first watering under intercropping and sole plantings, mineral N fertilizer was applied at a rate of 35.7 kg per hectare of soybeans as ammonium nitrate (33.5% N). The total number of rhizobia (colony-forming units, or "cfu") in the rhizosphere of maize roots after 30 days from maize planting was determined according to Black, 1965). The incubation conditions were 30°C/2 for three days, the culture medium was yeast extract mannitol agar, and the counting technique was the dilution plate count method. Soil samples for nematode populations were collected from the rhizosphere of soybean plants at a depth of 20 to 30 cm using the method described by Coyne et al. (2007). Nematode populations were collected from the soybean rhizosphere to calculate the total nematode count (cfu/kg soil) after 60 days from planting. All samples were obtained at the General Organization for Agriculture Equalization Fund, ARC, Giza, Egypt. At harvest, soybean seed yield per hectare (t) was calculated by converting the total weight of each plot to tons per hectare (t/ha). Maize grain yield per hectare (t) was calculated by converting the total weight of each plot to tons per hectare (t/ha). LER defines the ratio of area needed under sole cropping to one of intercropping at the same management level to produce an equivalent yield (Mead and Willey, 1980). It is calculated as follows: LER = (Yab/Yaa) + (Yba/Ybb), Where: Yaa = Pure stand yield of crop a (maize), Ybb = Pure stand yield of crop b (soybean), Yab = Intercrop yield of crop a (maize), and Yba = Intercrop yield of crop b (soybean). To compare the means of the traits being studied, all collected data underwent statistical analysis of variance (Gomez and Gomez, 1984) and tests for the least significant differences at a significance level of 5% (Freed, 1991).

12.2 Total count of rhizobia in the rhizosphere of maize roots

Careful selection of soybean cultivars for intercropping with maize is essential to maximize the benefits of rhizobia populations for soil remediation. In all studies, the total count of rhizobia in the rhizosphere of maize roots was higher under intercropping with soybean compared to maize sole planting (Fig. 12.10). Intercropping led to an increase in the total count of rhizobia in the rhizosphere of intercropped maize with the soybean cultivar Giza 22 (7.1×10^5, 8.2×10^5, 7.9×10^5, 6.9×10^5, and 7.5×10^5) compared to maize sole planting (2.4×10^4, 2×10^4, 3.5×10^4, 4.4×10^4, and 2.7×10^4) in 2012, 2016, 2018, 2019, and 2024, respectively. The total count of rhizobia in the rhizosphere of maize roots was higher when intercropped with the soybean cultivar Giza 22 compared to other soybean cultivars. This increase can be attributed to the specific symbiotic relationship between maize and Giza 22, which promotes the growth and colonization of rhizobia in the rhizosphere. Intercropping with the Giza 22 soybean cultivar shows promise in enhancing rhizobia populations in the maize rhizosphere, leading to improved nitrogen fixation and overall plant health. This symbiotic relationship may also positively impact crop yield and soil fertility, making it a potential strategy for efficient soil remediation of heavy metals through enhanced rhizobia populations. Similarly, intercropping led to an increase in the total count of rhizobia in the rhizosphere of intercropped maize with the soybean cultivar Giza 35 (5.5×10^5, 4.9×10^5, and 5.5×10^5) compared to maize sole planting (3.3×10^4, 4.0×10^4, and 2.9×10^4) in 2018, 2019, and 2024, respectively. On the other hand, intercropping led to a decrease in the total count of rhizobia in the rhizosphere of intercropped maize with the soybean cultivar Giza 111 (5.0×10^5, 4.1×10^5, and 4.9×10^5) compared to maize sole planting (3.5×10^4, 3.9×10^4, and 3.3×10^4) in 2012, 2016, and 2024, respectively. The total count of rhizobia in the rhizosphere of maize roots was lower when intercropped with the soybean cultivar Giza 111 due to differences in

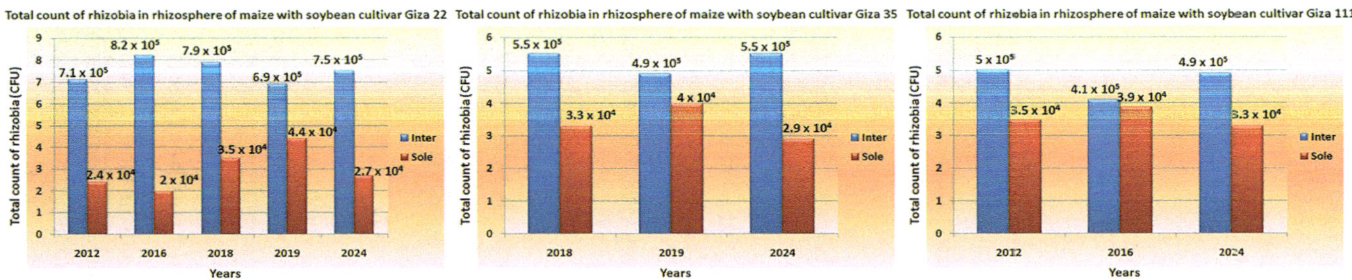

FIG. 12.10 Total count of rhizobia in the rhizosphere of maize roots under intercropping and sole plantings, 2012–2024.

root exudates and compatibility between the two plant species. Lower rhizobia counts in the rhizosphere may result in reduced absorption of soil heavy metals by maize roots, potentially leading to decreased soybean and maize yields. Therefore, considering both the compatibility of plant species and their ability to support beneficial microbial populations is crucial for sustainable agricultural practices.

12.3 Total count of nematodes in the rhizosphere of soybean roots

Plant-plant competition significantly influences the dynamics and composition of nematode populations (Tilman, 1988). The ecological environment created by intercropping (Giza 22 with S.C. 166) likely reduces negative competitive pressure between the intercrops, both above and below ground (Abdel-Galil et al., 2025a). In all studies, the total count of nematodes in the rhizosphere of soybean roots was lower under intercropping with maize as compared to soybean sole planting (Fig. 12.11). Intercropping led to a reduction in the total count of nematodes in the rhizosphere of intercropped soybean cultivar Giza 22 by 13.12%, 21.56%, 17.24%, 4.14%, and 17.21% in 2012, 2016, 2018, 2019, and 2024, respectively, compared to soybean sole planting, with an average decrease of 14.65% over the years. Similarly, intercropping led to a reduction in the total count of nematodes in the rhizosphere of intercropped soybean cultivar Giza 35 by 22.42%, 6.12%, and 15.82% in 2018, 2019, and 2024, respectively, compared to soybean sole planting, with an average decrease of 14.78% over the years. Intercropping soybean cultivar Giza 22 or Giza 35 with maize has been shown to enhance resistance to nematode infection and promote the translocation of photosynthates and metabolites between the intercrops. This practice also contributes to improving soil structure and fertility by diversifying the root systems and nutrient uptake of both crops. Meanwhile, intercropping led to a reduction in the total count of nematodes in the rhizosphere of intercropped soybean cultivar Giza 111 by 22.83%, 9.15%, and 13.33% in 2012, 2016, and 2024, respectively, compared to soybean sole planting, with an average decrease of 15.10% over the years. The growth and development of soybean cultivar Giza 111 under intercropping with maize were negatively impacted by the ability of nematode communities to absorb and store heavy metals in their tissues, which increased their population (Abdel-Galil et al., 2025a).

12.4 Soybean seed yield per hectare (t)

In all studies, the soybean cultivar Giza 22 consistently outperformed other cultivars in terms of seed yield per hectare, whether in intercropping or sole plantings (Fig. 12.10). Intercropping led to a reduction in the seed yield of soybean cultivar Giza 22 by 58.06%, 52.12%, 51.26%, 63.14%, and 51.31% compared to sole planting in 2012, 2016, 2018, 2019, and 2024, respectively, with

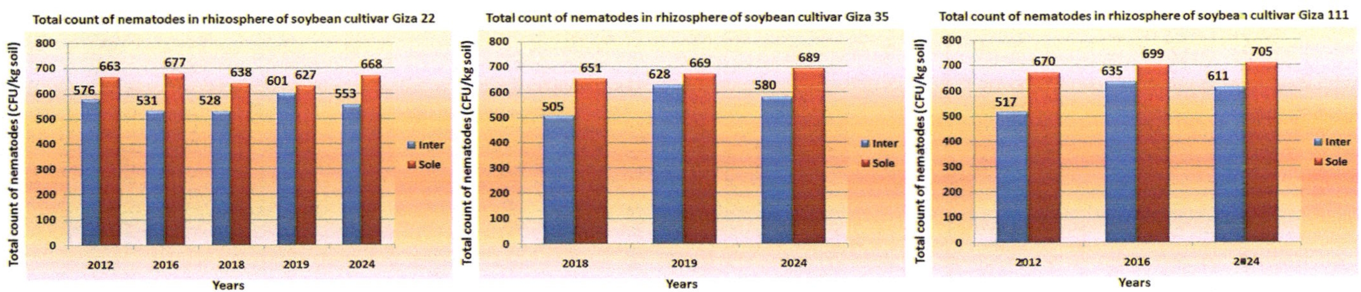

FIG. 12.11 Total count of nematodes in the rhizosphere of the tested soybean roots under intercropping and sole plantings, 2012–2024.

an average decrease of 55.17% over the years. Notably, the soybean cultivar Giza 22 exhibited a lower decrease in seed yield under intercropping conditions compared to the other cultivars, suggesting its ability to benefit from soil heavy metals in growth, metabolism, and physiological processes. The tolerance of soybean cultivars to shading by maize plants and their ability to uptake heavy metals from the soil, particularly evident in soybean cultivar Giza 22, may hold the key to optimizing intercropping strategies for improved yields and environmental sustainability. Further investigation is required to elucidate the specific mechanisms that enable soybean cultivar Giza 22 to maintain higher yields in intercropping scenarios. Meanwhile, soybean cultivar Giza 111 also experienced a decrease in seed yield by 63.77%, 55.14%, and 55.55% in 2012, 2016, and 2024, respectively, compared to soybean sole planting, with an average decrease of 58.15% over the years. Similarly, the seed yield of soybean cultivar Giza 35 decreased by 63.95%, 62.69%, and 59.21% in 2018, 2019, and 2024, respectively, compared to soybean sole planting, with an average decrease of 61.95% over the years. The lower seed yield reduction in Giza 111 compared to Giza 35 may be attributed to genetic differences and varying tolerance to environmental stresses (Abdel-Wahab et al., 2024b, 2025e). Giza 111 appears to have been selectively bred (Abdel-Wahab et al., 2019d) for increased resilience and productivity in challenging conditions, leading to a higher seed yield in comparison to Giza 35. Soybean cultivar Giza 35 may not be ideal for intercropping because it has lower tolerance to shading and a limited ability to absorb heavy metals from the soil. However, intercropping soybean cultivar Giza 35 with maize showed a lower ability to respond to increased soil heavy metal absorption compared to growing soybean cultivar Giza 35 alone. These findings suggest that soybean cultivar Giza 35 is less adaptable for intercropping, underscoring the importance of choosing the appropriate soybean cultivar for successful intercropping systems (Fig. 12.12).

12.5 Maize grain yield per hectare

In all studies, maize plants intercropped with soybean cultivar Giza 22 outperformed maize plants intercropped with the other soybean cultivars in terms of grain yield per hectare in intercropping. Meanwhile, the grain yield of maize plants was consistent in sole planting (Fig. 12.13). The grain yield of maize plants intercropped with soybean cultivar Giza 35 decreased by 6.93%, 22.16%, and 3.89% on average in 2018, 2019, and 2024, respectively, compared to maize sole planting, with an average decrease of 10.99% over the years. This indicates that Giza 35 may possess distinctive traits that enable it to withstand heavy metal stress more effectively and promote the growth of maize plants in intercropping systems. Further research is needed to uncover the specific mechanisms that allow maize plants intercropped with Giza 35 to maintain higher yields in intercropping scenarios. Additionally, investigating the impact of intercropping with Giza 35 on soil health and fertility could contribute to

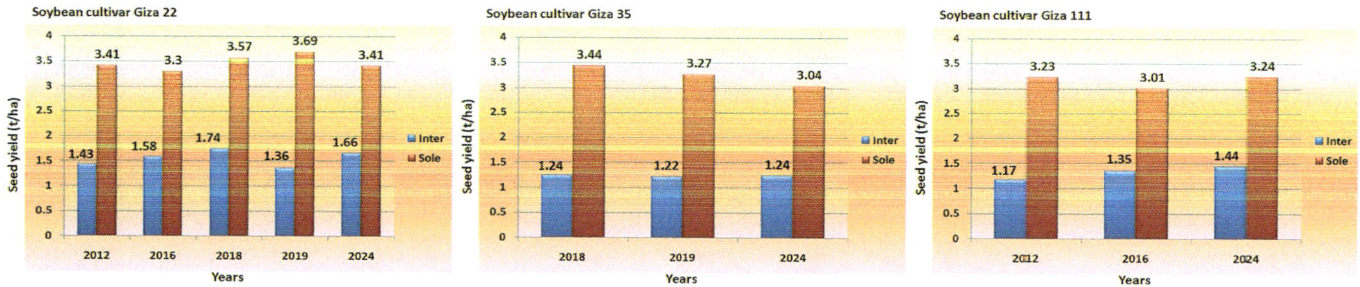

FIG. 12.12 Seed yield of the tested soybean cultivars in intercropping and sole plantings, 2012–2024. *(Source: Metwally, A.A., Shafik, M.M., El-Habbak, K.E., Abdel-Wahab, S.I., 2012. Yield and soybean characters under some intercropping patterns with corn. Soybean Res. 10, 24–42, Abdel-Wahab, T.I., Abdel-Rahman, R.A., 2016. Response of some soybean cultivars to low light intensity under different intercropping patterns with maize. Int. J. Appl. Agric. Sci. 2 (2), 21–31, Metwally, A.A., Safina, S.A., Abdel-Wahab, T.I., Abdel-Wahab, S.I., Hefny, Y.A.A., 2018. Productivity of soybean varieties under intercropping culture with corn in Egypt. Soybean Res. 16 (1&2), 63–77, Abdel-Wahab, T.I., Abdel-Wahab, E.I., Taha, A.M., Adel, M.M., Hussein, H.M., 2019c. Varietal response of soybean to applied irrigation water and insects incidence under different intercropping systems with maize. Res. Crops 20 (Issue Suppl), S1–S25, and Metwally, A.A., Saleh, N.A., Abdel-Wahab, E.I., Hefny, Y.A.A., 2024. Intercropping some soybean genotypes with corn for producing soybean seeds, quality and land equivalent ratios. Asian J. Biol. Sci. 17 (3), 331–350.)*

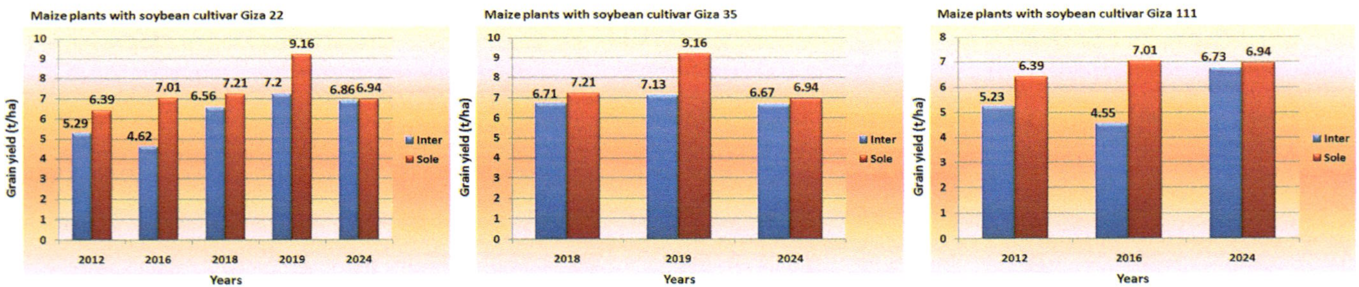

FIG. 12.13 Grain yield of maize plants intercropped with the tested soybean cultivars and sole planting, 2012–2024. *(Source: Metwally, A.A., Shafik, M.M., El-Habbak, K.E., Abdel-Wahab, S.I., 2012. Yield and soybean characters under some intercropping patterns with corn. Soybean Res. 10, 24–42, Abdel-Wahab, T.I., Abdel-Rahman, R.A., 2016. Response of some soybean cultivars to low light intensity under different intercropping patterns with maize. Int. J. Appl. Agric. Sci. 2 (2), 21–31, Metwally, A.A., Safina, S.A., Abdel-Wahab, T.I., Abdel-Wahab, S.I., Hefny, Y.A.A., 2018. Productivity of soybean varieties under intercropping culture with corn in Egypt. Soybean Res. 16 (1&2), 63–77, Abdel-Wahab, T.I., Abdel-Wahab, E.I., Taha, A.M., Adel, M.M., Hussein, H.M., 2019c. Varietal response of soybean to applied irrigation water and insects incidence under different intercropping systems with maize. Res. Crops 20 (Issue Suppl), S1–S25, and Metwally, A.A., Saleh, N.A., Abdel-Wahab, E.I., Hefny, Y.A.A., 2024. Intercropping some soybean genotypes with corn for producing soybean seeds, quality and land equivalent ratios. Asian J. Biol. Sci. 17 (3), 331–350.)*

long-term sustainability in agriculture. Meanwhile, intercropping led to a reduction in the grain yield of maize plants intercropped with soybean cultivar Giza 22 by 17.21%, 34.09%, 9.01%, 21.39%, and 1.15% compared to sole planting in 2012, 2016, 2018, 2019, and 2024, respectively, compared to maize sole planting, with an average decrease of 16.57% over the years. Similarly, maize plants intercropped with soybean cultivar Giza 111 also experienced a decrease in grain yield by 18.15%, 35.09%, and 3.02% on average in 2012, 2016, and 2024, respectively, compared to maize sole planting, with an average decrease of 18.75% over the years. Intercropping soybean cultivars Giza 22 or Giza 111 with maize resulted in lower soil heavy metal absorption into maize tissues, positively affecting soil heavy metal levels due to the efficient heavy metal absorption capabilities of these soybean cultivars.

12.6 Land equivalent ratio

The LER values were obtained by analyzing data from sole plantings of both crops. According to Vandermeer (1989), an LER greater than 1.00 indicates a yield advantage, while an LER less than 1.00 indicates a yield loss. An LER of 1.00 suggests no gain or loss. The LER serves as an additional metric for evaluating intercropping systems. Over the years, intercropping has consistently shown a significant increase in LER, highlighting its potential for sustainable agricultural practices. The collected data aligned well with the LER concept, showing that intercropping soybean cultivar Giza 22 with maize resulted in a higher LER compared to other treatments (Fig. 12.14). Intercropping soybean cultivar Giza 22 with maize led to an increase in LER by 24%, 12%, 39%, 16%, and 46% on average in 2012, 2016, 2018, 2019, and 2024, respectively, compared to sole planting, with an average increase of 27.40% over the years. Similarly, intercropping soybean cultivar Giza 35 with maize led to an increase in LER by 29%, 15%, and 37% on average in 2018, 2019, and 2024, respectively, compared to sole planting, with an average increase of 27.00% over the years. The complementary relationship between soybean cultivars Giza 22 or Giza 35 and maize in resource utilization and growth patterns enhances overall productivity in intercropping systems, resulting in increased LER. These findings indicate that intercropping soybean cultivars Giza 22 or Giza 35 with maize holds promise for optimizing land use efficiency and boosting crop yield. Meanwhile, intercropping soybean cultivar Giza 111 with maize led to an increase in LER by 18%, 8%, and 40% on average in 2012, 2016, and 2024, respectively, compared to sole planting, with an average increase of 22.00% over the years. The intercompetition between soybean cultivar Giza 111 and maize may have negatively impacted the overall productivity of both crops in certain years. Further research is needed to understand the underlying mechanisms of these interactions and optimize intercropping strategies for maximum yield potential.

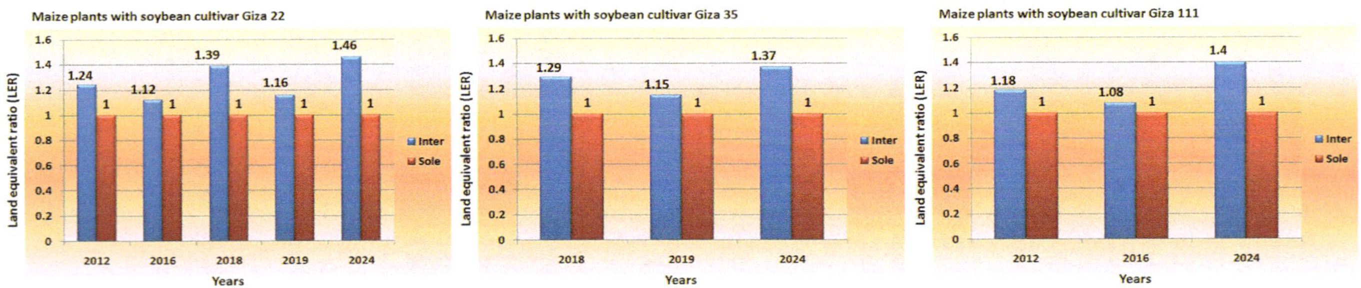

FIG. 12.14 LER of intercropping three soybean cultivars with maize, 2012–2024. *(Source: Metwally, A.A., Shafik, M.M., El-Habbak, K.E., Abdel-Wahab, S.I., 2012. Yield and soybean characters under some intercropping patterns with corn. Soybean Res. 10, 24–42, Abdel-Wahab, T.I., Abdel-Rahman, R.A., 2016. Response of some soybean cultivars to low light intensity under different intercropping patterns with maize. Int. J. Appl. Agric. Sci. 2 (2), 21–31, Metwally, A.A., Safina, S.A., Abdel-Wahab, T.I., Abdel-Wahab, S.I., Hefny, Y.A.A., 2018. Productivity of soybean varieties under intercropping culture with corn in Egypt. Soybean Res. 16 (1&2), 63–77, Abdel-Wahab, T.I., Abdel-Wahab, E.I., Taha, A.M., Adel, M.M., Hussein, H.M., 2019c. Varietal response of soybean to applied irrigation water and insects incidence under different intercropping systems with maize. Res. Crops 20 (Issue Suppl), S1–S25, and Metwally, A.A., Saleh, N.A., Abdel-Wahab, E.I., Hefny, Y.A.A., 2024. Intercropping some soybean genotypes with corn for producing soybean seeds, quality and land equivalent ratios. Asian J. Biol. Sci. 17 (3), 331–350.)*

12.7 $LER_{Synergy}$

$LER_{Synergy}$ demonstrates the power of synergistic effects by combining the strengths of different components in intercropping to achieve better results than using each component alone. This method enhances performance, efficiency, and overall effectiveness in reaching desired outcomes. $LER_{Synergy}$ indicates whether there is a synergistic effect or not. When the combined effect of rhizobia and nematode populations is balanced, this results in increased efficacy or potency in achieving a desired outcome. This can lead to reduced intercompetition between soybean and maize, promoting a more harmonious coexistence and contributing to a sustainable and balanced ecosystem. In the 2012 season, rhizobia populations increased by 2.9×10^9, while nematode populations decreased by 13.12% in the maize and Giza 22 rhizosphere, respectively. In the 2016 season, rhizobia populations increased by 4.1×10^9, while nematode populations decreased by 21.56% in the maize and Giza 22 rhizosphere, respectively. In the 2018 season, rhizobia populations increased by 2.2×10^9, while nematode populations decreased by 17.24% in the maize and Giza 22 rhizosphere, respectively. In the 2019 season, rhizobia populations increased by 1.5×10^9, while nematode populations decreased by 4.14% in the maize and Giza 22 rhizosphere, respectively. In the 2024 season, rhizobia populations increased by 2.7×10^9, while nematode populations decreased by 17.21% in the maize and Giza 22 rhizosphere, respectively. Meanwhile, rhizobia populations increased by 1.6×10^9, while nematode populations decreased by 22.42% in the maize and Giza 35 rhizosphere, respectively, in the 2018 season. In the 2019 season, rhizobia populations increased by 1.2×10^9, while nematode populations decreased by 6.12% in the maize and Giza 35 rhizosphere, respectively. In the 2024 season, rhizobia populations increased by 1.8×10^9, while nematode populations decreased by 15.82% in the maize and Giza 35 rhizosphere, respectively. On the other hand, rhizobia populations increased by 1.4×10^9, while nematode populations decreased by 22.83% in the maize and Giza 111 rhizosphere, respectively, in the 2012 season. In the 2016 season, rhizobia populations increased by 1.0×10^9, while nematode populations decreased by 9.15% in the maize and Giza 111 rhizosphere, respectively. In the 2024 season, rhizobia populations increased by 1.4×10^9, while nematode populations decreased by 13.33% in the maize and Giza 111 rhizosphere, respectively. When rhizobia populations exceed their individual effect, this indicates that the symbiotic relationship between the rhizobia and the intercrops is optimized, leading to increased N fixation and plant growth. When nematode populations do not exceed their individual effect, it means that the nematodes are unable to reach a critical mass where their combined impact becomes significant. This could be due to high competition with rhizobia in the intercrops' rhizosphere. This suggests that when rhizobia and nematode populations are balanced, there is potential for both increased N fixation and plant growth without the negative effects of nematode damage. This delicate balance is crucial for increasing intercrop yield.

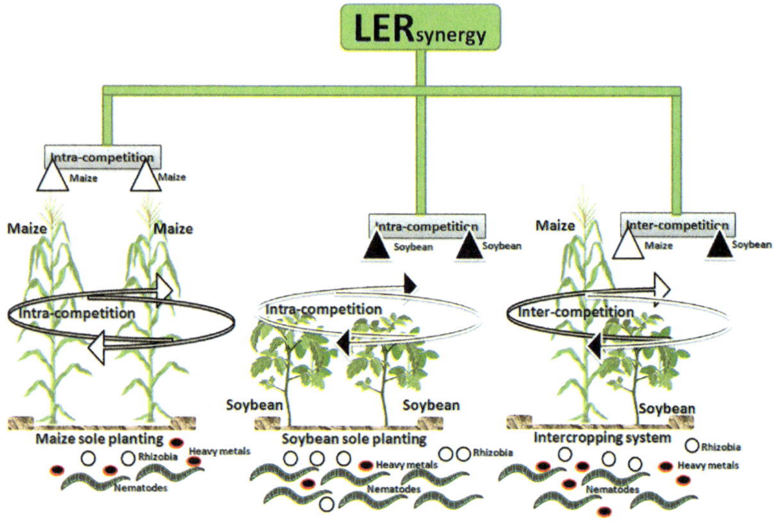

FIG. 12.15 $LER_{Synergy}$ of intercropping soybean with maize and sole plantings of both crops.

The high intercompetition observed between soybean cultivars Giza 22 or Giza 35 and maize resulted in higher $LER_{Synergy}$ when these cultivars were intercropped with maize (Fig. 12.15). This led to increased heavy metal uptake in both species and lower nematode populations in the rhizosphere of soybean roots, indicating improved heavy metal uptake and root health in the intercropped system. These results highlight the potential for a mutually beneficial relationship between soybean cultivars Giza 22 or Giza 35 and maize in agricultural practices, suggesting that intercropping these cultivars with maize can enhance heavy metal uptake efficiency. $LER_{Synergy}$ values less than one, on the other hand, indicate an antagonistic impact, in which the total effect of heavy metals is less than the sum of their individual effects, resulting in a reduction in the effectiveness or potency of reaching a goal. When there is less synergistic impact, intercompetition between Giza 111 and maize or intra-competition within the same species may become more intense as they try to outperform one another. The Giza 111 cultivar may have a trade-off between nitrogen fixation and nematode resistance because its rhizobia were lower and its nematode populations were higher than those of the other cultivars. By storing these heavy metals in nematode tissues, a higher nematode population in the rhizosphere of intercropped Giza 111 inhibited the absorption of heavy metals from the soil to maize and soybean in intercropping systems. Changes in metal dynamics and their distribution depend on nematode populations in the environment, which may be influenced by this factor.

12.8 Conclusion

$LER_{Synergy}$ demonstrates the power of synergistic effects by combining the strengths of different components in intercropping to achieve better results than using each component alone. $LER_{Synergy}$ analysis indicates that the soybean cultivar Giza 111 is not well-suited for intercropping in heavy metal-polluted soils, resulting in unsustainable practices. Sustainable agriculture hinges on choosing the appropriate soybean cultivar for successful intercropping with maize in heavy metal-affected soils.

AI disclosure

During the preparation of this work, the author(s) used ChatGPT to improve the English language. After using this tool/service, the author(s) reviewed and edited the content as needed and take(s) full responsibility for the content of the publication.

References

Abdel-Galil, A.M., Abdel-Wahab, S.I., Abdel-Wahab, T.I., 2014a. Compatibility of some maize and soybean varieties for intercropping under sandy soil conditions. Soybean Res. 12 (special issue), 22–44.

Abdel-Galil, A.M., Abdel-Wahab, S.I., Abdel-Wahab, T.I. 2025b. Intercropping: balancing productivity and environmental health. In: International Scientific Conference on the Axiology of International Climate Change Law, MS Teams, 30 June 2025. Institute for Life, Environment and Climate Science, Poland.

Abdel-Galil, A.M., Abdel-Wahab, S.I., Abdel-Wahab, T.I., 2025a. Role of soil microbes in reducing soybean—parasitic nematodes in soybean cultivars when intercropped with corn cultivars in sandy soil. In: Singh, K.P., Singh, N.K., T, A. (Eds.), Soybean Production Technology. Springer, Singapore, pp. 99–113. (Chapter 6). doi:10.1007/978-981-97-8104-1_6.

Abdel-Galil, A.M., Abdel-Wahab, T.I., Abdel-Wahab, S.I., 2014b. Productivity of four soybean varieties as affected by intercropping and corn planting geometry. Soybean Res. 12 (1), 36–58.

Abdel-Galil, A.M., Abdel-Wahab, T.I., Abdel-Wahab, S.I., 2014c. Maize productivity under intercropping with four soybean varieties and maize planting geometry. Middle East J. Agric. Res. 3 (2), 346–352.

Abdel-Wahab, E.I., Abdel-Wahab, S.I., Abdel-Wahab, T.I., 2025d. Advanced soybean breeding techniques to alleviate biotic and aboitic stresses under intercropping. In: Zohry, A.A., Ouda, S.A. (Eds.), Resilient Agroecosystems: Innovations in Cropping Systems and Climate Change. Springer , Singapore. pp. 95–115 (Chapter 6). doi:10.1007/978-981-96-9630-7_6.

Abdel-Wahab, E.I., Mohamed, M.Kh.A., Baheeg, M.A., Abdel-Rahman, S.F., Naroz, M.H., 2024b. Response of some soybean genotypes to insect infestation under three mineral nitrogen fertilizer rates. Agric. Sci. Dig. 44 (1), 122–138.

Abdel-Wahab, E.I., Naroz, M.H., Abd El-Rahman, S.F., 2019d. Potential of some soybean varieties for resistance to lima bean pod borer (*Etiella zinckenella*) under field conditions. Res. Crops 20 (2), 389–398.

Abdel-Wahab, E.I., Naroz, M.H., Abd El-Rahman, S.F., 2025e. Impact of planting dates on yield and resistance of soybean varieties to soybean stem fly (*Melanagromyza sojae*) in Egypt. Sci. Rep. 15, 32599.

Abdel-Wahab, S.I., Abdel-Wahab, E.I., 2020a. Competitive and facilitative effects of intercropping some soybean varieties with corn under different soybean plant densities. Plant Arch. 20 (2), 1631–1639.

Abdel-Wahab, S.I., Abdel-Wahab, E.I., Taha, A.M., Saied, S.M., Naroz, M.H., 2019b. Evaluation of intercropped soybean cultivars with corn for water consumption and soybean mosaic virus infection under different soybean plant densities. Res. Crops. 20 (Issue Suppl), S26–S46.

Abdel-Wahab, S.I., Abdel-Wahab, T.I., Abdel-Wahab, E.I. , 2025a. Mitigation of shading stress on soybean varieties through intercropping with maize in Egypt. In: Zohry, A.A., Ouda, S.A. (Eds.), Resilient Agroecosystems: Innovations in Cropping Systems and Climate Change. Springer, Singapore, pp. 79–94. (Chapter 5). doi:10.1007/978-981-96-9630-7_5.

Abdel-Wahab, S.I., Abdel-Wahab, T.I., Abdel-Wahab, E.I., 2025b. Innovative cropping systems to maximize the use of available natural resources. In: Zohry, A.A., Ouda, S.A. (Eds.), Resilient Agroecosystems: Innovations in Cropping Systems and Climate Change. Springer, Singapore, pp. 33–53. (Chapter 3). doi:10.1007/978-981-96-9630-7_3.

Abdel-Wahab, T.I., Abdel-Rahman, R.A., 2016. Response of some soybean cultivars to low light intensity under different intercropping patterns with maize. Int. J. Appl. Agric. Sci. 2 (2), 21–31.

Abdel-Wahab, T.I., Abdel-Wahab, E.I., 2020b. Interspecies interactions dynamics between soybean and corn as affected by different soybean varieties. Int. J. Adv. Sci. Technol. 29 (11s), 2864–2876.

Abdel-Wahab, T.I., Abdel-Wahab, E.I., Taha, A.M., Adel, M.M., Hussein, H.M., 2019c. Varietal response of soybean to applied irrigation water and insects incidence under different intercropping systems with maize. Res. Crops. 20 (Issue Suppl), S1–S25.

Abdel-Wahab, T.I., Abdel-Wahab, S.I., Abdel-Wahab, E.I., 2019a. Benefits of intercropping legumes with cereals. Integr. J. Conf. Proc. 1 (2), ICP.000510.2019.

Abdel-Wahab, T.I., Abdel-Wahab, S.I., Abdel-Wahab, E.I., 2024a. Biological engineering and its relationship to nematode resistance. In: Chaudhary, K.K., Meghvansi, M.K., Siddiqui, S. (Eds.), Sustainable Management of Nematodes in Agriculture, vol. 2: Role of Microbes—Assisted Strategies, Sustainability in Plant and Crop Protection. Springer Nature, Switzerland, pp. 383–408 (Chapter 15).

Abdel-Wahab, T.I., Abdel-Wahab, S.I., Abdel-Wahab, E.I., 2025c. Enhancing the efficiency of light interception in soybean and maize intercropping system. In: Zohry, A.A., Ouda, S.A. (Eds.), Resilient Agroecosystems: Innovations in Cropping Systems and Climate Change. Springer, Singapore, pp. 55–77. (Chapter 4). doi:10.1007/978-981-96-9630-7_4.

Alissa, E.M., Ferns, G.A., 2011. Heavy metal poisoning and cardiovascular disease. J. Toxicol. 2011, 870125.

Angon, P.B., Islam, M.S., KC, S., Das, A., Anjum, N., Poudel, A., Suchi, S.A., 2024. Sources, effects and present perspectives of heavy metals contamination: soil, plants and human food chain. Heliyon. 10 (7), e28357.

Aryal, M., 2024. Phytoremediation strategies for mitigating environmental toxicants. Heliyon. 10 (19), e38683.

Berti, W.R., Cunningham, S.D., 2000. Phytostabilization of metals. In: Raskin, I., Ensley, B.D. (Eds.), Phytoremediation of Toxic Metals: Using Plants to Clean-up the Environment. John Wiley & Sons, Inc., New York, NY, pp. 71–88.

Black, C.A., 1965. Methods of soil analysis: Part 2. In: Chemical and Microbiological Properties. American Society of Agronomy, Madison, Wisconsin, USA.

Chauvin, C., Trambolho, M., Hedde, M., Makowski, D., Cérémonie, H., Jimenez, A., Villenave, C., 2020. Soil nematodes as indicators of heavy metal pollution: a meta-analysis. Open J. Soil Sci. 10, 579–601.

Coyne, D.L., Nicol, J.M., Claudius-Cole, B., 2007. Practical plant nematology: a field and laboratory guide. In: SP-IPM Secretariat. International Institute of Tropical, Ibadan.

Danovaro, R., Corinaldesi, C., Illuminati, S., Willis, T.J., Gambi, C., 2023. Bioaccumulation and biomagnification of heavy metals in marine micro-predators. Commun. Biol. 6, 1206.

El-Shamy, M.A., Abdel-Wahab, T.I., Abdel-Wahab, S.I., Ragheb, S.B., 2015. Advantages of intercropping soybean with maize under two maize plant distributions and three mineral nitrogen fertilizer rates. Adv. Biosci. Bioeng. 3 (4), 30–48.

Elik, Ü., Gül, Z., 2025. Accumulation potential of lead and cadmium metals in maize (*Zea mays* L.) and effects on physiological-morphological characteristics. Life. 15 (2), 310.

Freed, R.D., 1991. MSTATC Microcomputer Statistical Program. Michigan State University, East Lansing, Michigan, USA.

Galal Jr, S., Abd El-Rasool, S.F., 1962. Possibilities of intercropping corn and soybean in Egypt. Official Report Tech., Comm. for Oil Crops, Ministry of Agric., Egypt.

Galal Jr, S., Abdalla, M.M.F., Metwally, A.A., 1983. Intensifying land and nutrient equivalent ratios by intercropping corn and soybean in Egypt. Soybean in tropical and subtropical cropping systems. In: Proc. Symp. Tsukubo, Japan, pp. 101–106.

Galal Jr, S., Hindi, L., Abdalla, M.M.F., Metwally, A.A., 1979. Soybean and corn yields under different intercropping patterns. In: World Soybean Research, Conf. II-Raleigh, North Carolina, p. 69.

Gomez, K.A., Gomez, A.A., 1984. Statistical Procedures for Agricultural Research, second ed. John Wiley and Sons, Toronto, ON, Canada.

Heng, Y.Y., Asad, I., Coleman, B., Menard, L., Benki-Nugent, S., Were, F.H., Karr, C.J., McHenry, M.S., 2022. Heavy metals and neurodevelopment of children in low and middle-income countries: a systematic review. PLoS ONE. 17 (3), e0265536.

Liu, C., Safitri, R., Van Leeuwen, S., Ozturk, B., Girzadas, D., Christoff, E., Krampe, C., 2025. Impacts of biodiversity-positive intercropping systems on food quality, safety and the consumer acceptance: a case study of intercropped wheat. J. Agric. Food Res. 21, 101881.

Mead, R., Willey, R.W., 1980. The concept of a "land equivalent ratio" and advantages in yields from intercropping. Exp. Agric. 16, 217–228.

Metwally, A.A., Abdel-Wahab, T.I., Abdel-Wahab, S.I., 2019a. Increasing land and water use efficiencies by intercropping summer legumes with corn in Egypt. Agric. Biol. Res. 35 (2), 6–10.

Metwally, A.A., Safina, S.A., Abdel-Wahab, E.I., Abdel-Wahab, S.I., Abdel-Wahab, T.I., 2021a. Screening thirty soybean genotypes under solid and intercropping plantings in Egypt. J. Crop Sci. Biotechnol. 24, 203–220.

Metwally, A.A., Safina, S.A., Abdel-Wahab, T.I., Abdel-Wahab, S.I., 2019b. Growing of twenty soybean genotypes in solid and intercropping systems with corn. Res. Crops. 20 (Issue Suppl), S47–S57.

Metwally, A.A., Safina, S.A., Abdel-Wahab, T.I., Abdel-Wahab, S.I., Hefny, Y.A.A., 2018. Productivity of soybean varieties under intercropping culture with corn in Egypt. Soybean Res. 16 (1&2), 63–77.

Metwally, A.A., Safina, S.A., Saleh, N.A., 2021b. The productivity of intercropping some soybean varieties with corn under low levels of irrigation water. Plant Cell Biotechnol. Mol. Biol. 22 (69&70), 285–300.

Metwally, A.A., Saleh, N.A., Abdel-Wahab, E.I., Hefny, Y.A.A., 2024. Intercropping some soybean genotypes with corn for producing soybean seeds, quality and land equivalent ratios. Asian J. Biol. Sci. 17 (3), 331–350.

Metwally, A.A., Shafik, M.M., El-Habbak, K.E., Abdel-Wahab, S.I., 2009. Yield and land equivalent ratio of intercropped soybean with maize under different intercropping patterns and high population densities. Egypt. J. Agron. 31 (2), 199–222.

Metwally, A.A., Shafik, M.M., El-Habbak, K.E., Abdel-Wahab, S.I., 2012. Yield and soybean characters under some intercropping patterns with corn. Soybean Res. 10, 24–42.

Oldroyd, G.E., 2013. Speak, friend, and enter: signalling systems that promote beneficial symbiotic associations in plants. Nat. Rev. Microbiol. 11, 252–264.

Rai, P.K., Lee, S.S., Zhang, M., Tsang, Y.F., Kim, K., 2019. Heavy metals in food crops: health risks, fate, mechanisms, and management. Environ. Int. 125, 365–385.

Shafshak, S.E., Shams El-Din, G.M., Hassan, M.Z., Mohamed, M.S.A., 1997. Evaluation of six soybean genotypes under different population densities and two sowing dates. Ann. Agric. Sci. Moshtohor 35 (1), 115–130.

Taha, A.M., Abdel-Wahab, E.I., 2024. Water used by soybean and maize intercropping patterns as affected by different soybean cultivars and plant population. J. Soils Crops. 34 (1), 29–39.

Tilman, D., 1988. Plant Strategies and the Dynamics and Structure of Plant Communities. Princeton University Press, Princeton.

Vandermeer, J.H., 1989. Intercropping: ecological principles and applications. In: Altieri, M.A., Liebman, M. (Eds.), Agroecology: Scientific Basis of Sustainable Agriculture. Cambridge University Press, Cambridge, UK, pp. 145–168.

Wang, S., Liu, C., Yang, G., Ma, S., Shao, D., 2024. Intercropping can accelerate the phytoremediation of Cd-contaminated soil. Sci. Total Environ. 956, 177350.

Williams, M., 2019. Geology and soils. In: The Nile Basin: Quaternary Geology, Geomorphology and Prehistoric Environments. Cambridge University Press. pp. 33–58.

Wu, Y., Zhang, X., Shen, L., 2011. The impact of urbanization policy on land use change: a scenario analysis. Cities. 28 (2), 147–159.

Yan, A., Wang, Y., Tan, S.N., Mohd Yusof, M.L., Ghosh, S., Chen, Z., 2020. Phytoremediation: a promising approach for revegetation of heavy metal-polluted land. Front. Plant Sci. 11, 513099.

Zhi, Y., Sun, T., Zhou, Q., Leng, X., 2020. Screening of safe soybean cultivars for cadmium contaminated fields. Sci. Rep. 10 (1), 1–12.

Chapter 13

Quantum effects of metal nanoparticles on cellular toxicodynamics

Kavita Kushwah[a], Charu Gupta[a], and Mahendra K. Gupta[b]
[a]*School of Studies in Microbiology, Jiwaji University, Gwalior, Madhya Pradesh, India*
[b]*School of Studies in Botany, Jiwaji University, Gwalior, Madhya Pradesh, India*

13.1 Introduction

The term "nanotechnology" was first popularized by Norio Taniguchi in 1974. Nanotechnology is the formulation and management of matter at dimensions ranging from 1 to 100 nm. Nanoparticles (NPs) are considered to be the main components of the nanotechnology field due to their high surface area-to-volume ratio and the higher percentage of atoms and molecules at the boundaries (Shrivastava et al., 2024).

The most common application of NPs is in medical science; therefore, the properties of NPs affect their behavior inside any living organism. The shape and size of NPs impact their flow and targeting in vivo (Moghimi and Hunter, 2001; Patil et al., 2024). Another characteristic of NPs is the charge, their degradation rate, the release of drugs that are loaded within NPs (Dunne et al., 2000), and also specific cell signaling at the target site (Jiang et al., 2008). Any minute changes in the above-mentioned properties are the main source of changes in NP behavior inside living organisms.

Manufacturing metal NPs (MNPs) by physical or chemical methods on a large scale for industrial and household applications, and their extensive use, can lead to adverse consequences for living organisms. In this chapter, we discuss how NPs are absorbed, distributed, metabolized, and exhibit toxic effects within cells.

In this chapter, we focus on only three MNPs: silver oxide, copper oxide, and zinc oxide, to study their quantum effects in the cellular environment (Table 13.1).

The Metallome in Motion. https://doi.org/10.1016/B978-0-443-44299-5.00013-4

TABLE 13.1 Summary of the different characterizations of nanoparticles.

Parameters	Instrument used
Particle size & size distribution	Zetasizer, photon correlation spectroscopy, mercury porosimetry, laser diffractometry
Particle morphology	Scanning electron microscopy (SEM), transmission electron microscopy (TEM), atomic force microscopy (AFM)
Charge determination	Laser droplet anemometry, Zeta potentiometer
Surface hydrophobicity	Water contact angle measurements, rose bangle (dye) binding, hydrophobic interaction chromatography, X-ray photoelectron spectrometry
Chemical analysis of surface	Static secondary ion mass spectrometry
Carrier drug interaction	Differential scanning calorimetry
Nanoparticle dispersion stability	Critical flocculation temperature
Release profile	In vitro release characteristics under physiological and sink conditions
Drug stability	Bioassay of a drug extracted from nanoparticles, chemical analysis of the drug

13.1.1 Features of CuO nanoparticles

CuO NPs are characterized by their small size (1–100 nm) and p-type semiconducting behavior which means that they have an excess of positive charge carriers (Cava, 1990; Tranquada et al., 1995). They also possess a monoclinic crystal structure. CuO NPs have the unique property of improving fluid viscosity and enhancing thermal conductivity (Namburu et al., 2007). They exhibit an extremely high surface area and crystal morphology, which contribute to their antimicrobial activity (Pan et al., 2010).

13.1.2 Features of ZnO NPs

ZnO NPs have a unique combination of properties, including high chemical and thermal stability, strong antimicrobial activity, and tunable optical properties. Moreover, they are biocompatible for biomedical research. They also have a large surface area-to-volume ratio, which, in turn, helps in catalysis and adsorption.

13.1.3 Features of AgO NPs

AgO NPs possess unique properties, most notably their strong antimicrobial activity and optical characteristics. Due to their large surface area-to-volume

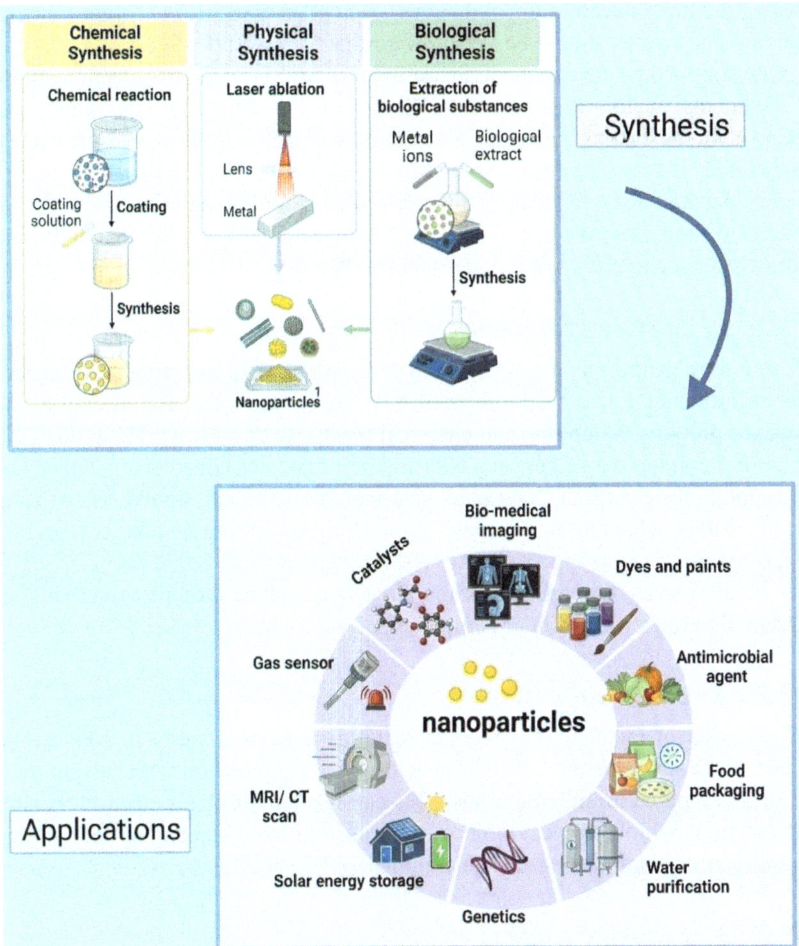

FIG. 13.1 Diagrammatic representation of the synthesis and applications of NPs.

ratio, their unique optical behavior as well as their increased reactivity, this phenomenon is known as localized surface plasmon resonance (Fig. 13.1).

13.2 Fundamental quantum effects of NPs

This chapter will provide an overview of the toxicodynamics of NPs with reference to their core components and mechanisms of toxicity.

13.2.1 Leading causes

The fundamental factors for NPs are chemical composition, dose, and exposure routes, in addition to nanosize, nanosurface, dissolution,quantum effects, nanostructure, concentration and aggregation (Yan et al., 2011). Immaculately, the leading causes should be very low so that they do not adversely affect the organisms or their environment; therefore, it is very essential to know how these fundamental factors influence the NPs' toxicity. In terms of ZnO, CuO, and AgO NPs, the leading causes are size, surface, dissolution, and exposure routes. When the NP sizes are equal to or below the excitation Bohr radius, their energy levels become discrete, altering optical, catalytic, and redox properties as compared to their original size. This effect increases their surface reactivity and ability to generate reactive oxygen species (ROS).

13.2.1.1 Surface characteristics

Size is one of the novel properties of NPs, which acts as a fundamental factor in influencing the toxic effects of NPs. Size is directly proportional to the surface property, solubility, and chemical reactivity of NPs, which, in turn, can modify the interactions between NPs and biomolecules (Zhao et al., 2007). For example, any change in NP radius size may alter the cell uptake rates (Yang et al., 2009), which affects toxicity. As a result, it will not be phagocytized by macrophages.

Smaller size is responsible for more reactive surface sites, promoting higher interaction rates with cellular components.

13.2.1.2 Dissolution

Dissolution of metal ions is another leading cause of toxicity in NPs due to their larger surface area, which allows for greater interaction with solvent molecules compared to bulk materials. This can result in stronger electron transfer interactions with biological molecules because of band gap and surface charge modifications, amplifying toxicodynamics.

13.2.1.3 Exposure routes

Different exposure routes can result in various effects. However, MNPs can enter the body via intratracheal, skin, oral routes, etc. (Yan et al., 2011). Particle deposition can be influenced by diffusion motion, which in turn affects the NP characteristics and physiology. Lesions may form due to the translocation of NPs into the blood or other organs from the respiratory tract (Kwan et al., 2008; Gieser et al., 2005). Meanwhile, some studies have shown that CuO, ZnO, and AgO NPs also cause eosinophilic to severely cytotoxic inflammation, which results in asthma and other allergic problems.

13.2.2 Toxicodynamic of NPs

The quantum effect of NPs is mainly dependent on the interactions between NPs and biomolecules, and the main reasons for its toxicity are protein unfolding (Chatterjee et al., 2010), enzymatic activity loss, and thiol cross-linking.

CuO, ZnO, and AgO NPs diffuse across the membrane easily due to their small size and the presence of positive ions on the surface of the NPs. At the same time, ion channels and transporter proteins allow NPs to pass through the plasma membrane. However, some NPs enter through "endocytosis" membrane bound the NPs to form the vesicles and transport NPs into cells. Cu^{2+}, Zn^{2+}, Ag^{2+} solute from NPs can enter cell by transport or ion/voltage—gated channels (Ho et al., 2010; Colvin, 2003). These ions can stimulate the production of ROS, and a high number of ROS can lead to oxidative stress and damage to cellular components such as DNA, proteins, and lipids. Moreover, these ions have the tendency to form chelates with biomolecules or displace metal ions in specific metalloproteins, leading to functional protein inactivation. Cu^{2+}, Zn^{2+}, Ag^{2+} Ag^{2+} ions released by NPs may increase their localized density and disrupt cellular metal cation homeostasis, resulting in cell toxicity.

13.2.2.1 ZnO NPs

ZnO NPs have significant cellular toxicodynamic effects due to their nanoscale properties, which lead to the interaction with and disruption of biological systems. The following are the mechanisms of toxicity of ZnO NPs (Fig. 13.2).

Cellular uptake and dissolution

ZnO NPs are readily taken up by diverse cell types, including human intestinal, alveolar epithelial, and endothelial cells (Fernández-Bertólez et al., 2024). The generation of large amounts of ROS, such as superoxide (O_2^-) and hydroxyl (OH^-) radicals, occurs due to the excitation of ZnO NPs. These species are responsible for oxidative stress and damage to cellular organelles such as mitochondria, membranes, DNA, and proteins (Figs. 13.3 and 13.4).

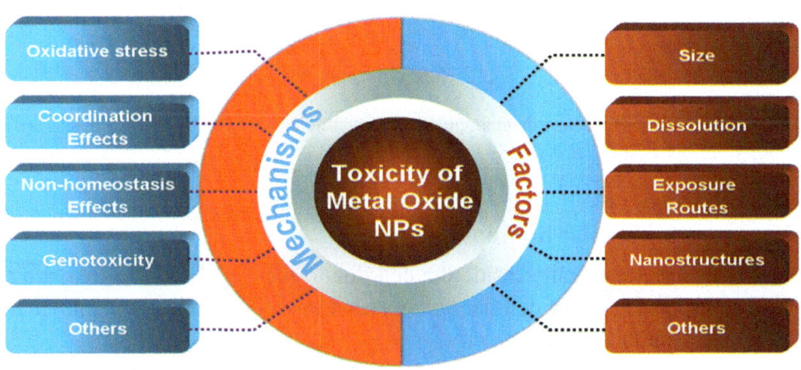

FIG. 13.2 Diagrammatic representation of mechanisms and factors of nanoparticles.

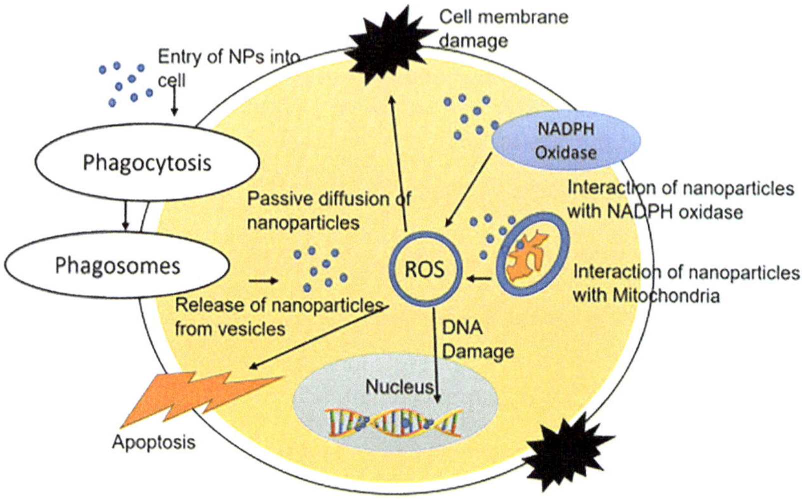

FIG. 13.3 A cellular diagram presents nanoparticle entry pathways leading to reactive oxygen species generation and damage.

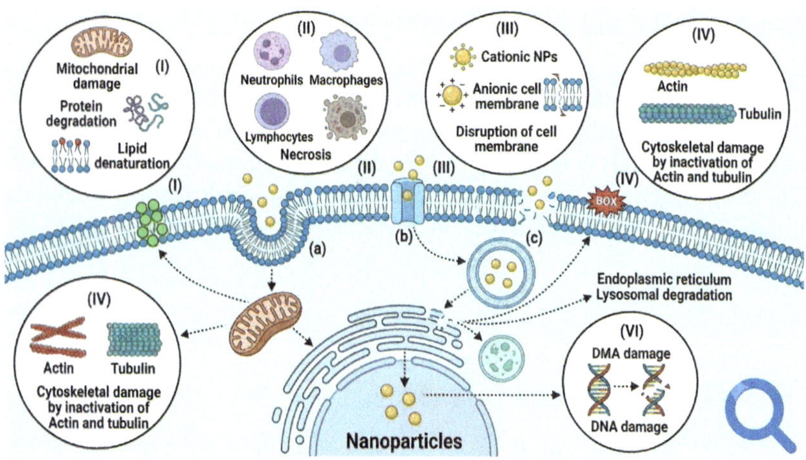

FIG. 13.4 A cellular pathway diagram presents nanoparticle induced damage mechanisms across multiple organelles and systems.

Disruption of cellular homeostasis

ZnO NPs distribute easily inside the cell due to increased surface area, which leads to the disruption of cellular homeostasis, such as signaling and enzymatic pathways, resulting in cytotoxicity.

In addition, impairment of the mitochondrial membrane leads to energy imbalance and, ultimately, apoptosis.

13.2.3 CuO NPs

Because of their unique quantum and nanoscale properties, CuO NPs significantly influence biological interactions and toxicological profiles.

13.2.3.1 Enhanced ROS generation and oxidative stress

The bandgap energy increases due to quantum confinement when the size of CuO NPs decreases. Their redox characteristics and chemical reactivity may be directly impacted by the changed electronic band structures that arise from this (Borgohain et al., 2000). Additional alterations to the band edges of the NPs may be brought about by exposure to biological settings; breakdown in bodily fluids or cell culture conditions can result in a significant rise in bandgap energy (up to 107% has been recorded) (Paruthi et al., 2021).

13.2.3.2 Genotoxicity and cytotoxicity

When ROS are produced, DNA and cellular structures sustain direct oxidative damage, which results in necrosis and apoptosis. Because of heightened quantum effects, the cytotoxicity and genotoxicity are more noticeable than those of larger or bulk CuO (Abudayyak et al., 2020; Karlsson et al., 2009).

13.2.4 Ago NPs

When a NP's size becomes close to the electron's Fermi wavelength, quantum effects occur, resulting in changes to electronic structures, surface plasmon resonance, and quantum confinement. These effects can boost surface reactivity, promote interactions with cellular biomolecules, and increase the generation of ROS in AgO NPs. At the nanoscale, silver oxide (AgO) NPs display unique quantum phenomena that significantly affect how they interact with biological systems. These quantum effects impact AgO NP reactivity, uptake, and subsequent toxicodynamic pathways in cells. They are caused by a high surface-area-to-volume ratio and altered electron configurations.

13.2.4.1 Dose dependency

As the amount of Ag in AgO nanocomposites increases, so does their toxicity. Effects are mild at low concentrations but cause considerable oxidative stress and cytotoxicity in a variety of cell types (both in vitro and in vivo) at higher concentrations (Neto et al., 2024). The majority of cytotoxic reactions, including DNA damage and cell death, are linked to oxidative stress brought on by AgO NP-induced ROS, a process that is closely related to quantum electron transfer mechanisms (Waktole, 2023; Kim et al., 2009).

TABLE 13.2 Quantum effect of nanoparticles on living cells.

Effect category	Quantum nanoparticle impact	Cellular consequences
Cellular uptake	Enhanced, pathway-dependent, quantum size/charge regulated	Accumulation, altered trafficking, possible overload
Intracellular ROS	Increased ROS due to surface states and quantum properties	Oxidative stress, cell damage, or adaptation
Metabolic disturbance	Lipid and energy metabolism alterations	Lipid droplet formation, altered mitochondrial activity
Genetic response	Changes in the expression of death/survival genes	Apoptosis, necrosis, altered proliferation
Nonlinear toxicity	Dose- and size-dependent	Variable toxicity, hormesis at low doses

13.2.4.2 Impacts on mitochondria

AgO NPs' interactions with mitochondria may be influenced by quantum effects, which could alter electron transport, modify energy production, and enhance the creation of ROS (Nunn et al., 2016).

13.2.4.3 Cellular communication

According to new theories in quantum biology, nonclassical cell signaling responses to NPs may be caused by quantum coherence or entanglement, which could have an impact on bystander effects and gene regulation (Matarèse et al., 2023) (Table 13.2).

13.3 Conclusion

It is concluded that NPs possess greater toxicity compared to micro-ones. The dissolution motion of metal ions from metal oxide NPs is the main cause of toxicity. The main toxicodynamics of NPs, such as oxidative stress, coordination effects, and nonhomeostasis effects, were discussed, and this will open up avenues for the applications of NPs in many fields, including biomedicine and catalysis.

Alternative methods of synthesis of NPs, such as the green synthesis of NPs using microorganisms like bacteria and fungi, will reduce toxicity. Controlling NP diameter (Zhang and Monteiro-Riviere, 2009) and surface modification should decrease toxic effects (Abdelhay et al., 2012).

NPs have special physicochemical characteristics that significantly impact cellular toxicodynamics because of quantum effects. By precisely targeting and altering cellular processes, these effects—which depend on size, shape, and surface chemistry—can both increase toxicity and open up new biological applications. It is essential to comprehend these quantum behaviors in order to fully utilize the therapeutic potential of nanomaterials and ensure their safety (Rivolta et al., 2012; Zhang and Monteiro-Riviere, 2009; Gladkovskaya et al., 2015).

Quantum phenomena that are intrinsic to nanomaterials profoundly influence the toxicodynamics of AgO at the cellular level. Critical cellular functions are disrupted, ROS-mediated toxicity is promoted, AgO's biochemical reactivity is increased, and new quantum-based signaling effects that are not entirely explained by conventional theories may be introduced. Comprehending these mechanisms is essential for creating safe nanomaterials and reducing harmful biological effects.

References

Abdelhay, M.H., Gazy, A.A., Shaalan, R.A., Ashour, H.K., 2012. Validated stability-indicating HPLC and HPTLC methods for the determination of ritonavir in bulk powder and in capsules. J. Food Drug Anal. 20 (4), 26.

Abudayyak, M., Guzel, E., Özhan, G., 2020. Cupric oxide nanoparticles induce cellulartoxicity in liver and intestine cell lines. Adv. Pharm. Bull. 10 (2), 213–220. doi:10.34172/apb.2020.025.

Borgohain, K., Singh, J.B., Rao, M.V.R., Shripathi, T., Mahamuni, S., 2000. Quantum size effects in CuO nanoparticles. Phys. Rev. B Condens. Matter 61 (16), 11093–11096. doi:10.1103/physrevb.61.11093.

Bruna, T., Maldonado-Bravo, F., Jara, P., Caro, N., 2021. Silver nanoparticles and their antibacterial applications. Int. J. Mol. Sci. 22 (13), 7202. doi:10.3390/ijms22137202.

Carlson, C., Hussain, S.M., Schrand, A.M., Braydich-Stolle, L.K., Hess, K.L., Jones, R.L., Schlager, J.J., 2008. Unique cellular interaction of silver nanoparticles: size-dependent generation of reactive oxygen species. J. Phys. Chem. B 112 (43), 13608–13619. doi:10.1021/jp712087m.

Cava, R.J., 1990. Structural chemistry and the local charge picture of copper oxidesuperconductors. Science. 247 (4943), 656–662. doi:10.1126/science.247.4943.656.

Chatterjee, T., Chakraborti, S., Joshi, P., Singh, S.P., Gupta, V., Chakrabarti, P., 2010. The effect of zinc oxide nanoparticles on the structure of the periplasmic domain of the Vibrio cholerae ToxR protein. FEBS J. 277 (20), 4184–4194. doi:10.1111/j.1742-4658.2010.07807.x.

Chibber, S., Ansari, S.A., Satar, R., 2013. New vision to CuO, ZnO, and TiO2 nanoparticles: their outcome and effects. J. Nanopart. Res. 15 (4). doi:10.1007/s11051-013-1492-x.

Collins, D., Luxton, T., Kumar, N., Shah, S., Walker, V.K., Shah, V., 2012. Assessing the impact of copper and zinc oxide nanoparticles on soil: a field study. PLoS ONE. 7 (8), e42663. doi:10.1371/journal.pone.0042663.

Colvin, V.L., 2003. The potential environmental impact of engineered nanomaterials. Nat. Biotechnol. 21 (10), 1166–1170. doi:10.1038/nbt875.

Dang, F., Huang, Y., Wang, Y., Zhou, D., Xing, B., 2021. Transfer and toxicity of silver nanoparticles in the food chain. Environ. Sci. Nano 8 (6), 1519–1535. doi:10.1039/d0en01190h.

Das, S., Srivastava, V.C., 2018. An overview of the synthesis of CuO-ZnO nanocomposite for environmental and other applications. Nanotechnol. Rev. 7 (3), 267–282. doi:10.1515/ntrev-2017-0144.

Dunne, M., Corrigan, O., Ramtoola, Z., 2000. Influence of particle size and dissolution conditions on the degradation properties of polylactide-co-glycolide particles. Biomaterials. 21 (16), 1659–1668. doi:10.1016/s0142-9612(00)00040-5.

Fernández-Bertólez, N., Alba-González, A., Touzani, A., Ramos-Pan, L., Méndez, J., Reis, A.T., Quelle-Regaldie, A., Sánchez, L., Folgueira, M., Laffon, B., Valdiglesias, V., 2024. Toxicity of zinc oxide nanoparticles: cellular and behavioural effects. Chemosphere. 363, 142993. doi:10.1016/j.chemosphere.2024.142993.

Gaillet, S., Rouanet, J., 2014. Silver nanoparticles: their potential toxic effects after oral exposure and underlying mechanisms—a review. Food Chem. Toxicol. 77, 58–63. doi:10.1016/j.fct.2014.12.019.

Gieser, H., Wolf, H., Iberl, F., 2005. Comparing arc-free capacitive coupled transmission line pulsing CC-TLP with standard CDM testing and CDM field failures. In: Interessengemeinschaft Electro Static Discharge (ESD-Forum) 2005.

Gladkovskaya, O., Greaney, P., Gun'ko, Y.K., O'Connor, G.M., Meere, M., Rochev, Y., 2015. An experimental and theoretical assessment of quantum dot cytotoxicity. Toxicol. Res. 4 (5), 1409–1415. doi:10.1039/c5tx00149h.

Gunawan, C., Lim, M., Marquis, C.P., Amal, R., 2014. Nanoparticle–protein Corona complexes govern the biological fates and functions of nanoparticles. J. Mater. Chem. B 2 (15), 2060. doi:10.1039/c3tb21526a.

Heim, J., Felder, E., Tahir, M.N., Kaltbeitzel, A., Heinrich, U.R., Brochhausen, C., Mailänder, V., Tremel, W., Brieger, J., 2015. Genotoxic effects of zinc oxide nanoparticles. Nanoscale. 7 (19), 8931–8938. doi:10.1039/c5nr01167a.

Ho, H.H., Swennen, R., Van Damme, A., 2010. Distribution and contamination status of heavy metals in estuarine sediments near Cua Ong Harbor, Ha Long Bay, Vietnam. Geol. Belg.

Ingle, A.P., Duran, N., Rai, M., 2013. Bioactivity, mechanism of action, and cytotoxicity of copper-based nanoparticles: a review. Appl. Microbiol. Biotechnol. 98 (3), 1001–1009. doi:10.1007/s00253-013-5422-8.

Jiang, W., Kim, B.Y.S., Rutka, J.T., Chan, W.C.W., 2008. Nanoparticle-mediated cellular response is size-dependent. Nat. Nanotechnol. 3 (3), 145–150. doi:10.1038/nnano.2008.30.

Karlsson, H.L., Gustafsson, J., Cronholm, P., Möller, L., 2009. Size-dependent toxicity of metal oxide particles—a comparison between nano- and micrometer size. Toxicol. Lett. 188 (2), 112–118. doi:10.1016/j.toxlet.2009.03.014.

Kim, S., Choi, J.E., Choi, J., Chung, K., Park, K., Yi, J., Ryu, D., 2009. Oxidative stress-dependent toxicity of silver nanoparticles in human hepatoma cells. Toxicol. In Vitro. 23 (6), 1076–1084. doi:10.1016/j.tiv.2009.06.001.

Kreyling, W.G., Semmler-Behnke, M., Möller, W., 2006. Health implications of nanoparticles. J. Nanopart. Res. 8 (5), 543–562. doi:10.1007/s11051-005-9068-z.

Kumar, P., Fennell, P., Robins, A., 2010. Comparison of the behaviour of manufactured and other airborne nanoparticles and the consequences for prioritising research and regulation activities. J. Nanopart. Res. 12 (5), 1523–1530. doi:10.1007/s11051-010-9893-6.

Kwan, V.S., John, O.P., Robins, R.W., Kuang, L.L., 2008. Conceptualizing and assessing self-enhancement bias: a componential approach. J. Pers. Soc. Psychol. 94 (6), 1062.

Lamas, B., Breyner, N.M., Houdeau, E., 2020. Impacts of foodborne inorganic nanoparticles on the gut microbiota-immune axis: potential consequences for host health. Part. Fibre Toxicol. 17 (1). doi:10.1186/s12989-020-00349-z.

Li, L., Zhou, D., Peijnenburg, W.J., Van Gestel, C.A., Jin, S., Wang, Y., Wang, P., 2011. Toxicity of zinc oxide nanoparticles in the earthworm, Eisenia fetida and subcellular fractionation of Zn. Environ. Int. 37 (6), 1098–1104. doi:10.1016/j.envint.2011.01.008.

Markiewicz, M., Kumirska, J., Lynch, I., Matzke, M., Köser, J., Bemowsky, S., Docter, D., Stauber, R., Westmeier, D., Stolte, S., 2018. Changing environments and biomolecule coronas: consequences and challenges for the design of environmentally acceptable engineered nanoparticles. Green Chem. 20 (18), 4133–4168. doi:10.1039/c8gc01171k.

Matarèse, B.F.E., Rusin, A., Seymour, C., Mothersill, C., 2023. Quantum biology and the potential role of entanglement and tunneling in non-targeted effects of ionizing radiation: a review and proposed model. Int. J. Mol. Sci. 24 (22), 16464. doi:10.3390/ijms242216464.

Moghimi, S.M., Hunter, C., 2001. Capture of stealth nanoparticles by the body's defences. Crit. Rev. Ther. Drug Carrier Syst. 18 (6), 24. doi:10.1615/critrevtherdrugcarriersyst.v18.i6.30.

Moore, M., 2006. Do nanoparticles present ecotoxicological risks for the health of the aquatic environment? Environ. Int. 32 (8), 967–976. doi:10.1016/j.envint.2006.06.014.

Namburu, P.K., Kulkarni, D.P., Misra, D., Das, D.K., 2007. Viscosity of copper oxidenanoparticles dispersed in ethylene glycol and water mixture. Exp. Therm. Fluid Sci. 32 (2), 397–402. doi:10.1016/j.expthermflusci.2007.05.001.

Neal, A.L., 2008. What can be inferred from bacterium–nanoparticle interactions about the potential consequences of environmental exposure to nanoparticles? Ecotoxicology. 17 (5), 362–371. doi:10.1007/s10646-008-0217-x.

Neto, J.R.D.C., Franco, P.I.R., Braga, Y.L.L., De Oliveira, J.F., Perini, H.F., Albuquerque, L.F.D., Martins, D.B., Helmo, F.R., Andrade, A.A., Miguel, M.P., Celes, M.R.N., Rocha, T.L., Silva, A.C.A., Machado, J.R., Da Silva, M.V., 2024. Toxicity assessment of new AG-ZNO/AGO nanocomposites: an in vitro and in vivo approach. J. Funct. Biomater. 15 (3), 51. doi:10.3390/jfb15030051.

Nunn, A.V., Guy, G.W., Bell, J.D., 2016. The quantum mitochondrion and optimal health. Biochem. Soc. Trans. 44 (4), 1101–1110. doi:10.1042/bst20160096.

Olejnik, M., Kersting, M., Rosenkranz, N., Loza, K., Breisch, M., Rostek, A., Prymak, O., Schürmeyer, L., Westphal, G., Köller, M., Bünger, J., Epple, M., Sengstock, C., 2020. Cell-biological effects of zinc oxide spheres and rods from the nano- to the microscale at sub-toxic levels. Cell Biol. Toxicol. 37 (4), 573–593. doi:10.1007/s10565-020-09571-z.

Palza, H., Galarce, N., Bejarano, J., Beltran, M., Caviedes, P., 2017. Effect of copper nanoparticles on the cell viability of polymer composites. Int. J. Polym. Mater. 66 (9), 462–468. doi:10.1080/00914037.2016.1252343.

Pan, P., Hu, C., Yang, W., Li, Y., Dong, L., Zhu, L., et al., 2010. The direct pyrolysis and catalytic pyrolysis of Nannochloropsis sp. residue for renewable bio-oils. Bioresour. Technol. 101 (12), 4593–4599.

Paruthi, A., Brown, J.M., Panda, E., Gautam, A.R.S., Singh, S., Misra, S.K., 2021. Transformation in band energetics of CuO nanoparticles as a function of solubility and its impact on cellular response. NanoImpact. 22, 100324. doi:10.1016/j.impact.2021.100324.

Patil, V., Suryawanshi, N.S., Bokhad, M.N., Parsodkar, V.J., Narhe, A.S., 2024. Engineered nanomaterials in plant protection: their controlled, site-directed delivery and phytotoxicity. Curr. Bot. 7–24. doi:10.25081/cb.2024.v15.7906.

Pulit-Prociak, J., Banach, M., 2016. Silver nanoparticles—a material of the future … ? Open Chem. 14 (1), 76–91. doi:10.1515/chem-2016-0005.

Rai, M., Yadav, A., Gade, A., 2008. Silver nanoparticles as a new generation of antimicrobials. Biotechnol. Adv. 27 (1), 76–83. doi:10.1016/j.biotechadv.2008.09.002.

Rajput, V., Minkina, T., Sushkova, S., Behal, A., Maksimov, A., Blicharska, E., Ghazaryan, K., Movsesyan, H., Barsova, N., 2019. ZnO and CuO nanoparticles: a threat to soil organisms, plants, and human health. Environ. Geochem. Health 42 (1), 147–158. doi:10.1007/s10653-019-00317-3.

Rivolta, I., Panariti, N., Miserocchi, N., 2012. The effect of nanoparticle uptake on cellular behavior: disrupting or enabling functions? Nanotechnol. Sci. Appl. 87. doi:10.2147/nsa.s25515.

Shrivastava, N., Shrivastava, V., Tomar, R.S., Jyoti, A., 2024. Toxic effects of copper oxide nanoparticles on chlorella vulgaris. Int. J. Environ. Health Eng. 13 (1). doi:10.4103/ijehe.ijehe_3_22.

Silver nanoparticles, n.d. Google Books. Available from: https://books.google.co.in/books?hl=en&lr=&id=_xaaDwAAQBAJ&oi=fnd&pg=PR7&dq=silver+nanoparticles&ots=_gHr06tbgQ&sig=XgusvCV-vvijkzlwo7PwtDnG-N0&redir_esc=y#v=onepage&q=silver%20nanoparticles&f=false.

Simonin, M., Cantarel, A.A.M., Crouzet, A., Gervaix, J., Martins, J.M.F., Richaume, A., 2018. Negative effects of copper oxide nanoparticles on carbon and nitrogen cycle microbial activities in contrasting agricultural soils and in presence of plants. Front. Microbiol. 9. doi:10.3389/fmicb.2018.03102.

Singh, S., 2018. Zinc oxide nanoparticles impacts: cytotoxicity, genotoxicity, developmental toxicity, and neurotoxicity. Toxicol. Mech. Methods 29 (4), 300–311. doi:10.1080/15376516.2018.1553221.

Spence, A.R., Hopkins, G.R., Neuman-Lee, L.A., Smith, G.D.S., Brodie, E.D., French, S.S., 2016. Detrimental effects of zinc oxide nanoparticles on amphibian life stages. J. Exp. Zool. A Ecol. Genet. Physiol. 325 (7), 415–424. doi:10.1002/jez.2026.

Sturikova, H., Krystofova, O., Huska, D., Adam, V., 2018. Zinc, zinc nanoparticles and plants. J. Hazard. Mater. 349, 101–110. doi:10.1016/j.jhazmat.2018.01.040.

Summer, M., Ashraf, R., Ali, S., Bach, H., Noor, S., Noor, Q., Riaz, S., Khan, R.R.M., 2024. Inflammatory response of nanoparticles: mechanisms, consequences, and strategies for mitigation. Chemosphere. 363, 142826. doi:10.1016/j.chemosphere.2024.142826.

Tranquada, J. M., Sternlieb, B.J., Axe, J.D., Nakamura, Y., Uchida, S.I., 1995. Evidence for stripe correlations of spins and holes in copper oxide superconductors. Nature 375 (6532), 561–563.

Upadhyaya, H., 2017. Physiological impact of Zinc nanoparticle on germination of rice (Oryza sativa L) seed. J. Plant Sci. Phytopathol. 1 (2), 062–070. doi:10.29328/journal.jpsp.1001008

Vimercati, L., Cavone, D., Caputi, A., De Maria, L., Tria, M., Prato, E., Ferri, G.M., 2020. Nanoparticles: an experimental study of zinc nanoparticles toxicity on marine crustaceans. General overview on the health implications in humans. Front. Public Health. 8. doi:10.3389/fpubh.2020.00192.

Waktole, G., 2023. Toxicity and molecular mechanisms of actions of silver nanoparticles. J. Biomater. Nanobiotechnol. 14 (03), 53–70. doi:10.4236/jbnb.2023.143005.

Yan, X.J., Xu, J., Gu, Z.H., Pan, C.M., Lu, G., Shen, Y., et al., 2011. Exome sequencing identifies somatic mutations of DNA methyltransferase gene DNMT3A in acute monocytic leukemia. Nat. Genet. 43 (4), 309–315.

Yang, S., Cao, L., Luo, P.G., Lu, F., Wang, X., Wang, H., Meziani, M.J., Liu, Y., Qi, G., Sun, Y., 2009. Carbon dots for optical imaging in vivo. J. Am. Chem. Soc. 131 (32), 11308–11309. doi:10.1021/ja904843x.

Zhang, L.W., Monteiro-Riviere, N.A., 2009. Mechanisms of quantum dot nanoparticle cellular uptake. Toxicol. Sci. 110 (1), 138–155. doi:10.1093/toxsci/kfp087.

Zhao, H.A.O., Wayne, S.J., Glibkowski, B.C., Bravo, J., 2007. The impact of psychological contract breach on work-related outcomes: a meta-analysis. Pers. Psychol. 60 (3), 647–680.

Zheng, H., Mortensen, L., Ravichandran, S., Bentley, K., Delouise, L., 2017. Effect of nanoparticle surface coating on cell toxicity and mitochondria uptake. J. Biomed. Nanotechnol. 13 (2), 155–166. doi:10.1166/jbn.2017.2337.

Zhou, K., Wang, R., Xu, B., Li, Y., 2006. Synthesis, characterization and catalytic propertiesof CuO nanocrystals with various shapes. Nanotechnology. 17 (15), 3939–3943. doi:10.1088/0957-4484/17/15/055.

Further reading

Annangi, B., Rubio, L., Alaraby, M., Bach, J., Marcos, R., Hernández, A., 2015. Acute and long-term in vitro effects of zinc oxide nanoparticles. Arch. Toxicol. 90 (9), 2201–2213. doi:10.1007/s00204-015-1613-7.

Athira, S., Prajitha, N., Mohanan, P., 2018. Interaction of Nanoparticles with Central Nervous System and its Consequences.

Bayade, G., Wu, M.R., Massicotte, R., Deryabin, D.G., Yahia, L., 2021. Biocidal properties of copper nanoparticles. Eng. Biomater. 24 (159). doi:10.34821/eng.biomat.159.2021.2-17.

Bondarenko, O., Juganson, K., Ivask, A., Kasemets, K., Mortimer, M., Kahru, A., 2013. Toxicity of Ag, CuO and ZnO nanoparticles to selected environmentally relevant test organisms and mammalian cells in vitro: a critical review. Arch. Toxicol. 87 (7), 1181–1200. doi:10.1007/s00204-013-1079-4.

Brun, E., Roselli, C.S., 2014. Could nanoparticle Corona characterization help for biological consequence prediction? Cancer Nanotechnol. 5 (1). doi:10.1186/s12645-014-0007-5.

Chapter 14

Risk assessment and modeling of metal transfer in food chains

Akansha and Aditi Rikhari
Department of Nutrition and Dietetics, SSAHS, Sharda University, Greater Noida, India

14.1 Introduction

Toxic metals pose enduring environmental and health challenges due to their persistence, nonbiodegradability, and ability to accumulate in living organisms. Unlike organic pollutants, metals cannot be degraded but instead cycle indefinitely through ecosystems, becoming more concentrated at higher trophic levels (Bjerregaard et al., 2021a, 2021b). Anthropogenic activities—industrial emissions, mining, fossil-fuel combustion, and agricultural inputs—have drastically altered the natural geochemical balance, increasing environmental metal loads and subsequent exposure risks to wildlife and humans (Tchounwou et al., 2012).

Metals are introduced into the environment via atmospheric deposition, wastewater discharges, soil contamination, and aquatic sedimentation. Once introduced, they undergo complex biogeochemical transformations, affecting their bioavailability and toxicity (Ali et al., 2019). Through bioaccumulation and trophic transfer, metals become integrated into food webs, leading to chronic exposure even in populations distant from pollution sources.

Risk assessment and modeling frameworks are vital tools for understanding and predicting these transfer processes. By integrating environmental chemistry, ecology, toxicology, and quantitative modeling, researchers can evaluate the fate and transport of metals, estimate exposure levels, and identify vulnerable populations. These assessments inform environmental policy, public health guidelines, and risk-management strategies (USEPA, 2020; WHO, 2017).

14.2 Key toxic metals in food chains

14.2.1 Lead (Pb)

Lead contamination remains pervasive due to its historical and ongoing industrial use. Pb strongly binds to soil particles, reducing its mobility but increasing exposure for grazing animals and soil-ingesting fauna (Alloway, 2013).

The Metallome in Motion. https://doi.org/10.1016/B978-0-443-44299-5.00012-2

TABLE 14.1 Summary of physicochemical properties, sources, and biological impacts of Pb, Hg, Cd, As, and Cr.

Element	Physicochemical properties	Common sources	Biological impacts
Lead (Pb)	• Atomic number: 82—Soft, malleable, heavy metal—Poor electrical conductor	• Paints and pigments—Batteries—Plumbing materials—Mining and smelting activities	• Neurotoxicity—developmental delays in children—kidney and liver damage
Mercury (Hg)	• Atomic number: 80—Liquid at room temperature—High vapor pressure	• Industrial emissions—Coal combustion—Thermometers—Fish (methylmercury)	• Neurotoxic effects—Impaired motor function—Kidney damage
Cadmium (Cd)	• Atomic number: 48—Soft, bluish-white metal—Corrosion-resistant	• Batteries (Ni–Cd)—Cigarette smoke—Industrial waste—Fertilizers	• Nephrotoxicity—Bone demineralization—Carcinogenic
Arsenic (As)	• Atomic number: 33—Metalloid—Exists in organic and inorganic forms	• Pesticides—Contaminated water—Mining—Wood preservatives	• Skin lesions—Carcinogenic—Cardiovascular and neurotoxic effects
Chromium (Cr)	• Atomic number: 24—Hard, steel-gray metal—Exists mainly as Cr(III) and Cr(VI)	• Stainless steel production—Leather tanning—Dyes and pigments	• Cr(VI) is carcinogenic—Respiratory issues—Skin irritation

In aquatic environments, it accumulates in sediments and transfers through benthic organisms to higher trophic levels (Jarvis et al., 2020). Chronic Pb exposure leads to neurodevelopmental deficits, renal dysfunction, and cardiovascular disease, with children being the most vulnerable (Needleman, 2004). Table 14.1.

14.2.2 Mercury (Hg)

Mercury exists in several forms—elemental, inorganic, and organic—with methylmercury being the most neurotoxic. Microbial methylation in aquatic systems leads to its rapid accumulation in fish, particularly apex predators such as tuna and swordfish (Selin, 2009). Human dietary exposure through seafood consumption is the predominant pathway (Basu et al., 2018). Methylmercury causes neurotoxicity, cognitive impairment, and developmental abnormalities (Grandjean and Landrigan, 2014).

14.2.3 Cadmium (Cd)

Cadmium contamination arises from industrial emissions, mining, and phosphate fertilizers (Satarug et al., 2010). It is readily taken up by plants, particularly cereals and leafy vegetables, resulting in dietary exposure (Clemens and Ma., 2016). Chronic exposure leads to renal dysfunction, osteomalacia, and carcinogenicity (Joint FAO/WHO Expert Committee on Food Additives, 2011). Historical incidents such as Itai-Itai disease exemplify Cd's ecological and human toxicity (Nordberg et al., 2018).

14.2.4 Arsenic (As)

Arsenic occurs naturally but is intensified by anthropogenic activities such as mining and pesticide use (Naujokas et al., 2013). Inorganic forms—arsenite (As^{3+}) and arsenate (As^{5+})—are the most toxic. Flooded rice cultivation enhances arsenic (As) uptake, posing dietary risks (Meharg, Zhao, 2012). Long-term exposure is associated with cancers of the skin, bladder, and lung (IARC, 2012).

14.2.5 Chromium (Cr)

Chromium exists mainly as trivalent [Cr(III)] and hexavalent [Cr(VI)] species. Cr(VI) is highly toxic and carcinogenic, released from industrial activities such as tanning and electroplating (Rahman and Singh, 2019). Exposure leads to oxidative stress, DNA damage, and organ toxicity.

14.2.6 Sources and environmental pathways

Metal pollutants arise from both natural sources (volcanic activity, weathering) and human activities such as mining and combustion (Alloway, 2013). These metals circulate among environmental compartments—soil, water, and air—before entering food chains (Ali et al., 2019). Fig. 14.1.

14.3 Pathways of metal entry into food chains

14.3.1 Soil–plant system dynamics

The soil–plant interface constitutes a major terrestrial pathway for metal entry (Adriano, 2001). Root uptake is influenced by soil pH, organic matter, and redox potential (Clemens et al., 2013). Certain plant species, known as hyperaccumulators, concentrate metals in their tissues and are valuable both for phytoremediation and risk studies (Van der Ent et al., 2013).

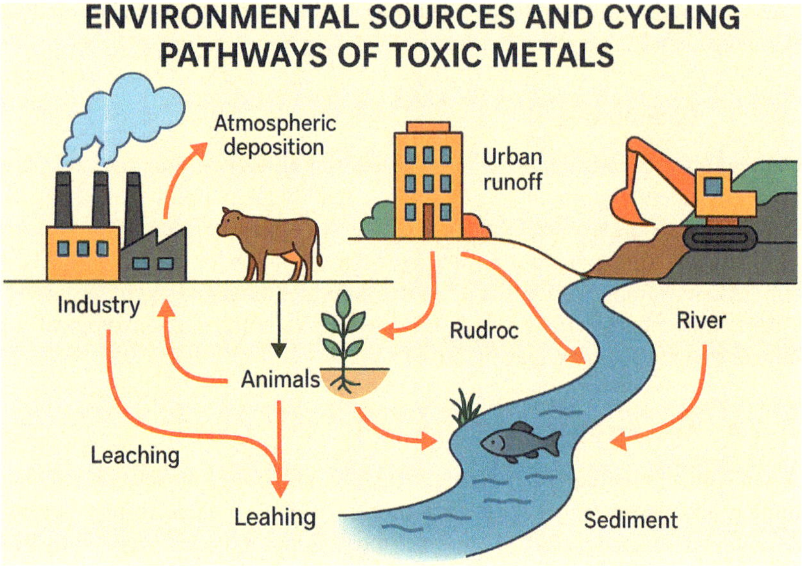

FIG. 14.1 Environmental sources and cycling pathways of toxic metals.

14.3.2 Aquatic uptake via algae and plankton

Aquatic organisms absorb metals either as dissolved ions or via particulates (Wang and Rainbow, 2008). Phytoplankton accumulate metals that are then transferred to zooplankton and fish, leading to significant biomagnification (Basu et al., 2018).

14.3.3 Airborne deposition and foliar absorption

Atmospheric deposition contributes to terrestrial contamination. Metals can deposit onto plant surfaces or penetrate leaves through stomata, particularly near industrial zones (Pacyna and Pacyna, 2001; Lu et al., 2011).

14.3.4 Transfer across trophic levels

Bioaccumulation and biomagnification lead to metal transfer through successive trophic levels (Newman, 2015). Predatory species exhibit the highest concentrations, posing substantial ecological and human health risks (Bjerregaard et al., 2021a).

14.4 Environmental factors influencing metal transfer

14.4.1 Metal speciation and valence states

Speciation determines a metal's toxicity and mobility. For example, Cr(VI) is more toxic than Cr(III); methylmercury is far more bioavailable than inorganic mercury (Sparks, 2003; Basu et al., 2018).

14.4.2 Soil and water chemistry

Soil pH, redox conditions, and organic matter content control metal solubility. Acidic conditions enhance the solubility of Cd and Pb, increasing plant uptake (Adriano, 2001). Similarly, redox-driven microbial methylation governs mercury dynamics in aquatic ecosystems (Selin, 2009).

14.4.3 Bioavailability and mobility

Total metal concentration is often a poor indicator of biological impact. Bioavailability—dictated by complexation, sorption, and mineral association—is a key metric in risk assessment (Luoma and Rainbow, 2008).

14.4.4 Species-specific uptake traits

Organisms differ in their capacity to absorb and retain metals. For example, rice efficiently accumulates As compared to other grains (Meharg and Zhao, 2012), while predatory fish biomagnify Hg more than herbivorous species (Basu et al., 2018). Table 14.2.

14.5 Metrics for quantifying metal transfer

Quantifying how toxic metals move through environmental compartments and biological systems requires standardized metrics that capture absorption, retention, and trophic propagation. These metrics—bioconcentration factor (BCF), bioaccumulation factor (BAF), biomagnification factor (BMF), and trophic transfer factor (TTF)—provide quantitative measures that help researchers assess exposure risks, compare contaminant loads across species, and develop predictive models for ecological and human health assessments. Together, these indices form the foundation for mechanistic and probabilistic approaches to contaminant fate modeling in ecosystems.

14.5.1 Bioconcentration factor

The BCF quantifies the ratio between the concentration of a metal in an organism and its concentration in the surrounding abiotic medium, typically water or sediment.

$$\mathrm{BCF} = \frac{C_{\mathrm{organism}}}{C_{\mathrm{medium}}}$$

BCF reflects **direct uptake** through respiration or surface absorption without considering dietary inputs. For aquatic organisms, a high BCF indicates efficient permeation of metals across gills or epithelial tissues, as well as limited efflux or metabolic detoxification. Metals such as mercury and cadmium often exhibit high BCF values due to their strong affinity for proteins and limited

TABLE 14.2 Factors affecting metal bioavailability and species-specific uptake.

Factor category	Specific factors	How it affects metal bioavailability/ uptake
Environmental chemistry	pH	Low pH increases metal solubility → higher bioavailability
	Redox potential (Eh)	Controls valence state (e.g., As(III) vs. As(V)) → changes mobility and toxicity
	Organic matter	Forms complexes with metals; can increase or decrease uptake depending on the species
	Water hardness (Ca^{2+}, Mg^{2+})	Competes with metals for biological binding sites → lower uptake
	Salinity	Alters metal speciation and affects uptake, especially in aquatic organisms
Soil/sediment properties	Cation exchange capacity	Higher CEC binds more metals → reduces plant/animal uptake
	Clay content	Clays adsorb metals, reducing mobility but increasing long-term persistence
	Sediment grain size	Fine sediments accumulate more metals → higher exposure for benthic species
Biological/ species-specific factors	Feeding strategy	Filter feeders (mussels) accumulate more metals than predators/ herbivores
	Respiratory surface characteristics	High gill surface area → greater uptake (e.g., fish)
	Gut physiology	Differences in digestion, pH, and enzymes alter absorption efficiency
	Metal detoxification ability	Species with high metallothionein levels excrete metals more effectively
	Life stage/size	Juveniles often show higher uptake due to rapid growth and metabolic rate
Metal-specific properties	Chemical form (speciation)	Determines solubility, toxicity, and the ability to cross membranes
	Lipophilicity	Fat-soluble metals/metalloids accumulate more in tissues (e.g., methylmercury)
	Binding affinity	Strong affinity for proteins affects bioaccumulation and organ distribution

Factor category	Specific factors	How it affects metal bioavailability/uptake
Environmental exposure conditions	Temperature	Higher temperature increases metabolic rate → higher uptake
	Dissolved oxygen	Low oxygen changes redox conditions and increases the mobility of some metals.
	Competing ions	Other metals or nutrients (e.g., Zn, Ca) reduce uptake by competition

excretion pathways (Wang et al., 2020). BCF is widely used for screening-level ecological risk assessments and regulatory classification of hazardous substances.

14.5.2 Bioaccumulation factor

The BAF expands upon the BCF by incorporating **all exposure routes**, including water, sediment, suspended particulates, and food.

$$\mathrm{BAF} = \frac{C_{\mathrm{organism}}}{C_{\mathrm{environment\ (all\ routes)}}}$$

BAF provides a more holistic measure of total body burden, especially for species that feed actively and can accumulate metals through their diet. This index is particularly relevant for benthic feeders, such as mollusks and crustaceans, that ingest contaminated sediments (Zhang et al., 2019). High BAF values often reflect long-term retention mechanisms, such as the binding of metals to metallothioneins or incorporation into tissues (e.g., liver, kidney, exoskeleton). BAF is, therefore, essential in long-term exposure assessments and human health risk analysis for seafood consumers.

14.5.3 Biomagnification factor

The BMF evaluates the extent to which metal concentrations increase from one trophic level to the next.

$$\mathrm{BMF} = \frac{\mathrm{C}_{\mathrm{predator}}}{\mathrm{C}_{\mathrm{prey}}}$$

A BMF greater than 1 indicates **biomagnification**, where metals accumulate to higher levels in predators than in their food sources. This phenomenon is characteristic of metals such as methylmercury and certain organometallic complexes that exhibit high assimilation efficiency and slow elimination rates (Bjerregaard et al., 2021a). BMF is particularly useful for assessing risks in apex predators, including humans, who occupy higher trophic positions in aquatic food webs. It is also used to compare biomagnification tendencies across ecosystems and evaluate ecological vulnerability.

14.5.4 Trophic transfer factor

The TTF quantifies the ratio of metal concentration in a predator relative to the prey it consumes:

$$\mathrm{TTF} = \frac{C_{\text{predator}}}{C_{\text{diet}}}$$

Although similar to BMF, TTF is often used in **controlled feeding studies** or field assessments where prey composition is known. TTF accounts for assimilation efficiency (the proportion of ingested metal retained) and dietary habits. TTF helps identify the relative contribution of prey species to metal burdens in predators and is essential for constructing accurate food web models (Ali and Khan, 2019).

14.5.5 Integration of indices in probabilistic models

Modern risk assessment frameworks frequently integrate BCF, BAF, BMF, and TTF into **probabilistic exposure models** that simulate metal transfer across entire ecosystems. Techniques such as Bayesian hierarchical modeling, Markov chain Monte Carlo simulations, and Monte Carlo–based uncertainty analysis capture natural variability in environmental concentrations, feeding rates, metabolism, and trophic structure.

Probabilistic models allow researchers to:

- Estimate contaminant burdens at multiple trophic levels
- Predict long-term accumulation trajectories
- Assess human dietary exposure risks
- Incorporate uncertainty and environmental heterogeneity

Recent work by Sanaei et al. (2021) demonstrates how these indices, when combined with trophic web data, help predict metal transfer patterns across aquatic ecosystems under different contamination scenarios. Such models are increasingly used by regulatory agencies and environmental managers to guide monitoring strategies and inform risk mitigation policies (see Table 14.3).

14.6 Toxicological impacts across the food chain

14.6.1 Sublethal and lethal effects in wildlife

Toxic metals exert a wide spectrum of adverse effects on wildlife, ranging from subtle physiological disturbances to lethal outcomes. Sublethal effects are particularly concerning because they impair key biological functions—such as

TABLE 14.3 Comparative definitions and equations of BCF, BAF, BMF, and TTF.

Metric	Full name	Definition	Equation	Key feature
BCF	Bioconcentration factor	Ratio of chemical concentration in an organism to water (excluding diet)	$BCF = \frac{C_{organism}}{C_{water}}$	No dietary exposure; uptake from water only
BAF	Bioaccumulation factor	Ratio of chemical concentration in an organism to the environment (water + diet)	$BAF = \frac{C_{organism}}{C_{environment}}$	Includes all uptake routes (water + food)
BMF	Biomagnification factor	Ratio of chemical concentration in a predator to its prey	$BMF = \frac{C_{predator}}{C_{prey}}$	Trophic transfer from one level to the next
TTF	Trophic transfer factor	Ratio of concentration between any two trophic levels	$TTF = \frac{C_{consumer}}{C_{diet}}$	Generalized form of BMF across the food web

growth, reproduction, and behavior—even at concentrations below those that cause mortality. These impacts accumulate over time and can destabilize population dynamics and ecological balance.

Birds are highly sensitive to metals like mercury (Hg), lead (Pb), cadmium (Cd), and arsenic (As), with effects often linked to the bioaccumulation of methylmercury through aquatic food webs. Chronic mercury exposure disrupts **avian reproductive success**, reducing hatchability by impairing embryo development and causing shell thinning. Neurobehavioral impairments—such as altered song patterns, compromised flight coordination, and diminished predator avoidance—have been documented even at relatively low exposure levels (Gall et al., 2015). These neurological disturbances reduce survival and mating competitiveness, resulting in long-term population-level consequences.

Fish are similarly vulnerable. Metals such as Cd, Cu, and Hg impair **gill function**, disrupt osmoregulation, reduce feeding efficiency, and alter endocrine pathways. Even sublethal concentrations can cause developmental deformities, diminished growth rates, and decreased reproductive output. In severe cases, acute exposure results in mortality through respiratory failure or systemic toxicity.

Invertebrates, including mollusks, crustaceans, and insects, serve as both ecological indicators and essential trophic links. Metals interfere with molting processes, enzymatic activity, immune function, and reproductive cycles. Because many invertebrates are sediment-dwellers, they experience chronic exposure to contaminated substrates, resulting in mortality events and reduced ecosystem services such as nutrient cycling.

Overall, wildlife toxicity is shaped by metal type, exposure duration, trophic position, and organism physiology. Sublethal effects often precede visible population declines, making early detection essential for conservation and ecological risk assessment.

14.6.2 Toxicity in livestock

Livestock represent a critical interface between environmental contamination and human food systems. Grazing animals, especially cattle, sheep, and goats, are routinely exposed to metals through soil, pasture grasses, and contaminated water sources. Chronic exposure facilitates bioaccumulation in soft tissues (e.g., liver, kidney), bones, and edible products such as milk.

Studies have shown that cattle feeding on metal-contaminated pastures accumulate **lead (Pb)** and **cadmium (Cd)** in significant quantities within milk and internal organs (Miclean et al., 2019). This is particularly concerning because:

- **Lead** interferes with hemoglobin synthesis, neuromuscular function, and calcium homeostasis in cattle, often resulting in anemia, decreased weight gain, reproductive impairment, and behavioral symptoms such as head pressing and ataxia.

- **Cadmium** induces kidney damage, disrupts mineral metabolism, and suppresses immune function, leading to chronic health issues in livestock.

Because dairy products constitute a major dietary component for human populations, metal transfer from livestock to humans poses substantial public health risks. Milk contaminated with Pb or Cd contributes to cumulative exposure in vulnerable groups, including children and pregnant women, heightening concerns about long-term health outcomes. Moreover, contaminated organ meats (e.g., liver, kidney) often exhibit metal concentrations that exceed food safety limits, creating additional exposure pathways for rural and agricultural communities.

Thus, livestock toxicity serves as both an environmental warning system and a direct concern for food safety governance.

14.6.3 Chronic health effects in humans

Human exposure to toxic metals arises through multiple pathways—diet, drinking water, occupational contact, inhalation of polluted air, and dermal interaction with contaminated soils or products. Over time, these exposures contribute to chronic diseases that disproportionately affect communities near industrial zones, mining regions, and metal-contaminated farmlands.

Neurotoxicity:

- **Lead (Pb)** damages the central nervous system, leading to cognitive deficits, reduced IQ in children, motor dysfunction, and behavioral changes.
- **Mercury (Hg)** exposure—especially methylmercury—affects sensory, motor, and cognitive functions, with pronounced impacts on fetal neurological development. Long-term exposure is linked to impaired memory, tremors, and vision/hearing disturbances.

Nephrotoxicity:

Cadmium (Cd) accumulates in the kidney cortex with a biological half-life exceeding 10–30 years. Chronic exposure leads to proximal tubule dysfunction, impaired glomerular filtration, proteinuria, and ultimately, chronic kidney disease.

Carcinogenicity:

- **Arsenic (As)** and **hexavalent chromium (Cr VI)** are classified as Group 1 human carcinogens
- Arsenic in drinking water is associated with cancers of the skin, bladder, lung, and liver
- Chromium VI exposure increases the risk of lung cancer, respiratory diseases, and DNA damage due to its strong oxidizing properties

Epidemiological studies consistently show elevated morbidity and mortality rates in **agricultural communities** and populations residing near industrial or mining activities (Sarker et al., 2022). Chronic low-dose exposure—often unnoticed—results in cumulative toxicity that manifests as cardiovascular disease, endocrine disruption, infertility, developmental delays in children, and weakened immune function.

Human health risks are further amplified by the dietary intake of contaminated crops, livestock products, and fish, establishing strong connections between environmental metal contamination and public health burdens.

14.7 Modeling approaches for metal transfer and risk prediction

Quantitative modeling provides essential tools for understanding how metals move through ecosystems, accumulate in organisms, and translate into health risks for wildlife and humans. Modern risk assessment relies on a suite of complementary modeling frameworks—ranging from simple mass-balance equations to advanced probabilistic and network-based simulations. These approaches collectively enable researchers to integrate environmental chemistry, toxicokinetics, ecology, and human exposure pathways into holistic predictive systems.

14.7.1 Mass balance and compartmental models

Mass balance models are grounded in the principle of **conservation of mass**, asserting that the total quantity of a metal entering an environmental system must equal the sum of what is stored, transferred, and lost. These models quantify metal fluxes between major environmental compartments—**soil, water, sediment, vegetation, and biota**—allowing researchers to track how contaminants move and accumulate over time.

Mathematically, mass balance equations often take the form:

$$\text{Input} - \text{Output} + \text{Generation} - \text{Degradation} = \Delta\text{Storage}$$

For metals, degradation is negligible because they are nonbiodegradable; thus, the model emphasizes retention and movement.

Compartmental models build on this framework by dividing ecosystems into a series of connected compartments, each characterized by specific transfer coefficients, uptake rates, and elimination parameters. These models facilitate **long-term projections**, enabling the simulation of how metals shift from abiotic reservoirs to organisms and eventually through food webs. Because of their structured design, compartmental models are widely used in both ecological and human health contexts to estimate steady-state concentrations and biological half-lives (Ali and Khan, 2019).

14.7.2 Monte Carlo simulations

Environmental systems exhibit high variability and uncertainty, stemming from fluctuating contaminant concentrations, differences in organism behavior, and natural heterogeneity in exposure. **Monte Carlo simulations** address this uncertainty by performing repeated random sampling across probability distributions of key parameters, such as ingestion rates, BCFs, exposure duration, and body weight.

Instead of single-point estimates, Monte Carlo analysis produces **probabilistic output distributions**, providing:

- Confidence intervals for exposure doses
- Probability of exceeding toxic thresholds
- Quantification of uncertainty and model sensitivity

Sanaei et al. (2021) demonstrated the effectiveness of Monte Carlo approaches in evaluating human health risks associated with the consumption of contaminated aquatic food. Their findings highlight how probabilistic modeling can capture real-world variability far better than deterministic methods.

14.7.3 Ecological network models

Ecological network models simulate the movement of metals through complex **food webs**, capturing the trophic relationships among primary producers, consumers, predators, and detritivores. These models integrate:

- Species interaction matrices
- Dietary preferences
- Trophic transfer efficiencies
- Biomagnification and bioaccumulation rates
- Predator–prey dynamics

By considering the **structure of entire food webs**, ecological network models reveal **nonlinear amplification** of metals at higher trophic levels, where small increases in lower-level contamination can result in disproportionately large metal burdens in apex predators (Shetty et al., 2025).

These models are particularly useful for predicting risks to endangered species, assessing ecosystem vulnerability, and identifying trophic bottlenecks where interventions (e.g., sediment remediation) may have the greatest benefits.

14.7.4 Exposure and dose–response models

Exposure and dose–response models form the backbone of human health risk assessment. They quantify how much of a metal individuals are exposed to and how this dose translates into adverse health effects. These models integrate environmental concentrations with human behavior patterns such as dietary habits, inhalation rates, and water consumption.

The key outputs include:

- Estimated daily intake
- Hazard quotient (HQ)
- Target hazard index (THI)

The **HQ** is calculated as:

$$HQ = \frac{\text{Estimated Exposure Dose}}{\text{Reference Dose (RfD)}}$$

An **HQ > 1** signals that exposure exceeds safe levels and may lead to adverse health effects. The **THI** aggregates HQ values across multiple metals or pathways, providing a cumulative toxicity indicator (Sarker et al., 2022). Dose–response models, therefore, help translate environmental contamination into meaningful health risk metrics for communities.

14.7.5 Integrative models

Modern environmental assessments increasingly rely on **hybrid integrative modeling frameworks** that combine elements of biogeochemical cycling, toxicokinetics, ecological interactions, and probabilistic analysis. These integrative models provide a more comprehensive understanding of metal fate because they address multiple dimensions simultaneously:

- Environmental transport processes
- Chemical speciation and bioavailability
- Organism physiology
- Exposure heterogeneity
- Population-level effects

By merging biogeochemical models with toxicokinetic–toxicodynamic frameworks, researchers can simulate not only **where metals move** but also **how organisms absorb, transform, and respond to them**. This enhances predictive accuracy across complex and variable ecosystems (Ali and Khan, 2019).

Such hybrid approaches are essential for addressing real-world scenarios where metal contamination interacts with climate variability, land-use change, and biodiversity loss.

14.8 Applications in regulatory risk assessment and management

As heavy metal contamination increasingly threatens global food security and human health, regulatory agencies have begun to rely heavily on modeling frameworks to establish exposure standards, assess risks, and implement management strategies. These modeling tools—ranging from mass-balance simulations to probabilistic exposure assessments—enable policymakers to translate scientific data into effective regulatory limits and mitigation interventions.

14.8.1 Integration in regulatory frameworks

International agencies such as the **World Health Organization**, the **Food and Agriculture Organization**, and the **United States Environmental Protection Agency** rely extensively on modeling outputs to inform environmental and food safety standards. Metal transfer models, including trophic transfer simulations, compartmental analyses, and human exposure assessments, provide the quantitative basis required to set:

- Permissible daily intakes
- Provisional tolerable weekly intakes
- Maximum residue limits for food commodities
- Reference dose (RfD) values for chronic exposure

Shetty et al. (2025) emphasize that regulatory bodies increasingly integrate ecological network models and bioaccumulation simulations to refine guidelines for fisheries, agricultural soils, and contaminated watersheds. By using predictive modeling outputs, regulatory agencies are better equipped to anticipate long-term accumulation, assess high-risk populations, and design evidence-based environmental limits.

14.8.2 Development of exposure thresholds

The establishment of safe exposure thresholds requires consideration of variability in human consumption patterns, environmental concentrations, and biological susceptibility. Traditional deterministic thresholds provide only a narrow safety margin and do not reflect real-world diversity.

To address these limitations, agencies such as the **European Food Safety Authority** have adopted **Monte Carlo–based probabilistic modeling** frameworks. These models allow regulators to:

- Generate full distributions of possible exposure levels
- Identify high-risk subpopulations (children, pregnant women, agricultural workers)
- Incorporate variability in ingestion rates, body weight, and environmental metal concentrations
- Assess cumulative exposure from multiple metals or exposure pathways

Sanaei et al. (2021) demonstrate that probabilistic approaches significantly improve the robustness of threshold-setting by quantifying uncertainty and capturing extreme exposure events. Such models form the basis for updated RfDs, benchmark dose modeling, and cumulative risk limits.

14.8.3 Risk management strategies

Risk management translates scientific assessment into actionable interventions to reduce metal exposure in agricultural systems, livestock, and human populations. Effective strategies target both **source reduction** and **uptake mitigation**.

Commonly applied strategies include:

14.8.3.1 Phytoremediation

Using hyperaccumulator plants (*Brassica juncea*, *Pteris vittata*) to extract heavy metals from contaminated soils is an eco-friendly approach that reduces soil metal reservoirs over time, thereby improving long-term food safety.

14.8.3.2 Crop rotation and varietal selection

Rotating crops with lower metal uptake capability or selecting cultivars genetically predisposed to exclude metals from edible tissues is a method that reduces metal concentrations in staple foods without altering agricultural productivity.

14.8.3.3 Soil amendments and pH adjustment

The addition of lime, organic matter, biochar, or phosphate compounds immobilizes metals by altering soil chemistry.

- Higher soil pH reduces metal solubility
- Organic amendments bind metals, reducing plant uptake

Ali and Khan (2019) emphasize that combining field-level management with modeling allows policymakers to identify which interventions will be most effective under specific climatic or soil conditions.

14.8.4 Policy implications

Integrating metal transfer modeling into policy frameworks has significant implications for public health protection and sustainable agriculture. Effective policy adoption ensures:

14.8.4.1 Evidence-based food safety regulations

Modeling outputs guide the development of national standards for crop residues, irrigation water quality, and livestock feed safety.

14.8.4.2 Early warning systems

Predictive modeling supports surveillance programs that detect emerging contamination hotspots before metal levels reach hazardous thresholds.

14.8.4.3 *Sustainable agricultural management*

Policies informed by ecological and toxicokinetic models promote soil health, reduce pollution exposure, and enhance long-term food system resilience.

14.8.4.4 *Targeted risk mitigation*

By identifying high-risk communities—such as mining-adjacent villages or industrial agriculture zones—governments can prioritize interventions where they are most needed.

Sarker et al. (2022) confirm that policy frameworks incorporating predictive exposure models are more successful in reducing environmental health burdens, particularly in rural or agriculture-dependent populations.

14.9 Challenges and future directions

Persistent challenges in assessing metal transfer and ecological risk arise largely from the absence of comprehensive long-term datasets, which limits the ability to detect temporal trends, evaluate chronic exposure, and validate predictive models across ecosystems. Many existing datasets are geographically restricted, short in duration, or methodologically inconsistent, making cross-study comparisons difficult and reducing confidence in ecological risk assessments (Ali et al., 2019). Moreover, species differ significantly in their physiological traits, feeding behaviors, metabolic rates, and detoxification capacities, resulting in high variability in biological responses to the same metal concentrations. This interspecific variation complicates the creation of universal toxicity thresholds and necessitates species- or guild-specific models that increase analytical complexity.

Climate change further amplifies uncertainty by modifying environmental parameters such as temperature, precipitation, and redox conditions, which directly influence metal speciation and mobility. Warmer temperatures, altered hydrological cycles, and extreme climatic events can accelerate the release of metals from soils and sediments, reshape food-web interactions, and heighten bioaccumulation risks for both aquatic and terrestrial organisms. These dynamic processes underscore the need for flexible and predictive modeling approaches capable of capturing nonlinear and climate-driven fluctuations.

To address these limitations, the integration of machine learning, big-data analytics, and real-time environmental monitoring offers promising pathways for improving predictive precision (Vallero, 2021). Machine learning algorithms can analyze large, heterogeneous datasets, identify hidden patterns, and enhance forecasting capability. Future research should, therefore, focus on developing harmonized global standards, establishing ecologically relevant threshold values, and designing open, interactive modeling platforms that support transparent and collaborative risk assessment.

14.10 Conclusion

Toxic metals continue to threaten environmental and human health through persistent accumulation in food chains. Effective risk assessment and modeling are essential to predict exposure, identify vulnerable species, and support evidence-based regulation. Advances in ecological modeling, computational power, and environmental monitoring promise a more integrated understanding of metal transfer and its long-term ecological impacts. By bridging chemistry, biology, and data science, the next generation of models will better protect both ecosystem integrity and public health.

References

Adriano, D.C., 2001. Trace Elements in Terrestrial Environments. Springer.

Ali, H., Khan, E., 2019. Trophic transfer, bioaccumulation, and biomagnification of heavy metals in aquatic ecosystems: a review. Environ. Chem. Lett. 17 (2), 945–957.

Ali, H., Khan, E., Ilahi, I., 2019. Environmental chemistry and ecological toxicity of heavy metals. Chemosphere 236, 124–125.

Alloway, B.J., 2013. Heavy Metals in Soils. Springer.

Basu, N., Scheuhammer, A.M., Chan, H.M., 2018. Metals and neurotoxicity. Environ. Res. 167, 123–146.

Bjerregaard, P., Andersen, O., Rankin, K., 2021a. Metals, Toxicology, and Ecology. CRC Press.

Bjerregaard, P., Kyhn, M., Damgaard, C.F., 2021b. Bioaccumulation and biomagnification of mercury in aquatic food webs. Ecotoxicology 30 (3), 427–443.

Clemens, S., Aarts, M., Thomine, S., Verbruggen, N., 2013. Plant transporter mechanisms for metal detoxification. Trends Plant Sci. 18 (12), 734–742.

Clemens, S., Ma, J.F., 2016. Toxic heavy metals and plants. Annu. Rev. Plant Biol. 67, 489–532.

Gall, J.E., Boyd, R.S., Rajakaruna, N., 2015. Transfer of heavy metals through terrestrial food webs: a review. Environ. Monit. Assess. 187 (4), 201–218.

Grandjean, P., Landrigan, P.J., 2014. Neurobehavioural effects of developmental toxicity. Lancet Neurol. 14744422. 13 (3), 330–338. doi:10.1016/s1474-4422(13)70278-3.

IARC, 2012. Arsenic, Metals, Fibres and Dusts. International Agency for Research on Cancer.

Jarvis, T., et al, 2020. Lead bioavailability and soil contamination. Sci. Total Environ. 715, 136–144.

Joint, FAO, World Health Organization and WHO Expert Committee on Food Additives, 2011. Evaluation of certain food additives and contaminants: seventy-fourth [74th] report of the Joint FAO/WHO Expert Committee on Food Additives. World Health Organization.

Lu, X., Wang, L., Li, L., Lei, K., Huang, L., Kang, D., 2011. Airborne heavy metals and crop contamination. Environ. Pollut. 159 (10), 2575–2585.

Luoma, S.N., Rainbow, P.S., 2008. Metal Contamination in Aquatic Environments. Cambridge University Press.

Meharg, A., Zhao, F., 2012. Arsenic and Rice, Springer.

Miclean, M., Cadar, O., Levei, E.A., Roman, C., 2019. Heavy metal accumulation in cattle reared in areas with environmental contamination. Environ. Sci. Pollut. Res. 26 (23), 23937–23947.

Naujokas, M.F., et al, 2013. The global health burden of arsenic. Environ. Health Perspect. 121 (3), 295–302.

Needleman, H., 2004. Lead Poisoning. Annu. Rev. Med. 0066-4219. 55 (1), 209–222. doi:10.1146/annurev.med.55.091902.103653.

Newman, M.C., 2015. Fundamentals of Ecotoxicology, CRC Press.

Nordberg, G., Fowler, B., Nordberg, M., 2018. Handbook on the Toxicology of Metals, Academic Press.

Pacyna, E., Pacyna, J., 2001. Atmospheric deposition of heavy metals. Water Air Soil Pollut. 115, 105–113.

Rahman, Z., Singh, V., 2019. Chromium in the environment. Environ. Sci. Pollut. Res. 26, 11319–11330.

Sanaei, F., Aminiyan, M.M., Ardestani, M.M., 2021. Probabilistic modeling of heavy metal bioaccumulation and human health risk assessment in aquatic ecosystems. Environ. Sci. Pollut. Res. 28 (12), 14532–14545.

Sarker, M.N.I., Islam, M.M., Rahman, M.M., 2022. Environmental exposure to heavy metals and its human health impacts: a systematic review. Environ. Sci. Pollut. Res. 29 (2), 2755–2773.

Satarug, S., Garrett, S.H., Sens, M.A., Sens, D.A., Cadmium,, 2010. Environmental exposure, and health outcomes. Environ. Health Perspect. 0091-6765. 118 (2), 182–190. doi:10.1289/ehp.0901234.

Selin, N.E., 2009. Global biogeochemical cycling of mercury: a review. Annu. Rev. Environ. Resour. 1543-5938. 34 (1), 43–63. doi:10.1146/annurev.environ.051308.084314.

Shetty, S., Ramanathan, A., Pillai, P., 2025. Ecological network analysis for evaluating trophic transfer and amplification of heavy metals in aquatic food webs. Ecotoxicol. Environ. Saf. 270, 115678.

Sparks, D., 2003. Environmental Soil Chemistry, Academic Press.

Tchounwou, P.B., Yedjou, C.G., Patlolla, A.K., Sutton, D.J. 2012. Heavy metal toxicity and the environment. EXS. 1023294X. (101), 133–164. doi: 10.1007/978-3-7643-8340-4_6.

USEPA, 2020. Human Health Risk Assessment Guidelines. U.S. Environmental Protection Agency.

Vallero, D., 2021. Environmental Pollutants and Control, Elsevier.

Van der Ent, A., Baker, A., Reeves, R., Pollard, A., 2013. Hyperaccumulator plants. New Phytol. 199 (2), 341–360.

Wang, Q., Chen, M., Li, Y., 2020. Bioconcentration and toxicokinetics of cadmium and lead in aquatic organisms: a review. Sci. Total Environ. 708, 135107.

Wang, W.X., Rainbow, P.S., 2008. Metal Uptake and Metabolism in Aquatic Invertebrates, CRC Press.

WHO, 2017. Guidelines for drinking-water quality: first addendum to the fourth edition edition.

Zhang, L., Wang, Y., Zhou, Q., 2019. Bioaccumulation and trophic transfer of heavy metals in aquatic food webs: implications for human health. Environ. Pollut. 249, 109–118.

Chapter 15

Chronic dietary metal exposure: Mechanisms of toxicity and implications for human health

Ashok Kumar Sah[a], Anushka Sharma[b], Rahul Kumar[b], Prem Shankar Mishra[b], Rakhi Mishra[c], and Nasiruddin Khan[d]
[a]*Department of Medical Laboratory Sciences, College of Applied and Health Sciences, A' Sharqiyah University, Ibra, Oman*
[b]*Faculty of Pharmacy, Vidya University, Meerut, India*
[c]*Noida Institute of Engineering & Technology (Pharmacy Institute), Greater Noida, India*
[d]*Department of Food Sciences, College of Applied and Health Sciences, A' Sharqiuah University, Ibra, Oman*

15.1 Introduction

Naturally occurring metals are found in the earth's crust, and the levels of these metals in the environment might differ by location. The characteristics of metals and the influence of environmental factors dictate their distribution in the environment (Garrett, 2000; H. Bradl, 2005; Sheng et al., 2012; H. B. Bradl, 2005; Runnells et al., 1992). About 30 metals and metalloids, out of the 92 naturally occurring elements, have the potential to be harmful to people. Metallic elements having an atomic weight higher than 40.04 (the atomic mass of Ca) are classified as heavy metals (HMs). Both natural and man-made sources can release HMs into the environment (Appenroth, 2009; Duffus, 2002). These sources include soil erosion, mining, industrial discharge, urban runoff, sewage effluents, pesticides or disease-control agents applied to plants, fallout from air pollution, and the earth's natural weathering. The majority of people are exposed to these harmful substances mostly through their diet (food and water), even though other people are exposed primarily at work. There is typically a cyclical sequence to the poisoning of people, industry, soil, water, food, and the atmosphere (Xu et al., 2024; Sonone et al., 2020; Mishra et al., 2018). Although toxicity and the associated risk to human health are evidently dependent on concentration, it is well recognized that extended exposure to comparatively low levels of HMs and metalloids can yield detrimental effects. As a result, concerns

The Metallome in Motion. https://doi.org/10.1016/B978-0-443-44299-5.00014-6

regarding human exposures, intakes, and absorption of HMs have grown, primarily in the industrialized world (Morais et al., 2012).

The severity of HM poisoning is becoming more widely acknowledged in many emerging nations, especially China and India (Meharg, 2004; Cheng, 2003). Human and animal bodies are known to suffer from a number of negative consequences when dietary materials are contaminated by chemicals and nonessential elements such as HMs (D'Souza and Peretiatko, 2002). Because they are so common and difficult to eliminate from the body, human populations may be susceptible to health issues. Since metals can evade regulatory systems, including homeostasis, transport, compartmentalization, and binding to specific cell constituents, they can have detrimental and even lethal effects. By displacing necessary components from their proper locations, HMs can disrupt biological processes. It has been found that the primary cause of the oxidative destruction of biological macromolecules is metal binding to nuclear proteins and DNA (Flora et al., 2008). Symptoms aid in identifying the pollutant because they are frequently the first signs of contamination. Metal toxicity manifests as sleepiness, emotional instability, melancholy, kidney and liver difficulties, central nervous system disorders, visual anomalies, and intellectual disabilities or dementia in children (de Carvalho Machado and Dinis-Oliveira, 2023; Jan et al., 2011). In conclusion, metal exposure poisoning is a clinically dangerous medical condition that has a greater impact on increasing the rate of morbidity and mortality if it is not identified or treated appropriately (Jan et al., 2015).

There are numerous safeguards in place to keep individuals safe by preventing them from consuming potentially dangerous metal ions. European nations invest significantly in preventing the public from absorbing metals, from identifying contamination during food preparation to monitoring endogenous levels of metal ions in meals and beverages (Hida et al., 2002, 2000; Sarkar and Li, 2006). The removal of metal ions from the body is the subject of extensive research and development from a medical perspective. Researchers have developed techniques to address hazardous metal ions since the use of As during World War I (Piazza et al., 2009; Raffoul et al., 2007). More recently, attempts have been made to eliminate deposits from the brain and counteract the oxidative stress caused by redox-active metal ions. The latter approach focuses on chelators that reverse any potential negative effects by producing mimetics of antioxidant enzymes after chelating the labile redox-active metal ion. It's interesting to note that typical dietary components like catechins make excellent prodrug chelators for antioxidants. Target hazard quotients (THQ) were developed by the United States Environmental Protection Agency (EPA) to calculate the potential health risks associated with extended exposure to chemical pollutants. Estimating the health risks associated with exposure to HMs found in seafood and, in one case, breast milk is the aim of the few THQ studies on foods that have been published. Furthermore, debates about the mechanism of aging have centered on dietary metal ions. Because they are thought to encourage oxidative stress, redox-active metal ions like Cu(I)/(II) and Fe(II)/(III) are particularly linked to the free radical theory of aging (Sunilson et al., 2009). Metal ions, however, can interfere with normal tissue and cell function in a number of ways, such as altering membrane potentials and interacting with proteins and other biomolecules, in addition to generating radicals. Reports on the detrimental health impacts of extended exposure to dietary metals are compiled in this study (Mudgal et al., 2010).

15.2 Sources of dietary metals

15.2.1 Contaminated water and soil

HMs, including mercury, lead, arsenic, chromium, cadmium, and thallium, are necessary for biological metabolism but can be hazardous in larger amounts. They can find their way into aquatic environments through both natural and man-made sources, including sewage, landfill leaching, storm runoff, shipping, port operations, and the atmosphere (Jaishankar et al., 2014). In addition, they can enter the body through drinking water, food, and the air. Because metals are bioaccumulative—that is, they build up over time in living organisms—they have the potential to harm or even destroy biota. In aquatic species, the toxicity of HMs is significantly influenced by temperature, turbidity, dissolved oxygen, alkalinity, hardness, and pH (Jakimska-Nagórska et al., 2011; Stankovic and Stankovic, 2013). Although they are necessary for cellular metabolism, HMs such as mercury, lead, arsenic, chromium, cadmium, and thallium can be hazardous in higher concentrations. They enter the body through the air, food, and drinking water. They can also enter aquatic environments through natural and man-made sources such as sewage, landfill leaching, storm runoff, shipping, port operations, and the atmosphere. Because metals build up over time in living organisms, they can have detrimental impacts on biota and can be fatal. Both natural and man-made sources can introduce HMs into surface water systems. Volcanic eruptions, sea-salt sprays, forest fires, weathering of metal-containing rocks, and natural weathering processes are among the geological and natural phenomena that could cause the release of metals from their native states into various environmental sections (Armah et al., 2010) (Table 15.1).

HMs and metalloids are regarded as agricultural soil contaminants because high soil concentrations of these elements may harm crop health and yield (Shahid et al., 2015). They can build up in the soil and remain there for a very long time if plants don't absorb them or flush them out. In addition, they don't deteriorate easily (Wuana and Okieimen, 2011; Ali et al., 2019). High concentrations of Ni, Cd, Hg, Cu, Cr, As, Pb, and Zn found in agricultural soils can be harmful to plants. Among them, at almost all pollution levels, Cr, Cd, Hg, As, and Pb are extremely poisonous and detrimental to plants (Tiwari and Lata, 2018; Singh et al., 2016). While the overstandard rate of soil pollution is 16.1%, the overstandard rates for Cr, Cd, As, Pb, and Hg are 1.10%, 1.50%, 1.60%, 2.70%, and 7.00%, respectively.

TABLE 15.1 Sources of metals in contaminated water.

S. no.	Metals/ contaminants	Mechanism of contamination	Health impacts	References
1.	Sulfuric acid (H_2O_2), HCl, HF, ash-metals	Ash falls into water bodies; acidification and turbidity	Biodiversity loss, low pH, life toxicity	(Rudnik, 2024)
2.	Pesticides, fertilizers, and drug residues	Runoff from fields and farms into surface water	Bioaccumulation in the food chain, carcinogen exposure, and eutrophication	(Rose, 2023; Ray and Shaju, 2023)
3.	Pb, Hg, Cd. As, Zn	Acid mine drainage and waste rock erosion	Contaminated groundwater, health risks	(Obasi and Akudinobi, 2020)
4.	Ni, Cr, Cd, Zn, Cu, Pb	Effluent discharge containing plating chemicals	Soil and water pollution, carcinogenic effects	(Liu et al., 2011; Aendo et al., 2022)
5.	Pb, Cd, Hg, As, Ni, BFRs	Improper disposal leads to leaching into water	Skin, respiratory, immune, and endocrine disorders	(Obuzor and Onyedikachi, 2023; Lawati et al., 2024)
6.	Pb, Cd, Hg, PAHs, pathogens	Leaching from medical waste dumping	Infectious diseases and groundwater toxicity	(Lodhi et al., 2024)

HM buildup in soil can reduce soil fertility, quality, and agricultural production. According to some research, it might even be detrimental to the health of people and animals (Zang et al., 2017; Fei et al., 2020). Given how quickly the economy and culture are evolving, a number of HMs in contaminated soil pose a problem for both the environment and the general populace. In soil ecosystems, the HMs Hg, Cd, Cu, Zn, Ni, Pb, As, and Cr are commonly present as pollutants. This kind of contamination is widespread, harmful from a biological perspective, and pervasive in the soil environment. Approximately 5 million sites across the globe have soil HM concentrations over the acceptable level (Li et al., 2019). Arsenic, cadmium, lead, and mercury are the four most hazardous metals in the environment, according to the EPA (Robert and Mari, 2003). The main causes of HM deposition in soil are human production activities such as chemical manufacturing, mineral mining, and the use of agricultural fertilizers (Tang et al., 2019). Several studies have shown that natural sources of HMs in the environment often have minor impacts compared to anthropogenic activities (Dixit et al., 2015; Xu et al., 2024).

15.2.2 Food crops and seafood

Vegetables provide protein, vitamins, iron, calcium, and other elements that are typically lacking, making them vital dietary components (Ebabhi and Adebayo, 2022). In addition, they serve as buffers for the acidic compounds created during digestion. However, they contain a variety of hazardous and important substances in varying amounts. Vegetable metal buildup could directly endanger human health. Among the crops whose HM toxicity was evaluated were Chinese cabbage, winter greens, pakchoi, and celery (Cao et al., 2024; Zhang et al., 2018). Vegetables collect metals from contaminated soils and from deposits on various vegetable portions exposed to air in polluted settings. Reports indicate that approximately half of the typical dietary intake of lead, cadmium, and mercury comes from plants (Galal-Gorchev, 1993; de Vries et al., 2007).

Due to the lack of an efficient method of elimination, prolonged low-level intakes of HMs are detrimental to both humans and other species. Metals are taken up by vegetables through absorption from contaminated soils and deposits on vegetable sections that are exposed to air from polluted settings. Temperature, moisture content, organic matter, pH, and nutrient availability all affect how HMs are absorbed and accumulate in plant tissues (Tangahu et al., 2011). Plant species also affect the accumulation of HMs, and plant absorption or soil-to-plant metal transfer variables regulate how well plants absorb metals (Khan et al., 2008). By obstructing essential plant functions, including photosynthesis, mitosis, and water absorption, a very low lead content might result in toxic symptoms such as brown short roots, stunted foliage, wilting of older leaves, and dark green leaves (Bhattacharyya et al., 2008). On the other hand, high lead concentrations in soils may lower soil productivity. In addition to causing chlorosis, poor plant development, and low yield, HMs can cause metabolic problems, decreased nutrient uptake, and a reduced capacity to fix molecular nitrogen in leguminous plants (Guala et al., 2010; Onakpa et al., 2018).

Consequently, due to their high nutritional content, seafood products are regarded as essential to our diet. They might, nevertheless, also serve as transporters of biotic and abiotic contamination. Toxic trace elements are among the most significant abiotic pollutants. To describe the ingredients and assess the risk of consuming food containing them, numerous studies have been carried out. A study showed how a mother's diet of seafood largely affected the neurobehavioral function of children (ages 7–14) exposed to CH3Hg in utero (Choi and Grandjean, 2012; Driscoll et al., 2013). Fish and canned goods contain high levels of cadmium (Cd), making seafood a significant source of the metal in the human diet. Shellfish have the highest amounts, especially bivalves, which can have up to 10 mg/kg fw (Saher and Kanwal, 2019). Generally speaking, crustaceans have lower amounts of Cd than bivalves; nevertheless, products made from brown crab flesh have greater levels, up to 8 mg/kg fw. Algal concentrations in dry seaweed range from 0.02 to 4.82 mg/kg dw (Yuan, 2007). Arsenic levels in fish are normally <5 mg/kg fw, although higher levels have been found in some samples available to consumers (Olmedo et al., 2013). Arsenobetaine (AB), the most prevalent As species in fish and shellfish, accounts for about 70% of most fish and crustaceans. The majority of seafood samples have lead (Pb) levels below the current legal limit, making Pb the least worrisome trace element. Pb levels in seaweeds and their derivatives are comparable to those in other fisheries products (Guo et al., 2023; Chiocchetti et al., 2017).

15.2.3 Food processing and packaging

One of the main ways that the general public is exposed to dangerous metals or metalloids throughout their lives is through the consumption of contaminated food. Industrial processing, packaging, and postharvest handling can all introduce metals into food (Acharya, 2024; Gerster-Bentaya, 2015). Metal alloys used in processing equipment can cause nickel, chromium, or tin to be present in food items. Despite increased regulation, preservatives and additives may still contain lead, arsenic, or mercury compounds. Metal cans can release tin, lead, and cadmium, especially when they come into contact with acidic foods like tomato sauce and fruit juice. Plastic packaging may release trace metals because it is manufactured using dyes and stabilizers. Aluminum foil and containers may come into contact with hot, acidic, or salty foods, increasing the likelihood that aluminum may leach. Inadequate processing and packaging are major contributors to dietary metal consumption from processed and convenience foods (Jellesen et al., 2006; Tetteh, 2022; Reilly, 2008; Mohammad et al., 2018).

The amount of cadmium ingested through diet is influenced by both food consumption patterns and cadmium levels in foods. Cereals, vegetables, grains, roots, potatoes, and other plant foods are the primary sources of dietary cadmium intake; their mean cadmium concentrations are generally <0.03 mg/kg. Recent research has also demonstrated a strong link between urinary cadmium and tofu consumption (Adams et al., 2011). Consuming large amounts of kidney, certain mushrooms, and bivalve mollusks will also significantly increase cadmium exposure. According to Italian research, toddlers and children consumed more cadmium than adults, primarily because they consumed more food per kilogram of body weight at younger ages (Fowler et al., 2015).

15.3 Absorption and bioaccumulation

Dietary metals can enter the body through contaminated food and drink, where they can interact with biological molecules and travel to different organs. Their toxicity can persist for long periods of time due to their delayed clearance, which relies on metabolic fate, bioaccumulation capacity, and absorption effectiveness (Sonone et al., 2020).

Through direct contact with contaminated media or indirect ingestion of contaminated food, pollutants can enter the bodies of living organisms. Bioaccumulation occurs when the rate of pollutant absorption surpasses the rate of pollutant removal. Consequently, the contaminant accumulates inside the organism after becoming trapped there. The process by which hazardous metals or chemical compounds form bonds inside a cell structure is known as HM bioaccumulation. Numerous exposure pathways (diet and solution) and geochemical effects on bioavailability influence metal bioaccumulation. Because metals are not digested, metal bioaccumulation is especially useful as an exposure indicator (Chojnacka, 2010). However, one useful integrative indicator of species exposure to chemicals in polluted habitats is bioaccumulation (Mondal et al., 2018). The process of bioaccumulation depends on the bioactivity of biomass. For metabolic processes to absorb contaminants, cells must be alive. The entire cell absorbs metal ions during bioaccumulation. The same mechanisms that allow nutrients to enter cells can also allow metals to enter living organisms. Metals and vital minerals like calcium and magnesium are absorbed by unicellular organisms.

There are two stages to the bioaccumulation process. In the initial stage, metal ions adhere to the cell surface. This early stage is devoid of metabolic activity. Afterward, metal ions are added to the cell. Only when the cells are metabolically active can the second stage of this process be completed. If the ideal circumstances for organism growth in the second stage are preserved, the amount of biomass rises. This makes it possible for more metal ions to bind (Zabochnicka-Świątek and Krzywonos, 2014; Nnaji et al., 2023). In human organisms, the competition of metal ions for protein-binding sites impedes molecular mobility and chemical reaction catalysis. Metal selectivity, which should be investigated at the single-protein level, is linked to the makeup of the immediate environment surrounding the metal-binding site (Barber-Zucker et al., 2017; Young and Xiao, 2021). Understanding metal-mediated protein-protein interactions is necessary to comprehend the molecular details of how HMs affect human health. Metal homeostasis in cells is maintained by proteins called metallothioneins (MTs), cysteine-rich metal-binding peptides like glutathione (GSH), and phytochelatins (PCs) found in microorganisms and plants. In response to various forms of stress, protective proteins known as MTs are produced. Because of their biophysicochemical resemblance to calcium, magnesium, and other divalent minerals, cadmium and lead can either imitate or replace important metals at certain locations. However, Pb(II) and Cd(II) are lethal to mammalian cells because they cannot mediate some essential processes (Srivastava and Kowshik, 2013; Kern et al., 2000).

When cadmium ions cause the phospholipase C (PLC)-IP3 pathway to release Ca(II) from endoplasmic reticulum storage, reactive oxygen species (ROS) may be generated. This can damage the kidneys by increasing intracellular Ca(II) levels, triggering mitogen-activated protein kinase, and altering the roles of ion transporters in renal cells (Kosiba et al., 2020). Cd(II) neurotoxicity has been associated with decreased mitochondrial membrane potential and the cleavage of the caspase-9 and caspase-3 proteases (Gu et al., 2018). Because of its hazardous, particularly neurotoxic, properties, lead is still one of the most researched toxic elements. Lead ions disrupt synapse formation and may result in problems in epigenetic processes by blocking voltage-activated and receptor-operated calcium channels in human and invertebrate neurons (Garza-Lombó et al., 2018).

Since there are numerous ways that metal exposure might occur, it is challenging to accurately quantify intakes in order to identify minute rates of absorption in human individuals. The interpretation of balance investigations can be complicated by the biliary secretion of some metals (Robson, 2003; Sexton et al., 1995). Homeostatic control governs the physiological disposition of important metals, including absorption, and can vary between species. Metal absorption can differ significantly among human populations due to a variety of factors, including the chemical form of the metal, the environmental matrix in which it is ingested, the contents of the gastrointestinal tract, diet, nutritional status, age, and, in some cases, genotype (Diamond et al., 1998).

The duodenum is the main site of intestinal absorption of lead, while the isolated rat gut exhibits the maximum absorption and serosal lead transfer activity (Conrad and Barton, 1978). The precise processes of absorption are unclear; however, they could include active transport or diffusion between cells (paracellular) or across intestinal epithelial cells (transcellular). Measurements of the net flow kinetics of lead in different intestines have led to the inference of saturable processes. Based on research using the isolated rat gut, Aungst and Fung developed a kinetic model of lead transport that forecasts both saturable and nonsaturable lead transport pathways (Aungst and Fung, 1981). It is anticipated that the saturable pathway will predominate, except at comparatively high concentrations that correspond to exceptionally large intakes. Because the paracellular pathway is extremely permeable to larger cations like Cs' and Rb +, the higher ionic radius of the PbZ + ion cannot account for the lower expected contribution of the nonsaturable pathway for lead relative to calcium. Even though the exact mechanism of the lead nonsaturable pathway is unknown, a paracellular pathway can be inferred by comparisons to calcium and other inorganic cations. Lead's potential ability to cross cell membranes and pass through cation channels is intriguing, despite the lack of evidence. An L-type Ca" channel was recently discovered in the apical membranes of cultured rabbit proximal tubule cells, indicating a "leaky" transporting epithelium that resembles the duodenum. Lead has also been reported to enter excitable cells via voltage-gated L-type Ca" channels (Kasten-Jolly and Lawrence, 2018).

Depending on their chemical characteristics, binding affinities, and interactions with proteins, metals enter the bloodstream and are subsequently transported to different organs. The long biological half-lives of several metals cause bioaccumulation over time (Hontela and Lacroix, 2006). Either the free ionic form or protein-bound complexes that circulate to tissues are the two ways in which blood and plasma are transported. Because of the high expression of metallothionein, metals such as copper, arsenic, and cadmium accumulate in the liver, which is a significant location for accumulation and detoxification. The accumulation of cadmium in the renal cortex causes long-term kidney damage (Yan and Allen, 2021). Lead becomes a long-term storage site and stores strontium in bone by replacing calcium in hydroxyapatite. Lead and methylmercury subsequently penetrate the blood-brain barrier and have neurological effects. Arsenic and mercury are helpful indicators that are deposited in keratin-rich tissues, and adipose tissue can collect lipophilic organometallic substances (Martinez-Morata et al., 2023). The dynamics of bioaccumulation entail a slow accumulation that frequently doesn't show symptoms right away and might occur under stressful circumstances (Spacie et al., 2020).

15.4 Mechanisms of toxicity

Chronic exposure to dietary metals triggers a series of molecular and cellular reactions that are responsible for their hazardous properties. The toxicological consequences of metal exposure are determined by the metal species, the amount and duration of exposure, and the host's nutritional and genetic state. The key processes include oxidative stress, mitochondrial malfunction, DNA and protein damage, and alterations in enzymatic and hormonal activity (Fig. 15.1).

15.4.1 Oxidative stress

The homeostasis of metal ions is one of the many biological processes in which metals are essential. Oxidative degradation of biological macromolecules can result from metal binding to protein sites or metal replenishment due to a breakdown in metal-ion homeostasis (Bertini and Cavallaro, 2008; Halliwell and Gutteridge, 1990). This mechanism interferes with signal transduction pathways to modulate gene expression and is implicated in a number of diseases, including anemia and neurological conditions like Parkinson's and Alzheimer's. Iron, copper, chromium, and cobalt are examples of redox-active metals that help keep cells' redox states within precise physiological bounds (Valko et al., 2016). A disturbance of metal homeostasis can change calcium and sulfhydryl homeostasis, affect DNA bases, increase lipid peroxidation, and cause unchecked metal-mediated production of harmful free radicals. Humans can also be exposed to redox-inert metals such as arsenic and cadmium, which

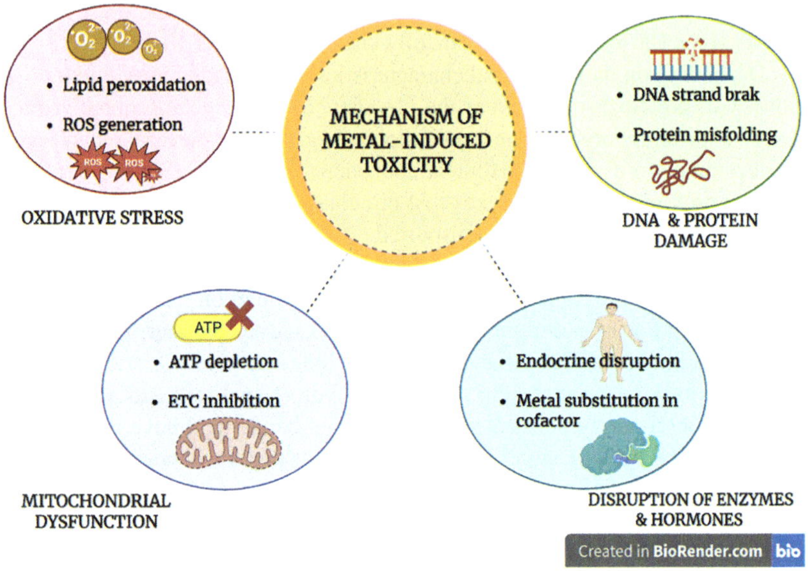

FIG. 15.1 Various mechanisms of metal-induced toxicity.

are poisonous at low doses and have no recognized biological purpose (Speisky et al., 2008).

Although iron is an essential nutrient, too much of it can be harmful. Numerous proteins react to iron levels and stressors, making iron homeostasis a complex process. Iron is stored in proteins like ferritin and hemosiderin and is attached to cytochromes, hemoglobin, myoglobin, and iron-containing enzymes. Iron regulatory proteins control the intake and storage of iron in cells, and their dysregulation can be detrimental (Eisenstein and Blemings, 1998). Iron and oxidative stress are tightly related. An iron and copper redox pair determines the redox state of the cell, and homeostatic processes control iron release and limit excessive iron intake. Free iron can promote the production of harmful reactive free radicals, and iron overload can result in extensive organ damage. Excess superoxide anion radicals and iron overload can result from mutations in iron-uptake regulators and superoxide dismutase enzymes. Excess superoxide causes iron-containing molecules like ferritin to release "free iron" while under in vivo stress. Highly reactive hydroxyl radicals are produced by the Fenton reaction and can harm tissues (Ganz, 2003; Jomova and Valko, 2011).

In addition, copper is a necessary trace metal in living organisms, a cofactor of numerous enzymes engaged in redox reactions, and an electron transporter in biological systems. The biliary tract is the main excretory route, and copper is absorbed from the diet and stored in the liver (Linder and Hazegh-Azam, 1996). Through Fenton-like processes and reduced GSH levels, copper can cause oxidative stress and catalyze the production of ROS. Through ROS, it can potentially result in base oxidation and DNA strand breakage. The strong cellular antioxidant GSH also serves as a substrate for enzymes that eliminate ROS. It is essential for the metabolism and detoxification of intracellular copper (Mattie and Freedman, 2004; Prousek, 2007). By directly chelating the metal, copper toxicity can be reduced, which otherwise raises ROS levels. Cardioprotective qualities may be impacted by copper oxidation of high-density lipoprotein and low-density lipoprotein. Selenium and vitamin E help guard against copper toxicity and lipid peroxidation. While copper deficiency makes cells more vulnerable to oxidative damage, smoking raises copper plasma levels and lipid peroxidation. Lipid oxidation and DNA fragmentation can be brought on by the strong cytotoxic oxidizing agent peroxynitrite anion (Hillstrom et al., 2003).

15.4.2 Mitochondrial dysfunction

By primarily producing the superoxide anion, mitochondria transform 0.2–2% of the oxygen that cells absorb into ROS (Requejo et al., 2010). The disproportionation of superoxide anions in the mitochondrial respiratory chain is a key source of ROS. The primary source of ROS in mitochondria is the electron transport chain. At least three different superoxide dismutase isoenzymes, including manganese, copper, and zinc forms, are found in mammalian tissues (Brand, 2010). The dismutation of $O_2^{\bullet -}$ to O_2 and H_2O_2 is catalyzed in large part by superoxide dismutase (SOD). Nitric oxide (NO°) is a crucial oxidative biological signaling molecule, and GSH peroxidase and catalase eliminate hydrogen peroxide. Nitric oxide synthases (NOS) produce NO° enzymatically, which can lead to lipid peroxidation and DNA fragmentation (Yon et al., 2008).

Chromium (Cr) is a chemical widely utilized in a variety of sectors, including steel, alloys, cast iron, chrome, paints, metal coatings, and wood treatments. It has harmful and cancer-causing effects on both people and animals and is a major source of allergic dermatitis (Stohs et al., 2001). Workplace exposure to excessive levels of chromium, mainly in the valence forms Cr(VI) and Cr(III), can cause lung cancer, occupational asthma, pulmonary fibrosis, and chronic bronchitis (Mertz, 1969). Exposure to Cr(VI) dramatically reduces the activity of essential mitochondrial processes, impairing oxygen reduction and causing oxidative stress. Research has indicated that exposed groups have considerably greater levels of total blood Cr, SOD, lipid peroxidation, and DNA damage than unexposed groups. Cross-linking processes are mostly linked to Cr(III) toxicity, which results in multiform DNA damage. Numerous DNA lesions, such as Cr-DNA adducts, DNA-protein cross-links, DNA-DNA cross-links, and oxidative damage, are caused by chromium within cells (Rossi et al., 1988). Exposure to Cr(VI) in vivo causes cell disruption, cytochrome *c* release, mitochondrial instability, and cell death (Sahin et al., 2003).

A prevalent industrial and environmental pollutant, lead (Pb) is poisonous and poses a health risk to the general public due to its environmental persistence.

Pb accumulates in the liver, kidney, and brain, where it causes harmful biochemical effects (Patrick, 2006). Pb has a severe neurotoxic effect, especially on the developing brain, as evidenced by behavioral abnormalities, learning disabilities, hearing loss, and cognitive impairments in both humans and experimental animals. Pb-induced toxicity has been explained by a number of processes, although none have been clearly defined. One of the key mechanisms underlying Pb's harmful effects is oxidative stress. Lead-related oxidative stress has demonstrated antioxidant capacity when treated with tocopherol and ascorbic acid. Pb is also known to cause oxidative damage, limit hemoglobin formation, and alter the proteins and lipids in red blood cell membranes (Buettner, 1993). The direct impact of Pb on membrane lipids and mitochondrial dysfunction, as well as the pro-oxidative effect of δ-ALA, may be two separate causes of Pb-induced oxidative damage (Rodriguez et al., 2012).

15.4.3 DNA and protein damage

HMs are regarded as possible toxicants because they can interfere with various cellular processes, increasing susceptibility to various diseases by changing the expression patterns of many genes and interfering with the function of several important proteins (Ademuyiwa et al., 2010). For instance, human exposure to lead raises the levels of the detoxifying genes heme oxygenase-1 (HO-1) in renal tubule cells and alpha-GSH S-transferase (GSTA1) excreted in the urine (Garçon et al., 2004). In contrast, mercury causes the kidneys to produce more hydrogen peroxide and alters renal HO-1 expression, which leads to renal damage. Furthermore, 8-oxoguanine DNA-glycosylase 1 (OGG1), a gene implicated in the excision repair of 8-hydroxy-2′-deoxyguanosine (8-OHdG), a biomarker for DNA damage, is inhibited by the well-known human carcinogen Cd (Chevillard et al., 1998).

Saleh Bakheet et al.'s study examined how detoxifying, xenobiotic-metabolizing, and DNA repair genes in Mahd Ad-Dahab city were affected by prolonged exposure to HMs, including lead, cadmium, and mercury. Forty healthy male citizens and twenty healthy individuals from Riyadh city participated in the study. Significantly lower detoxifying gene mRNA expression levels and a corresponding decrease in xenobiotic-metabolizing gene expression were observed in the HM-exposed group. Notably, only the levels of the DNA repair genes OGG1 and 8-OHdG were significantly inhibited in the cadmium-exposed group (Al Bakheet et al., 2013).

15.4.4 Disruption of enzymes and hormones

One of the main ways that long-term exposure to dietary metals might be harmful is by impairing hormone and enzyme activity. By attaching to enzyme active sites or substituting vital trace elements required as cofactors, metals interact with biological systems (Zhang and Gladyshev, 2009). In addition to causing metabolic disturbances and chronic endocrine disruption, enzymatic activity is altered or interrupted. Certain metals, such as lead, mercury, cadmium, and arsenic, are particularly "sticky" with the sulfhydryl (-SH) groups of proteins and undergo conformational changes that impair the activity of enzymes (Manna and Firdous, 2025). For instance, lead contaminates heme-producing enzymes (such as ferrochelatase and δ-aminolevulinic acid dehydratase), which eventually interferes with hemoglobin synthesis and might cause anemia. Mercury binds covalently to thiol-containing enzymes, ceasing important antioxidant enzymatic processes (e.g., GSH peroxidase, thioredoxin reductase) and increasing oxidative stress. Cadmium is described as replacing zinc in metalloproteins and biochemical pathways (e.g., superoxide dismutase), which can further damage cellular defense mechanisms (Chamoli and Karn, 2024).

Metals can cause endocrine disruption in addition to enzymatic inhibition by acting on hormonal pathways. There is strong evidence that cadmium functions as a "metalloestrogen," binding to estrogen receptors and triggering genes that respond to estrogen (Chedrese et al., 2006). Breast and endometrial cancer are two examples of hormone-dependent malignancies that may be exacerbated by this activation. Through changes in receptor expression and downstream gene transcription, arsenic modifies the signaling pathways for thyroid and glucocorticoid hormones, resulting in metabolic disturbance (Miki, 2023). Lead disrupts neurotransmitter release, affects calcium-dependent transmission in neurons, and ultimately impacts neuroendocrine function. Mercury also modifies the activity of the hypothalamic-pituitary-adrenal axis, which influences developmental processes and the stress response. Absolutely, one of the main pathways of metal poisoning is the disruption of the hormonal and enzymatic systems. Enzymes essential to endocrine signaling networks and transcriptional activator pathways are disrupted by metals. Because it will have quantifiable effects on metabolism, reproduction, growth, and brain function, the "reach" of metal effects on an individual increases dramatically when these systems are affected (Henson et al., 2016). Chronic illnesses like reproductive toxicity, metabolic problems, and hormone-related cancers, as well as acute risks like anemia, are caused by ongoing disruption. For prevention, we need to strengthen regulations around dietary metals and provide dietary assistance (Gibson et al., 2000).

15.5 Biomarkers of exposure and toxicity

Biomarkers are of essence when conducting assessments of human exposure to dietary metals, as well as evaluating their related toxicological effects. They present an objective representation of both internal exposure and early and midpoint biological effects, as well as potential health outcomes, and thus fill in the gap between environmental exposure and clinical manifestation. Such biomarkers are especially essential when dealing with certain metals, e.g., lead, arsenic, cadmium, and mercury, which have long biological half-lives and a propensity to bioaccumulate in different tissues.

15.5.1 Blood, urine, and hair analysis

Blood and urine continue to be the most accepted matrices to monitor exposure to metals. Lead, cadmium, and mercury in blood are agreed upon as reflecting acute and on-going or recent exposure, and thus the integrity of circulating and toxic potential (Freeland-Graves et al., 2012). Urinary analysis can be especially useful in assessing exposure to metals excreted in urine, e.g., cadmium and arsenic, and is commonly used in occupational and environmental health investigations.

Nail and hair samples will serve as another noninvasive biomarker, showing a more prolonged exposure to metals such as arsenic, mercury, and lead. It is possible, due to their low growth rates and structure that is rich in keratin, that hair and nails act as historical indicators of exposure and are particularly useful in epidemiological studies as well as in forensic examinations. However, extraneous contamination and individual variability in hair growth can serve as confounding factors, with individual hair analysis requiring standardized methods of collection and analysis (Martinez-Morata et al., 2023; CHAN, 2023).

15.5.2 Recent advances in biomonitoring

Biomonitoring has become significantly more sensitive, specific, and broad due to technological advances. ICP-MS and AAS are now the gold standard methods for determining trace metals at extremely low levels in populations (Ogidi et al., 2024). With subcellular to cellular resolution, new techniques like synchrotron-based X-ray fluorescence and laser ablation inductively coupled plasma-mass spectrometry are becoming widely used and enable high-level detailed mapping of metal distribution within tissues (Wang et al., 2011).

At the molecular level, biomarkers of oxidative stress, such as 8-hydroxy-2-deoxyguanosine, expression of metallothionein, and epigenetic changes, are becoming popular signatures of early metal-induced toxicity (Oros et al., 2025). Such biomarkers provide a clue about the mechanism that connects exposure to other detrimental health outcomes. Beyond this, there is potential, as system-level insights into metal toxicity are becoming available through the use of high-throughput omics studies, e.g., metabolomics, proteomics, and transcriptomics, to apply these insights in the context of precision risk assessment. Altogether, the combination of the classical blood/urine/hair matrices with the use of advanced molecular/imaging biomarkers is a complete approach to dietary metal exposure monitoring. This amalgamation enhances the power of exposure measurement and helps to forecast the chemical impacts early on, and hence plays the role of prevention and treatment medicine (Hurst and Martin, 2017; Sah et al., 2025).

15.6 Risk factors and vulnerable populations

The dietary toxic impacts of metals do not occur consistently among the population. Distribution varies because of age, nutritional status, socioeconomic conditions, and occupational involvement, which pose varying risk profiles (Hejna

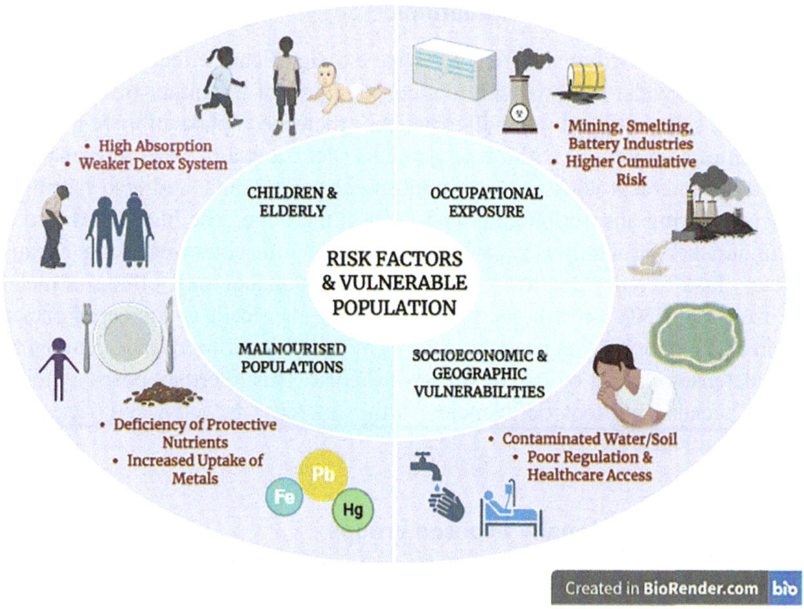

FIG. 15.2 Various risk factors and vulnerable populations.

et al., 2018). It is crucial to identify vulnerable populations to devise specific measures for public health and regulation (Fig. 15.2).

15.6.1 Children and the elderly

Because of faster absorption rates in the gastrointestinal tract, limited detoxification mechanisms at an earlier age, and greater food consumption per unit of weight, children are disproportionately exposed to dietary metals (Huang et al., 2025). Lead and arsenic cross the placenta and may alter neurodevelopment, leading to learning disabilities, behavioral problems, reduced intelligence quotient (IQ), and cognitive deficits (Kaur et al., 2021). In the early stages of exposure, mercury and cadmium have been linked to poor growth, immune dysregulation, and subsequent lifelong metabolic effects (Wang et al., 2021).

However, the elderly population is exposed to different complications associated with age-related impairment. Acute bioavailability, decreased renal clearance, altered intestinal absorption, and life-long exposure—all these predispose the patient to metal toxicity. Impacts of neurodegeneration: Chronic exposure to redox-active metals like copper and iron has been linked to neurodegenerative diseases, including Alzheimer's and Parkinson's disease, which exacerbate oxidative stress in aging brains (Jomova et al., 2025).

15.6.2 Malnourished populations

Deficiencies: Nutritional deficiencies have a significant effect on the toxicity caused by metals. Persons with low consumption of important trace elements like zinc, selenium, and iron will experience increased uptake of toxic metals as a result of competition with these elements (Peraza et al., 1998). For example, cadmium interacts with zinc at the intestinal transporters, and lead resembles calcium during absorption and deposition in the bone. The high risk faced by malnourished populations in low- and middle-income countries occurs because dietary insufficiency aggravates both the absorption and toxic effects of metals (Elizabeth, 2020). Protein-energy malnutrition also leads to increased urinary excretion of detoxifying proteins, such as metallothionein and GSH, leaving the cell defenses against oxidative stress weakened. This interplay poses a vicious cycle because nutrient deficiencies further increase toxicity, and vice versa (Patel and Patel, 2017).

15.6.3 Occupationally exposed groups

Some occupational categories are exposed to a particularly high risk because of the direct or indirect intake of metals with food. Persons engaged in the mining, metallurgy, pesticide-intensive agriculture, battery manufacturing, and recycling of electronic waste industries often have high levels of metals in their blood and urine (Mahaffey et al., 1975). The idea of take-home exposure, with respect to the contamination of household food and water, further poses a danger to family members, particularly children. There is also a risk of chronic dietary mercury and cadmium exposure for workers in the seafood industry and populations relying on fishing in contaminated waters. In industrial areas, the additive effects of dietary and inhalational exposures are worse because the exposures interact to cause more health outcomes than in the general population (Feron et al., 2002).

15.6.4 Socioeconomic and geographic vulnerabilities

Other factors that determine the level of risk include socioeconomic status and geography. People in rural or industrially polluted regions might consume foods and water containing higher levels of metals due to a lack of infrastructure and government control (Birley and Lock, 1998). The total burden of metal toxicity in these communities is exacerbated by limited access to healthcare, safe food, and nutritional supplementation. A combination of these vulnerable groups demonstrates the heterogeneity of risk relative to dietary metals. Identifying such populations is essential for the development of adequate surveillance schemes, enforcement of regulations, and the targeted distribution of nutritional and medical interventions to the population groups at greatest risk (Nsubuga et al., 2011).

15.7 Preventive measures and management

Future prevention and management of dietary metal exposure must incorporate a close combination of nutritional strategies, public health policies, and therapeutic responses. With metals continuing to bioaccumulate when they refuse to leave the environment and cause harm to its ability to sustain life, this has created a difficult task not only to minimize exposure to these toxins but also to address the associated health effects in those who have already been affected (Maynard, 2000).

15.7.1 Dietary strategies and nutritional interventions

Dietary interventions are a first line of metal toxicity defense. Proper nutrition, involving the consumption of essential and necessary micronutrients like calcium, zinc, selenium, and iron, inhibits the absorption of toxic metals because they compete for the same transporters (Peraza et al., 1998). Routinely, adequate dietary calcium lowers gastrointestinal absorption of lead, and zinc reduces cadmium intake. Selenium also acts as a defense mechanism since it forms nontoxic compounds with mercury and arsenic, thus decreasing their availability (Raza et al., 2021).

Such foods specifically include antioxidants, especially those rich in vitamins C and E, carotenoids, and polyphenols, which boost cellular antioxidant defense mechanisms or counteract the production of ROS occurring during oxidative stress induced by metals. Green leafy vegetables, fruits, and phytochemicals have been examined in relation to their protective effects, extending to catechins and flavonoids (Randhawa et al., 2015). Probiotics and dietary fibers could also be useful by binding toxic metals in the gut and facilitating their fecal elimination (Abdel-Megeed, 2021).

Interventions based on the nutritional supplementation of at-risk groups—particularly children, pregnant women, and the undernourished—have proven useful in reducing markers of exposure and increasing resilience to toxicity (Torkelsen, 1985). Nutritional interventions cannot solve the problem of high-exposure environments, even though they should be supported by comprehensive interventions of a systemic character.

15.7.2 Public health regulations and guidelines

The major flaw that should be addressed with strong regulatory frameworks is reducing the level of contamination at its source. On a smaller scale, international agencies such as the Food and Agriculture Organization and the World Health Organization have established upper limits for exposure to hazardous metals in food and water (Othman, 2007). In a similar manner, national control authorities such as the United States Food and Drug Administration and the European Food Safety Authority consistently revise the levels of safety and risk evaluation procedures (Chatzopoulou et al., 2020).

Prevention is effective when there is strict control of agricultural soils, water used to irrigate crops, fertilizers, and pesticides to ensure metals do not pass into the food chain. Better management of industrial waste, pollution abatement methods, and tightening up of effluent-based regulations are essential in curbing environmental pollution (Hines, 2013).

There is a role of publicity campaigns too. Training communities on the sources of exposure, safe methods of cooking, and the dangers of eating or drinking dirty food and water strengthens individuals so that they can protect themselves (Bisset, 1980). Long-term prevention depends especially on the implementation of policies that facilitate safer food processing activities, sustainable farming, and more regular monitoring of those populations that are at high risk.

15.7.3 Role of chelators and antioxidants

Chelation therapy is still one of the fundamental treatments for metal poisoning. Examples of such sequestering agents include ethylenediaminetetraacetic acid (EDTA), dimercaptosuccinic acid (DMSA), and 2,3-dimercapto-1-propanesulfonic acid (DMPS), which bind metals in circulation and excrete them through urine (Blanusa et al., 2005). These treatment modalities are especially applicable in acute poisoning but are also being evaluated for low levels of chronic exposures. Chelators are limited by a lack of specificity, as they bind to essential metals, and by side effects such as nephrotoxicity and vitamin/mineral deficiencies. As a result, interest in natural chelating agents—some of which are found in PCs, polyphenols, and sulfur-containing amino acids—is beginning to emerge as a safer and long-term solution in research (Eckhardt et al., 2013).

Antioxidants provide complementary interventions, where they reduce the effects of oxidation and rebalance the redox. Antioxidants such as Vitamin C, Vitamin E, N-acetylcysteine, and alpha-lipoic acid have also been found to alleviate lipid peroxidation, damage to DNA, and mitochondrial malfunction caused by exposure to metals. Recently, it has been observed that a combination-therapy (chelators and antioxidants) might be superior to the individual therapy options in alleviating systemic toxicity (Liu et al., 2025).

15.7.4 Integrative and future approaches

Recent discoveries in the area of personalized medicine are transforming preventive and curative approaches. Interventions identified through biomarkers can be used to individualize diet and pharmacological treatment of patients according to their exposure patterns and genetic profiles (Rodríguez-Antona and Taron, 2015). Omics technologies, such as metabolomics and epigenomics, are likely to hone these tactics so that early signs of toxicity and recovery can be identified. Future perspectives also focus on greener remediation

TABLE 15.2 Key insights on biomarkers, vulnerable populations, and preventive measures in dietary metal toxicity.

Category	Main points	Highlights
Biomarkers	• Blood/urine: recent exposure • Hair/nails: long-term record • Molecular markers: oxidative stress, metallothionein, epigenetics	Combining classical and molecular biomarkers improves accuracy
Vulnerable populations	• Children: high absorption, neurodevelopmental risks • Elderly: reduced clearance • Malnourished: nutrient deficiencies ↑ uptake • Workers: mining, e-waste, agriculture	Risk is shaped by age, nutrition, and occupation
Preventive measures	• Nutrition: Zn, Ca, Se, antioxidants • Regulations: food safety, pollution control • Medical: chelators + antioxidants • Future: personalized nutrition, phytoremediation	Integrative prevention is most effective

options involving phytoremediation of soils contaminated with metals or bioremediation of metallurgically contaminated soils, which minimize the addition of metals into the food chain (Patra et al., 2020). Integration of environmental, nutritional, and occupational health frameworks at the policy level can be used as a combined measure to overcome population-level risks. A concise overview of biomarkers, risk groups, and preventive approaches is provided in Table 15.2. Combined application of dietary optimization, strict laws concerning the exposure to metals, and treatment advancements offer a comprehensive approach to establishing a dietary metal poisoning burden. Prevention is the best, most cost-effective, and sustainable method in the management of this issue, yet there must always be sustained investments in biomonitoring, research, and educating people about this issue to serve as a long-term safeguard for human health (Babafemi et al., 2024; Batzias and Siontorou, 2006).

15.8 Conclusion and future perspectives

Chronic exposure to dietary toxic metals is a long-overlooked and continuing risk to people worldwide. Contaminated foodstuffs and drinking water play a major role in introducing metals (arsenic, cadmium, lead, and mercury) into the human body, contributing to their bioaccumulation and the appearance of toxic effects through oxidative stress, perturbed mitochondrial functions, DNA and protein damage, and altered enzymatic and hormonal functions. These mechanistic findings help explain why such exposure is associated with a wide range of disorders, including neurodegenerative diseases, cardiovascular disease, cancer, and developmental abnormalities. Exposure and toxicity have been better understood through the use of reliable biomarkers. Early toxicity is diagnostically assessed using classical matrices, such as blood, urine, and hair, alongside the application of new molecular and imaging biomarkers, which are becoming increasingly precise in elucidating early toxicity and underlying pathways. This progress highlights the value of biomonitoring, not only for identifying high-risk individuals but also for determining interventions at both clinical and population levels. The recognition of vulnerable groups—children, the elderly, malnourished individuals, and those occupationally exposed—underscores the diversity in risk and the need for specific preventative strategies. These populations are at significantly increased risk due to physiological, nutritional, or environmental factors that enhance metal absorption and intoxication. Addressing these disparities requires not only scientific innovation but also an equity-oriented public health policy.

Preventive and management approaches are required to work on multipronged fronts. Nutritional interventions, such as micronutrient supplementation and antioxidant rich diets, can inhibit absorption and counter oxidative effects. On the social level, strict food safety measures, farming processes, and industrial discharges have to be introduced to curb environmental pollution. In clinical practice, chelation therapy and antioxidant supplementation have continued to offer certain value, though it is possible that safer, more naturalized, or more selective modulators will be found in the future.

Future opportunities include the application of improved technologies in the field of omics, personalized medicine, and sustainable remediation measures that could aid in more accurate exposure estimation and intervention. Longitudinal cohort studies that would help clarify dose-response relationships, as well as follow-up on long-term health outcomes in different populations, are required. Just as importantly, international regulatory standards will need to be harmonized, and investment in public education efforts will be needed to minimize the worldwide impact of dietary metal toxicity. To sum up, dietary metals are a complex and multidimensional health risk that requires an interdisciplinary approach, entailing scientific, medical, regulatory, as well as societal interventions. By combining biomarker-based surveillance, targeting risk groups, and holistic prevention activities, it is feasible to reduce the threats of the long-term effects of metal exposure and protect human health for future generations.

References

Abdel-Megeed, R.M., 2021. Probiotics: a promising generation of heavy metal detoxification. Biol. Trace Elem. Res. 199 (6), 2406–2413.

Acharya, S., 2024. Heavy Metal Contamination in Food: sources, Impact, and Remedy. In: Food Safety and Quality in the Global South. Springer Nature Singapore, Singapore, pp. 233–261.

Adams, S.V., Newcomb, P.A., Shafer, M.M., Atkinson, C., Bowles, E.J.A., Newton, K.M., Lampe, J.W., 2011. Sources of cadmium exposure among healthy premenopausal women. Sci. Total Environ. 409 (9), 1632–1637.

Ademuyiwa, O., Agarwal, R., Chandra, R., Behari, J.R., 2010. Effects of sub-chronic low-level lead exposure on the homeostasis of copper and zinc in rat tissues. J. Trace Elem. Med. Biol. 24 (3), 207–211.

Aendo, P., Netvichian, R., Thiendedsakul, P., Khaodhiar, S., Tulayakul, P., 2022. Carcinogenic risk of Pb, Cd, Ni, and Cr and critical ecological risk of Cd and Cu in soil and groundwater around the municipal solid waste open dump in central Thailand. J. Environ. Public Health 2022 (1), 1–12.

Al Bakheet, S.A., Attafi, I.M., Maayah, Z.H., Abd-Allah, A.R., Asiri, Y.A., Korashy, H.M., 2013. Effect of long-term human exposure to environmental heavy metals on the expression of detoxification and DNA repair genes. Environ. Pollut. 181, 226–232.

Ali, H., Khan, E., Ilahi, I., 2019. Environmental chemistry and ecotoxicology of hazardous heavy metals: environmental persistence, toxicity, and bioaccumulation. J. Chem. 2019 (1), 1–14.

Appenroth, K.J., 2009. Definition of "heavy metals" and their role in biological systems. In: Soil Heavy Metals. Springer, Berlin, Heidelberg, pp. 19–29.

Armah, F.A., Obiri, S., Yawson, D.O., Onumah, E.E., Yengoh, G.T., Afrifa, E.K., Odoi, J.O., 2010. Anthropogenic sources and environmentally relevant concentrations of heavy metals in surface water of a mining district in Ghana: a multivariate statistical approach. Journal of Environmental Science and Health Part A 45 (13), 1804–1813.

Aungst, B.J., Fung, H.L., 1981. Kinetic characterization of in vitro lead transport across the rat small intestine: mechanism of intestinal lead transport. Toxicology and Applied Pharmacology 61 (1), 39–47.

Babafemi, O.P., Ajani, T.F., Binuyo, M.O., Ajagbe, A.O., Owonibi, S.K., Ogwu, M.C., 2024. Biomonitoring for sustainable development. In: Biomonitoring of Pollutants in the Global South. Springer Nature Singapore, Singapore, pp. 191–239.

Barber-Zucker, S., Shaanan, B., Zarivach, R., 2017. Transition metal binding selectivity in proteins and its correlation with the phylogenomic classification of the cation diffusion facilitator protein family. Sci. Rep. 7 (1), 1–12. doi:10.1038/s41598-017-16777-5.

Batzias, F.A., Siontorou, C.G., 2006. A knowledge-based approach to environmental biomonitoring. Environmental Monitoring and Assessment 123 (1), 167–197.

Bertini, I., Cavallaro, G., 2008. Metals in the "omics" world: copper homeostasis and cytochrome c oxidase assembly in a new light. JBIC Journal of Biological Inorganic Chemistry 13 (1), 3–14.

Bhattacharyya, P., Chakrabarti, K., Chakraborty, A., Tripathy, S., Powell, M.A., 2008. Fractionation and bioavailability of Pb in municipal solid waste compost and Pb uptake by rice straw and grain under submerged condition in amended soil. Geosciences Journal 12 (1), 41–45.

Birley, M.H., Lock, K., 1998. Health and peri-urban natural resource production. Environ. Urban. 10 (1), 89–106.

Bisset, A. (1980). *Implementation of water pollution control measures: theory and practice* (Doctoral dissertation, Durham University).

Blanusa, M., Varnai, V.M., Piasek, M., Kostial, K., 2005. Chelators as antidotes of metal toxicity: therapeutic and experimental aspects. Curr. Med. Chem. 12 (23), 2771–2794.

Bradl, H. (Ed.), 2005. Heavy Metals in the Environment: Origin, Interaction and Remediation, Vol. 6. Elsevier.

Bradl, H.B., 2005. Sources and origins of heavy metals. In: Interface Science and Technology, Vol. 6. Elsevier, pp. 1–27.

Brand, M.D., 2010. The sites and topology of mitochondrial superoxide production. Exp. Gerontol. 45 (7-8), 466–472.

Buettner, G.R., 1993. The pecking order of free radicals and antioxidants: lipid peroxidation, α-tocopherol, and ascorbate. Arch. Biochem. Biophys. 300 (2), 535–543.

Cao, C., Liang, B.Y., Yang, Y., Ren, D., Tang, Q.H., Wang, C.W., Wang, J., 2024. Temporal variations in absorption and translocation of heavy metal (loid) s in pak choi (Brassica rapa L.) under open-field and greenhouse cultivation. Ecotoxicol. Environ. Saf. 281, 1–9.

Chamoli, A., Karn, S.K., 2024. The effects of mercury exposure on neurological and cognitive dysfunction in human: a review. In:Mercury Toxicity Mitigation: Sustainable Nexus Approach, pp. 117–135.

CHAN, Y.N. (2023). Future Perspective on Elemental Analysis of Non-invasive Samples for Biomonitoring-From Advanced Analytical Methods to Data Analysis.

Chatzopoulou, S., Eriksson, N.L., Eriksson, D., 2020. Improving risk assessment in the European food safety authority: lessons from the European Medicines Agency. Frontiers in Plant Science 11, 349.

Chedrese, P.J., Piasek, M., Henson, M.C., 2006. Cadmium as an endocrine disruptor in the reproductive system. Immunology, Endocrine & Metabolic Agents-Medicinal ChemistryCurrent Medicinal Chemistry-Immunology, Endocrine & Metabolic Agents) 6 (1), 27–35.

Cheng, S., 2003. Heavy metal pollution in China: origin, pattern and control. Environ. Sci. Pollut. Res. 10 (3), 192–198.

Chevillard, S., Radicella, J.P., Levalois, C., Lebeau, J., Poupon, M.F., Oudard, S., Boiteux, S., 1998. Mutations in OGG1, a gene involved in the repair of oxidative DNA damage, are found in human lung and kidney tumours. Oncogene 16 (23), 3083–3086.

Chiocchetti, G., Jadan-Piedra, C., Velez, D., Devesa, V., 2017. Metal (loid) contamination in seafood products. Crit. Rev. Food Sci. Nutr. 57 (17), 3715–3728.

Choi, A.L., Grandjean, P., 2012. Human health significance of dietary exposures to methylmercury. In:Environmental Chemistry and Toxicology of Mercury, vol. 1, pp. 545–568. doi:10.1002/9781118146644.

Chojnacka, K., 2010. Biosorption and bioaccumulation–the prospects for practical applications. Environment International 36 (3), 299–307.

Conrad, M.E., Barton, J.C., 1978. Factors affecting the absorption and excretion of lead in the rat. Gastroenterology 74 (4), 731–740.

D'Souza, C., Peretiatko, R., 2002. The nexus between industrialization and environment: a case study of Indian enterprises. Environmental Management and Health 13 (1), 80–97.

de Carvalho Machado, C., Dinis-Oliveira, R.J., 2023. Clinical and forensic signs resulting from exposure to heavy metals and other chemical elements of the periodic table. J. Clin. Med. 12 (7), 2591.

de Vries, W., Römkens, P.F.A.M., Schütze, G., 2007. Critical soil concentrations of cadmium, lead, and mercury in view of health effects on humans and animals. In:Reviews of Environmental Contamination and Toxicology, vol. 191. Springer, New York, NY, pp. 91–130. doi:10.1007/978-0-387-69163-3_4.

Diamond, G.L., Goodrum, P.E., Felter, S.P., Ruoff, W.L., 1998. Gastrointestinal absorption of metals. Drug Chem. Toxicol. 21 (2), 223–251.

Dixit, R., Wasiullah, X., Malaviya, D., Pandiyan, K., Singh, U.B., Sahu, A., Paul, D., 2015. Bioremediation of heavy metals from soil and aquatic environment: an overview of principles and criteria of fundamental processes. Sustainability 7 (2), 2189–2212.

Driscoll, C.T., Mason, R.P., Chan, H.M., Jacob, D.J., Pirrone, N., 2013. Mercury as a global pollutant: sources, pathways, and effects. Environ. Sci. Technol. 47 (10), 4967–4983.

Duffus, J.H., 2002. " Heavy metals" a meaningless term?(IUPAC Technical Report). Pure Appl. Chem. 74 (5), 793–807.

Ebabhi, A., Adebayo, R., 2022. Nutritional values of vegetables. Veg. Crops-Health Benefits Cultiv. 1839699485, 1–11.

Eckhardt, S., Brunetto, P.S., Gagnon, J., Priebe, M., Giese, B., Fromm, K.M., 2013. Nanobio silver: its interactions with peptides and bacteria, and its uses in medicine. Chemical Reviews 113 (7), 4708–4754.

Eisenstein, R.S., Blemings, K.P., 1998. Iron regulatory proteins, iron responsive elements and iron homeostasis. J. Nutr. 128 (12), 2295–2298.

Elizabeth, K.E., 2020. Micronutrient disorders in tropics. In:IAP Textbook of Tropical Diseases, vol. 1, p. 92.

Fei, X., Lou, Z., Xiao, R., Ren, Z., Lv, X., 2020. Contamination assessment and source apportionment of heavy metals in agricultural soil through the synthesis of PMF and GeogDetector models. Sci. Total Environ. 747, 141293.

Feron, V.J., Cassee, F.R., Groten, J.P., van Vliet, P.W., van Zorge, J.A., 2002. International issues on human health effects of exposure to chemical mixtures. Environmental Health Perspectives 110 (suppl 6), 893–899.

Flora, S.J.S., Mittal, M., Mehta, A., 2008. Heavy metal induced oxidative stress & its possible reversal by chelation therapy. Indian J. Med. Res. 128 (4), 501–523.

Fowler, B.A., Alexander, J., Oskarsson, A., 2015. Toxic metals in food. In: Handbook on the Toxicology of Metals. Academic Press. pp. 123–140.

Freeland-Graves, J., Kodama, H., Klimis-Zacas, D., Hunt, C., Vienna, I.S.T.E.R.H., McClung, A.J., Karakas, S., 2012. Trace elements in health and disease: essentiality, toxicity. J Trace Elem Med Biol 26, 149–152.

Galal-Gorchev, H., 1993. Dietary intake, levels in food and estimated intake of lead, cadmium, and mercury. Food Additives & Contaminants 10 (1), 115–128.

Ganz, T., 2003. Hepcidin, a key regulator of iron metabolism and mediator of anemia of inflammation. Blood 102 (3), 783–788.

Garçon, G., Leleu, B., Zerimech, F., Marez, T., Haguenoer, J.M., Furon, D., Shirali, P., 2004. Biologic markers of oxidative stress and nephrotoxicity as studied in biomonitoring of adverse effects of occupational exposure to lead and cadmium. J. Occup. Environ. Med. 46 (11), 1180–1186.

Garrett, R.G., 2000. Natural sources of metals to the environment. Hum. Ecol. Risk Assess. 6 (6), 945–963.

Garza-Lombó, C., Posadas, Y., Quintanar, L., Gonsebatt, M.E., Franco, R., 2018. Neurotoxicity linked to dysfunctional metal ion homeostasis and xenobiotic metal exposure: redox signaling and oxidative stress. Antioxidants & Redox Signaling 28 (18), 1669–1703.

Gerster-Bentaya, M., 2015. Urban agriculture's contributions to urban food security and nutrition. In:Cities and Agriculture: Developing Resilient Urban Food Systems, vol. 1, pp. 139–161.

Gibson, R.S., Hotz, C., Temple, L., Yeudall, F., Mtitimuni, B., Ferguson, E., 2000. Dietary strategies to combat deficiencies of iron, zinc, and vitamin A in developing countries: development, implementation, monitoring, and evaluation. Food and Nutrition Bulletin 21 (2), 219–231.

Gu, J., Dai, S., Liu, Y., Liu, H., Zhang, Y., Ji, X., Shi, H., 2018. Activation of Ca2+-sensing receptor as a protective pathway to reduce Cadmium-induced cytotoxicity in renal proximal tubular cells. Sci. Rep. 8 (1), 1092.

Guala, S.D., Vega, F.A., Covelo, E.F., 2010. The dynamics of heavy metals in plant–soil interactions. Ecol. Model. 221 (8), 1148–1152.

Guo, Y., Lundebye, A.K., Li, N., Ergon, Å., Pang, S., Jiang, Y., Aakre, I., 2023. Comparative assessment of food safety regulations and standards for arsenic, cadmium, lead, mercury and iodine in macroalgae used as food and feed in China and Europe. Trends Food Sci. Technol. 141, 1–11.

Halliwell, B., Gutteridge, J.M., 1990. Role of free radicals and catalytic metal ions in human disease: an overview. Methods Enzymol. 186, 1–85.

Hejna, M., Gottardo, D., Baldi, A., Dell'Orto, V., Cheli, F., Zaninelli, M., Rossi, L., 2018. Nutritional ecology of heavy metals. Animal 12 (10), 2156–2170.

Henson, M.C., Piasek, M., Chedrese, P.J., Castracane, V.D., 2016. Metal toxicity in mammalian reproduction. In: Endocrine Toxicology. CRC Press. pp. 270–293.

Hida, T., Kozaki, K.I., Ito, H., Miyaishi, O., Tatematsu, Y., Suzuki, T., Takahashi, T., 2002. Significant growth inhibition of human lung cancer cells both in vitro and in vivo by the combined use of a selective cyclooxygenase 2 inhibitor, JTE-522, and conventional anticancer agents. Clinical Cancer Research 8 (7), 2443–2447.

Hida, T., Kozaki, K.I., Muramatsu, H., Masuda, A., Shimizu, S., Mitsudomi, T., Takahashi, T., 2000. Cyclooxygenase-2 inhibitor induces apoptosis and enhances cytotoxicity of various anticancer agents in non-small cell lung cancer cell lines. Clin. Cancer Res. 6 (5), 2006–2011.

Hillstrom, R.J., Lynch, S.M., Yacapin-Ammons, A.K., 2003. Vitamin C inhibits lipid oxidation in human HDL. J. Nutr. 133 (10), 3047–3051.

Hines, N.W., 2013. History of the 1972 Clean water act: the story behind how the 1972 act became the capstone on a decade of extraordinary environmental reform. Geo. Wash. J. Energy & Envtl. L 4, 80.

Hontela, A., Lacroix, A., 2006. Heavy Metals. Oxford University Press, UK, pp. 356–374.

Huang, N., Wang, B., Liu, S., Wang, K., Wang, R., Liu, F., Chen, C., 2025. Cadmium exposure in infants and children: toxicity, health effects, dietary risk assessment and mitigation strategies. Crit. Rev. Food Sci. Nutr. 65 (26) , 5085–5107. doi:10.1080/10408398.2024.2403036.

Hurst, H.E., Martin, M.D., 2017. Toxicology, Pharmacology and Therapeutics for Dentistry (Seventh Edition), Mosby, vol. 1, pp. 603–620. doi:10.1016/B978-0-323-39307-2.00040-0.

Jaishankar, M., Tseten, T., Anbalagan, N., Mathew, B.B., Beeregowda, K.N., 2014. Toxicity, mechanism and health effects of some heavy metals. Interdiscip. Toxicol. 7 (2), 60.

Jakimska-Nagórska, A., Konieczka, P., Skóra, K., Namieśnik, J., 2011. Bioaccumulation of metals in tissues of marine animals, part I: the role and impact of heavy metals on organisms. Pol. J. Environ. Stud. 20, 1117–1125.

Jan, A.T., Ali, A., Haq, Q.M.R., 2011. Glutathione as an antioxidant in inorganic mercury induced nephrotoxicity. Journal of Postgraduate Medicine 57 (1), 72–77.

Jan, A.T., Azam, M., Siddiqui, K., Ali, A., Choi, I., Haq, Q.M.R., 2015. Heavy metals and human health: mechanistic insight into toxicity and counter defense system of antioxidants. Int. J. Mol. Sci. 16 (12), 29592–29630.

Jellesen, M.S., Rasmussen, A.A., Hilbert, L.R., 2006. A review of metal release in the food industry. Materials and Corrosion 57 (5), 387–393.

Jomova, K., Alomar, S.Y., Valko, R., Nepovimova, E., Kuca, K., Valko, M., 2025. The role of redox-active iron, copper, manganese, and redox-inactive zinc in toxicity, oxidative stress, and human diseases. EXCLI Journal 24, 880–954.

Jomova, K., Valko, M., 2011. Advances in metal-induced oxidative stress and human disease. Toxicology 283 (2-3), 65–87.

Kasten-Jolly, J., Lawrence, D.A., 2018. The cationic (calcium and lead) and enzyme conundrum. Journal of Toxicology and Environmental Health, Part B 21 (6-8), 400–413.

Kaur, I., Behl, T., Aleya, L., Rahman, M.H., Kumar, A., Arora, S., Akter, R., 2021. Role of metallic pollutants in neurodegeneration: effects of aluminum, lead, mercury, and arsenic in mediating brain impairment events and autism spectrum disorder. Environ. Sci. Pollut. Res. 28 (8), 8989–9001.

Kern, M., Wisniewski, M., Cabell, L., Audesirk, G., 2000. Inorganic lead and calcium interact positively in activation of calmodulin. Neurotoxicology 21 (3), 353–363.

Khan, S., Cao, Q., Zheng, Y.M., Huang, Y.Z., Zhu, Y.G., 2008. Health risks of heavy metals in contaminated soils and food crops irrigated with wastewater in Beijing, China. Environ. Pollut. 152 (3), 686–692.

Kosiba, A.A., Wang, Y., Chen, D., Wong, C.K.C., Gu, J., Shi, H., 2020. The roles of calcium-sensing receptor (CaSR) in heavy metals-induced nephrotoxicity. Life Sci. 242, 117183. doi:10.1016/j.lfs.2019.117183.

Lawatı, A.A., Hashmı, L.A., Aswamı, H.A., Hadhrami, A.A., Chin, K.Y., Sirasanagandla, S.R., Das, S., 2024. Deleterious Biological Effects of Endocrine Disruptors: an Insight into Human Health Risks. Endocrine, Metabolic & Immune Disorders-Drug Targets (Formerly Current Drug Targets-Immune, Endocrine & Metabolic Disorders) 24 (13), 1471–1479.

Li, C., Zhou, K., Qin, W., Tian, C., Qi, M., Yan, X., Han, W., 2019. A review on heavy metals contamination in soil: effects, sources, and remediation techniques. Soil and Sediment Contamination: An International Journal 28 (4), 380–394.

Linder, M.C., Hazegh-Azam, M., 1996. Copper biochemistry and molecular biology. The American Journal of Clinical Nutrition 63 (5), 797S–811S.

Liu, J., Zhang, X.H., Tran, H., Wang, D.Q., Zhu, Y.N., 2011. Heavy metal contamination and risk assessment in water, paddy soil, and rice around an electroplating plant. Environ. Sci. Pollut. Res. 18 (9), 1623–1632.

Liu, Y.E., Wu, G., Feng, L., Li, J., Xia, Y., Guo, W., Zhao, K., 2025. Harnessing Antioxidants in Cancer Therapy: opportunities, Challenges, and Future Directions. Antioxidants 14 (6), 674.

Lodhi, T., Rohatgi, R., Pathak, S.R., 2024. Biomedical Wastes as Environmental Toxicants. In: Bioremediation of Environmental Toxicants. CRC Press. pp. 73–84.

Mahaffey, K.R., Corneliussen, P.E., Jelinek, C.F., Fiorino, J.A., 1975. Heavy metal exposure from foods. Environ. Health Perspect. 12, 63–69.

Manna, S., Firdous, S.M., 2025. Unravelling the developmental toxicity of heavy metals using zebrafish as a model: a narrative review. BioMetals 38 (2) , 419–463. doi:10.1007/s10534-025-00671-z.

Martinez-Morata, I., Sobel, M., Tellez-Plaza, M., Navas-Acien, A., Howe, C.G., Sanchez, T.R., 2023. A state-of-the-science review on metal biomarkers. Curr. Environ. Health Rep. 10 (3), 215–249.

Mattie, M.D., Freedman, J.H., 2004. Copper-inducible transcription: regulation by metal-and oxidative stressresponsive pathways. Am. J. Physiol.-Cell Physiol. 286 (2), C293–C301.

Maynard, R.L., 2000. Environmental toxicants: human exposures and their health effects. Occup. Environ. Med. 57 (7), 503. doi:10.1136/oem.57.7.503c .

Meharg, A.A., 2004. Arsenic in rice–understanding a new disaster for South-East Asia. Trends Plant Sci. 9 (9), 415–417.

Mertz, W., 1969. Chromium occurrence and function in biological systems. Physiol. Rev. 49 (2), 163–239.

Miki, Y., 2023. Hormone-dependent cancers: new aspects on biochemistry and molecular pathology. Int. J. Mol. Sci. 24 (13), 1–4. doi:10.3390/ijms241310830.

Mishra, S., Bharagava, R.N., More, N., Yadav, A., Zainith, S., Mani, S., Chowdhary, P., 2018. Heavy metal contamination: an alarming threat to environment and human health. In: Environmental Biotechnology: For Sustainable Future. Springer Singapore, Singapore, pp. 103–125.

Mohammad, A.M., Chowdhury, T., Biswas, B., Absar, N., 2018. Food poisoning and intoxication: a global leading concern for human health. In: Food Safety and Preservation. Academic Press. pp. 307–352.

Mondal, K., Ghosh, S., Haque, S., 2018. A review on contamination, bioaccumulation and toxic effect of cadmium, mercury and lead on freshwater fishes. Int. J. Zool. Stud 3 (2), 153–159.

Morais, S., Costa, F.G., Pereira, M.D.L., 2012. Heavy metals and human health. Environ. Health–Emerg. Issues Pract. 10 (1), 227–245.

Mudgal, V., Madaan, N., Mudgal, A., Singh, R.B., Mishra, S., 2010. Effect of toxic metals on human health. Open Nutraceuticals J. 3 (1), 94–99.

Nnaji, N.D., Onyeaka, H., Miri, T., Ugwa, C., 2023. Bioaccumulation for heavy metal removal: a review. SN Appl. Sci. 5 (5), 125.

Nsubuga, P., White, M.E., Thacker, S.B., Anderson, M.A., Blount, S.B., Broome, C.V., Trostle, M. (2011). Public health surveillance: a tool for targeting and monitoring interventions.

Obasi, P.N., Akudinobi, B.B., 2020. Potential health risk and levels of heavy metals in water resources of lead–zinc mining communities of Abakaliki, southeast Nigeria. Appl. Water Sci. 10 (7), 1–23.

Obuzor, G.U., Onyedikachi, U.B., 2023. Chemical leaching into food and the environment poses health hazards. In: Modernity in Health and Disease Diagnosis: The Account from STEM Women. Springer Nature Switzerland, Cham, pp. 129–148.

Ogidi, O.I., Onwuagba, C.G., Richard-Nwachukwu, N., 2024. Biomonitoring tools, techniques and approaches for environmental assessments. In: Biomonitoring of Pollutants in the Global South. Springer Nature Singapore, Singapore, pp. 243–273.

Olmedo, P., Pla, A., Hernández, A.F., Barbier, F., Ayouni, L., Gil, F., 2013. Determination of toxic elements (mercury, cadmium, lead, tin and arsenic) in fish and shellfish samples. Risk assessment for the consumers. Environment International 59, 63–72.

Onakpa, M.M., Njan, A.A., Kalu, O.C., 2018. A review of heavy metal contamination of food crops in Nigeria. Ann. Glob. Health 84 (3), 488.

Oros, A., Coatu, V., Damir, N., Danilov, D., Ristea, E., Lazar, L., 2025. Molecular Mechanisms and Biomarker-Based Early-Warning Indicators of Heavy Metal Toxicity in Marine Fish. Fishes 10 (7), 339.

Othman, N.M., 2007. Food safety in Southeast Asia: challenges facing the region. Asian Journal of Agriculture and Development 4 (2), 83–92.

Patel, J., Patel, A., 2017. The role of nutritional factors in pathogenesis of diseases. In: Nutrigenomics and Nutraceuticals. CRC Press. pp. 483–514.

Patra, D.K., Pradhan, C., Patra, H.K., 2020. Toxic metal decontamination by phytoremediation approach: concept, challenges, opportunities and future perspectives. Environ. Technol. Innov. 18, 100672. doi:10.1016/j.eti.2020.100672 .

Patrick, L., 2006. Lead toxicity, a review of the literature. Part I: exposure, evaluation, and treatment. Altern. Med. Rev. 11 (1), 2–22.

Peraza, M.A., Ayala-Fierro, F., Barber, D.S., Casarez, E., Rael, L.T., 1998. Effects of micronutrients on metal toxicity. Environ. Health Perspect. 106 (suppl 1), 203–216.

Piazza, G.A., Keeton, A.B., Tinsley, H.N., Gary, B.D., Whitt, J.D., Mathew, B., Reynolds, R.C., 2009. A novel sulindac derivative that does not inhibit cyclooxygenases but potently inhibits colon tumor cell growth and induces apoptosis with antitumor activity. Cancer Prev. Res. 2 (6), 572–580.

Prousek, J., 2007. Fenton chemistry in biology and medicine. Pure Appl. Chem. 79 (12), 2325–2338.

Raffoul, J.J., Sarkar, F.H., Hillman, G.G., 2007. Radiosensitization of prostate cancer by soy isoflavones. Current Cancer Drug Targets 7 (8), 759–765.

Randhawa, M.A., Khan, A.A., Javed, M.S., Sajid, M.W., 2015. Green leafy vegetables: a health promoting source. In: Handbook of Fertility. Academic press. pp. 205–220.

Ray, S., Shaju, S.T., 2023. Bioaccumulation of pesticides in fish resulting toxicities in humans through food chain and forensic aspects. Environmental Analysis, Health and Toxicology 38, e2023017.

Raza, A., Hussain, S., Javed, R., Hafeez, M.B., Hasanuzzaman, M., 2021. Antioxidant defense systems and remediation of metal toxicity in plants. In: Approaches to the Remediation of Inorganic Pollutants. Springer Singapore, Singapore, pp. 91–124.

Reilly, C., 2008. Metal Contamination of Food: Its Significance for Food Quality and Human Health, John Wiley & Sons.

Requejo, R., Chouchani, E.T., Hurd, T.R., Menger, K.E., Hampton, M.B., Murphy, M.P., 2010. Measuring mitochondrial protein thiol redox state. In: Methods in Enzymology, Vol. 474. Academic Press, pp. 123–147.

Robert, G., Mari, G., 2003. Human health effects of metals. In: *US Environmental Protection Agency Risk Assessment Forum, Washington, DC*, vol. 23, pp. 1–49. https://www.epa.gov/sites/default/files/2014-11/documents/human_health_effects.pdf.

Robson, M., 2003. Methodologies for assessing exposures to metals: human host factors. Ecotoxicol. Environ. Saf. 56 (1), 104–109.

Rodríguez-Antona, C., Taron, M., 2015. Pharmacogenomic biomarkers for personalized cancer treatment. J. Intern. Med. 277 (2), 201–217.

Rodriguez, B.L., Curb, J.D., Davis, J., Shintani, T., Perez, M.H., Apau-Ludlum, N., Harrigan, R.C., 2012. Use of the dietary supplement 5-aminiolevulinic acid (5-ALA) and its relationship with glucose levels and hemoglobin A1C among individuals with prediabetes. Clin. Transl. Sci. 5 (4), 314–320.

Rose, M., 2023. Pollutants, residues and other contaminants in foods obtained from marine and fresh water. In: Present Knowledge in Food Safety. Academic Press. pp. 128–141.

Rossi, S.C., Gorman, N., Wetterhahn, K.E., 1988. Mitochondrial reduction of the carcinogen chromate: formation of chromium (V). Chem. Res. Toxicol. 1 (2), 101–107.

Rudnik, E., 2024. Review on gallium in coal and coal waste materials: exploring strategies for hydrometallurgical metal recovery. Molecules 29 (24), 5919.

Runnells, D.D., Shepherd, T.A., Angino, E.E., 1992. Metals in water. Determining natural background concentrations in mineralized areas. Environmental Science & Technology 26 (12), 2316–2323.

Sah, A.K., Elshaikh, R.H., Shalabi, M.G., Abbas, A.M., Prabhakar, P.K., Babker, A.M., Agarwal, S., 2025. Role of artificial intelligence and personalized medicine in enhancing hiv management and treatment outcomes. Life 15 (5), 745.

Saher, N.U., Kanwal, N., 2019. Assessment of some heavy metal accumulation and nutritional quality of shellfish with reference to human health and cancer risk assessment: a seafood safety approach. Environ. Sci. Pollut. Res. 26 (5), 5189–5201.

Sahin, K., Sahin, N., Kucuk, O., 2003. Effects of chromium, and ascorbic acid supplementation on growth, carcass traits, serum metabolites, and antioxidant status of broiler chickens reared at a high ambient temperature (32 C). Nutrition Research 23 (2), 225–238.

Sarkar, F.H., Li, Y., 2006. Using chemopreventive agents to enhance the efficacy of cancer therapy. Cancer Research 66 (7), 3347–3350.

Sexton, K., Callahan, M.A., Bryan, E.F., 1995. Estimating exposure and dose to characterize health risks: the role of human tissue monitoring in exposure assessment. Environmental Health Perspectives 103 (suppl 3), 13–29.

Shahid, M., Khalid, S., Abbas, G., Shahid, N., Nadeem, M., Sabir, M., Dumat, C., 2015. Heavy metal stress and crop productivity. In: Crop Production and Global Environmental Issues. Springer International Publishing, Cham, pp. 1–25.

Sheng, J., Wang, X., Gong, P., Tian, L., Yao, T., 2012. Heavy metals of the Tibetan top soils: level, source, spatial distribution, temporal variation and risk assessment. Environ. Sci. Pollut. Res. 19 (8), 3362–3370.

Singh, S., Parihar, P., Singh, R., Singh, V.P., Prasad, S.M., 2016. Heavy metal tolerance in plants: role of transcriptomics, proteomics, metabolomics, and ionomics. Front. Plant Sci. 6, 1143.

Sonone, S.S., Jadhav, S., Sankhla, M.S., Kumar, R., 2020. Water contamination by heavy metals and their toxic effect on aquaculture and human health through food Chain. Lett. Appl. NanoBioSci. 10 (2), 2148–2166.

Spacie, A., McCarty, L.S., Rand, G.M., 2020. Bioaccumulation and bioavailability in multiphase systems. In: Fundamentals of Aquatic Toxicology. CRC Press. pp. 493–521.

Speisky, H., Gómez, M., Carrasco-Pozo, C., Pastene, E., Lopez-Alarcón, C., Olea-Azar, C., 2008. Cu (I)–Glutathione complex: a potential source of superoxide radicals generation. Bioorganic & Medicinal Chemistry 16 (13), 6568–6574.

Srivastava, P., Kowshik, M., 2013. Mechanisms of metal resistance and homeostasis in haloarchaea. Archaea 2013 (1), 1–16.

Stankovic, S., Stankovic, A.R., 2013. Bioindicators of toxic metals. Green Mater. Energy Prod. Depollut. 3, 151–228. https://hero.epa.gov/reference/6709147/.

Stohs, S.J., Bagchi, D., Hassoun, E., Bagchi, M., 2001. Oxidative mechanisms in the toxicity of chromium and cadmium ions. J. Environ. Pathol. Toxicol. Oncol. 19 (3), 201–213.

Sunilson, J.A.J., Rejitha, G., Anandarajagopal, K., Amitava Das, A.D., Muthappan, M., Promwichit, P. (2009). Cytotoxic effect of Cayratia carnosa leaves on human breast cancer cell lines.

Tang, J., Zhang, J., Ren, L., Zhou, Y., Gao, J., Luo, L., Chen, A., 2019. Diagnosis of soil contamination using microbiological indices: a review on heavy metal pollution. J. Environ. Manage. 242, 121–130.

Tangahu, B.V., Sheikh Abdullah, S.R., Basri, H., Idris, M., Anuar, N., Mukhlisin, M., 2011. A review on heavy metals (As, Pb, and Hg) uptake by plants through phytoremediation. Int. J. Chem. Eng. 2011 (1), 1–31.

Tetteh, H. (2022). *Convenience food and its packaging effect on human health a case study of Bantama market* (Doctoral dissertation, University of Education, Winneba).

Tiwari, S., Lata, C., 2018. Heavy metal stress, signaling, and tolerance due to plant-associated microbes: an overview. Front. Plant Sci. 9, 452.

Torkelsen, S.E., 1985. Cross-national Social Work: A Residential Model for Homeless Children in Guatemala (Orphans, Model Adaptation, Organizational, Locality Development, Exchange Theory), City University of New York.

Valko, M., Jomova, K., Rhodes, C.J., Kuča, K., Musílek, K., 2016. Redox-and non-redox-metal-induced formation of free radicals and their role in human disease. Arch. Toxicol. 90 (1), 1–37.

Wang, H.A., Grolimund, D., Van Loon, L.R., Barmettler, K., Borca, C.N., Aeschlimann, B., Gunther, D., 2011. Quantitative chemical imaging of element diffusion into heterogeneous media using laser ablation inductively coupled plasma mass spectrometry, synchrotron micro-X-ray fluorescence, and extended X-ray absorption fine structure spectroscopy. Anal. Chem. 83 (16), 6259–6266.

Wang, Z., Sun, Y., Yao, W., Ba, Q., Wang, H., 2021. Effects of cadmium exposure on the immune system and immunoregulation. Front. Immunol. 12, 1–15. doi:10.3389/fimmu.2021.695484.

Wuana, R.A., Okieimen, F.E., 2011. Heavy metals in contaminated soils: a review of sources, chemistry, risks and best available strategies for remediation. Int. Sch. Res. Not. 2011 (1), 1–20. doi:10.5402/2011/402647.

Xu, W., Jin, Y., Zeng, G., 2024. Introduction of heavy metals contamination in the water and soil: a review on source, toxicity and remediation methods. Green Chem. Lett. Rev. 17 (1), 1–25. doi:10.1080/17518253.2024.2404235.

Yan, L.J., Allen, D.C., 2021. Cadmium-induced kidney injury: oxidative damage as a unifying mechanism. Biomolecules 11 (11), 1575.

Yon, J.M., Baek, I.J., Lee, S.R., Jin, Y., Kim, M.R., Nahm, S.S., Nam, S.Y., 2008. The spatio-temporal expression pattern of cytoplasmic Cu/Zn superoxide dismutase (SOD1) mRNA during mouse embryogenesis. J. Mol. Histol. 39 (1), 95–103.

Young, T.R., Xiao, Z., 2021. Principles and practice of determining metal–protein affinities. Biochemical Journal 478 (5), 1085–1116.

Yuan, Y.V., 2007. 11 Marine Algal. Mar. Nutraceuticals Funct. Foods 259, 1–20.

Zabochnicka-Świątek, M., Krzywonos, M., 2014. Potentials of biosorption and bioaccumulation processes for heavy metal removal. Pol. J. Environ. Stud. 23 (2), 551–561.

Zang, F., Wang, S., Nan, Z., Ma, J., Zhang, Q., Chen, Y., Li, Y., 2017. Accumulation, spatio-temporal distribution, and risk assessment of heavy metals in the soil-corn system around a polymetallic mining area from the Loess Plateau, northwest China. Geoderma 305, 188–196.

Zhang, W., Chen, Y., Qi, Y., Hong, C., 2018. Seasonal variations of mercury levels and human health risk in vegetables from Arid Oasis (Shihezi city), Xinjiang, Northwest China. Human and Ecological Risk Assessment: An International Journal 24 (1), 122–136.

Zhang, Y., Gladyshev, V.N., 2009. Comparative genomics of trace elements: emerging dynamic view of trace element utilization and function. Chemical Reviews 109 (10), 4828–4861.

Chapter 16

Regulation of metal contaminants in food and ecosystems: Global perspectives

Vandana Singh[a], Ankush Verma[b], Amit Pratap Singh Chouhan[b], Anmol Kumar[c], and Shabir Ahmad Padder[d]

[a]*Department of Microbiology, Sharda School of Allied Health Sciences, Sharda University, Greater Noida, Uttar Pradesh, India*

[b]*Department of Radiology, School of Allied Health Sciences, Galgotias University, Greater Noida, Uttar Pradesh, India*

[c]*Department of Radiology, Santosh Medical College, Ghaziabad, Uttar Pradesh, India*

[d]*Govt. Degree College Kilam, Kulgam, Jammu and Kashmir, India*

16.1 Introduction

The contamination of food and ecosystems with toxic metals has emerged as a critical global concern, transcending geographical boundaries and impacting populations across diverse socioeconomic strata. Unlike organic pollutants that may degrade over time, metals are persistent elements that cannot be destroyed, only transformed or redistributed, making their long-term management particularly challenging. The ubiquity of metals in the Earth's crust, combined with extensive anthropogenic activities, has created a complex web of contamination pathways that affect agricultural systems, water resources, and ultimately human food supplies. The significance of this issue is underscored by the World Health Organization's (WHO) estimates that exposure to heavy metals contributes to millions of disability-adjusted life years lost annually, with particularly severe impacts on children's cognitive development and adults' cardiovascular and renal health (FAO/WHO, 2021; Al-Musharraf and Rahman, 2025).

The regulatory landscape governing metal contaminants is characterized by a patchwork of international guidelines, regional standards, and national regulations that often reflect varying risk assessments, analytical capabilities, and socioeconomic priorities. This fragmentation creates challenges for global trade, consumer protection, and environmental management, particularly as food supply chains become increasingly internationalized. The

The Metallome in Motion. https://doi.org/10.1016/B978-0-443-44299-5.00017-1

EU's comprehensive approach under the General Food Law Regulation, the United States' multiagency framework involving the Food and Drug Administration (FDA) and Environmental Protection Agency (EPA), and the Codex Alimentarius Commission's international standards represent different philosophical approaches to risk management, each with distinct strengths and limitations (European Commission, 2022; U.S. Food and Drug Administration, 2023; Codex Alimentarius Commission, 2023; Aslam et al., 2023).

This chapter aims to provide a comprehensive synthesis of current knowledge on metal contaminant regulation, examining the scientific foundations that inform policy decisions, the practical challenges of implementation, and the emerging trends that will shape future regulatory approaches (Fig. 16.1). In addition, the chapter also analyzes the full spectrum of considerations, from source identification and environmental behavior to human health impacts and mitigation strategies. The scope encompasses both essential metals that become toxic at elevated concentrations and nonessential metals that pose risks at any exposure level. Particular attention is given to regulatory harmonization efforts, the balance between protection and practicality in standard setting, and the special challenges faced by developing countries in implementing effective monitoring and enforcement programs.

The global perspective adopted in this chapter reflects the reality that metal contamination does not respect political boundaries, and effective management requires international cooperation, knowledge sharing, and capacity building. Through comparative analysis of regulatory frameworks and examination of successful case studies, the chapter identifies persistent gaps in the

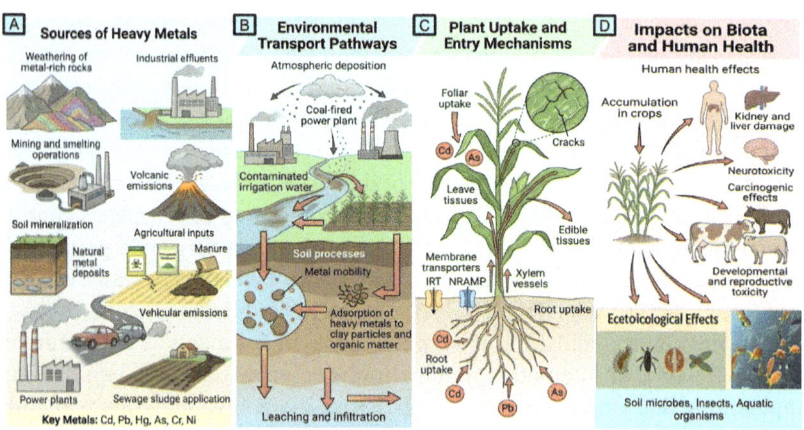

FIG. 16.1 This visual synthesis illustrates the global distribution of heavy metal contamination, the varying stringency of regional regulatory frameworks, and the environmental pathways through which metals like lead and cadmium move from industrial and natural sources into food systems, ultimately impacting human health and ecosystems.

current system and provides recommendations for more coherent and effective approaches to protecting food safety and environmental health worldwide. This comprehensive treatment aims to serve as a valuable resource for researchers, policymakers, and practitioners working to address one of the most complex environmental health challenges of our time.

16.2 Types and toxicological characteristics of metal contaminants

16.2.1 Essential and nonessential metals

For the purpose of human and environmental health, metals can be classified into two broad categories. Essential metals such as Fe, Zn, Cu, Mn, and Se are involved in enzymatic mechanisms, structures, and metabolic pathways. However, these elements can also be toxic at concentrations higher than what is physiologically needed, illustrating the well-known fact that toxicity depends on dose. The therapeutic window of essential metals varies widely across species and populations, making it difficult to develop common regulatory norms. For example, selenium deficiency results in Keshan disease, whereas excessive levels induce selenosis with classical features such as hair loss, nail brittleness, and neurological effects (Haq et al., 2023).

Nonessential metals, on the other hand, do not have an established biological role and can exert harmful effects even at low concentrations. And, of course, there are the old poisonous heavy metals: lead, cadmium, mercury, and arsenic, which above all have been the subject of extensive regulation in view of their established toxicity and environmental persistence. The line between essential and nonessential metals has become increasingly blurred as burgeoning information suggests that different metals interact with each other in a complex manner in biological systems. For instance, cadmium can disturb Zn-enzyme systems, and lead can compete with Ca to be bound in bone tissue, as indicated by the cross-correlation of metal toxicology (Chowdhury et al., 2024).

16.2.2 Toxic heavy metals of concern (Pb, Cd, Hg, As, Cr)

Lead (Pb) remains one of the most concerning environmental contaminants, despite significant historical successes in regulating exposure from gasoline and paint. The neurotoxicity of lead is especially significant in children, with cognitive deficits occurring at levels as low as 5 μg/dL. The similar calcium–metal behavior enables it to pass through the blood-brain barrier, thus disrupting neurotransmitter systems, synaptogenesis, and myelination. In adults, chronic exposure to lead is associated with hypertension, renal failure, and reproductive toxicity, with new reports highlighting its effect on cardiovascular mortality at doses previously thought to be safe in terms of occupational exposure levels (Singh et al., 2025).

Cadmium (Cd) is found to be selectively toxic to the kidneys, leading to proximal tubular damage and possible subsequent renal failure upon chronic exposure. Its long biological half-life allows the gradual accumulation of the metal in organs such as the kidney cortex. The International Agency for Research on Cancer (IARC's), WHO inclusion of cadmium in the category for carcinogenicity is based primarily on the solid association between occupational exposure and lung cancer, though it has also been positively associated with bone demineralization and fractures (Jaishankar et al., 2023).

Mercury (Hg) is found in several species with different toxicological characteristics. The CNS is most affected by exposure to elemental mercury vapor; however, inorganic compounds of mercury tend to affect the kidneys and intestinal tract. The organic form that bio accumulates in aquatic food webs, methylmercury, is especially neurotoxic and results in severe functional deficits among fetuses and children. The Minamata incident in Japan, which swept the nation with its disastrous impact, proved how serious the adverse effects of methylmercury can be and prompted a regulatory response at the international level, such as the enactment of the Minamata Convention on Mercury. The metal can chelate sulfhydryl groups in proteins, thereby inhibiting enzymes and cellular signaling pathways systemically (Singh et al., 2025)

Arsenic (As), which is a metalloid, can be considered in discussions of toxic metals because it possesses similar environmental characteristics and health effects. Inorganic arsenic compounds are highly carcinogenic and strongly linked with skin, bladder, and lung cancers via oral exposure and inhalation. Prolonged arsenic exposure also leads to characteristic skin lesions, peripheral neuropathy, and cardiovascular disease. The broad biological impacts of the metal are due to its inhibition of cellular respiration and disruption of DNA methylation patterns (Singh et al., 2025)

Chromium (Cr) shows opposite toxicological characteristics depending on its oxidation state. Chromium(III) is an essential trace element and a cofactor in glucose metabolism; however, compounds containing hexavalent chromium are acknowledged as occupational carcinogens, primarily affecting the lungs through inhalation. The high solubility and cellular uptake of hexavalent chromium enable its interaction with DNA, leading to mutations and chromosomal damage. The extensive industrial applications of the metal in plating, pigment manufacturing, and wood treatment have resulted in numerous cases of environmental contamination, warranting clean-up efforts with attention paid by regulatory authorities to the associated risks (Kabir et al., 2024).

16.2.3 Bioaccumulation, biomagnification, and toxicity mechanisms

Bioaccumulation refers to the progressive buildup of metals in individual organisms over time, resulting from the net balance between uptake and elimination rates. This process is particularly pronounced for metals with long biological half-lives, such as cadmium and lead, which can accumulate in specific target organs over decades of low-level exposure. The concept of bioaccumulation underlies many regulatory approaches that establish tolerable daily intake values based on chronic exposure scenarios rather than acute toxicity thresholds. Biomagnification (BMF) describes the increasing concentration of metals as they move up trophic levels in food webs. While this phenomenon is most pronounced for organic compounds like dichloro-diphenyl-trichloroethane (DDT), certain metals, particularly mercury and arsenic, demonstrate significant BMF potential in aquatic ecosystems. Methylmercury's strong binding to proteins and limited excretion efficiency results in concentration increases of up to tenfold between trophic levels, explaining why predatory fish species often exceed regulatory limits even when environmental concentrations appear low. The molecular mechanisms underlying metal toxicity involve multiple pathways that often act synergistically. Oxidative stress represents a common mechanism, as many metals undergo redox cycling and generate reactive oxygen species that damage cellular components. Protein dysfunction occurs through direct binding to sulfhydryl groups in critical enzymes and structural proteins, while DNA damage results from direct metal-DNA interactions and indirect oxidative stress. Disruption of calcium homeostasis, interference with essential metal metabolism, and activation of stress response pathways further contribute to the complex toxicological profiles of metal contaminants (Khan et al., 2023).

16.3 Sources of metal contamination

16.3.1 Natural geogenic sources

Nearly all metals in the environment originate from natural geological processes and can be found at extremely variable concentrations, depending on bedrock compos ition, soil-forming processes, and geochemical situations. Ultramafic and mafic rocks have high levels of nickel, chromium, and cobalt, while sulfide ore deposits create localized enrichments of lead, zinc, and copper. Weathering of these deposits gradually releases these metals into soils and surface water, forming natural background loadings, even in amounts that can sometimes exceed statute-based guidelines and interfere with source apportionment studies. Another important natural source is volcanism, which releases significant amounts of metal into the atmosphere during an eruption. Plutonic plume research has shown higher concentrations of arsenic, mercury, and other toxic heavy metals that can travel thousands of kilometers before they are deposited, such as during the Icelandic (2010) Eyjafjallajökull eruption, which, for instance, injected ~30,000 tons of iron in addition to a plethora of other metals into the atmosphere, degrading air quality and numerous European soil systems suitable for agriculture. Background levels, being variable, require a regional to location-specific approach to regulation, which takes geological heterogeneity into account in deriving Environmental Quality Standards (Kumar et al., 2021).

16.3.2 Human impact and industrial sources

Industries are the main source of metal contamination in most populated areas, where metal mining and smelting activities are major contributors to environmental loadings. The mining industry produces enormous volumes of waste rock and tailings with high metal content that, if not managed properly, could lead to contaminated surface water and ground water as a result of acid mine drainage. Anthropogenic industrial manufacturing activities discharge a wide range of metals through point source discharges and diffuse atmospheric releases. Chromium, nickel, and zinc are discharged as effluents in wastewater streams from metal plating industries, while lead and cadmium are found in particulate matter released during cement production. The electronics manufacturing industry, though increasingly regulated, has traditionally used lead-based solders and a variety of toxic metals to manufacture components, and these areas are often hotspots for localized contamination near the manufacturing facility. Agricultural activities also constitute a major anthropogenic source, often due to the use of phosphate fertilizers, which are naturally contaminated with cadmium. Cadmium can build up in the soil over time when fertilizer is applied on a long-term basis, and this has been shown to occur in Europe and North America, with European studies documenting rising levels of cadmium in farming soils during the last century. Pesticide residues, and particularly arsenical applications historically used in orchard crops, cause long-term soil contamination and crop uptake even decades after the last application (Li et al., 2025).

16.3.3 New sources: E-waste, nanomaterials and urban runoff

E-waste has become a significant new source of metallic contamination, especially in developing countries that accept much of the world's e-waste and where informal recycling is on the rise. Discarded electronics are a rich source of valuable metals (such as copper, gold, and silver) and hazardous substances (like lead-based solder, mercury, and cadmium). Exposure during inappropriate recycling can result in serious environmental problems. High levels of metal contamination have been reported in the soils and water bodies surrounding informal e-waste recycling operations in China, India, and Ghana, with evidence of bio-magnification within local food chains resulting in adverse health impacts to exposed populations (Muhammad, 2023). Novel contamination pathways are created by nanotechnology applications as engineered nanomaterials enter the environment via multiple entry points. Ag nanoparticles (NPs), which are used as antimicrobials in consumer products, can be converted to $Ag+$ in aquatic systems, and TiO2 NPs from sunscreens tend to sediment, where they may impact benthic organisms. Regulation of nanomaterials is limited because the environmental fate, transformation, and toxicity at ecosystem-relevant concentrations remain elusive (Muhammad, 2023). Urban runoff is a diffuse but significant source of metal pollution, especially in heavily populated urban regions. Copper, zinc, and antimony are released into urban dust from vehicle brake wear, whereas tire wear adds zinc and cadmium to the dust. Stormwater infrastructures can accumulate these pollutants during storms and release pulse inputs to the receiving waters, which in some cases may exceed acute toxicity limits for aquatic organisms. Green infrastructure practices and better stormwater management for these urban sources of metal are becoming more prevalent; however, the standardization of regulations for urban runoff continues to vary from jurisdiction to jurisdiction (Muhammad, 2023).

16.4 Transport and fate of metals in the environment

16.4.1 Metal behavior in soil, water, and sediment systems

Metals' environmental behaviors are guided by intricate geobiological processes controlling their mobility, bioavailability, and fate in ecosystems. Metal solubility is primarily controlled by soil pH. Most cationic metals, which include cadmium, lead, and zinc, are more mobile under acidic conditions because competition for binding sites with hydrogen ions becomes greater. The redox potentials are important in controlling the speciation of environmentally sensitive elements such as As and Cr, under reducing conditions, arsenic is most mobile as As(III) (arsenite); on the contrary, chromium is immobilized as Cr(III). The latter controls are seasonal and related to land-use changes, resulting in changes over time in metal availability, which makes monitoring for compliance somewhat complicated (Rahman and Singh, 2024).

Soil organic matter has two opposing effects on soil metal fate, acting as a sink via complexation reactions (binding by organic matter) and as a source via microbial mineralization (release of bound metals). Humic and fulvic acids possess a large number of functional groups that strongly bind metals, decreasing their bioavailability and leachable potential. What is known about the stability of these metal-organic complexes under different environments suggests that the accommodation and unbundling processes can be sensitive to factors such as pH and ionic strength, which might result in metal release. Metal immobilization by clay minerals can occur through metal binding to some of the mineral phases, such as cation exchange capacity and specific adsorption mechanisms, which coalesce to form deposits with variable charge clays, such as kaolinite, and permanent charge clays, such as montmorillonite. In aquatic systems, metal speciation plays a role in influencing environmental behaviors and toxicities. Metals present in dissolved forms may occur as free ions, simple or larger complexes, including colloids, and they differ in bioavailability. The particulate-bound metals are normally deposited in the sediments and may be permanently buried or re-dissolved under varying redox conditions. Deposition of sediments from the water column on to surfaces transiently stabilizes metals, while resuspension by storm events and dredging can be a source of metal contamination in the water column downstream (Rahman and Singh, 2024).

16.4.2 Regulations of uptake and translocation in plants

Metal uptake in plants is mediated by several mechanisms, but root absorption is the major route for the majority of food crops (Fig. 16.2). Roots use both active and passive uptake systems, the expression of which is controlled by membrane transport proteins that can transport essential metals into root cells, while nonessential elements may enter roots through nonspecific channels. This rhizosphere environment, which is distinctive because of the high microbial population and root exudate release, provides special chemical conditions whereby metal bioavailability may be either enhanced or decreased by changes in pH and other factors such as organic acid secretion and redox reactions.

Translocation of metals from roots to shoots is highly variable among elements and species. For instance, cadmium and zinc are relatively mobile elements in the majority of plants, where they accumulate at concentrations in edible tissues that might surpass legislated upper limits. Lead, on the other hand, exhibits restricted translocation in most plants; however, many hyperaccumulator species are capable of accumulating and transporting lead efficiently. Arsenic exhibits intermediate behavior with arsenate mimicking phosphate and entering via phosphorus transporters, but it can also enter through aquaporin channels in the case of arsenite. Metal accumulation patterns are

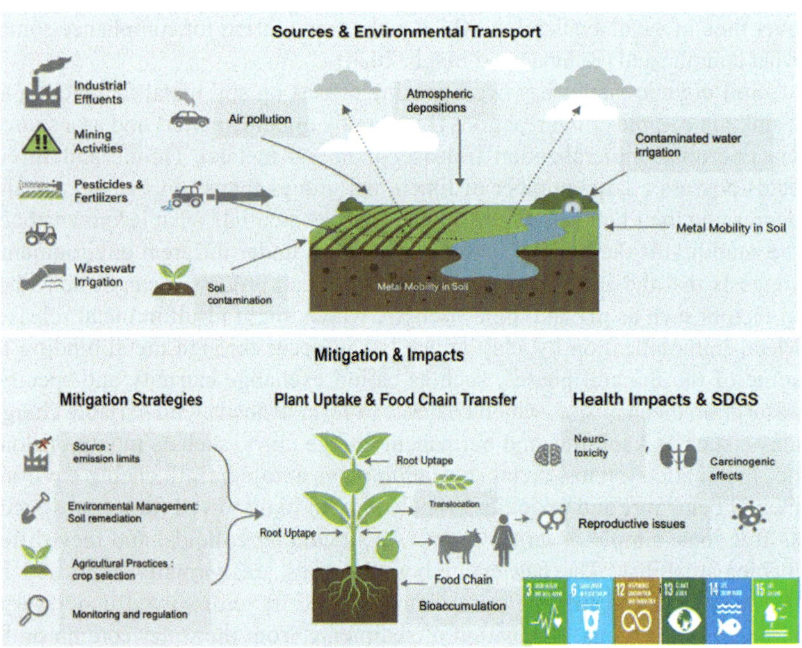

FIG. 16.2 Integrated framework showing mitigation strategies from source to consumer, depicting the continuum of intervention points, including industrial emission controls, agricultural best practices, remediation technologies, food processing controls, and consumer protection measures.

highly influenced by genetic factors and vary substantially among crop varieties and wild relatives. Low-cadmium wheat genotypes and low-arsenic rice varieties, which possess genetic traits that restrict uptake or increase transport to shoots while limiting translocation to grain by maximizing sequestration into nonedible parts of plants, have been developed through crop breeding approaches. Such genetic strategies act synergistically with crop management practices to minimize metal exposure via the food chain, the effectiveness of which is dependent on environmental conditions and the availability of metals (Singh et al., 2025).

16.4.3 Trophic transfer in terrestrial and aquatic eco-systems

The trophic transfer of metals is complex, and its pathways are based on element-specific bioaccumulation factors as well as the structure of the ecosystem. In the terrestrial environment, invertebrates are known to accumulate metals from soils and pore water, acting as a vector for the transfer of metals to predators at higher trophic levels, i.e., birds and small mammals. In general, metals tend to biomagnify across trophic levels for metals with low elimination rates and high assimilation efficiency; however, the extent of BMF can differ widely between ecosystems as well as for different metal species. Marine Food Webs Marine food webs show stronger BMF, especially for mercury and methylmercury. The methylation of inorganic mercury by sulfate-reducing bacteria in anoxic sediments stimulates the formation of methylmercury, a bioavailable form that is highly efficient at being bioaccumulated through binding to proteins and low rates of excretion. Laboratory and field studies in freshwater and marine ecosystems have found that mercury concentrations typically increase by 7–10-fold for each step up the food chain; this gradient is consistent with observations of human health determinants of top predatory fish species that frequently exceed safe consumption advice despite apparently low ambient water concentrations. The BMFs could differ different among metals due to their chemical speciation and biological response. Bioaccumulation of essential metals such as copper and zinc is usually restricted due to the regulatory homeostatic mechanisms in organisms, whereas nonessential metals like mercury and arsenic have higher potential than other trophic levels (Alengebawy, et. al., 2021). It is this variability that has implications for both risk assessment methodologies and, subsequently, the design of regulatory measures, which need to take into account not just concentrations in the environment but also food web dynamics when setting protective standards.

16.5 Metal contaminants in food systems

16.5.1 Plant-based foods

The plant-contaminated food is considered to be an ultimate exposure route for most metal contaminants, especially in vegetarian populations. Among cereal grains, there is differential accumulation according to the cultivation environment, such as irrigated water quality and application of fertilizers. Rice shows a specific ability to accumulate arsenic, including flooded agricultural practices that favor arsenic mobility in paddy soils. The levels of arsenic in rice reported in surveys from a number of Asian countries range from 0.05 to >0.4 mg/kg, with high regional variation reflecting underlying groundwater concentrations and agricultural practices. Both root uptake and atmospheric deposition are efficient ways for cadmium and lead to accumulate in leafy vegetables. Urban-grown or near-industrial-origin leafy vegetables and salad leaf crops, e.g., spinach, lettuce, etc., are reported to accumulate levels exceeding the limits prescribed for lead and cadmium. The large surface area of leaf tissues may allow for direct deposition from the air, and efficient translocation from roots has the potential to concentrate metals in edible organs. This is confirmed by studies of lead and cadmium accumulation in potato tubers, where the former accumulates primarily in the peel tissues and the latter is more evenly distributed throughout the tuber (Briffa et al., 2020). Metal content varies among legumes and nuts, mainly due to species-specific uptake systems and growth environments. Cadmium can be rapidly and extensively accumulated by peanuts and other groundnuts, especially in acidic soils without sufficient organic matter. For tree nuts, metal levels are generally lower than for ground-grown crops, though almond orchards historically treated with arsenic-containing pesticides may still show elevated levels decades after the cessation of application.

16.5.2 Animal-derived foods

Animal products contribute significantly to dietary metal exposure through bioaccumulation in livestock. The liver and kidney are the primary organs responsible for accumulating Cd and Pb, with levels generally about 5–10 times higher than those found in the muscle of the same animal. These offal products are typically consumed in smaller amounts than muscle meat but can contribute disproportionately to the total dietary intake of potentially toxic elements (PEs) especially in communities with high offal consumption. Dairy is also a significant exposure pathway, particularly for lead and cadmium. For example, cows grazing on contaminated pastures can have elevated metal concentrations in their milk, resulting from both feed contamination and transfer from the mammary gland. In some industrial areas, lead levels in milk have been reported to exceed 0 · 1 mg/kg, but regulatory actions and environmental improvements have reduced lead content in many developed countries. Eggs, however, present a mixed exposure profile; generally speaking, albumen has lower metal concentrations than yolk due to differences in protein binding and lipid content. Eggs produced in free-range systems may contain higher concentrations of lead and cadmium because the chickens have direct contact with soil, and these levels tend to increase. On the other hand, computerized feeding systems using controlled feed ingredients can reduce metal contamination, but it is also possible that new contamination pathways are introduced through feed additives and mineral supplementation if they are not properly regulated (Briffa et al., 2020).

16.5.3 Fish, fish products, and other seafood productions

Fish and seafood represent the dominant exposure pathway for methylmercury, with predatory species accumulating the highest concentrations due to BMF through aquatic food webs. Mercury content is particularly high in tuna, swordfish, and shark, while small pelagic fish generally contain significantly lower levels. Regional trends show that emission patterns of mercury are reflected on the ground, marking higher levels of Hg in industrial areas as well as gold-mining regions. The filter-feeding and sedentary nature of marine bivalves, such as mussels and oysters, render them good bioindicators of metal contamination in coastal areas. They can efficiently accumulate cadmium, lead, and arsenic from the suspended and dissolved phases, sometimes reaching levels of concern for human consumption in polluted coastal areas. With the development of marine aquaculture, it has brought with it the issue of increased potential for contamination has arisen, with differences in feed quality and site conditions influencing metal accumulation in cultivated fish species. The metal content in freshwater fish varies greatly depending on the quality of local water and sediment contamination. Species species that feed close to the bottom, e.g., carp and catfish, contain more sediment-bound metals like lead and arsenic, in contrast to pelagic-feeding fish, which contain higher mercury levels due to bioaccumulation. The rapid growth of freshwater fish culture in Asia offers an example of new exposure scenarios, wherein fish reared in polluted water bodies may accumulate enhanced levels of heavy metals, leading to their bioaccumulation. This constitutes a call for better monitoring and regulatory control (Rai et al., 2021).

16.5.4 Processed food and materials in contact with food

The use of processed products has also increased exposure to other metal sources, such as raw material choices, processing equipment, and packaging. Cocoa-based products, especially dark chocolate, often show high cadmium content as a consequence of soil characteristics in the main growing areas. In 2019, the EU set a maximum cadmium regulation for chocolate products. This decline pathway is increasingly being understood, and appropriate regulations are being established. Another significant source of metal exposure is food contact materials, particularly due to the migration of aluminum, antimony, and lead from cooking equipment, packaging, or processing machinery. Aluminum pots and pans can also be a significant source of dietary aluminum, particularly when used to prepare acidic foods. Tin-plated cans and equipment with lead-soldering joints could also pose off-flavor problems, as constituents from the can leach into foods during processing or storage, requiring stringent material specifications and migration testing. Particular attention should be given to food for infants and young children, as they are more susceptible to metal neurotoxicity (Kumar et al., 2022). Infant rice cereal can often have problematic levels of arsenic, and fruit juice products may be high in lead and cadmium due to contaminated raw ingredients and process equipment. This growing concern is evident in the development of specific and more stringent standards proposed for infant foods, with varying enforcement between regulatory jurisdictions.

Data compiled from monitoring studies (2018–2023).

16.6 Human exposure and health risk assessment

16.6.1 Dietary exposure pathways

Dietary exposure is the primary route of human exposure to most metal contaminants and generally accounts for more than 90% of total intake for elements such as lead, cadmium, and arsenic in nonoccupationally exposed populations. There has been a major development in the methods for assessing exposure over the past two decades, evolving from overall food concentration measurements to the use of sophisticated probabilistic models that include consumption patterns, bioavailability factors, and population variability. Cereal grains, vegetables, and seafood continue to be identified within total diet studies in various regions as the predominant contributors of metals to the diet, but individual contributions differ based on cultural food preferences and dietary behaviors. Differences in dietary exposure among geographical areas are a composite of both contamination and consumption patterns. Rice-dominated diets increase exposure to arsenic in Asian populations, while exposure to cadmium increases with wheat and potato consumption among European populations. These regional discrepancies require targeted risk assessment practices and regulatory standards based on local dietary patterns, rather than intercontinental common denominators, which could overprotect or underprotect specific population subgroups.

Special diets may have a unique pattern of exposure that needs to be considered separately. Increased cadmium exposure is more common among vegetarians and vegans, who depend on higher consumption of plant foods compared to high consumers in fish-eating populations, where methylmercury exposure has been elevated. Another critical target group is infants and young children, who consume more (in mg) of food per mass of body weight and have developing organs that heighten sensitivity to exposure to heavy metals. Breast-fed infants typically show lower metal exposure than formula-fed infants, though maternal contamination status can transfer metals through breast milk, creating exposure trade-offs that complicate public health recommendations.

16.6.2 Toxicokinetics and adverse effects on health

The toxicokinetic behavior of metals determines internal dose and target organ exposure, influencing both the nature and severity of health effects. Lead demonstrates complex distribution patterns, with approximately 95% of the body burden residing in bone tissue, where it can serve as an endogenous source of exposure for decades after the initial exposure (Barbosa et al., 2005). Bone lead mobilization during pregnancy, lactation, and osteoporosis creates periods of increased internal exposure that can affect sensitive populations even when external exposure has been controlled.

Cadmium accumulation primarily targets the kidney cortex, where progressive binding to metallothionein proteins creates a long-term reservoir that gradually releases cadmium over decades (Nordberg et al., 2021). The development of proteinuria and decreased glomerular filtration rate represents key biomarkers of cadmium-induced renal dysfunction, with these effects typically appearing after cumulative exposures exceeding 200 μg/g creatinine in the kidney cortex. The long latency period between exposure and observable effects creates challenges for regulatory standard-setting, as protection must be based on preventing accumulation rather than responding to observed health impacts.

Methylmercury's toxicokinetics are characterized by efficient gastrointestinal absorption (95%), strong binding to sulfhydryl groups in proteins, and slow elimination, with a biological half-life of approximately 50 days in humans (Sunderland, 2007). The developing nervous system shows particular vulnerability due to the disruption of neuronal migration, synapse formation, and neurotransmitter systems. Prenatal exposure through maternal fish consumption can cause measurable reductions in IQ and language development at maternal hair mercury concentrations as low as 1 μg/g, highlighting the need for protective standards that account for developmental sensitivity.

Arsenic toxicokinetics involve complex methylation pathways that can both detoxify and activate arsenic species, depending on individual metabolic capacity. The efficiency of arsenic methylation varies among populations due to genetic polymorphisms and nutritional status, influencing individual susceptibility to arsenic-induced health effects (Naujokas et al., 2013). Skin lesions, cardiovascular disease, and various cancers represent major health outcomes associated with chronic inorganic arsenic exposure, with dose-response relationships that vary by endpoint and population characteristics.

16.6.3 Sensitive subpopulations and long-term risk assessment

Groups with high sensitivity need to be taken into account in risk assessment and in the establishment of regulatory standards. Children are believed to be particularly susceptible to lead and methylmercury neurotoxicity because of their developing nervous systems, greater gastrointestinal absorption rates, and more frequent hand-to-mouth activity. Blood lead levels as low as 5 mc g/dL have been linked to demonstrable cognitive deficits in children, and as a result of this "threshold" being adjusted downward over time based on evolving scientific understanding of vulnerability, regulations continue to drive down acceptable exposure thresholds. Another vulnerable group of people is pregnant women, who are more susceptible due to physiological changes in iron absorption and distribution that are made to a greater extent toward the growing fetus. Mobilization of bone lead during pregnancy may generate an internal exposure, which may affect fetal development independent of the external maternal exposure to lead. On the other hand, enhanced absorption of cadmium in the gut due to elevated gastrointestinal iron absorption during pregnancy may lead to interesting interactions between nutritional status and metal toxicology. Genetic influences appear to be strong determinants of both intra- and inter-individual variability in susceptibility to metals. Polymorphisms of the genes coding for metal transporters, detoxifying enzymes, and DNA repair systems can determine personal susceptibility to metal exposure. These genetic differences account for some of the variation in health effects between similar exposure groups and present a challenge to the establishment of regulatory levels that are equally protective across all segments of the population. Cumulative exposure to several metals and their interactions need to be taken into account when evaluating long-term risk. Metals may have additive, synergistic, or antagonistic effects, depending on their toxicological pathways and exposure. For instance, the combined exposure to lead and cadmium can cause more pronounced renal toxicity than either metal alone, whereas sufficient zinc supply may offer some protection against Cd-induced lesions. Such complex interactions require a global risk assessment strategy that considers the entire suite of contaminants rather than individual metals in isolation.

The pathways model of exposure depicts the multiple paths by which metal contaminants move from sources to human targets. Metals are released into the environment through industrial emissions, agricultural uses, and natural weathering; they undergo geochemical transformations and transport within environmental matrices. Soil pollution causes the uptake of metals and their accumulation in crops, while water contamination induces exposure through fish consumption. Impacts of atmospheric deposition result in contamination at the level of both terrestrial and aquatic systems, generating intricate exposure networks that require integrated regulatory strategies. The framework identifies key control points for regulation that can effectively reduce human exposure, including source reduction, environmental quality control, food safety standards, and consumer advice.

16.7 Detection and monitoring analytical strategies

16.7.1 Established instrumental methods

Conventional instrumental methods continue to serve as the workhorses for metal analysis in compliance monitoring and risk assessment. Despite these advances, Atomic Absorption Spectroscopy (AAS) remains a low-cost technique for simple metal analysis. A flame AAS is best suited to measurements of higher concentrations, while metals present at lower levels may be considered trace-level and measured via graphite furnace AAS, which offers greater sensitivity compared to the flame system (Yan et al., 2020). The major limitations of the technique are that it is useful only for single-element analysis, and detection limits are high compared with other current technologies. However, these limitations have been adequate for regulatory purposes as improvements in background correction and atomization systems have been made further.

Inductively coupled plasma (ICP) optical emission spectroscopy provides multielement capability at moderate levels of sensitivity for most regulatory monitoring requirements. The strong sample-handling capacity and moderate running costs of the technique qualify it to be part of high-throughput screening programs. However, the detection limits of some elements may be too high to satisfy the strictest regulatory conditions, particularly for trace metals in food matrices, whose concentrations can often be <10 μg/kg. In addition, matrix effects may lead to spectral interferences and require careful method development and validation in complex matrices.

ICP Mass Spectrometry (ICP-MS) is a leading technology for low-level trace metal analysis; the method offers extraordinary sensitivity, multielement detection capabilities, and isotopic measurements as well. The capacity of the technique to determine several elements at once makes it particularly suited to chemistry for comprehensive monitoring programs and risk assessment. Newer developments, such as collision/reaction cell technology, high-resolution features, and automatic sample introduction systems, have both enhanced performance and minimized interferences. Nevertheless, the expensive machinery cost and the requirement of skilled technical personnel limit its utilization within some regulatory laboratories, especially in underdeveloped countries.

16.7.2 Rapid screening and sensor - based approaches

Rapid screening methods have been developed in response to the demand for high-throughput testing and field-deployable diagnostics. Portable X-ray fluorescence spectrometry allows rapid screening of metal contaminants in the field, such as in soil, food products, and environmental samples, providing real-time data used to assist sampling protocols and regulatory actions. The method does not achieve all of the regulatory detection limits; however, its nondestructive nature and rapid analysis make it useful for prescreening and source identification.

Electrochemical sensors represent a promising candidate for onsite detection of metals, and their sensitivity and selectivity are enhanced by advances in nanomaterials fabrication as well as microfabrication technology. Stripping voltammetry procedures allow the determination of lead, cadmium, and mercury at sub-ppb levels, applying low-cost, simple instrumentation that can be employed in field conditions (Zwolak et al., 2019). Biosensor methodologies with biological recognition units offer selectivity advantages, but the key aspects—sensor stability and the influence of matrices—still need to be addressed due to the complexity of food analysis samples.

Colorimetric test strips and portable assay kits offer easy-to-use screening for regulatory agencies and community monitoring. Although they are less quantitative than laboratory-based approaches, portable devices allow rapid decision-making regarding which samples should be collected for confirmatory analysis. The latest advancements in smartphone-based detection systems have made colorimetric methods more accessible and quantitative, which could be exploited by citizen science and community-level surveillance projects.

16.7.3 Progress in metal speciation and trace analysis

Speciation analysis has become essential in metal risk assessment, since toxicology greatly depends on the chemical form of an element. High-performance liquid chromatography linked to ICP-MS separates and quantifies individual metal species, providing a differentiation between inorganic forms of arsenic that have higher toxicity associated with them as compared to organic types, including arsenobetaine (Abdullahi and Sani, 2020). Similarly, the speciation of mercury can distinguish between methylmercury and inorganic forms of mercury, which is necessary to accurately assess the risk of contamination of the food supply.

ICP-MS is a game-changing technique for NP analysis that allows detection and characterization of NPs containing metals in environmental and food samples. The method offers size distributions and concentration measurements on particles that are needed to understand nanomaterial behavior and potential risk (Bereda, 2025). It is important that their concentration kinetics be studied because, as engineered nanomaterials are introduced into food systems and the environment by diverse application means, equilibrium may not be achieved rapidly.

Isotope ratio analysis can provide effective tools to apportion sources and track pathways of metal contamination. Isotope ratios of lead can differentiate between sources of contamination (industrial, automotive, and natural), and stable isotope methods can track metal cycling. Such methods are of vital use for developing focused legislative actions and assessing the efficiency of interventions (Komárek et al., 2008).

Standardization of detection methods is a key issue in harmonized regulatory enforcement. Standard methods and validation protocols have been established by international organizations such as AOAC International (Association of Official Analytical Chemists), the International Organization for Standardization (ISO), and the International Union of Pure and Applied Chemistry (IUPAC) to ensure that results are comparable between laboratories and regions. Membership in proficiency testing and/or accreditation to ISO/IEC 17025 promotes data quality and acceptance of results; however, the extent of implementation varies across geographic regions and regulatory authorities (AOAC International, 2019).

16.8 International and regional regulatory frameworks

16.8.1 International guidelines and standards (FAO/WHO, Codex Alimentarius)

The Codex Alimentarius Commission, established jointly by the Food and Agriculture Organization (FAO) and the WHO, serves as the primary international body for developing food safety standards, including maximum levels for metal contaminants. Codex standards are developed through consensus among member countries, incorporating scientific risk assessments from the Joint FAO/WHO Expert Committee on Food Additives (JECFA) and considerations of fair trade practices (Codex Alimentarius Commission, 2023). The committee's risk assessments establish provisional tolerable weekly intakes (PTWIs) for various metals, which serve as scientific foundations for national regulatory standard-setting worldwide (Bouida et al., 2022).

JECFA's evaluation process involves a comprehensive review of toxicological data, exposure assessments, and analytical methodology to establish health-based guidance values. Recent decades have seen the progressive tightening of these values as scientific understanding of metal toxicity has improved, with the withdrawal of PTWI for lead in 2010 and cadmium in 2010 reflecting the recognition that no safe exposure levels exist for these nonessential metals (JECFA, 2011). This evolution demonstrates the dynamic nature of scientific understanding and the necessity for regulatory frameworks that can adapt to new evidence while maintaining practical implementation considerations (Kuhangana et al., 2024).

The Codex process involves multiple committees working on different aspects of food safety, with the Codex Committee on Contaminants in Foods specifically addressing metal contaminants. Standard setting follows an eight-step procedure requiring multiple rounds of review and comments from member countries and observer organizations (FAO/WHO, 2021). This inclusive process ensures broad international acceptance but can also slow standard development in response to emerging contaminants. The resulting standards serve as reference points for World Trade Organization (WTO) dispute resolution and facilitate international trade while protecting consumer health.

16.8.2 European Union regulations

The United States employs a multiagency framework for metal contaminant regulation, with the FDA taking primary responsibility for food safety standards and the EPA addressing environmental aspects and drinking water contaminants. The FDA's action levels and guidance documents establish enforceable limits for metal contaminants in various food commodities, though these standards often focus on specific high-concern products rather than providing comprehensive coverage across all food categories (Table 16.1) (U.S. Food and Drug Administration, 2023). The FDA's regulatory approach has historically emphasized enforcement actions against contaminated products rather than establishing comprehensive preventive standards. However, recent initiatives, including the Food Safety Modernization Act (FSMA), have shifted focus toward preventive controls and hazard analysis throughout the food supply chain (Taylor, 2018). This evolution reflects a growing recognition that effective metal contaminant control requires systematic approaches rather than reactive enforcement actions. The EPA's Clean Water Act and Safe Drinking Water Act establish environmental quality standards that indirectly affect food contamination levels. The agency's water quality criteria for metals and maximum contaminant levels for drinking water represent important components of the overall regulatory framework (United States Environmental Protection Agency, 2021). Coordination between FDA and EPA responsibilities remains challenging, with overlapping jurisdiction and different approaches to risk assessment sometimes creating regulatory gaps or inconsistencies (Laoye et al., 2025).

Values represent maximum limits for the specified commodities. The term "action level" indicates the FDA enforcement threshold rather than an absolute prohibition. Empty cells indicate that no specific standard has been established.

TABLE 16.1 Representative metal concentrations (mg/kg fresh weight) in various food categories across different regions.

Food category	Metal	Europe	North America	Asia	Africa	Regulatory limit
Rice	As	0.15	0.20	0.30	0.25	0.20–0.30
Wheat	Cd	0.08	0.10	0.15	0.12	0.10–0.20
Leafy Vegetables	Pb	0.12	0.15	0.25	0.20	0.10–0.30
Root Vegetables	Cd	0.05	0.08	0.10	0.09	0.05–0.10
Beef Muscle	Pb	0.03	0.04	0.06	0.05	0.05–0.10
Fish (predatory)	Hg	0.8	1.0	1.2	0.9	0.5–1.0
Shellfish	Cd	0.5	0.8	1.0	0.7	0.5–1.0
Milk	Pb	0.02	0.03	0.04	0.03	0.02–0.05

16.8.3 Regulatory approaches in the United States

The United States employs a multiagency framework for metal contaminant regulation, with the FDA taking primary responsibility for food safety standards and the EPA addressing environmental aspects and drinking water contaminants. The FDA's action levels and guidance documents establish enforceable limits for metal contaminants in various food commodities, though these standards often focus on specific high-concern products rather than providing comprehensive coverage across all food categories (U.S. Food and Drug Administration, 2023). The FDA's regulatory approach historically emphasizes enforcement actions against contaminated products rather than establishing comprehensive preventive standards. However, recent initiatives, including the FSMA, have shifted focus toward preventive controls and hazard analysis throughout the food supply chain (Taylor, 2018). This evolution reflects a growing recognition that effective metal contaminant control requires systematic approaches rather than reactive enforcement actions (Al-Musharraf and Rahman, 2025). The EPA's Clean Water Act and Safe Drinking Water Act establish environmental quality standards that indirectly affect food contamination levels. The agency's water quality criteria for metals and maximum contaminant levels for drinking water represent important components of the overall regulatory framework. Coordination between FDA and EPA responsibilities remains challenging, with overlapping jurisdiction and different approaches to risk assessment sometimes creating regulatory gaps or inconsistencies (Li et al., 2025).

16.8.4 Regulatory overviews in Asia, Africa and Latin America

Asian countries demonstrate diverse regulatory approaches, reflecting varying economic development, trade relationships, and scientific capacity (Table 16.2). China has developed comprehensive food safety standards through the National Food Safety Standard system, with maximum levels for contaminants established based on JECFA assessments and national monitoring data (NHFPC, 2022). Japan's regulatory framework combines Codex standards with additional protective measures, reflecting high consumer expectations and sophisticated risk assessment capabilities. India's Food Safety and Standards Authority has progressively strengthened metal contaminant standards, though implementation challenges remain due to diverse agricultural systems and varying monitoring capacity across regions (FSSAI, 2021).

African regulatory systems face unique challenges, including limited analytical infrastructure, diverse food production systems, and variable implementation capacity. The African Continental Free Trade Area's harmonization efforts aim to create unified standards that facilitate trade while protecting consumer health, though resource constraints and capacity limitations affect implementation. Regional economic communities, including ECOWAS and SADC, have developed common standards, but national variations persist based on local priorities and enforcement capabilities (Ondrasek et al., 2025).

TABLE 16.2 Maximum levels (mg/kg) for selected metal contaminants in food commodities across major regulatory frameworks.

Food Commodity	Metal	Codex Alimentarius	European Union	United States (FDA)	China	Australia/ New Zealand	Japan
Cereals							
Rice (polished)	Pb	0.2	0.2	0.2 (action level)	0.2	0.2	0.2
Rice (polished)	Cd	0.4	0.2	–	0.2	0.1	0.2
Wheat	Pb	0.2	0.2	0.2 (action level)	0.2	0.2	0.2
Wheat	Cd	0.2	0.1	–	0.1	0.1	0.1
Vegetables							
Leafy vegetables	Pb	0.3	0.3	0.3 (action level)	0.3	0.3	0.3
Root vegetables	Pb	0.1	0.1	0.1 (action level)	0.1	0.1	0.1
Root vegetables	Cd	0.1	0.05	–	0.1	0.1	0.1
Tomatoes	Pb	0.1	0.1	0.1 (action level)	0.1	0.1	0.1
Animal products							
Meat (bovine)	Pb	0.1	0.1	0.1 (action level)	0.2	0.1	0.1
Meat (bovine)	Cd	0.05	0.05	–	0.1	0.05	0.05
Milk	Pb	0.02	0.02	0.02 (action level)	0.05	0.02	0.02
Milk	Cd	–	0.02	–	0.05	0.02	0.02

Fish							
Fish (general)	Hg	0.5	0.5	1.0 (action level)	0.5	0.5	0.4
Predator fish	Hg	1.0	1.0	1.0 (action level)	1.0	1.0	0.8
Infant foods							
Infant formula	Pb	0.02	0.02	0.02 (action level)	0.02	0.02	0.02
Infant formula	Cd	0.01	0.01	–	0.01	0.01	0.01
Infant cereals	Pb	0.2	0.2	0.2 (action level)	0.2	0.2	0.2
Processed foods							
Fruit juices	Pb	0.05	0.05	0.05 (action level)	0.05	0.05	0.05
Canned foods	Sn	150	50	50 (action level)	150	200	150

Latin American countries demonstrate regulatory approaches influenced by both Codex standards and major trading partners' requirements. Brazil's National Health Surveillance Agency (ANVISA) has established comprehensive contaminant standards that often exceed Codex requirements, reflecting strong domestic consumer protection goals. The Mercosur common market has developed harmonized standards among member countries, though implementation varies based on national infrastructure and enforcement priorities. Chile and Mexico have developed sophisticated risk assessment systems that inform national standard-setting, though capacity for ongoing monitoring and enforcement remains variable across the region (Scutarașu and Trincă, 2023; Singh et al., 2023).

Comparison showing the diversity of regulatory approaches across global regions.

16.9 Comparative assessment of regulatory limits

16.9.1 Maximum allowable limits in food commodities

The regulatory limits of metal contaminants differ considerably among regions, mainly due to differences in risk assessment methods, dietary habits, and practical application. Lead standards present some of the largest differences, with maximum levels for lead in leafy vegetables varying from 0.1 mg/kg in the EU to up to 0.3 mg/kg in Codex and further up to 0.4 mg/kg in some Asian countries. These differences are a result of both scientific incompleteness in assessing low-dose toxicity and considerations of feasibility for compliance by producers within the different agricultural systems.

This diversity is also reflected in cadmium standards, especially for food crops such as staple foods, where levels can vary widely as a function of natural variations in soil characteristics. The EC's established MRL of 0.20 mg/kg for rice in husk is contrasted by Codex, which has set its limit at 0.40 mg/kg, and China, which permits variations according to types of rice (Yaseen, 2021). These variations can pose barriers to trade and complicate global trade, particularly for smallholder farmers in developing countries who may not have access to low-cadmium varieties or soil amendments.

Mercury guidelines indicate more international consistency, particularly for species of fish already known to be toxic on the basis of scientific evidence. The major regulatory jurisdictions have established maximum levels of about 0.5–1.0 mg/kg in predatory fish, which can again be traced back to a common interpretation of JECFA reviews. However, the implementation varies; some countries set limit values by species, while others use uniform ones for fish. This coherence stems from the well-documented scientific agreement on mercury toxicity and the broad-based international support that already exists through the Minamata Convention on Mercury.

Regulations governing arsenic content are the most variable due to complicated speciation and scientific developments. Inorganic arsenic limits for rice vary from 0.20 mg/kg in the EU to 0.30 mg/kg in Codex, whereas other countries apply a total arsenic limit without distinguishing between the toxic inorganic and less toxic organic forms. The difficulties involved in speciation analysis contribute to these differences, and some regulatory authorities lack not have the capacity necessary to operate inorganic arsenic-specific monitoring networks.

16.9.2 Environmental quality standards for soil and water

There is even greater international variation in environmental quality standards for metals in agricultural soils compared to food, reflecting disparities in geological baseline levels, farming methods, and policy priorities. Threshold values for agricultural soils in the EU vary between 1–3 mg/kg (cadmium) and 50–300 mg/kg (lead), depending on soil pH and use. These criteria are intended to avoid crop uptake above food standards, allow for differences in background levels, and address the practical difficulties of application (Zaynab et al., 2022).

The soil environmental quality standard for China provides the risk screening (RS)values for agricultural land, which are defined as different values in consideration of soil type, land use, and contaminants. The values are classified as RS levels that require additional investigation, or risk intervention levels that will trigger the need for corrective action, demonstrating a tiered approach to reflect practical considerations in implementation. This approach accepts background variation while setting clear-cut triggers for when intervention is required. In the United States, there are no such broad federal standards for soil metals in agriculture; state regulations and site-specific risk assessments are used. This method represents the Australian focus on site-specific risk rather than uniform national standards, but it may lead to disparities in protection among states and territories.

The pattern of variability across metals for water quality standards also mirrors the differences in the sensitivities of aquatic ecosystems, water uses, and policy concerns. The Water Framework Directive of the EU prescribes water quality standards, for instance regarding these metal priority substances, in the form of numerical values for various kinds of water bodies. In the United States, metals criteria designated for aquatic life are linked to use designations of aquatic life and hardness parameters under the Clean Water Act, recognizing water chemistry that affects metal bioavailability and toxicity (FAO/WHO, 2021).

16.9.3 Regulatory harmonization and trade considerations

Lack of regulatory harmonization is a major obstacle to international trade in food, as nonharmonized requirements are used to create technical barriers to trade (Table 16.3). In the WTO's Sanitary and Phytosanitary Agreement, the rights of countries to set their level of protection are acknowledged, but standardization at an international level is nevertheless solicited through entities such as Codex Alimentarius. Still, differences in the way jurisdictions assess risks, their capacity to act on responses, and the priorities of consumer protection mean that standards may remain different across jurisdictions.

TABLE 16.3 Comparison of regulatory bodies and their key mandates across regions.

Region	Primary Regulatory Body	Key Legislation/ Standard	Mandate Scope	Risk Assessment Approach	Standard Setting Frequency
International	Codex Alimentarius	General Standards for Contaminants	Global trade harmonization	JECFA scientific evaluations	Every 4–5 years
European Union	EFSA/EC	Regulation (EC) No 1881/2006	Comprehensive food safety	Precautionary principle, EFSA opinions	Regular reviews (2–3 years)
United States	FDA/EPA	Food Safety Modernization Act	Food safety, environmental protection	Agency-specific risk assessments	As needed, case-by-case
China	NHFPC	GB 2762 National Food Safety Standard	Domestic food safety	JECFA-based with national data	Periodic updates
Japan	MHLW	Food Sanitation Act	Domestic food safety	Conservative approach, high protection	Regular reviews
India	FSSAI	Food Safety and Standards Act	Domestic food safety	Codex-based with national adaptation	Periodic updates
Brazil	ANVISA	RDC No. 42/2013	Domestic food safety	Conservative, consumer protection	Regular reviews
Africa	Various national bodies	Diverse national standards	National food safety	Variable, often Codex-based	Irregular updates

The effects of trade are especially pronounced for developing countries, which may not have the technical capabilities to comply with higher standards demanded in key export markets. Academic research on African agricultural exports has revealed rejection rates of 5–15% on account of contaminant violations, equating to financial losses in the millions per annum. These rejections are felt most strongly by smallholders, who do not have access to the testing labs or quality control processes that would help ensure compliance.

The equivalence concept offers a basis to acknowledge different regulatory strategies that achieve commensurable levels of protection (Alengebawy et al., 2021). EU equivalence with trading partners is a means to access markets while simultaneously retaining food safety aims. Similarly, the United States' Foreign Supplier Verification Program under FSMA 28 requires importers to ensure that foreign suppliers adhere to comparable safety standards, thereby promoting regulatory alignment. Capacity building is a fundamental element in these efforts, and international organizations provide technical aid to developing countries to improve their regulatory systems. FAO and WHO are strengthening countries' capacity to develop risk assessment competencies, establish monitoring systems, and enforce measures. These initiatives aim to mitigate disparities in regulatory implementation while recognizing that standards must be adapted to local circumstances and capacities.

Values are expressed as mg/kg fresh weight unless otherwise specified. Dashes indicate that no specific standard has been established. Data reflect regulations as of 2023.

16.10 Management and mitigation strategies

16.10.1 Prevention and source control

Prevention of metal contamination at the source represents the most cost-effective and sustainable approach to protecting food safety and environmental quality. Industrial emission controls have been largely successful in lowering the amount of metal deposition from air to land, as evidenced by lead emissions showing some potential for regulation when deposited from gasoline and paint (Briffa et al., 2020). In the agricultural sector, control at the source has been considered to restrict metal input through fertilizer quality standards, pesticide restrictions, and irrigation water management. Outcomes such as the creation and application of low-cadmium phosphate fertilizers are one notable success. The banning of arsenic pesticides and lead arsenate for use in agriculture, where they were applied as pesticides, has also helped to decrease contamination inputs. However, there are still concerns about metal levels because metals added over many years remain in the soil (Briffa et al., 2020).

Advances in waste management have brought new opportunities for source reduction. Legitimate landfill operations (including leachate collection systems) prevent metal pollution from entering groundwater, and hazardous waste incineration facilities equipped with effective air pollution control systems result in the destruction of organic pollutants along with metal containment for safe disposal (Kumar et al., 2022). The increasing adoption of circular economy strategies and waste prevention contributes to reducing potential sources of metal release through more efficient use of resources and enhanced material recovery.

Best management practices in the mining industry have been shown to be successful in reducing metal emissions into the environment. Contemporary mine waste controls, such as tailings impoundments, water treatment plants, and active reclamation practices, have helped lower the amount of metal that reaches runoff from mines. To guide responsible mining that achieves minimal environmental metal impact while maximize economic benefits, the International Council on Mining and Metals has developed an enabling sustainable development framework.

16.10.2 Remediation strategies for polluted ecosystems

There are a number of soil remediation processes that can be used for treating contaminated soils and sediments, and the choice of technology will depend on various site-specific factors (extent of contamination, contaminant levels, intended land use). Phytoremediation utilizes metal-accumulating plants to extract or immobilize metals in metal-contaminated soils, and among them are hyperaccumulator species capable of accumulating these elements thousands of times higher than background concentrations. Although phytoremediation is a cost-effective and green remediation technology, the long-term periods required for large-scale applications, as well as the disposal of the contaminated plant biomass at highly polluted sites that need immediate treatment, can limit its implementation.

The application of soil amendments offers a viable remediation strategy through the immobilization of metals with reduced bioavailability. Liming has been shown to increase soil pH, thereby decreasing the solubility and plant uptake of cationic metal species, while phosphate application can be used to form insoluble minerals such as pyromorphite. Organic matter additives, such as compost and biochar, enhance metal binding through complexation reactions, leading to a decrease in the mobility and bioavailability of metals. Such in-situ stabilization strategies tend to require continuous surveillance but can mitigate potential exposure while preserving the ability of the soil to remain productive for agriculture (Kadlec and Wallace, 2009).

Constructed wetlands are cost-efficient treatment systems for the remediation of metal-polluted waters, using natural removal mechanisms such as sedimentation, plant accumulation, and microbial changes. Approximately 50–90% reduction of metals in contaminated waters can be achieved by wetland systems, generally depending on design parameters, metallic species, and hydraulic loading rates. Ecological services from wetland creation, such as habitat provision and carbon sequestration, add to the sustainability of remediation efforts (Kadlec and Wallace, 2009).

Different strategies have been applied utilizing microbes to convert metal species or increase immobilization through bioremediation methods. Metals can be bio-precipitated as insoluble sulfides by sulfate-reducing bacteria, and some fungi are able to remove metals via the biosorption process. These biotechnological methods are of high interest since they have shown the potential to assist in situ metal-contamination without causing side-effects, unlike commonly implemented remediation technologies. Successful engineering applications may depend on careful management and understanding of site-specific conditions and microbial community dynamics (Gadd, 2010).

16.10.3 Sustainable food production and monitoring schemes

Sustainable farming systems can result in lower metal uptake and can be used to maintain productivity and environmental quality. Cultivation of crops with specific metal accumulation attributes reduces reduce the transfer of contaminants to edible parts. For instance, it has been demonstrated that the adoption of low-cadmium wheat cultivars or cultivars of fruit crops with limited metal translocation both represent valid options to decrease contamination risks while preserving agricultural feasibility. In addition, avoiding flood irrigation of arsenic-affected soils can lower the mobilization and accumulation of arsenic in rice plants (Grant et al., 2008).

There are also advanced technologies in precision agriculture that make it feasible to submit applications targeting management practices (reduction of metal exposure) as well as stimulate resource use. Cadmium inputs can be prevented by variable-rate soil testing, and the mobilization of metals in vulnerable areas can be reduced with site-specific irrigation management. The model-based, data-driven solutions achieve maximum land use efficiency that balances food production and environmental protection, suggesting the promise of technology integration for sustainable food systems (Zhang et al., 2018).

Surveillance programs supply crucial information required for risk analysis, surveillance compliance, and source identification. Integrated monitoring networks that include environmental, food, and human monitoring provide a comprehensive view of the contamination pathways and potential exposures (Fig. 16.2). The EU's coordinated monitoring programs under the Rapid Alert System for Food and Feed (RASFF) demonstrate the value of integrated surveillance systems for the rapid detection and response to contamination incidents.

Capacity enhancement and technology transfer remain vital to the successful application in developing areas. Training analytical personnel and providing equipment to monitoring laboratories, as well as offering technical assistance for establishing regulatory capacity, can strengthen local capabilities in managing the risks of metal contamination. Global models, such as those of the International Atomic Energy Agency's collaborative centers and FAO capacity-building programs are useful in strengthening global food safety systems;

however, context-specific strategies tailored to local situations and priorities are required.

The mitigation model identifies several levers through which intervention reduces metal exposure across the entire food chain. Prerelease source control measures, such as industrial emissions laws, chemical controls, and waste management, act to reduce the release of contaminants at the front end. Management of the environment through remediation technology, land use planning, and water quality protection is decreasing both the level of environmental metals and their transport into agricultural systems. Control of food production and processing, which includes planting, irrigation, and processing equipment, can preserve agricultural products, ensuring that the transfer of metals is kept to a minimum in food. Consumer protection steps—such as surveillance actions, standard implementation, and public information—are yet another set of final mechanisms that prevent food-related risks in the supply chain. This integrative approach is based on the understanding that the management of metal contaminants with respect to food safety cannot be addressed by strategies targeting single points in the food chain but rather requires coordination across several components and actors.

16.11 Emerging challenges and future trends

16.11.1 Effects of climate change on metal mobility

Climate change is dramatically affecting metal behavior in the environment, with several mechanisms interplaying. Elevated temperatures could increase the solubility and biological availability of metals, leading to faster metal release from contaminated soils or sediments. The warming trends already being observed have particularly significant impacts in cold regions, as permafrost thaw may release metals hitherto immobilized into aquatic systems and open up new pathways for exposure to human populations in the north, which are reliant on traditional foods. In addition, metal transport and distribution may also be affected in various directions by changing precipitation patterns. More regular extreme-rainfall increases erosion and transfer of contaminants from pollution structures into the food sector or canals. On the other hand, extended dry periods can increase levels of these metals in arable soil by reducing leaching and increasing evapotranspiration, which may raise the risk to biota and humans from crop up take. Furthermore, land subsidence and sea level rise introduce more challenges for the migration of metals in coastal areas, such as salt water intrusion and increased frequency of flooding. Saltwater intrusion has the potential to mobilize metals occluded within sediments as a result of ion exchange processes, with enhanced inundation by coastal flooding re-suspending contaminated sediments and transporting them onto agricultural land. The consequences are most alarming for low-lying agricultural areas and small-island developing states, whose coastlines provide crucial food production for food security.

16.11.2 Nanotechnology and novel contaminants

The increased use of nanotechnology has led to new scenarios of contamination that are not covered by current regulations. Manufactured nanomaterials (MNMs), such as silver NPs, titanium dioxide (TiO_2), and quantum dots, are being utilized increasingly in industries as components of consumer products, food packaging, or agricultural pesticides. These products may degrade in the environment to form ionic metals or create new pathways of exposure that are not sufficiently addressed by existing regulations. The behavior of nanomaterials is markedly dissimilar from that of metal species in solution, exhibiting different transport, bioavailability, and toxicity. NPs can traverse body barriers and concentrate in certain organs, forming exposure pathways that are not accounted for in standard risk evaluations. Existing analytical methods are typically unable to accurately identify and characterize NPs in complex matrices, creating significant gaps in risk analysis and regulation. Furthermore, compliance with nanomaterial contamination regulations remains inconsistent globally, as some countries respond on a case-by-case basis while others prefer to act only after receiving scientific evidence to adjust standards. There is some guidance available for the risk assessment of nanomaterials under the EU's Registration, Evaluation, Authorisation and Restriction of Chemicals (REACH) regulation, but its implementation is hindered by a scarcity of data and methodological uncertainties. Global collaboration through organizations such as the Organisation for Economic Co-operation and Development (OECD) Working Party on MNMs endeavors to create harmonized testing and risk assessment strategies.

16.11.3 Gaps and next steps in regulation

Existing regulatory schemes have significant limitations with respect to emerging contaminants, as well as cumulative exposures and vulnerable populations. Targeting single metals and particular food items does not take into account realistic exposure situations, which include several contaminants in complex food substances. Such a reductionist view could miscalculate mixture effects and lead to unintended impacts, such as the situation where, by decreasing one contaminant, we indirectly increase another. Despite increasing evidence of metal mixtures' additivity and synergy, cumulative risk assessment approaches for metal mixtures are poorly developed. The complicated interrelationships of essential and nonessential metals, as well as individual susceptibility factors, can make it difficult to establish protective standards that are applicable to realistic exposure scenarios. More advanced mixture toxicity models and probabilistic exposure estimates must be considered in future regulation. Furthermore, the current regulatory paradigms often provide insufficient protection for vulnerable populations such as children, pregnant women, and subsistence consumers. There is a lack of consideration for increased susceptibility, unique exposure patterns, or dietary practices by different cultures that may result in higher risk among some groups. The future development of regulation will have to apply more sophisticated risk characterization approaches that safeguard the most vulnerable parts of society. Similarly, regulatory harmonization challenges will intensify as global trade expands and new contaminants emerge. The current patchwork of international standards creates trade barriers and unequal protection for consumers across different regions (WTO, 2021). Future directions must emphasize capacity building, technology transfer, and coordinated standard development to ensure equitable protection while facilitating international commerce in food products.

16.12 Case studies and global perspectives

16.12.1 EU cadmium standards and agricultural adaptation

The EU's progressive tightening of cadmium standards in food commodities offers a compelling case-study of regulatory implementation challenges along with adaptation strategies. The establishment of maximum levels for cadmium in cereals, vegetables, and other foods in 2001, followed by further reductions in 2014, required significant adjustments across the agricultural sector (European Commission, 2022). These regulatory changes prompted the development of low-cadmium crop varieties, the implementation of soil testing programs, and modifications to fertilizer application practices. The implementation process highlighted the importance of stakeholder engagement and phased approaches to regulatory change. Agricultural extension services provided technical assistance to farmers on cadmium management practices, while research programs developed an improved understanding of soil–plant transfer factors (Grant et al., 2008). The EU's Common Agricultural Policy incorporated support measures for farmers affected by contamination issues, demonstrating how regulatory changes can be balanced with economic considerations. Similarly, the long-term monitoring data emerging from this regulatory transition provides valuable insights into the effectiveness of different management approaches. Studies show that areas with comprehensive soil testing and targeted fertilizer management achieved the greatest reductions in crop cadmium levels, while regions with limited technical support continued to struggle with compliance (EFSA, 2012). This experience demonstrates the critical role of capacity building and technical assistance in successful regulatory implementation (Fig. 16.3).

16.12.2 China's response to soil metal contamination

China's comprehensive approach to addressing soil metal contamination represents one of the world's largest environmental remediation efforts. The publication of the national soil contamination survey in 2014 revealed that 16.1% of surveyed land exceeded standards for metal contaminants, prompting the development of the Soil Pollution Prevention and Control Action Plan (MEE, 2016). This ambitious program targets both pollution source control and remediation of contaminated sites, with a specific focus on agricultural land affecting food safety. The implementation strategy combines regulatory measures with

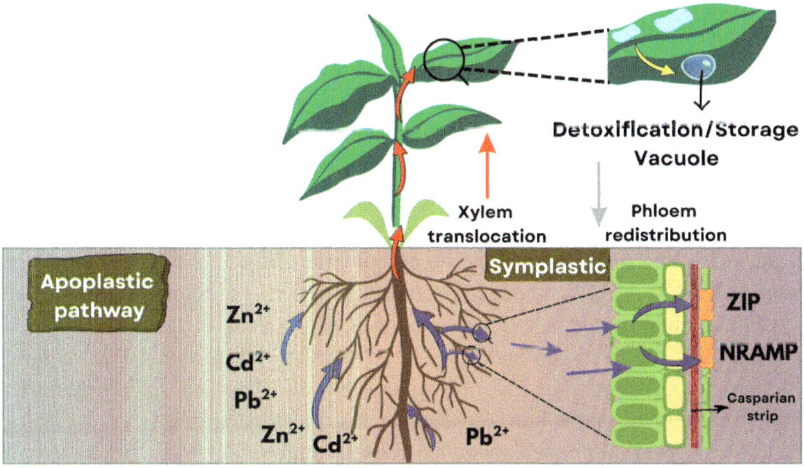

FIG. 16.3 Mechanism of metal uptake and translocation in plants.

technological innovation and market-based mechanisms. Strict environmental enforcement has reduced industrial emissions, while remediation demonstration projects showcase effective technologies for different contamination scenarios (Zhao et al., 2019). The development of soil pollution liability insurance and contamination liability transfer mechanisms creates financial incentives for pollution prevention and remediation. China's experience highlights the challenges of scaling up remediation efforts across vast areas with varying contamination levels and land use patterns. The country's investment in research and development of remediation technologies has accelerated innovation in areas including phytoremediation, soil washing, and in-situ stabilization (Mahar et al., 2016). However, technical capacity limitations and financial constraints continue to challenge implementation in less developed regions, demonstrating the need for differentiated approaches based on local conditions and capabilities.

16.12.3 Minamata convention and global mercury management

The Minamata Convention on Mercury, adopted in 2013 and entering into force in 2017, represents the first global treaty specifically addressing a metal contaminant (UNEP, 2017). The convention's comprehensive approach addresses all aspects of the mercury life cycle, from primary mining and trade to use in products and processes, emissions releases, and the environmentally sound management of mercury waste. This holistic framework provides a model for international coordination on metal contaminant management. The convention's implementation has already achieved significant successes in reducing mercury use and emissions. Phase-out timelines for mercury-containing products, including thermometers, batteries, and lighting, have accelerated the transition to alternatives, while best available technology requirements for industrial emissions have reduced environmental releases (UNEP, 2021). The convention's financial mechanism and capacity-building programs have supported implementation in developing countries, demonstrating how international cooperation can facilitate global environmental protection. Furthermore, ongoing challenges remain in addressing artisanal and small-scale gold mining, which represents the largest source of mercury emissions globally. The convention's approach to this issue combines the formalization of mining operations, mercury-free technology promotion, and public health protection measures (UNEP, 2021). The gradual progress in this sector illustrates the complexities of addressing contamination sources that are deeply embedded in cultural practices and economic livelihoods.

The global perspective map illustrates the spatial distribution of metal contamination challenges and regulatory responses worldwide (Table 16.4). Industrial regions in North America, Europe, and East Asia show historical contamination hotspots but also feature the most comprehensive regulatory frameworks and monitoring systems. Rapidly industrializing regions in South Asia, Latin America, and parts of Africa demonstrate increasing contamination pressures but variable regulatory implementation capacity. Mining regions in Central Africa, South America, and Australia show localized high contamination levels, while agricultural regions with intensive fertilizer use demonstrate diffuse contamination patterns. The map also illustrates international cooperation through regional trading blocs and pollution control agreements, demonstrating how regulatory approaches transcend national boundaries through collaborative initiatives and harmonization efforts (Table 16.5).

16.13 Conclusions

Metal pollution in food and the environment is a multidimensional problem that must be addressed globally through an integrated action across several levels of expertise. This in-depth review has demonstrated that significant advances have been made in understanding how metals behave, their effects on health, and how to manage responses. However, there remain considerable challenges to overcome before effective protection of public health and environmental quality can be fully established. Variety may be the spice of life, but when dealing with international regulation, it is no understatement to observe that varied responses in risk assessment and operation reflect legitimate differences as well as barriers and opportunities for learning. Major findings indicate that the success and quality of regulation heavily depend on scientific knowledge, technical capability, and stakeholder involvement. Effective regulatory undertakings combine evidence-based standards with recommendations for practical and efficient implementation, as practicable in local contexts. The EU's experience with cadmium control, China's national soil remediation initiative, and global mercury management under the Minamata Convention—which gained traction on both fronts only when supported by strengthened resources and political effort—illustrate what can be achieved when policy actions are adequately resourced and politically

Australian and New Zealand Food Authority (FSANZ)	Australia & New Zealand	Food Standards Australia New Zealand Act 1991, Standard 1.4.1	Pb, Cd, Hg, As, Sn, and Cr	Scientific assessment with public consultation and ministerial approval	State enforcement agencies, import inspections, and product recalls
Mercosur Food Safety Committee	Argentina, Brazil, Paraguay, Uruguay	Mercosur Technical Regulations on Food Contaminants	Pb, Cd, Hg, As, inorganic Sn	Harmonized regional standards based on Codex and scientific risk assessments	National enforcement agencies, regional market surveillance
African Union Commission	55 African Union member states	African Continental Free Trade Area (AfCFTA) sanitary and phytosanitary measures	Pb, Cd, Hg, As (based on Codex)	Adoption of Codex standards with regional adaptations	National enforcement, customs controls, and technical assistance programs
ASEAN Food Safety Authorities	10 ASEAN member states	ASEAN Guideline for Food Contaminant Limits	Pb, Cd, Hg, As, Sn	Regional harmonization based on Codex standards	National food safety agencies, mutual recognition arrangements

supported. Key deficiencies in the current regulatory landscape that must be addressed include the lack of consideration for cumulative exposure to multiple metals, insufficient protection for highly susceptible populations such as pregnant women and newborns, and inadequate resources to assess new contaminants such as nanomaterials. The potential impacts of climate change on metal mobility and bioavailability add yet another layer of uncertainty to a sector that requires adaptive approaches and robust regulatory regimes. The globalization of trade and increasingly complex food supply chains necessitate better international cooperation and harmonization to ensure consistent protection while facilitating trade. Suggestions for future regulatory development emphasize the importance of science-based, risk-appropriate mechanisms that are responsive to evolving data and sustainable in practice. Enhanced capacity building in less developed areas, more advanced analytical techniques for emerging compounds, and increasingly sophisticated methods to assess the toxic effects of mixtures will provide a more robust knowledge base. Greater combined use of environmental surveillance, food testing, and human biomonitoring data will enable improved risk characterization and more efficient targeting of intervention initiatives. Future research priorities include better understanding of low-dose metal effects, refinement of more sensitive biomarkers (either of exposure or effect), and improved modeling of the environmental behavior of metals under changing climate conditions. The rapid increase in the use of nanomaterials demands intensified efforts to develop detection methods, risk assessment strategies, and regulations suitable for these new potential pollutants. Finally, greater focus on environmental justice issues will help ensure that regulatory safeguards for metal contamination serve all populations equally, particularly those already burdened populations that suffer most disproportionately from such contamination.

References

Abdullahi, I.L., Sani, A., 2020. Welding fumes composition and their effects on blood heavy metals in albino rats. Toxicol. Rep. 7, 1495–1501. doi:10.1016/j.toxrep.2020.10.021.

Al-Musharraf, N., Rahman, M.A., 2025. Assessing heavy metal contamination in food: implications for human health and environmental safety. Toxics 13 (3). doi:10.3390/toxics13030333.

Alengebawy, A., Abdelkhalek, S.T., Qureshi, S.R., Wang, M.-Q., 2021. Heavy metals and pesticides toxicity in agricultural soil and plants: ecological risks and human health implications. Toxics 9 (3). doi:10.3390/toxics9030042.

AOAC International, 2019. Official Methods of Analysis of AOAC International, twenty first ed. AOAC International, Rockville, MD, USA.

Aslam, M.M., et al, 2023. Heavy metal contamination and its impact on the food chain: exposure, bioaccumulation, and risk assessment. Food Agric. Immunol. doi:10.1080/19476337.2024.2438726.

Barbosa, F., Tanus-Santos, J.E., Gerlach, R.F., Parsons, P.J., 2005. A critical review of biomarkers used for monitoring human exposure to lead: advantages, limitations, and future needs. Environ. Health Perspect. 113, 1669–1674.

Bereda, G., 2025. Toxicological impacts and mitigation strategies of food contaminants: a global perspective and comprehensive narrative review. Curr. Res. Toxicol. 9, 100268. doi:10.1016/j.crtox.2025.100268.

Bouida, L., Rafatullah, M., Kerrouche, M., Qutob, M., Alosaimi, A.M., 2022. Lead contamination: sources, fate, mechanism, health effects and remediation methods. Water 14 (21). doi.10.3390/w14213432.

Briffa, J., Sinagra, E., Blundell, R., 2020. Heavy metal pollution in the environment and their toxicological effects on humans. Heliyon 6 (9), e04691. doi:10.1016/j.heliyon.2020.e04691 (updated perspectives in 2023–2025 reviews).

Chowdhury, S., et al, 2024. Heavy metals in agricultural soils: sources, influencing factors, and remediation strategies. Toxics 12 (1). doi:10.3390/toxics12010063.

Codex Alimentarius Commission, 2023. General Standard for Contaminants and Toxins in Food and Feed (CXS 193-1995). Joint FAO/WHO Food Standards Programme, Rome.

EFSA, 2012. Cadmium dietary exposure in the European population. EFSA J. 10, 2551.

European Commission, 2022. Commission Regulation (EU) No 1881/2006 of 19 December 2006 setting maximum levels for certain contaminants in foodstuffs. Off. J. Eur. Union L364, 5–24.

FAO/WHO, 2021. Joint FAO/WHO Food Standards Programme. Codex Alimentarius Commission, Rome.

FSSAI, 2021. Food Safety and Standards (Contaminants, Toxins and Residues) Regulations, 2011. Food Safety and Standards Authority of India, New Delhi.

Gadd, G.M., 2010. Metals, minerals and microbes: geomicrobiology and bioremediation. Microbiology 156, 609–643.

Grant, C.A., Clarke, J.M., Duguid, S., Chaney, R.L., 2008. Selection and breeding of plant cultivars to minimize cadmium accumulation. Sci. Total Environ. 390, 301–310.

Haq, I.U., et al, 2023. Toxicological impacts, mitigation, and policy strategies of food contaminants: a global perspective and comprehensive narrative review. Preprints. doi:10.20944/preprints202510.2196.v1.

Jaishankar, M., et al, 2023. Heavy metal pollution in the environment and its impact on health: exploring green technology for remediation. Environ. Health Insights 17. doi:10.1177/11786302231201259.

JECFA (2011). Evaluation of Certain Food Additives and Contaminants. Seventy-third Report of the Joint FAO/WHO Expert Committee on Food Additives. WHO Technical Report Series, No. 960.

Kabir, M.A., et al, 2024. Review of regulatory reference values and background levels for heavy metals in the human diet. Regul. Toxicol. Pharmacol. 138, 105363. doi:10.1016/j.yrtph.2022.105009 (updated perspectives post-2020).

Kadlec, R.H., Wallace, S.D., 2009. Treatment Wetlands, 2nd. CRC Press, Boca Raton.

Khan, J., Shrivastava, R., Gupta, G., Singh, N.K., 2023. Heavy metal contamination in groundwater: environmental concerns and mitigation measures. In: Heavy Metal Toxicity: Environmental Concerns, Remediation and Opportunities. Springer Nature Singapore, Singapore, pp. 139–165.

Komárek, M., Ettler, V., Chrastný, V., Mihaljevič, M., 2008. Lead isotopes in environmental sciences: a review. Environ. Int. 34, 562–577.

Kuhangana, T.C., Bujiriri, G.L., Musa, B.B., Potgieter, N., Mushagalusa, E.F., Smis, S., 2024. Cottage industry as a source of high exposure to lead: a biomonitoring study among people involved in manufacturing cookware from scrap metal. Environ. Res. 250, 118493. doi:10.1016/j.envres.2024.118493.

Kumar, S., Prasad, S., Yadav, K.K., Shrivastava, M., Gupta, N., Nagar, S., Bach, Q.V., Kamyab, H., Khan, S.A., Yadav, S., Malav, L.C., Yadav, V.K., Khan, M.S., Cabral-Pinto, M.M.S.,

2022. Hazardous heavy metals contamination of vegetables and food chain: role of sustainable remediation approaches – a review. Environ. Res. 213. 113709. doi:10.1016/j.envres.2022.113709.

Kumar, V., et al, 2021. Toxic and heavy metals contamination assessment in soil and water to evaluate human health risk. Sci. Rep. 11. doi:10.1038/s41598-021-94616-4.

Laoye, B., Oyewole, O.I., Ogunfowokan, A.O., 2025. Heavy metal contamination: sources, health impacts, and sustainable mitigation strategies with insights from Nigerian case studies. F1000Research 14, 134. doi:10.12688/f1000research.160148.4.

Li, Y., Li, Y., Zhang, S., Gao, T., Gao, Z., Lai, C.W., Xiang, P., 2025. Global distribution, ecotoxicity, and treatment technologies of emerging contaminants in aquatic environments: a recent five-year review. Toxics 13 (8). doi:10.3390/toxics13080616.

Mahar, A., Wang, P., Ali, A., Awasthi, M.K., Lahori, A.H., Wang, Q., Li, R., Zhang, Z., 2016. Challenges and opportunities in the phytoremediation of heavy metals contaminated soils: a review. Ecotoxicol. Environ. Saf. 126, 111–121.

MEE, 2016. Soil Pollution Prevention and Control Action Plan. Ministry of Ecology and Environment, Beijing.

Muhammad, Q., 2023. Tackling heavy metal pollution: evaluating governance models and frameworks. Sustainability 15 (22). doi:10.3390/su152215863.

Naujokas, M.F., Anderson, B., Ahsan, H., Aposhian, H.V., Graziano, J.H., Thompson, C., Suk, W.A., 2013. The broad scope of health effects from chronic arsenic exposure: update on a worldwide public health problem. Environ. Health Perspect. 121, 295–302.

NHFPC, 2022. National Food Safety Standard for Maximum Levels of Contaminants in Foods. National Health Commission of the People's Republic of China, Beijing. GB 2762-2022.

Nordberg, G., Jin, T., Wu, X., Lu, J., Chen, L., Liang, Y., Lei, L., Hong, F., Bergdahl, I.A., Nordberg, M., 2021. Kidney dysfunction and cadmium exposure–revision of risk assessment and references values. Environ. Health Perspect. 129, 65001.

Ondrasek, G., Shepherd, J., Rathod, S., Dharavath, R., Rashid, M.I., Brtnicky, M., Shahid, M.S., Horvatinec, J., Rengel, Z., 2025. Metal contamination – a global environmental issue: sources, implications & advances in mitigation. RSC Adv. 15 (5), 3904–3927. doi:10.1039/d4ra04639k.

Rahman, Z., Singh, V.P., 2024. A review on estimation of heavy metals contamination in various food products. Int. J. Pharm. Sci. Res. Rev. 84 (11), 14–25.

Rai, P.K., Lee, S.S., Zhang, M., Tsang, Y.F., Kim, K.H., Lee, J.H., Ok, Y.S., 2021. Heavy metals in food crops: health risks, fate, mechanisms, and management. Environ. Int. 125, 478–493. doi:10.1016/j.envint.2019.01.067.

Scutarașu, E.C., Trincă, L.C., 2023. Heavy metals in foods and beverages: global situation, health risks and reduction methods. Foods 12 (18). doi:10.3390/foods12183340.

Singh, R., et al, 2025. Priority toxic metals arsenic, cadmium, mercury, and lead in ecosystems. Chem. Rev. Lett. https://www.chemrevlett.com/article_226760_fca1f046fe7e7db2206fed491ab21820.pdf.

Singh, V., Singh, N., Rai, S.N., Kumar, A., Singh, A.K., Singh, M.P., Sahoo, A., Shekhar, S., Vamanu, E., Mishra, V., 2023. Heavy metal contamination in the aquatic ecosystem: toxicity and its remediation using eco-friendly approaches. Toxics 11 (2). doi:10.3390/toxics11020147.

Sunderland, E.M., 2007. Mercury exposure from domestic and imported estuarine and marine fish in the U.S. seafood market. Environ. Health Perspect. 115, 235–242.

Taylor, M.R., 2018. The Food Safety Modernization Act: a new era for food safety regulation. Food Drug Law J. 73, 1–34.

U.S. Food and Drug Administration, 2023. Guidance for Industry: Action Levels for Poisonous or Deleterious Substances in Human Food and Animal Feed. U.S. Food and Drug Administration.

https://www.fda.gov/regulatory-information/search-fda-guidance-documents/guidance-industry-action-levels-poisonous-or-deleterious-substances-human-food-and-animal-feed.
UNEP, 2017. Minamata Convention on Mercury: Text and Annexes. United Nations Environment Programme, Geneva.
UNEP, 2021. Global Mercury Assessment 2018. United Nations Environment Programme, Nairobi.
United States Environmental Protection Agency, 2021. National Recommended Water Quality Criteria. U.S. Environmental Protection Agency. https://www.epa.gov/wqc/national-recommended-water-quality-criteria.
WTO, 2021. Understanding the WTO: Sanitary and Phytosanitary Measures. World Trade Organization, Geneva.
Yan, A., Wang, Y., Tan, S.N., Mohd Yusof, M.L., Ghosh, S., Chen, Z., 2020. Phytoremediation: a promising approach for revegetation of heavy metal-polluted land. Front. Plant Sci. 11 359. doi:10.3389/fpls.2020.00359 (2020+ ecosystem remediation).
Yaseen, Z.M., 2021. An insight into machine learning models era in simulating soil, water bodies and adsorption heavy metals: review, challenges and solutions. Chemosphere 277, 130126. doi:10.1016/j.chemosphere.2021.130126.
Zaynab, M., Al-Yahyai, R., Ameen, A., Sharif, Y., Ali, L., Fatima, M., Khan, K.A., Li, S., 2022. Health and environmental effects of heavy metals. J. King Saud Univ. Sci. 34 (1), 101653. doi:10.1016/j.jksus.2021.101653.
Zhang, H., Zhou, Y., Huang, J., Li, Y., Wang, Y., Gu, J., He, Z., 2018. Variation of heavy metal concentrations in vegetables and their associated soils with different cultivation types in Zhejiang Province, China. Environ. Sci. Pollut. Res. 25, 21816–21826.
Zhao, F.J., McGrath, S.P., Meharg, A.A., 2019. Arsenic as a food chain contaminant: mechanisms of plant uptake and metabolism and mitigation strategies. Annu. Rev. Plant Biol. 70, 109–132.
Zwolak, A., Sarzyńska, M., Szpyrka, E., Stawarczyk, K., 2019. Sources of soil pollution by heavy metals and their accumulation in vegetables: a review. Water Air Soil Pollut. 230(7), 164. doi:10.1007/s11270-019-4221-y (post-2020 review updates).

Chapter 17

Metallotoxicant-driven cellular dysregulation: Redox pathways in stress signalling and death program execution

Shrabani Das, Sateesh Alavala, Shaon Santaki, Pooja Yadav, Ravi Prakash Jamalpur, and Suresh Challa
Cell Biology Division, ICMR-National Institute of Nutrition, Hyderabad, Telangana, India

17.1 Introduction

Heavy metals (HMs) are a class of metals and metalloids with atomic weights between 63.5 and 200.6 and a high density, usually >4.5 g/cm^3. Because they may have hazardous effects, accumulate in living organisms, and persist over an extended period of time, they are regarded as important environmental pollutants. The route and duration of exposure, the quantity absorbed, and individual characteristics such as age, gender, and nutritional status all influence their harmful effects (Tchounwou et al., 2012).

HMs are broadly present throughout the biosphere and are naturally found in elements such as rocks, soil, and water. Their presence arises from both natural processes and human activities. Naturally, they are released through events like volcanic eruptions, tectonic shifts, hydrothermal processes, dust storms, wildfires, and the breakdown of rocks rich in metals. In addition, microbial activity can contribute to their release. Anthropogenic sources are extensive and include mining operations, industrial effluents, urban runoff, sewage discharge, soil erosion, pesticide and herbicide use in agriculture, water transported through metal pipes, traffic emissions, and combustion byproducts from coal-burning plants (Abd Elnabi et al., 2023).

After being introduced into the environment, toxic metal particles can persist for long durations. For instance, metals released into the air from mining operations may accumulate in floodplains and riverbank soils, remaining there for centuries. Globally, millions of individuals, especially in areas of North and South

The Metallome in Motion. https://doi.org/10.1016/B978-0-443-44299-5.00016-X

America and Asia, reside in regions where harmful residues from past or ongoing mining activities exist at potentially hazardous levels (Briffa et al., 2020).

There are many ways that HMs may enter the human body, including via the skin, inhaled air, and contaminated food or drink. By losing one or more electrons while inside the body, they interact with biological processes by creating metal cations that easily attach to nucleophilic sites on essential macromolecules. These interactions disrupt normal cellular functions and can result in acute or chronic toxicity, affecting multiple organ systems. Common health complications include neurological disorders, vascular damage, immune system dysfunction, renal impairment, and cancer (Jomova et al., 2025).

Oxidative stress (OS) stemming from the generation of reactive oxygen species (ROS) and reactive nitrogen species is a primary mechanism by which HMs cause toxicity. Radicals such as superoxide (O^{2-}), molecular oxygen (O_2), nitric oxide (NO), hydrogen peroxide (H_2O_2), and peroxyl (ROO•) radicals are formed in part by metals like arsenic (As) and lead (Pb). These reactive molecules cause cellular damage and compromise the antioxidant defense system by decreasing the functionality of key antioxidant enzymes, including glutathione peroxidases (GPx), catalase (CAT), superoxide dismutase (SOD), and glutathione transferases (GST), along with reduced levels of intracellular glutathione (GSH). Simultaneously, there is a notable rise in oxidative damage indicators such as MDA and H_2O_2 (Mansoor et al., 2023).

Beyond inducing OS, certain HMs also possess carcinogenic potential. Cadmium (Cd), for example, can attach to regulatory proteins involved in essential cellular processes like cell cycle progression, DNA repair and replication, and programmed cell death. Toxicogenomic analyses indicate that cadmium interferes with key transcription regulators such as activator protein 1 (AP-1), nuclear factor kappa B (NF-Kb), and the tumor suppressor p53. Disruption of these factors hampers the normal expression of protective genes, thereby promoting abnormal and unregulated cell growth (Davidova et al., 2024).

Given the broad health implications, numerous international agencies have established strict guidelines for the presence of HMs in the environment, food, and drinking water. While high-dose exposures can cause acute conditions like kidney failure, even low-dose, chronic exposures represent a hidden yet significant risk, potentially leading to long-term complications such as neuropsychiatric disorders (Mitra et al., 2022).

Taken together, the persistence of HMs in the environment and their ability to bioaccumulate pose a serious threat to public health and ecological stability. Among the diverse mechanisms of metal-induced toxicity, the development of OS stands out as a critical and unifying pathway. Through excessive production of reactive oxygen and nitrogen species, HMs disrupt redox balance, damage cellular macromolecules, impair antioxidant defenses, and trigger signaling cascades that promote inflammation, apoptosis, and disease. This chapter focuses on providing an in-depth exploration of the role of OS in mediating HM toxicity, highlighting molecular mechanisms, affected organ systems, and the implications for cytotoxicity. A better understanding of these processes may inform future strategies for prevention, detoxification, and therapeutic intervention.

17.2 Sources and routes of exposure to toxic metals

HMs are nonbiodegradable toxic substances emitted from both anthropogenic and natural sources (Qin et al., 2021). Some natural sources, such as fresh vegetables and fruits, contain higher concentrations of HMs, which may cause renal dysfunction, carcinogenesis, immunological imbalance, and even death due to their ability to bioaccumulate and biomagnify (Shamsudduha et al., 2020). Fertilizer or pesticides containing HMs, improper industrial effluent disposal, and polluted irrigation water allow HMs to enter the food chain and induce toxicity (Zakir et al., 2020). Arsenic affects the food chain through polluted irrigation water and inappropriate mining. Trophic transmission of HMs is a significant problem these days, as everyone indirectly ingests HMs by consuming fruits, vegetables, and other plant products grown on polluted soil (Subhavana et al., 2020). The spread of HMs from primary sources, such as pesticide-containing HMs, improper disposal of industrial effluent, mining, poultry manure, trace metals, rocks and minerals, and weathering, to food webs and adjoining ecosystems poses a serious threat to global food hygiene. Children and adults who consume raw cow milk and graze in polluted fields face the risk of toxicity and biomagnification (Boudebbouz et al., 2021). Petrochemicals pose threats to human health and the environment by accumulating HMs such as zinc, lead, cadmium, nickel, and copper from contaminated soil. Long-term consumption of contaminated food may lead to the accumulation of HMs in vital organs and bones, causing impairment of vital organs and bone-related problems. Consequently, HMs cause biomagnification at each trophic level after entering the food chain. Biomagnification refers to the toxicity, persistence, and capacity of HMs to enhance their detrimental effects at each successive trophic level. Their growing concentration, due to greater absorption than excretion and elimination, causes increased health risks, some of which are lethal, at each trophic level. Biomagnification can reduce the growth of plankton, crustaceans, and mollusks as well as diminish the photosynthetic ability and productivity of aquatic ecosystems. In addition, it may result in cytogenic damage, lower embryo viability in wild animals, mental retardation, cardiovascular issues, renal malfunction, and abnormalities in fish, birds, and mammals. Biomagnification, such as that seen in Hg-, As-, and Se-polluted water, can be observed from phytoplankton to invertebrates to fish, and finally to humans. MeHg concentrations have been shown to increase more than 50 times as it moves from copepods (*Calanus hyperboreus*) to seabirds (such as *Sterna paradisaea*). Bioaccumulation (the accumulation of HMs in an organism) of these HMs causes several health concerns in various organisms, including the following: Effects on Fish: Fish at higher trophic levels are more negatively impacted by HMs. Teratogenesis is induced by Hg, which reduces reproductive ability, damages tissues, genes, and proteins, and alters their ecological behavior. Enzymatic deficiency, hyperglycemia, and immune system dysfunction are all possible consequences. Se),lenium (Se when interacting with Hg, reduces embryo survival and fertility, as well as increases juvenile mortality. **Effects on birds**: Hg bioaccumulation in seabirds and waterbirds reduces flying capability due to Hg's strong affinity for keratin in feathers. Hg also impairs reproductive function in seabirds by affecting gonadotropin-releasing hormone. Weight loss, egg hatching, abnormalities (e.g., beak, eye, microphthalmia, and anophthalmia), and hydrocephalus development all impact reproduction. It lowers red blood cell synthesis and disrupts the endocrine system (Córdoba-Tovar et al., 2022). Effects on Humans: According to the World Health Organization, by eating mercury-contaminated fish, every 17th child in one thousand develops mental disorders in fishing areas of Colombia, China, Brazil, and Greenland. Ataxia, muscular weakness, numb limbs, and difficulties with speaking, chewing, and swallowing, as well as rapid and enhanced tendon reflexes, are all examples of neurological injury. Hg has various deleterious consequences, including renal impairment and hepatotoxicity. Mercury may also harm newborns through maternal exposure. As a result, health risks such as central nervous system (CNS) injury, gastrointestinal pain, and liver damage arise. Since it can readily cross the placenta, it can cause complications such as abortion, preterm delivery, stillbirth, and low birth weight when women consume contaminated water (Balali-Mood et al., 2021) as shown in Fig. 17.1.

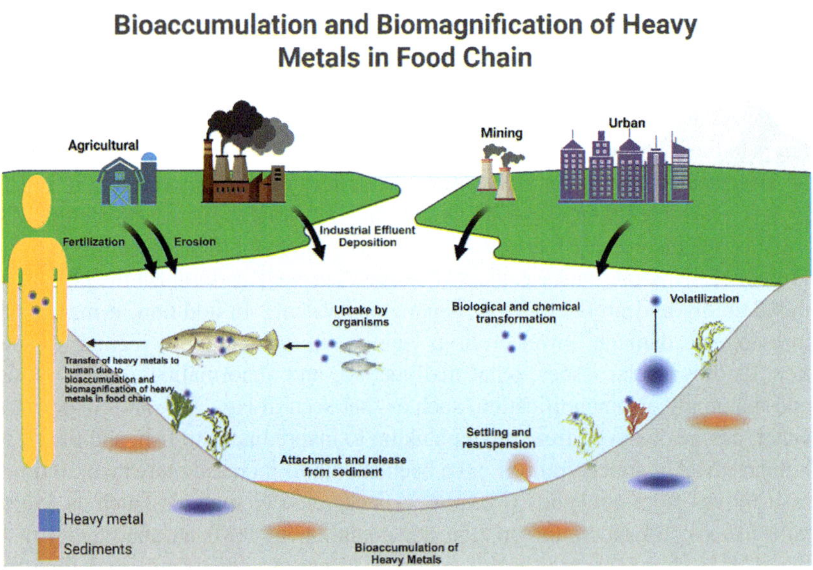

FIG. 17.1 The illustration shows heavy metal bioaccumulation and biomagnification in the food chain.

17.3 Oxidative stress as a central mediator of heavy metal toxicity: Insights from experimental models

HMs are well-established environmental toxicants that exert their deleterious effects primarily through the generation of ROS. These species are produced via auto-oxidative mechanisms, resulting in OS that damages vital cellular components. In addition, HMs can bind to functional groups such as carboxyl, histidyl, and thiol moieties in proteins or interact with molecules like GSH. Some also mimic essential functional groups, particularly phosphate groups, thereby altering protein structure and function and disrupting crucial signaling pathways (Wang et al., 2016). Lead (Pb) exposure during critical developmental periods poses significant neurotoxic risks. As demonstrated by Shilpa et al. 2021b), who exposure during the developmental period leads to elevated Pb accumulation in the brains of both wild-type and antioxidant-deficient *Drosophila melanogaster*. This was associated with increased ROS and lipid peroxidation (LPO), indicating heightened OS, along with a disrupted antioxidant defense system marked by reduced levels of SOD, CAT, and cytochrome P450. These alterations culminated in extensive brain vacuolation, neuropil disruption, oxidative DNA damage, and apoptosis, which are considered hallmark features of neurodegeneration. Pb buildup in the adult fly brain and behavioral traits resembling autism spectrum disorder (ASD) were also caused by exposure to Pb during the larval stage. These results highlight how Pb-induced OS contributes to the development of neurological defects and provide credence to the use of *Drosophila melanogaster* as a model organism to study the external influences of ASD (Shilpa et al., 2021a).

According to a similar study (Kataba et al., 2020), exposure to environmentally pertinent levels of lead caused neurobehavioral changes in larval zebrafish. These changes were accompanied by dysregulated expression of genes linked to OS (HO-1, Ucp2, CoxI) and impacted expression of proapoptotic (TP53) and antiapoptotic (Bcl-2) genes, indicating a possible involvement of lead in the occurrence of neurobehavioral conditions. (Xu et al., 2008), shown that oral exposure to lead acetate causes OS in mice, as shown by increased ROS and MDA levels and substantial DNA damage. Furthermore, a disruption in the Bax/Bcl-2 ratio and elevated expression of proteins like p53 and Bax indicate that OS-mediated apoptosis is a key factor in Pb-produced toxicity.

Numerous studies have shown that long-term exposure to arsenic (As) increases OS, mainly via lowering intracellular GSH levels (Li et al., 2002). Chattopadhyay et al. (2002) shown that exposure dramatically raises ROS and NO levels while lowering GSH content and SOD activity at the same time. This redox imbalance is associated with elevated LPO and a substantial decline in both DNA and protein synthesis. In BALB/c mice, oral administration of As induces OS characterized by macromolecular oxidation, depletion of antioxidant reserves, and upregulation of pro-inflammatory cytokines, ultimately contributing to the development of hepatic fibrosis. Furthermore, As has been shown to cause telomere shortening, Its considerable genotoxic potential is shown by chromosomal from beginning to end combinations and apoptotic death of cells (Das et al., 2005).

Similarly, in neurons, manganese (Mn) exposure has been shown to induce programmed cell death, characterized by DNA fragmentation and a decline in microtubule-associated protein 2 (MAP-2), a critical marker of neuronal integrity. In aquatic models such as goldfish, Mn exposure triggers OS, characterized by reduced antioxidant enzyme activities and increased LPO, underscoring both systemic and tissue-specific toxic effects (Vieira et al., 2012). Furthermore, developmental exposure to Mn has been associated with delayed growth and maturation, accompanied by elevated MDA levels, increased antioxidant enzyme activity, and upregulation of stress-related genes such as p53, along with enhanced expression of proinflammatory markers (Li et al., 2023b).

A strong environmental toxin, cadmium (Cd) causes oxidative damage and apoptosis, particularly in the early stages of development. Cd exposure in *Drosophila melanogaster* altered the expression of genes linked to apoptosis while raising the concentration of ROS and DNA damage (Yang et al., 2022). In human keratinocytes, Cd caused oxidative damage to DNA, lipids, and proteins by reducing CAT and GSH-Px levels (Nzengue et al., 2008). In male Wistar rats, Cd exposure led to testicular OS and toxicity (Imafidon et al., 2016). Cd changed the activity of enzymes linked to OS and increased ROS in microglial cells, indicating a possible involvement in neuroinflammation and neuronal damage (Yang et al., 2007). Furthermore, prolonged exposure to Cd in proximal tubule cells raised intracellular calcium and ROS, which depleted GSH and caused necrotic and apoptotic cell death (Wang et al., 2009).

Although copper (Cu) is an essential trace element, excessive exposure can lead to significant oxidative damage. Oral administration of copper sulfate ($CuSO_4$) in mice increased ROS, MDA, and DNA damage while suppressing antioxidant markers such as GSH, SOD, CAT, and GSH-Px, ultimately causing inflammatory responses and pulmonary apoptosis (Jian et al., 2020). Chronic Cu exposure in the liver elevated protein carbonylation and impaired antioxidant defense, alongside the upregulation of apoptotic markers, contributing to hepatocyte apoptosis (Liu et al., 2020).

Chronic exposure to mercuric chloride ($HgCl_2$) in adult rats caused mercury (Hg) accumulation in the brain, OS, as evidenced by increased LPO, decreased antioxidant levels, and motor deficits. These changes were associated with neuronal and astrocytic loss in the motor cortex via apoptosis and cytotoxicity (Teixeira et al., 2018).

Taken together, the evidence from various model organisms and experimental systems highlights OS as a central and conserved mechanism underlying HM toxicity, and the consistent involvement of OS across diverse biological contexts underscores its pivotal role in mediating the cellular and systemic consequences of HM exposure.

17.4 HM-induced oxidative stress and disruption of cellular signaling pathways

A study by Dey et al., demonstrated that chronic exposure to environmentally relevant concentrations of Pb activates the Nrf2/Keap1 signalling pathway while simultaneously impairs DNA repair mechanisms in zebrafish (Babiker et al., 2019). This was accompanied by elevated expression of tumour suppressor genes p53 and brca2, indicating a neurotoxic effect upon prolonged Pb exposure (Dey et al., 2025). Consistently, long-term Pb exposure has been shown to suppresses the heart's protective response to ischemia–reperfusion injury by elevating OS, disrupting the cardiac antioxidant balance, and promoting apoptosis in male rats. Moreover, Pb exposure has been associated with neurotoxicity in the cerebellum of Japanese quail, characterized by morphological deformities in neuroglial and Purkinje cells. It seems that this impact is mediated by dysregulation of the Nrf2/Keap1 signalling pathway, which disrupts glutathione metabolism, ultimately leading to impaired neurotransmission and neuronal apoptosis (Zhang et al., 2024).

Combinational exposure at levels pertinent to the environment of Pb and Cr was found to exacerbate hepatotoxicity and induce necrosis by disrupting the Nrf2-Keap1-ARE signaling pathway, characterized by elevated OS, depleted glutathione levels, and marked histopathological alterations (Sarkar et al., 2025b). In mice, combinational exposure to a high-fat diet and Pb led to significant suppression of Nrf2-mediated antioxidant defense proteins, resulting in CNS dysfunction characterized by impaired memory, learning abilities, and distorted locomotor activities (Zhang et al., 2021).

Similar perturbations have also been observed with As exposure at environmentally relevant levels. The significance of this pathway in reducing As-induced oxidative damage is highlighted by the fact that As concentration has been shown to cause OS, with increased MDA and the activation of Nrf2/Keap1 and its downstream effectors, such NQO1 and GCLC (Sun et al., 2022). However, chronic occupational As exposure has been associated with global DNA methylation, leading to functional suppression of the Nrf2 pathway and altered expression of its effectors, thereby implicating epigenetic mechanisms in the long-term toxicity (Janasik et al., 2018).

Likewise, prolonged Cu exposure has been reported to cause damage through oxidation and renal impairment via dysregulation of the Keap1/Nrf2-Msr signaling pathway, as evidenced by increased creatinine and carbamide levels and reduced activities of enzymes with antioxidant properties (Zhong et al., 2021). The protective role of Nrf2 was further demonstrated in a recent study by Li et al., where Nrf2 knockout mice, upon exposure to As and Cu, exhibited increased NLRP3 inflammasome formation and caspase-1 activation, underscoring the importance of Nrf2 in counteracting HM-induced apoptosis and pyroptosis (Li et al., 2023a).

Chronic exposure to Cd has also been shown to damage the antioxidant defense system, which is controlled by the Nrf2-Keap1 signaling pathway and its downstream effectors like HO-1, resulting in OS and promoting apoptosis (Choudhury et al., 2021). Similarly, Deng et al. reported that excessive exposure to Mn disrupts the Nrf2/Keap1/ARE signaling pathway, leading to OS, locomotor impairment, and neurodegeneration (Deng et al., 2015b). Furthermore, combinational treatment with Pb and Mn has been demonstrated to exaggerate oxidative damage and neuroinflammation via disruption of the Nrf2/HO-1/BDNF signaling axis. This was accompanied by increased APP expression and decreased occludin levels in the cerebral cortex of rats, suggesting compromised blood–brain barrier (BBB) integrity and enhanced neurotoxicity (Dooka et al., 2025).

Overexpression of heat shock proteins and inflammatory markers, along with exposure to Pb, has been demonstrated to cause metabolic impairment and severe liver damage (Mesalam et al., 2023). Continuous exposure to Pb in Wister rats has been associated with kidney damage via the ROS-driven MAPK/NF-κβ signaling axis, which leads to inflammation (Liu et al., 2012). Qi et al. demonstrated in a different study that prenatal exposure to As altered the PI3K/Akt/NF-κβ pathway in the hippocampus, leading to neurodevelopmental abnormalities, particularly during the postnatal period.

In microglial cells, Pb exposure has been reported to accelerate the expression of proinflammatory cytokines via upregulation of NF-kβ/ERK/Akt signalling pathway, cumulating in neuronal cell death via activation of caspase-3 (Kumawat et al., 2014). Similarly, in hippocampal neurons dose-dependent Pb exposure has been shown to trigger aberrant cell death via dysregulation of PI3K/Akt-Cyclin D1-CDK4 signalling axis (Li et al., 2008). In Swiss-albino male mice, Pb induced pulmonary inflammation was elevated expression of both proinflammatory and antiinflammatory cytokines such as NF-kβ, TNF-α, and IFN-γ respectively (Gupta and Sharma, 2025). Moreover, Pb exposure has been implicated in frenal damage via suppression of PI3k/Akt mRNA expression and in nephrotoxicity in Japanese quail by inhibiting PI3k/Akt, activating NF-κβ, and triggering apoptosis (Balaji et al., 2021; Zhang et al., 2023). Likewise, Alhusaini et al., has also been demonstrated Pb exposure induces inflammation and hepatotoxicity by upregulating NF-κβ, JNK and TNF-α, while suppressing the Akt/GSK-3β pathway, further contributing to OS and live damage (Alhusaini et al., 2019).

As exposure during the prenatal period has been associated with inflammation and renal fibrosis, mediated by NF-κβ/ERK1/2 signaling and epigenetic deregulation involving EZH2 and H3K27me3, leading to nephrotoxicity in offspring (Singh et al., 2025). Furthermore, As exposure during gestation has been shown to induce autophagy-mediated neuronal cell death through dysregulation of the PI3K/Akt/mTOR signaling pathway, along with upregulation of key autophagic markers, including Autophagy-Related Gene 5 (Atg5),

Autophagy-related 12 (Atg12), Beclin1, and Microtubule-associated protein light chain 3 (LC3), leading to developmental neurotoxicity in mice (Manthari et al., 2018). In swine, chronic Cd exposure triggered NLRP3-mediated inflammasome formation and pyroptosis via activation of the TRAF6/NF-κβ signaling axis, which was further associated with the correlation between pro-inflammatory and antiinflammatory cytokines (Cai et al., 2021). In Sprague-Dawley rats, coexposure to Cd and As enhanced the expression of NF-κβ and IL-1β, promoting hepatorenal inflammation (Cengiz et al., 2023) as shown in Table 17.1.

Similarly, Mn exposure has been shown to promote proinflammatory cytokine and chemokine production in alveolar and bronchial cells via stimulation of the ERK/NF-κB/p65 pathway, suggesting a link between Mn-induced cytotoxicity and respiratory disorders (Gandhi et al., 2025) as shown in Fig. 17.2.

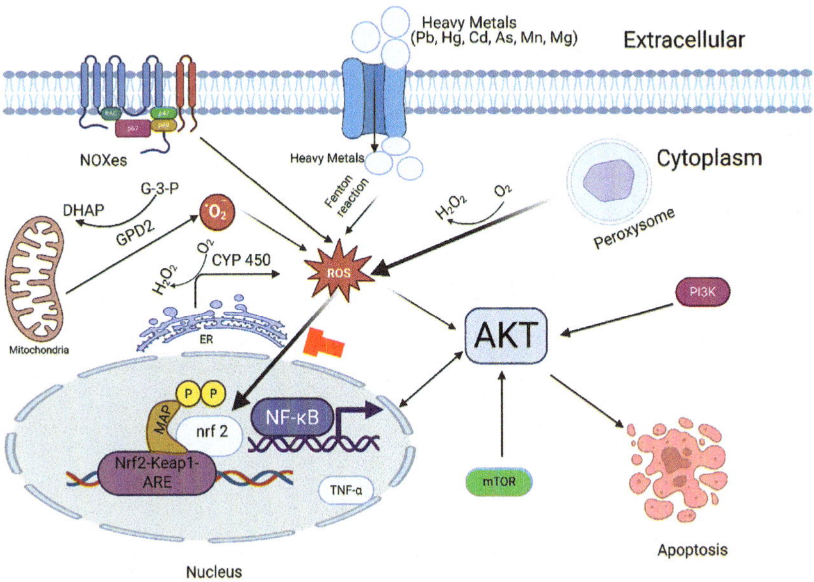

FIG. 17.2 Schematic representation of heavy metal-induced signaling pathways. Exposure to heavy metals activates multiple intracellular signaling cascades, including MAPK (ERK, JNK, and p38), NF-κB, PI3K/Akt, and Keap1-Nrf2 pathways. These signaling networks regulate cellular responses such as oxidative stress (OS), inflammation, apoptosis, and autophagy. Heavy metals trigger ROS generation, which, in turn, activates stress-responsive kinases and transcription factors (e.g., Nrf2 and NF-κB), leading to the release of antioxidant enzymes or proinflammatory cytokines. In parallel, disruption of mitochondrial and lysosomal function further amplifies oxidative damage and cell death signaling. The figure highlights key molecular mediators and downstream effectors associated with heavy metal toxicity. Schematic representation of heavy metal-induced signaling pathways.

TABLE 17.1 The HMs' effect on cellular signaling.

Heavy metals	Experimental procedures and treatments	Specific mechanisms and pathway(s)	Effect(s)	Reference (s)
Lead (Pb)	Adult Zebrafish (*Danio rerio*) Pb for 15 and 30 days. Zebrafish (*D. rerio*) Pb (2.5 + 5 + 10 ppb) + Cr (0.5 + 7 + 2 ppm) for 15, 30, and 60 days C57BL/6 J mice Pb (250 mg/L in drinking water) + high-fat diet for 12 weeks Wister RatPb (500 mg/L) for 75 days BV2 Microglial Cell and N2a neuroblastoma cell 1,5,10,25,50,100 uM for 24 h	Activation of the Nrf2/Keap1 signaling pathway, along with alterations in its downstream effector genes such as HO-1 and NQO1 ↑MDA ↓GSH ↑p53 and BRCA2 ↑ROS ↑LPO ↑Catalase ↓Glutathione ↑Necrosis ↓Keap1,ucp2 mRNA expression ↑nrf2,ho1,nqo1, and hsp70 mRNA expression ↑ROS ↓Nrf2, HO-1, NQO1 and SOD2 protein levels	Chronic Pb toxicity resulted in impairment of DNA repair mechanism, followed by excessive DNA damage and neurotoxicity. Combinational exposure to Pb and Cr for a prolonged period of time resulted in elevation of OS following hepatotoxicity via disruption of Nrf2/Keap1/ARE signaling pathway. Chronic Pb exposure, along with a high-fat diet, resulted in cognitive dysfunction via downregulation NRF2 signaling pathway in mice. Exposure to Pb resulted in inflammation and hepatotoxicity by modulating the expression of NF-κB. Pb exposure is reported to induce renal dysfunction by elevating OS and inflammation.	(Dey et al., 2024; Sarkar et al., 2025a)

	Swiss Albino male mice Pb (50 mg/kg body weight) for 30 days. Japanese quail (Coturnix japonica) Pb (500–1000 ppm) for 5 weeks	↑NF-kβ, TNF-α ↑HSP60, HSP 70 and HSP 90 ↓GSH, SOD, CAT, GPx ↑MDA, NO ↑TBARS ↑COX-2 ↑NF-kβ ↑TNF-α, IL-6 ↑pERK/pAkt ↑NF-kβ ↑Caspase-3 ↑NF-kβ ↑TNF-α ↑IL-6 ↓IFN-γ ↓IL-10 ↑NF-kβ ↓PI3k/Akt	In neuronal cells, Pb exposure led to the activation of microglial cells, resulting in neuroinflammation and apoptosis. Pb exposure is reported to elevate inflammation, resulting in pulmonary toxicity. Pb exposure manifests in nephrotoxicity via the elevation of OS, inflammation, and apoptosis.	

Continued

TABLE 17.1 The HMs' effect on cellular signaling—cont'd

Heavy metals	Experimental procedures and treatments	Specific mechanisms and pathway(s)	Effect(s)	Reference (s)
Arsenic (As)	Female adult ICR mice As (10–200ugL-1) for 30 days BALB/c mouse (0.4 ppm) for 15 days	↓ZnSOD ↓MnSOD ↓Metallothionein ↑MDA ↑ Nrf2/Keap1 ↑ HO-1 ↑NQO1 ↑GCLC ↑Serum creatinine ↓GFR ↑NF-kβ ↑TNF-α, IL-6	Chronic As exposure resulted in the activation of the Nrf2/Keap1 signaling pathway, along with its downstream effectors such as HO-1, NOQ1, and GCLC.	(Che et al., 2019)
Copper (Cu)	CD-1 rats Cu (30, 60, and 120 mg/kg body weight) for 24 weeks C57BL/6 wild-type and Nrf2-KO Mice Arsenic trioxide (0.05 mg/kg body weight) + (0.013 mg/kg body weight)	↓GSH, CAT, and Total Antioxidant Capacity ↑Nrf2/Keap1 ↓NQO1, SOD-1, TRX, MsrA, MsrB1, MsrB2 and MsrB3 mRNA ↑Nrf2/Keap1 signalling Pathway ↑NLRP3 formation ↑Caspase-3	Cu exposure has been reported to result in the activation of the Nrf2/Keap1-Msr signaling pathways along with its downstream effector genes as a compensatory mechanism to combat oxidative damage and nephrotoxicity. Combinational exposure to Cu and As resulted in the activation of the Nrf2/Keap1 signaling pathway and the induction of apoptosis and pyroptosis. However, Nrf2-KO further aggravated apoptosis and pyroptosis by downregulating the expression of antioxidants like CAT and HO-1	(Zhang et al., 2016)

Cadmium (Cd)	Heart Kidney Macrophage (HKM) of Channa punctatus Bloch $CdCl_2$ (1.96 mg/L) for 7 days Weaned Piglets 20 mg/kg $CdCl_2$ for 40 days	↓HO-1 ↑Caspase-3 ↑ Caspase-8 ↑ TNF-α ↑p53 ↑NLRP3 ↑Cas1, ↑ASC ↑IL-2, IL-6, IL-7 ↓IL-10 ↑TRAF6/Ikβ-α-NF-kβ	Cd exposure resulted in alteration in the Nrf2/Keap1 signaling pathway, which further resulted in alteration in the expression of cytochrome C and induction of apoptosis. In swine, Cd exposure resulted in the formation of inflammasomes, causing cerebral pyroptosis.	(Yao et al., 2021)
Manganese (Mn)	Kunming Mice $MgCl_2$ (12.5, 25, and 50 mg/kg body weight) for 2 weeks Cerebral Cortex of Rat Mn (0.564 mg/kg body weight) + Pb (20 mg/kg body weight) + Al (35 mg/kg body weight) for 90 days Human Normal Bronchial (BEAS-2B), adenocarcinoma alveolar (A549) epithelial cells, and murine macrophages (J774). Pb (0–1400 μM) for 24 h	↑Nrf2/Keap1/ARE ↑MDA ↓GSH ↓SOD ↓GPx, SOT, CAD ↑COX-2 and Caspase-3 ↑Nrf2 ↑MDA ↓BDNF, HO-1, Occludin ↑pERK1/2 ↑p65 ↑NF-kβ	Mn exposure resulted in the activation of the Nrf2/Keap1/ARE signaling pathway, which further led to neuronal degeneration, activation of astrocytes, and programmed cell death. Mixture of heavy metals containing Mn and Pb has been reported to aggravate OS, inflammation, and neurodegeneration via downregulating the Nrf2/HO-1/BDNF signaling axis. Mn exposure resulted in the induction of an inflammatory response by enhancing the expression of ERK/NF-κB.	(Deng et al., 2015a)

17.5 Molecular mechanisms of heavy metal-induced organelle dysfunction

17.5.1 Effect on mitochondria

Heavy metals have been widely implicated in mitochondrial dysfunction across diverse organ systems, contributing to their toxicological profiles and disease pathogenesis.

Lead (Pb) exposure has been shown to severely impair mitochondrial integrity, particularly in neurons. Chronic exposure to Pb has been reported to stimulate the opening of the mitochondrial permeability transition pore (MPTP), resulting in mitochondrial fragmentation and loss of mitochondrial membrane potential (MMP), which subsequently leads to oxidative damage and programmed cell death, considered hallmarks of Pb-induced neurotoxicity (Ye et al., 2020). Chronic exposure to Pb has also been shown to disrupt mitochondrial oxidative phosphorylation (OXPHOS), promoting a metabolic shift toward glycolysis. This metabolic reprogramming results in the loss of ATP synthesis and a decline in the production of synaptic proteins, thereby inhibiting neurite outgrowth and neurogenesis (Li et al., 2022). Similarly, prenatal and neonatal Pb exposure in female Wister rats has been associated with deficits in memory and learning, along with morphological abnormalities in synaptic mitochondria, including swelling and elongation (Gąssowska et al., 2016). Pb-induced hepatotoxicity has also been linked to impairment of mitochondrial function, characterized by disruption of mitochondrial respiratory chain complexes, opening of MPTP, collapse of MMP, and release of cytochrome *c* (Ma et al., 2017). Furthermore, it has been shown to aggravate mitochondrial localization of the fission protein Drp1, while reducing the colocalization of the fusion proteins Mitofusin 2 (MFN2) and Optic Atrophy 1 (OPA1) with mitochondria, thereby promoting mitochondrial fragmentation. Recent evidence has also demonstrated that Pb enhances PTEN-induced kinase 1 (PINK1)-driven ubiquitination and degradation of MFN2, a key mitochondrial fusion protein, thereby implicating Pb in the development of neurotoxicity (Zhang et al., 2022). Supporting these findings, Lalwani et al. reported that combinational exposure to Pb along with FCCP, a mitochondrial uncoupler, or Ruthenium Red, an inhibitor of the mitochondrial calcium uniporter (MCU), exacerbates cytotoxicity and apoptotic cell death by altering the MMP (Lalwani et al., 2023).

Similarly, manganese (Mn) exposure has been reported to result in mitochondrial fragmentation and loss of MMP through dysregulation of proteins associated with mitochondrial dynamics. This is accompanied by changes in the Bax/Bcl-2 ratio, followed by activation of the intrinsic apoptotic pathway, as evidenced by caspase-9 activation and increased release of caspase-3/7(Alaimo et al., 2013). Mn-induced exposure has also been shown to trigger the production of proinflammatory cytokines and the accumulation of α-synuclein by reducing mitochondrial mass, ATP production, and oxygen consumption rate, thereby implicating mitochondrial dysfunction in Mn-induced dopaminergic neurotoxicity (Sarkar et al., 2018). Notably, Mn has also been reported to disturb intermitochondrial connectivity by increasing the formation of mitochondrial nanotunnels and impairing axonal mitochondrial transport through the dysregulation of motor proteins such as Dynactin-1 (DCTN1) and Kinesin Family Member 5B (KIF5B), further contributing to neurodegenerative progression associated with Mn exposure.

In HEK-293 T cells, mercury (Hg), particularly $HgCl_2$ induces mitochondrial fission via dysregulation of the SIRT1/PGC-1α pathway, causing OS and nephrotoxicity.

Cadmium (Cd) has been widely implicated in mitochondrial dysfunction across various organ systems. In zebrafish, chronic exposure to Cd has been reported to disrupt hepatic lipid metabolism, as evidenced by the aberrant upregulation of genes associated with mitophagy, such as PINK1, PARKin, NIP3-like protein X (NIX), and LC3, along with a loss of MMP and decreased ATP production, indicating a potential link between Cd-induced mitophagy, mitochondrial dysfunction, and metabolic dysregulation (Pan et al., 2018). In rat proximal tubule cells, acute Cd exposure stimulates mitochondrial biogenesis, as evidenced by increased expression of Peroxisome proliferator-activated receptor gamma (PPARγ), a key regulator of mitochondrial biogenesis, and MFN 2, along with elevated mtDNA levels. These findings suggest an adaptive mitochondrial response to counteract Cd-induced nephrotoxicity (Nair et al., 2015). Conversely, chronic Cd exposure increases the risk of nephrotoxicity by disrupting mitochondrial homeostasis, primarily through the downregulation of proteins involved in the mitochondrial unfolded protein response and mitochondrial dynamics, ultimately leading to structural damage and mitochondrial dysfunction (Ge et al., 2019). Cd has also been shown to impair the male reproductive system by disrupting mitochondrial dynamics followed by mitophagy, thereby causing decreased recruitment of PINK1 and increased accumulation of LC3 and p62, resulting in apoptosis (Yi et al., 2022). In MN6 cells, Cd exposure leads to pancreatic β-cell toxicity by increasing mitochondrial ROS (mtROS) levels, which further lead to mitochondrial dysfunction, impaired insulin secretion, and inflammation (Hong et al., 2022).

Arsenic (As) exposure similarly disrupts mitochondrial integrity. In GC1 spermatogonial cells, chronic exposure to As damages mitochondrial functioning by impairing mitochondrial structure and inhibiting ATP-linked respiration and the respiratory control rate (Chen et al., 2020). Furthermore, As elevates mtROS and intracellular Ca^{2+} levels via mitochondria-ER crosstalk, thereby causing mitochondrial dysfunction, redox imbalance, and stimulation of potential apoptotic signaling (Cantoni et al., 2021). In primary mouse hepatocytes, As exposure has been associated with enhanced ROS production and activation of MPTP, resulting in programmed cell death (Santra et al., 2022). In rats, As exposure impairs mitochondrial respiration by disrupting the activity of complex II of the ETC and dysregulating mitochondrial SirT3 activity, which further results in increased OS, impaired glucose tolerance, insulin resistance, and the development of diabetes-like symptoms (Rezaei et al., 2019). Notably, individuals with nonclinical hyperglycemia may exhibit increased susceptibility to As-induced mitochondrial damage, characterized by increased MMP and cristae swelling, further accelerating diabetes development (Kalo and Rezaei, 2022).

Copper (Cu) toxicity has also been linked to significant mitochondrial impairment. In SHSY-5Y cells, Cu exposure has been shown to be involved in the excessive accumulation of mitochondrial Cu, impaired mitochondrial dehydrogenase levels, and depleted activity of complex I and complex V, along with pyruvate, subsequently leading to Cu-mediated mitochondrial damage in the occurrence of neurodegeneration (Arciello et al., 2005). Excessive Cu exposure has been shown to cause hepatotoxicity in chickens, characterized by an elevation in the expression of apoptotic proteins, along with a reduction in MMP (Yang et al., 2019). Cu overload in the hearts of mice has been reported to be associated with mitochondrial dysfunction, along with the loss of mitochondrial proteins, thereby causing apoptosis and further leading to cardiac injury (Pan et al., 2022). In cultured neurons and astrocytes, Cu exposure has been shown to reduce MMP, activate the MPTP, and cause the loss of ATP levels, which mainly indicates the role of Cu in the occurrence of neurotoxicity via an MPTP-dependent mechanism (Reddy et al., 2008). In pigs, excessive accumulation of dietary Cu has been demonstrated to induce mitochondria-mediated cell death by downregulating levels of mitochondrial fusion and antiapoptosis-related genes, including Mfn1, Mfn2, and Bcl-2, respectively (Hu et al., 2023).

Taken together, these studies suggest the significance of mitochondrial dysfunction and mitophagy in mediating the toxic effects of HMs across a wide range of biological systems, and a deeper understanding of these mitochondrial disruptions can provide critical insights into the biological consequences of HM exposure and highlight potential molecular targets for therapeutic intervention.

17.5.2 Effect on lysosome

HMs are extensively associated with the impairment of autophagic flux and the dysfunction of lysosomes in various organ systems, playing a significant role in their overall toxicity and involvement in disease development.

In PC12 cells, lead (Pb) exposure has been reported to cause alterations in lysosomal functioning by increasing lysosomal pH and reducing the number and size of lysosomes through the downregulation of LAMP1 expression. These alterations impair autophagy, leading to aberrant accumulation of autophagosomes (Gu et al., 2019). Similarly, in proximal tubular cells, Pb exposure induces nephrotoxicity by impairing lysosomal functioning, as evidenced by lysosomal alkalization resulting from suppression of the V-ATPase subunit, followed by increased lysosomal membrane permeabilization (LMP) and decreased lysosomal degradation capacity via downregulation of cathepsin B and D expression, implicating the role of Pb-mediated nephrotoxicity in LMP-mediated cell death (Song et al., 2017). In mice, high doses of Pb exposure have been demonstrated to cause excessive accumulation of lipid droplets in Sertoli cells due to impaired autophagic flux, characterized by lysosomal dysfunction and disrupted autophagosome-lysosome fusion (Guo et al., 2025).

Copper (Cu) dyshomeostasis has been implicated in the accumulation of oligomeric Aβ peptides and the progression of Alzheimer's disease, with lysosomal dysfunction and suppression of Transcription Factor EB (TFEB), a key transcription factor involved in lysosomal biogenesis (Tan et al., 2020). Furthermore, in MN9D dopaminergic neurons, CuCl2 exposure has been reported to impair lysosomal proteolytic activity, characterized by elevated cytosolic Ca^{2+} levels and compromised autophagic flux (Kim et al., 2024).

Chronic exposure to cadmium (Cd) has been associated with a decline in both mRNA and protein levels of TFEB. Conversely, chloroquine-induced compromised lysosomal functioning upregulates the expression of TFEB and its downstream targets, aimed at enhancing lysosomal biosynthesis and mitigating neurotoxicity (Pi et al., 2017). Cd exposure also promotes LMP and caspase-dependent cell death. Notably, TFE3 overexpression has been shown to protect against neurotoxicity by preserving the mitochondrial-lysosomal axis, a mechanism through which lysosomes influence mitochondria-driven apoptotic processes (Pi et al., 2018).

A current investigation has revealed that in microglial cells, manganese (Mn) exposure activates LRRK2 and its signaling effector, RAB10, contributes to the suppression of ALP, impairment of lysosomal functioning, aberrant release of cathepsin B into the cytosol, and formation of the inflammasome. These events culminate in the initiation of inflammation and promotion of neuronal damage (Pajarillo et al., 2023). Arsenic (As) exposure in dendritic cells has been shown to induce lysosomal dysfunction by downregulating Cathepsin L (CTSL) and Cathepsin (D) CTSD, thereby impairing autophagic flux. Interestingly, this defect can be rescued by TFEB overexpression, highlighting its therapeutic potential in As-induced cellular stress (Alcon et al., 2020). Chronic exposure to mercury (Hg), particularly in the form of methylmercury (MeHg), has been reported to impair lysosomal degradative function, leading to autophagosome accumulation and contributing to neurotoxicity (Zhao et al., 2020).

Collectively, these findings underscore the importance of lysosomal dysfunction and impaired autophagic flux as converging mechanisms underlying HM-induced cytotoxicity, highlighting the disruption of lysosomal acidification, membrane integrity, and proteolytic capacity across various cell types and organ systems (Lin et al., 2019) as shown in Table 17.2.

Collectively, these signify the importance of lysosomal dysfunction and impaired autophagic flux as converging mechanisms underlying HM-induced cytotoxicity, highlighting the disruption of lysosomal acidification, membrane integrity, and proteolytic capacity across various cell types and organ systems (Fig. 17.3).

TABLE 17.2 The HMs effect on cellular organelles.

Heavy Metals	Organelle	Key Mechanism	Molecular Markers	Cell/Tissue Type	Functional Outcome	Reference
Lead (Pb)	Mitochondria Endoplasmic Reticulum Lysosome	Mitochondrial fragmentation, Disrupted Mitochondrial dynamics MPTP opening, loss of MMP, impaired mitophagy, release of cytochrome *c*. Elevation of intracellular [Ca^{2+}] level Activation of Unfolded Protein Response (UPR) and Er-stress mediated apoptosis Increased lysosomal pH Lysosomal Membrane Permeabilization (LMP), Impaired Autophagy-Lysosome Fusion, LMP-mediated cell death	↓ATP production ↓OXPHOS ↓MFN2 ↓OPA ↑Drp1 ↓PINK1/PARKIN ↑GRP78 ↑PERK/eIF2α/ATF4/CHOP ↓Cyclin D ↓LC3I/LC3II ↑p62 ↑LAMP1 ↓vATPase ↓Cat B ↓Cat D	SHSY-5Y Neuroblastoma cell, Wister rat Astrocytes, Proximal Tubular Cell PC12 cell Proximal Tubular Cell	Impaired neurogenesis, neurotoxicity, hepatotoxicity, Apoptosis Neurotoxicity, Nephrotoxicity Nephrotoxicity Neurotoxicity	(Bihaqi et al., 2018)
Manganese (Mn)	Mitochondria Endoplasmic Reticulum Lysosome	Loss of MMP, Impaired mitochondrial dynamics and Elevated mitochondrial fragmentation Impaired autophagy-Lysosomal pathway (ALP), formation of NLRP3-mediated inflammasome	↓Oxygen Consumption Rate (OCR) ↓ATP production Impaired Bax/Bcl-2 ratio ↑caspase-9 ↑caspase 3/7 ↑LRRK2 and it's downstream effector RAB10 ↑ Cathepsin B in cytosol	Microglial cells	Neurotoxicity	(Hernández et al., 2021)

Continued

Cadmium (Cd)	Mitochondria Endoplasmic Reticulum Lysosome	Increased ER stress Downregulation of SIRT1/AMPK/Akt signalling axis Impaired lysosomal functioning, impaired lysosomal biogenesis Elevated LMP and Caspase-mediated cell death	↑GADD-153 ↑GRP78 ↑ATF6 ↑XBP1 ↓TFEB mRNA and protein level ↑ Caspase 3/7	SHSY-5Y neuroblastoma cell	Neurotoxicity Neurotoxicity	(Li et al., 2023a)
Arsenic (As)	Mitochondria Endoplasmic Reticulum Lysosome	Damaged Mitochondrial structure, Inhibited ATP-linked respiratory and respiratory control rate, swelling of mitochondrial cristae Impaired functioning of β-cells, increased expression of ER stress related proteins, cell death Impaired lysosomal functioning, impaired autophagic flux	↑mtROS ↑MMP ↑$[Ca^{2+}]i$ ↓mitoSIRT3 level ↓Complex II of ETC ↑GRP78 ↑GRP94 ↑CHOP ↑XBP1 ↑RyR2/IP3R/CaMkII ↓ Cathepsin D ↓ Cathepsin L	GC1 Spermatogonial cell Pancreatic Cell Dendritic cell	Apoptosis Apoptosis Neurotoxicity	(Woo et al., 2006)

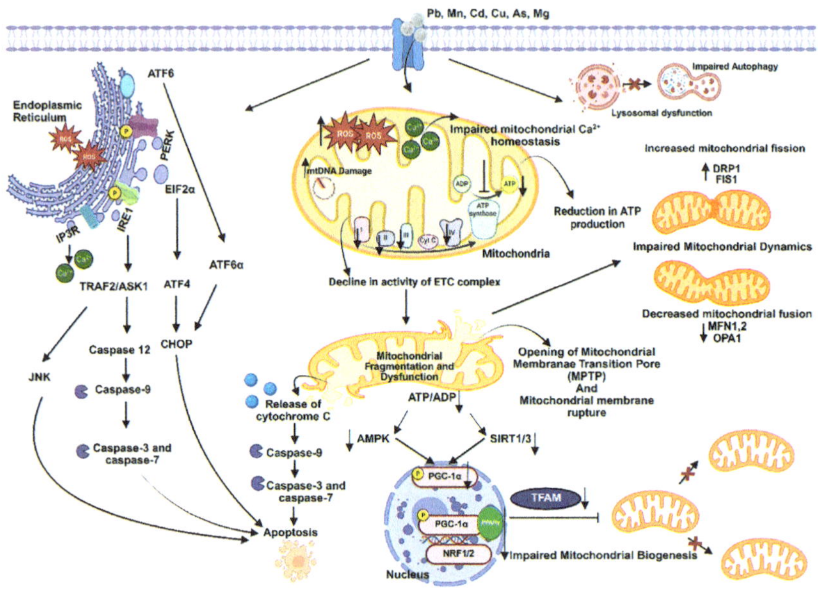

FIG. 17.3 Heavy metal-induced toxicity and associated organelle dysfunction. This schematic illustrates the impact of heavy metal exposure on key cellular organelles. Mitochondria exhibit impaired oxidative phosphorylation, increased ROS generation, and altered membrane potential. ER stress is triggered through disrupted protein folding and unfolded protein response (UPR) activation. Lysosomes display compromised acidification, autophagic flux impairment, and membrane permeabilization. Together, these dysfunctions contribute to cellular stress, inflammation, and apoptotic or necrotic cell death in response to toxic metal accumulation.

17.6 Specific metals and their OS mechanisms

Lead (Pb): This metal pollutes the environment by causing genotoxicity. It may be found in many industrial products, such as paint, batteries, fuel, pesticides, medicines, and cosmetics. Its negative effects on humans include nephrotoxicity, neurotoxicity, and reproductive toxicity. Humans may absorb lead through their skin, respiratory system, and digestive system. Lead is then carried by blood to the brain, liver, kidneys, testes, and other soft tissues. Lead attaches itself to the SH group of cysteine, the carboxyl group of glutamic or aspartic acid carboxylates, the OH group of tyrosine, the NH group of lysine, and the phosphate group, altering the function of enzymes on cell surfaces. In addition, lead may displace vital metal ions, including Ca, Fe, Zn, and Mg. This can lead to OS by disrupting the body's antioxidant defense system, which includes CAT and SOD. It also results in a reduction in and depletion of the GSH pool. Lead binds to the thiol group of GSH to inhibit it (Dobrakowski et al., 2022). OS forms via the upregulation ROS due to a depression of the antioxidant defense system. OS harms vital biological macromolecules, which may affect brain function. The energy metabolism, γ-aminobutyric acid-glutamine shuttle, and antioxidant system are among the neuroprotective and astroglial homeostatic systems that are adversely affected. Neuronal damage, impaired mitochondrial functions, oxidative burden, and apoptosis are all consequences of its promotion of astrocytic activation and neuroinflammation (Ghaderi et al., 2024). Lead is neurotoxic because it primarily targets multipotent cells called neural stem cells (NSCs). It may cross the BBB and replace Ca^{2+}, which affects how signals are sent in neurons. By activating calmodulin, Ca^{2+} triggers the release of neurotransmitters via the CaM kinase pathway. No further signal transmission takes place when lead is present because the Ca^{2+} channels are closed. In addition, the phospholipase C pathway and synaptic vesicle endocytosis are hindered, which affects information transfer and neuronal function. This results in the accumulation of neurotransmitters, leading to neurotoxicity and neurodegenerative disorders. Lead causes apoptosis by disrupting the mitochondria. Ca^{2+} accumulation occurs within cells because of lead's disruption of Ca^{2+} homeostasis and redox potential. When Ca^{2+} attaches itself to the mitochondrial transition pore, it opens, depolarizing the membrane and triggering the death effector proteins and cytochrome C-caspases, which in turn trigger cell death. The NMDA receptor is inhibited by lead noncompetitively, which results in the inhibition of synaptic plasticity reactions, making it impossible even if Ca^{2+} promotes it. In postsynaptic neurons, Mg^{2+} inhibits NMDA receptor channels, but these channels open in response to inputs from neurotransmitters. This has an impact on cognitive capacity. Apoptosis, neurotoxicity, and other illnesses are brought on by lead (Parithathvi et al., 2024).

Cadmium (Cd): Cadmium is emitted by the cadmium mining industry, batteries, and cigarette smoke. As a result, it pollutes the environment and workplace. Cd primarily affects the brain by accumulating in it, where it may readily cross the BBB, resulting in severe nerve poisoning, neurobehavioral consequences, and amyotrophic lateral sclerosis. In fetuses and children, it causes learning difficulties, cognitive abnormalities, and neurobehavioral attention problems. This is related to an incorrect distribution of mitochondria and aberrant mitochondrial dynamics (Tang et al., 2021). Cd causes female infertility by inducing granulosa cell death. Cd exposure causes mitochondrial malfunction in KGN cells, including decreased energy generation, increased ROS levels in cells, and increased Ca^{2+} concentration. OS stimulates the ASK1-p38 signaling pathway, causing KGN cells to die while preserving the functional characteristics of granulosa cells. It ultimately results in the aberrant development of follicles (Xu et al., 2021). Cd exposure may cause renal failure, blockage of arteries, hepatic damage, and male infertility. Ferroptosis is a type of programmed cell death that depends on iron. Ferroptosis induces Cd-induced damage to renal tubular epithelial cells. Ferroptosis is the process by which iron and lipid ROS accumulate. Heme oxygenase-1 (HO-1) converts heme into carbon monoxide (CO), Fe^{2+} and biliverdin. Upregulation of HO-1 leads to the buildup of Fe^{2+} ions and eventually ferroptosis (Lv et al., 2024).

Mercury (Hg): Mercury is a very hazardous HM with cardiotoxic effects. Human wellness may be affected by dietary changes. It may alter the neurological system, damage DNA and chromosomes, produce allergic responses, fatigue, and headaches, and have unfavorable reproductive consequences. Mercury interferes with cell proliferation by inhibiting DNA synthesis, altering gene expression, increasing OS, altering protein phosphorylation, inhibiting sulfhydryl-containing enzymes, increasing ROS production, and disrupting Ca^{2+} balance. It causes cytoplasmic calcium ion (Ca^{2+}) excess and endoplasmic reticulum (ER) Ca^{2+} depletion via Ca^{2+} regulatory malfunction in the ER, causing its stress and misfolded protein accumulation, resulting in cardiomyocyte death via the PERK pathway. Mercury has a negative impact on the developing CNS owing to OS and apoptotic processes. It alters NSC growth, resulting in reduced neuron count and microcephaly. It inhibits DNA synthesis and lowers the levels of cyclins in neurons. It also alters the levels of p16 and p21, which are cyclin-dependent kinase (CDK) inhibitors that arrest the cell cycle at the G1 phase. As a result, it inhibits the development of neurons. Methylmercury also influences cell signaling pathways that regulate brain progenitor cell development into astrocytes. When the JAK/STAT signaling system is activated, neural progenitor cells differentiate into astrocytes. However, methylmercury promotes this signaling pathway, which results in favoring gliogenesis over neurogenesis. As a result, it has the potential to impair brain development and function. Furthermore, metal-induced OS increases ROS, such as superoxides, which impair healthy brain development. OS also affects Ca^{2+} homeostasis by affecting Ca^{2+} entry through the membrane and protein phosphorylation (where Ca^{2+} acts as a second messenger). Increased intracellular Ca^{2+} levels may activate calcium-dependent enzymes and modify protein kinase activities, resulting in neurotoxicity. As a result, mercury influences healthy CNS development via a variety of mechanisms (Abbott and Nigussie, 2021). Mercury-induced OS also affects the mitochondria, leading to toxicity through reduced ATP generation from the MPTP, decreased state 3 and 3UDNP respiration, decreased mitochondrial potential, mitochondrial expansion, increased state 4 respiration, increased membrane fluidity, Cyt c release, and decreased mitochondrial permeability (Korotkov, 2023).

Arsenic (As): Arsenic (As) is a poisonous metalloid commonly found in the environment. It may be present in the air, water, soil, and foods, particularly shellfish. Arsenic is released into the environment through volcanic activity as well as human activities such as pesticide and herbicide production, semiconductor and germicide industries, metal smelting, and mining. Arsenic is primarily absorbed through inhalation and ingestion, and in pregnant women, a portion is transmitted to the fetus via the placenta. Arsenic causes the development of oxidized lipids, which generate bio-reactive molecules. ROS-mediated oxidative damage is a prevalent factor in arsenic toxicity. Organic arsenic is not as reactive as inorganic arsenic. Carcinogenic metal ions like arsenic and nickel generate redox reactions in biological systems. These processes create free radicals, which cause oxidative injury to vital biomolecules. The liver is the major target for arsenic poisoning. Prolonged exposure harms liver structure and function, alters metabolism, and causes toxic chemical build up, resulting in OS, inflammatory reactions, DNA damage, and other negative consequences. This exposure gradually causes liver damage, typically in the form of hepatomegaly, hepatitis, fibrosis, cirrhosis, and possibly cancer (Shao et al., 2024). As a comutagen, it prevents cells from responding to stimuli that can cause DNA damage, such as benzo[a]pyrene and UV rays. It alters the gene expression of those involved in reducing oxidative stress and repairing DNA damage, interfering with transcriptional activity. The shape of chromosomes is governed by cytosine methylation at CpG islands, which is critical for controlling transcription. When a methyl group is transferred to CpG dinucleotides at the fifth carbon of cytosine from SAM (S-adenosylmethionine), methylation occurs. However, SAM is also essential for the metabolism of arsenic. In the presence of abundant arsenite, arsenite methyltransferase (AS3MT) uses SAM to methylate arsenic rather than supporting cellular methylation processes. As a result, S-adenosylhomocysteine (SAH) accumulates in the cell, which inhibits SAM-dependent methyltransferase. Since AS3MT-mediated metabolism occurs primarily in the liver, this organ is the most affected. Aberrant cell proliferation occurs due to the repression of cell cycle-controlling genes such as p21. ROS-induced cell signaling also affects cell cycle progression and proliferation. Thus, hypomethylation increases chromosomal abnormalities, resulting in genetic instability and spontaneous mutations (Stößer et al., 2023).

Manganese (Mn): Mn is a trace element essential for several bodily functions. Dust, water, air, and activities such as mining, welding, and smelting expose the body to Mn. It aids in the functioning of glutamine synthetase and MnSOD. Mn is required daily for physiological functions (2.3 mg for males, 1.8 mg for females). However, persistent and increasing exposure to industrial and atmospheric Mn can lead to manganism, a neurological disorder affecting the brain's basal ganglia. Mn induces neurotoxicity through OS, mitochondrial malfunction, mitophagy, autophagy, inflammation, glutamate excitotoxicity, apoptosis, and epigenetic transformation. Higher Mn exposure increases reactive oxygen species (ROS, damaging brain cells. Mn restricts mitochondrial ATP synthesis, causing electron leakage and ROS production. It also reduces GSH production, weakening antioxidant defenses and exacerbating OS. Mitochondrial dysfunction, characterized by disrupted mitochondrial homeostasis and altered mitochondrial bioenergetics, results in necrotic or apoptotic cell death. By downregulating ocular atrophy protein 1 (Opa1) and mitofusin 2 (Mfn2) and upregulating dynamin-related protein 1 (Drp1), Mn disrupts the balance of mitochondrial fission and fusion, leading to mitochondrial malfunction and fragmentation. The activation of microglia and astrocytes due to mitochondrial dysfunction results in the production of pro-inflammatory mediators such as NOS2, TNF-α, and IL-1β, which, in nonprimate models, cause neuroinflammation and neuronal injury. Cytokine production is further exacerbated by astrocyte mitochondrial malfunction, intensifying neurotoxic effects. Mn also induces epigenetic modifications, particularly by altering histone acetylation through its influence on histone deacetylases and histone acetyltransferases. These changes lead to neurotoxicity by dysregulating gene expression (Pajarillo et al., 2022).

17.7 Current gaps and future directions

HMs produce ROS, which damage DNA, proteins, and lipids and cause metal-induced OS. Early identification, risk assessment, and therapy monitoring all benefit from the use of biomarkers. Damage to DNA caused by oxidation anti-oxidant enzyme activity, protein oxidation, and LPO. proteins that bind metals. Patterns of gene expression linked to OS. Without changing DNA sequences, metals may change the epigenome, which affects gene expression. This includes microRNAs as well as epigenetic modifications. Metals seldom work alone. Their toxicity to other environmental agents may be additive, antagonistic, or synergistic. Coexposure negative effects include organic solvents, pesticides, and air pollution. The Nrf2 pathway, inflammatory mediators, mitochondrial protectors, and chelation treatment are examples of therapeutic targets.

17.8 Conclusion

HMs cause cytotoxicity, mostly via OS. They alter the cellular redox equilibrium by producing ROS and depleting antioxidant defense systems. Redox-inactive metals harm mitochondria and block antioxidant enzymes, while redox-active metals produce ROS directly via Fenton and Haber-Weiss reactions. OS damages proteins, lipids, and DNA while activating stress signaling pathways such as NF-κB, MAPK, and Nrf2-Keap1-ARE. This promotes calcium imbalance, autophagy, mitochondrial malfunction, and, eventually, cell death. This chapter discusses new research into the processes by which metal-induced OS leads to cytotoxicity.

Acknowledgment

S.D. expresses gratitude to the University Grants Commission (UGC), New Delhi, India, for financial support through a Senior Research Fellowship. S.A. acknowledges the Anusandhan National Research Foundation (ANRF), New Delhi, India, for financial assistance via the National Postdoctoral Fellowship (PDF/2023/000639). The authors extend their thanks to the Director of the ICMR-National Institute of Nutrition, Hyderabad, for institutional support. We also acknowledge BioRender for facilitating the development of scientific illustrations used in this work.

References

Abbott, L.C., Nigussie, F., 2021. Mercury toxicity and neurogenesis in the mammalian brain. Int. J. Mol. Sci. 14220067. 22(14). Available from: https://www.mdpi.com/1422-0067/22/14/7520/pdf. doi:10.3390/ijms22147520.

Abd Elnabi, M.K., Elkaliny, N.E., Elyazied, M.M., Azab, S.H., Elkhalifa, S.A., Elmasry, S., Mouhamed, M.S., Shalamesh, E.M., Alhorieny, N.A., Elaty, A.E.A., Elgendy, I.M., Etman, A.E., Saad, K.E., Tsigkou, K., Ali, S.S., Kornaros, M., Mahmoud, Y.A.G., 2023. Toxicity of heavy metals and recent advances in their removal: a review. Toxics. 23056304. 11(7). Available from: http://www.mdpi.com/journal/toxics. doi:10.3390/toxics11070580.

Alaimo, A., Gorojod, R.M., Miglietta, E.A., Villarreal, A., Ramos, A.J., Kotler, M.L., 2013. Manganese induces mitochondrial dynamics impairment and apoptotic cell death: a study in human Gli36 cells. Neurosci. Lett. 18727972. 554, 76–81. doi:10.1016/j.neulet.2013.08.061.

Alcon, S.P., Gorojod, R.M., Kotler, M.L., 2020. Kinetic and protective role of autophagy in manganese-exposed BV-2 cells. Biochim. Biophys. Acta Mol. Cell Res. 1867(10), 118787.

Alhusaini, A., Fadda, L., Hasan, I.H., Zakaria, E., Alenazi, A.M., Mahmoud, A.M., 2019. Curcumin ameliorates lead-induced hepatotoxicity by suppressing oxidative stress and inflammation, and modulating akt/gsk-3β signaling pathway. Biomolecules. 2218273X. 9(11). Available from: https://www.mdpi.com/2218-273X/9/11/703/pdf. doi:10.3390/biom9110703.

Arciello, M., Rotilio, G., Rossi, L., 2005. Copper-dependent toxicity in SH-SY5Y neuroblastoma cells involves mitochondrial damage. Biochem. Biophys. Res. Commun. 327 (2), 454–459.

Babiker, F., Al-Kouh, A., Kilarkaje, N., 2019. Lead exposure induces oxidative stress, apoptosis, and attenuates protection of cardiac myocytes against ischemia–reperfusion injury. Drug Chem. Toxicol. 42 (2), 147–156.

Balaji, K., Vijayakumar, J., Sankaran, P.K., Senthilkumar, S., Vijayaraghavan, R., Selvaraj, J., Yuvaraj, M.F., 2021. Molecular studies on the nephroprotective potential of celastrus paniculatus against lead-acetate-induced nephrotoxicity in experimental rats: role of the pi3k/akt signaling pathway. Molecules. 14203049. 26(21). Available from: https://www.mdpi.com/1420-3049/26/21/6647/pdf. doi:10.3390/molecules26216647.

Balali-Mood, M., Naseri, K., Tahergorabi, Z., Khazdair, M.R., Sadeghi, M., 2021. Toxic mechanisms of five heavy metals: mercury, lead, chromium, cadmium, and arsenic. Front. Pharmacol. 16639812. 12. Available from: http://www.frontiersin.org/Pharmacology. doi:10.3389/fphar.2021.643972.

Bihaqi, S.W., Alansi, B., Masoud, A.M., Mushtaq, F., Subaiea, G.M., Zawia, N.H., 2018. Influence of early life lead (Pb) exposure on α-synuclein, GSK-3β and caspase-3 mediated tauopathy: implications on Alzheimer's disease. Curr. Alzheimer Res. 18755828. 15(12), 1114–1122. Available from: http://www.eurekaselect.com/164219. doi:10.2174/1567205015666180801095925.

Boudebbouz, A., Boudalia, S., Bousbia, A., Habila, S., Boussadia, M.I., Gueroui, Y., 2021. Heavy metals levels in raw cow milk and health risk assessment across the globe: a systematic review. Sci. Total Environ. 18791026. 751. Available from: http://www.elsevier.com/locate/scitotenv. doi:10.1016/j.scitotenv.2020.141830.

Briffa, J., Sinagra, E., Blundell, R., 2020. Heavy metal pollution in the environment and their toxicological effects on humans. Heliyon 6 (9), e04691.

Cai, J., Guan, H., Jiao, X., Yang, J., Chen, X., Zhang, H., Zheng, Y., Zhu, Y., Liu, Q., Zhang, Z., 2021. NLRP3 inflammasome mediated pyroptosis is involved in cadmium exposure-induced neuroinflammation through the IL-1β/IkB-α-NF-κB-NLRP3 feedback loop in swine. Toxicology. 0300483X. 453, 152720. doi:10.1016/j.tox.2021.152720.

Cantoni, O., Zito, E., Fiorani, M., Guidarelli, A., 2021. Arsenite impinges on endoplasmic reticulum-mitochondria crosstalk to elicit mitochondrial ROS formation and downstream toxicity. Semin. Cancer Biol. 1044579X. (76), 132–138. doi:10.1016/j.semcancer.2021.06.002.

Cengiz, M., Gür, B., Sezer, C.V., Cengiz, B.P., Gür, F., Bayrakdar, A., Ayhancı, A., 2023. Alternations in interleukin-1β and nuclear factor kappa beta activity (NF-kB) in rat liver due to the co-exposure of Cadmium and Arsenic: protective role of curcumin. Environ. Toxicol. Pharmacol. 18727077. 102. Available from: https://www.elsevier.com/locate/etap. doi:10.1016/j.etap.2023.104218.

Chattopadhyay, S., Bhaumik, S., Purkayastha, M., Basu, S., Chaudhuri, A.N., Gupta, S.D., 2002. Apoptosis and necrosis in developing brain cells due to arsenic toxicity and protection with antioxidants. Toxicol. Lett. 03784274. 136 (1), 65–76. doi:10.1016/S0378-4274(02)00282-5.

Che, W., Yang, M., Cheng, Y., Wu, M., Lan, Y., Zhang, H., 2019. Arsenic induces gender difference of estrogen receptor in AECII cells from ICR fetal mice. Toxicol. Vitro. 08872333. 56, 133–140. doi:10.1016/j.tiv.2019.01.014.

Chen, H., Liu, G., Qiao, N., Kang, Z., Hu, L., Liao, J., Yang, F., Pang, C., Liu, B., Zeng, Q., Li, Y., Li, Y., 2020. Toxic effects of arsenic trioxide on spermatogonia are associated with oxidative stress, mitochondrial dysfunction, autophagy and metabolomic alterations. Ecotoxicol. Environ. Saf. 01476513. 190, 110063. doi:10.1016/j.ecoenv.2019.110063.

Choudhury, C., Mazumder, R., Kumar, R., Dhar, B., Sengupta, M., 2021. Cadmium induced oxystress alters Nrf2-Keap1 signaling and triggers apoptosis in piscine head kidney macrophages. Aquat. Toxicol. 0166445X. 231, 105739. doi:10.1016/j.aquatox.2020.105739.

Córdoba-Tovar, L., Marrugo-Negrete, J., Barón, P.R., Díez, S., 2022. Drivers of biomagnification of Hg, As and Se in aquatic food webs: a review. Environ. Res. 10960953. 204. Available from: http://www.elsevier.com/inca/publications/store/6/2/2/8/2/1/index.htt. doi:10.1016/j.envres.2021.112226.

Das, S., Santra, A., Lahiri, S., Guha Mazumder, D.N., 2005. Implications of oxidative stress and hepatic cytokine (TNF-α and IL-6) response in the pathogenesis of hepatic collagenesis in chronic arsenic toxicity. Toxicol. Appl. Pharmacol. 0041008X. 204(1), 18–26. Available from: http://www.elsevier.com/inca/publications/store/6/2/2/9/5/1/index.htt. doi:10.1016/j.taap.2004.08.010.

Davidova, S., Milushev, V., Satchanska, G., 2024. The mechanisms of cadmium toxicity in living organisms. Toxics 12 (12), 875.

Deng, Y., Zhu, J., Mi, C., Xu, B., Jiao, C., Li, Y., Xu, D., Liu, W., Xu, Z., 2015a. Melatonin antagonizes Mn-induced oxidative injury through the activation of keap1–Nrf2–ARE signaling pathway in the striatum of mice. Neurotoxicity Res. 27 (2), 156–171.

Deng, Y., Zhu, J., Mi, C., Xu, B., Jiao, C., Li, Y., Xu, D., Liu, W., Xu, Z., 2015b. Melatonin antagonizes Mn-induced oxidative injury through the activation of keap1–Nrf2–ARE signaling pathway in the striatum of mice. Neurotoxicity Res. 27, 156–171.

Dey, K., Ghosh, D., Pilot, M., Pering, S.R., Roose, B., Deswal, P., Senanayak, S.P., Cameron, P.J., Islam, M.S., Stranks, S.D., 2024. Substitution of lead with tin suppresses ionic transport in halide perovskite optoelectronics. Energy Environ. Sci. 17 (2), 760–769.

Dey, K.K., Kamila, S., Das, T., Chattopadhyay, A., 2025. Chronic exposure to lead causes neurotoxicity by generating oxidative stress and inducing DNA damages in zebrafish brain: involvement of Nrf2-Keap1 regulation and DNA repair pathways. Biol. Trace Elem. Res. 15590720. 203(9), 4863–4875. Available from: https://www.springer.com/journal/12011. doi:10.1007/s12011-025-04534-z.

Dobrakowski, M., Machoń-Grecka, A., Nowak, P., Szczęsny, P., Maciejczyk, M., Kasperczyk, A., Pryzwan, T., Kasperczyk, S., 2022. The influence of erdosteine administration on lead-induced oxidative stress in rat muscle. Drug Chem. Toxicol. 0148-0545. 45 (1), 88–92. doi:10.1080/01480545.2019.1659810.

Dooka, B.D., Orish, C.N., Ezejiofor, A.N., Anyachor, C.P., Umeji, T.C., Nkpaa, K.W., Obasi, C.N., Cirovic, A., Cirovic, A., Orisakwe, O.E., 2025. Aluminum, lead and manganese mixture exacerbates oxidative stress, neuroinflammation, and apoptosis via downregulation of Nrf-2/HO-1/BDNF signaling pathway in rats. Biomarkers 30 (4), 1–16.

Gandhi, D., Bhandari, S., Maity, S., Mahapatra, S.K., Rajasekaran, S., 2025. Activation of ERK/NF-kB pathways contributes to the inflammatory response in epithelial cells and macrophages following manganese exposure. Biol. Trace Elem. Res. 15590720. 203(1), 127–138. Available from: https://www.springer.com/journal/12011. doi:10.1007/s12011-024-04154-z.

Gąssowska, M., Baranowska-Bosiacka, I., Moczydłowska, J., Frontczak-Baniewicz, M., Gewartowska, M., Strużyńska, L., Gutowska, I., Chlubek, D., Adamczyk, A., 2016. Perinatal exposure to lead (Pb) induces ultrastructural and molecular alterations in synapses of rat offspring. Toxicology. 0300483X. 373, 13–29. doi:10.1016/j.tox.2016.10.014.

Ge, J., Zhang, C., Sun, Y.C., Zhang, Q., Lv, M.W., Guo, K., Li, J.L., 2019. Cadmium exposure triggers mitochondrial dysfunction and oxidative stress in chicken (*Gallus gallus*) kidney via mitochondrial UPR inhibition and Nrf2-mediated antioxidant defense activation. Sci. Total Environ. 18791026. 689, 1160–1171. Available from: http://www.elsevier.com/locate/scitotenv. doi:10.1016/j.scitotenv.2019.06.405.

Ghaderi, S., Rashno, M., Sarkaki, A., Khoshnam, S.E., 2024. Sesamin mitigates lead-induced behavioral deficits in male rats: the role of oxidative stress. Brain Res. Bull. 03619230. 206, 110852. doi:10.1016/j.brainresbull.2023.110852.

Gu, X., Han, M., Du, Y., Wu, Y., Xu, Y., Zhou, X., Ye, D., Wang, H.L., 2019. Pb disrupts autophagic flux through inhibiting the formation and activity of lysosomes in neural cells. Toxicol. Vitro. 18793177. 55, 43–50. Available from: http://www.elsevier.com/locate/toxinvit. doi:10.1016/j.tiv.2018.11.010.

Guo, C., Wang, L., Cui, K., Zhang, G., Tan, Y., Chen, W., Wang, Y., Liu, J., Liu, W., Zhang, G., Zhou, Z., 2025. Lead causes lipid droplet accumulation by impairing lysosomal function and autophagic flux in testicular sertoli cells. Toxics. 23056304. 13(3). Available from: http://www.mdpi.com/journal/toxics. doi:10.3390/toxics13030175.

Guofeng, X., Liu, S., Huang, M., Jiang, X., Yang, M., 2021. Cadmium induces apoptosis of human granulosa cell line KGN via mitochondrial dysfunction-mediated pathways. Ecotoxicol. Environ. Saf. 01476513. 220, 112341. doi:10.1016/j.ecoenv.2021.112341.

Gupta, S., Sharma, V., 2025. Amelioration of lead nitrate induced pulmonary toxicity by Garlic essential oil in inflammatory markers of Swiss albino male mice. J. Appl. Nat. Sci. 2231-5209. 17 (1), 302–308. doi:10.31018/jans.v17i1.6237.

Hernández, R.B., de Souza-pinto, N.C., Kleinjans, J., van Herwijnen, M., Piepers, J., Moteshareie, H., Burnside, D., Golshani, A., 2021. Manganese-induced neurotoxicity through impairment of cross-talk pathways in human neuroblastoma cell line sh-sy5y differentiated with retinoic acid. Toxics. 23056304. 9(12). Available from: https://www.mdpi.com/2305-6304/9/12/348/pdf. doi:10.3390/toxics9120348.

Hong, H., He, H., Lin, X., Hayuehashi, T., Xu, J., Zhang, J., Xu, Y., Tong, T., Lu, Y., Zhou, Z., 2022. Cadmium exposure suppresses insulin secretion through mtROS-mediated mitochondrial dysfunction and inflammatory response in pancreatic beta cells. J. Trace Elem. Med. Biol. 18783252. 71. Available from: http://www.urbanfischer.de/journals/jtraceelm/trace.htm. doi:10.1016/j.jtemb.2022.126952.

Hu, Z., Liao, J., Zhang, K., Huang, K., Li, Q., Lei, C., Han, Q., Zhang, H., Guo, J., Hu, L., Pan, J., Li, Y., Tang, Z., 2023. Effects of long-term exposure to copper on mitochondria-mediated apoptosis in pig liver. Biol. Trace Elem. Res. 0163-4984. 201 (4), 1726–1739. doi:10.1007/s12011-022-03303-6.

Imafidon, C.E., Olatoye, T., Bamidele, F., Ojo, O., Ademoye, K., 2016. Cadmium-induced testicular toxicity, oxidative stress and histopathology in Wistar rats: sustained effects of polyphenol-rich extract of Vernonia amygdalina (Del.) leaf. J. Interdiscipl. Histopathol 4 (3), 54–62.

Janasik, B., Reszka, E., Stanislawska, M., Jablonska, E., Kuras, R., Wieczorek, E., Malachowska, B., Fendler, W., Wasowicz, W., 2018. Effect of arsenic exposure on NRF2-KEAP1 pathway and epigenetic modification. Biol. Trace Elem. Res. 0163-4984. 185 (1), 11–19. doi:10.1007/s12011-017-1219-4.

Jian, Z., Guo, H., Liu, H., Cui, H., Fang, J., Zuo, Z., Deng, J., Li, Y., Wang, X., Zhao, L., 2020. Oxidative stress, apoptosis and inflammatory responses involved in copper-induced pulmonary toxicity in mice. Aging. 1945-4589. 12 (17), 16867–16886. doi:10.18632/aging.103585.

Jomova, K., Alomar, S.Y., Nepovimova, E., Kuca, K., Valko, M., 2025. Heavy metals: toxicity and human health effects. Arch. Toxicol. 14320738. 99(1), 153–209. Available from: https://www.springer.com/journal/204. doi:10.1007/s00204-024-03903-2.

Kalo, M.B., Rezaei, M., 2022. In vitro toxic interaction of arsenic and hyperglycemia in mitochondria: an important implication of increased vulnerability in pre-diabetics. Environ. Sci. Pollut. Res. 16147499. 29(19), 28375–28385. Available from: https://link.springer.com/journal/11356. doi:10.1007/s11356-022-18513-7.

Kataba, A., Botha, T.L., Nakayama, S.M.M., Yohannes, Y.B., Ikenaka, Y., Wepener, V., Ishizuka, M., 2020. Acute exposure to environmentally relevant lead levels induces oxidative stress and neurobehavioral alterations in larval zebrafish (Danio rerio). Aquat. Toxicol. 18791514. 227. Available from: http://www.elsevier.com/wps/find/journaldescription.cws_home/505509/description#description. doi:10.1016/j.aquatox.2020.105607.

Kim, Y., Lee, Y., Choo, M., Yun, N., Cho, J.W., Oh, Y.J., 2024. A surge of cytosolic calcium dysregulates lysosomal function and impairs autophagy flux during cupric chloride–induced neuronal death. J. Biol. Chem. 1083351X. 300(1). Available from: https://www.sciencedirect.com/science/journal/00219258. doi:10.1016/j.jbc.2023.105479.

Korotkov, S.M., 2023. Mitochondrial oxidative stress is the general reason for apoptosis induced by different-valence heavy metals in cells and mitochondria. Int. J. Mol. Sci. 1422-0067. 24 (19), 14459. doi:10.3390/ijms241914459.

Kumawat, K.L., Kaushik, D.K., Goswami, P., Basu, A., 2014. Acute exposure to lead acetate activates microglia and induces subsequent bystander neuronal death via caspase-3 activation. NeuroToxicology. 18729711. 41, 143–153. Available from: http://www.elsevier.com/inca/publications/store/6/2/1/3/5/5. doi:10.1016/j.neuro.2014.02.002.

Lalwani, P., King, D.E., Morton, K.S., Rivera, N.A., Huayta, J., Hsu-Kim, H., Meyer, J.N., 2023. Increased cytotoxicity of Pb2+ with co-exposures to a mitochondrial uncoupler and mitochondrial calcium uniporter inhibitor. Environ. Sci. Process Impacts. 20507895. 25(11), 1743–1751. Available from: http://pubs.rsc.org/en/journals/journal/em. doi:10.1039/d3em00188a.

Li, C., Xing, T., Tang, M., Yong, W., D, Y., Deng, H., Wang, H., Wang, M., Chen, J., Ruan, D., 2008. Involvement of cyclin D1/CDK4 and pRb mediated by PI3K/AKT pathway activation in Pb2+-induced neuronal death in cultured hippocampal neurons. Toxicol. Appl. Pharmacol. 0041008X. 229 (3), 351–361. doi:10.1016/j.taap.2008.01.039.

Li, M., Cai, J.F., Chiu, J.F., 2002. Arsenic induces oxidative stress and activates stress gene expressions in cultured lung epithelial cells. J. Cell. Biochem. 87 (1), 29–38.

Li, X., Li, X., Xiang, C., Ye, F., 2022. Lead exposure represses mitochondrial metabolism by activation of heme-binding protein BACH1 in differentiated SH-SY5Y cell. Sci. Total Environ. 00489697. 853, 158665. doi:10.1016/j.scitotenv.2022.158665.

Li, Y., Zhong, G., He, T., Quan, J., Liu, S., Liu, Z., Tang, Z., Yu, W., 2023a. Effect of arsenic and copper in kidney of mice: crosstalk between Nrf2/Keap1 pathway in apoptosis and pyroptosis. Ecotoxicol. Environ. Saf. 266, 115542.

Li, Z., Shi, Y., Wang, Y., Qi, H., Chen, H., Li, J., Li, L., 2023b. Cadmium-induced pyroptosis is mediated by PERK/TXNIP/NLRP3 signaling in SH-SY5Y cells. China Environ. Toxicol. 15227278. 38(9), 2219–2227. Available from: http://onlinelibrary.wiley.com/journal/10.1002/(ISSN)1522-7278. doi:10.1002/tox.23861.

Lin, T., Ruan, S., Huang, D., Meng, X., Li, W., Wang, B., Zou, F., 2019. MeHg-induced autophagy via JNK/Vps34 complex pathway promotes autophagosome accumulation and neuronal cell death. Cell Death Dis. 2041-4889. 10(6). doi:10.1038/s41419-019-1632-z.

Liu, C.M., Sun, Y.Z., Sun, J.M., Ma, J.Q., Cheng, C., 2012. Protective role of quercetin against lead-induced inflammatory response in rat kidney through the ROS mediated MAPKs and NF κB pathway. Biochim. Biophys. Acta Gen. Subj. 18728006. 1820 (10), 1693–1703. doi:10.1016/j.bbagen.2012.06.011.

Liu, H., Guo, H., Jian, Z., Cui, H., Fang, J., Zuo, Z., Deng, J., Li, Y., Wang, X., Zhao, L., 2020. Copper induces oxidative stress and apoptosis in the mouse liver. Oxid. Med. Cell. Longev. 1942-0900. 2020, 1–20. doi:10.1155/2020/1359164.

Lv, Y.T., Liu, T.B., Li, Y., Wang, Z.Y., Lian, C.Y., Wang, L., 2024. HO-1 activation contributes to cadmium-induced ferroptosis in renal tubular epithelial cells via increasing the labile iron pool and promoting mitochondrial ROS generation. Chem. Biol. Interact. 18727786. 399. Available from: https://www.sciencedirect.com/science/journal/00092797. doi:10.1016/j.cbi.2024.111152.

Ma, L., Liu, J.Y., Dong, J.X., Xiao, Q., Zhao, J., Jiang, F.L., 2017. Toxicity of Pb2+ on rat liver mitochondria induced by oxidative stress and mitochondrial permeability transition. Toxicol. Res. 20454538. 6(6), 822–830. Available from: http://pubs.rsc.org/en/journals/journalissues/tx. doi:10.1039/c7tx00204a.

Mansoor, S., Ali, A., Kour, N., Bornhorst, J., AlHarbi, K., Rinklebe, J., El Moneim, D.A., Ahmad, P., Chung, Y.S., 2023. Heavy metal induced oxidative stress mitigation and ROS scavenging in plants. Plants. 2223-7747. 12 (16), 3003. doi:10.3390/plants12163003.

Manthari, R.K., Tikka, C., Ommati, M.M., Niu, R., Sun, Z., Wang, J., Zhang, J., Wang, J., 2018. Arsenic induces autophagy in developmental mouse cerebral cortex and hippocampus by inhibiting PI3K/Akt/mTOR signaling pathway: involvement of blood–brain barrier's tight junction proteins. Arch. Toxicol. 14320738. 92(11), 3255–3275. Available from: https://link.springer.de/link/service/journals/00204/index.htm. doi:10.1007/s00204-018-2304-y.

Mesalam, N.M., Ibrahim, M.A., Mousa, M.R., Said, N.M., 2023. Selenium and vitamin E ameliorate lead acetate-induced hepatotoxicity in rats via suppression of oxidative stress, mRNA of heat shock proteins, and NF-kB production. J. Trace Elem. Med. Biol. 18783252. 79. Available from: https://www.urbanfischer.de/journals/jtraceelm/trace.htm. doi:10.1016/j.jtemb.2023.127256.

Mitra, S., Chakraborty, A.J., Tareq, A.M., Emran, T.B., Nainu, F., Khusro, A., Idris, A.M., Khandaker, M.U., Osman, H., Alhumaydhi, F.A., Simal-Gandara, J., 2022. Impact of heavy metals on the environment and human health: novel therapeutic insights to counter the toxicity. J. King Saud Univ. Sci. 10183647. 34(3). Available from: http://www.sciencedirect.com/science/journal/10183647. doi:10.1016/j.jksus.2022.101865.

Nair, A.R., Lee, W.K., Smeets, K., Swennen, Q., Sanchez, A., Thévenod, F., Cuypers, A., 2015. Glutathione and mitochondria determine acute defense responses and adaptive processes in cadmium-induced oxidative stress and toxicity of the kidney. Arch. Toxicol. 14320738. 89(12), 2273–2289. Available from: https://www.link.springer.de/link/service/journals/00204/index.htm. doi:10.1007/s00204-014-1401-9.

Nzengue, Y., Steiman, R., Garrel, C., Lefèbvre, E., Guiraud, P., 2008. Oxidative stress and DNA damage induced by cadmium in the human keratinocyte HaCaT cell line: role of glutathione in the resistance to cadmium. Toxicology. 0300483X. 243 (1-2), 193–206. doi:10.1016/j.tox.2007.10.005.

Pajarillo, E., Kim, S., Digman, A., Dutton, M., Son, D.-S., Aschner, M., Lee, E., 2023. The role of microglial LRRK2 kinase in manganese-induced inflammatory neurotoxicity via NLRP3 inflammasome and RAB10-mediated autophagy dysfunction. J. Biol. Chem. 00219258. 299 (7), 104879. doi:10.1016/j.jbc.2023.104879.

Pajarillo, E., Nyarko-Danquah, I., Digman, A., Multani, H.K., Kim, S., Gaspard, P., Aschner, M., Lee, E., 2022. Mechanisms of manganese-induced neurotoxicity and the pursuit of neurotherapeutic strategies. Front. Pharmacol. 16639812. 13. Available from: http://www.frontiersin.org/Pharmacology. doi:10.3389/fphar.2022.1011947.

Pan, M., Cheng, Z.W., Huang, C.G., Ye, Z.Q., Sun, L.J., Chen, H., Fu, B.B., Zhou, K., Fang, Z.R., Wang, Z.J., Xiao, Q.Z., Liu, X.S., Zhu, F.Q., Gao, S., 2022. Long-term exposure to copper induces mitochondria-mediated apoptosis in mouse hearts. Ecotoxicol. Environ. Saf. 10902414. 234. Available from: http://www.elsevier.com/inca/publications/store/6/2/2/8/1/9/index.htt. doi:10.1016/j.ecoenv.2022.113329.

Pan, Y.X., Luo, Z., Zhuo, M.Q., Wei, C.C., Chen, G.H., Song, Y.F., 2018. Oxidative stress and mitochondrial dysfunction mediated Cd-induced hepatic lipid accumulation in zebrafish Danio rerio. Aquat. Toxicol. 18791514. 199, 12–20. Available from: http://www.elsevier.com/wps/find/journaldescription.cws_home/505509/description#description. doi:10.1016/j.aquatox.2018.03.017.

Parithathvi, A., Choudhari, N., Dsouza, H.S., 2024. Prenatal and early life lead exposure induced neurotoxicity. Hum. Exp. Toxicol. 43, 09603271241285523.

Pi, H., Li, M., Tian, L., Yang, Z., Yu, Z., Zhou, Z., 2017. Enhancing lysosomal biogenesis and autophagic flux by activating the transcription factor EB protects against cadmium-induced neurotoxicity. Sci. Rep. 20452322. 7. Available from: https://www.nature.com/srep/index.html. doi:10.1038/srep43466.

Pi, H., Li, M., Xie, J., Yang, Z., Xi, Y., Yu, Z., Zhou, Z., 2018. Transcription factor E3 protects against cadmium-induced apoptosis by maintaining the lysosomal-mitochondrial axis but not autophagic flux in Neuro-2a cells. Toxicol. Lett. 18793169. 295, 335–350. Available from: https://www.elsevier.com/locate/toxlet. doi:10.1016/j.toxlet.2018.07.015.

Qin, G., Niu, Z., Yu, J., Li, Z., Ma, J., Xiang, P., 2021. Soil heavy metal pollution and food safety in China: effects, sources and removing technology. Chemosphere. 00456535. 267, 129205. doi:10.1016/j.chemosphere.2020.129205.

Reddy, P.V., Rao, K.V.R., Norenberg, M.D., 2008. The mitochondrial permeability transition, and oxidative and nitrosative stress in the mechanism of copper toxicity in cultured neurons and astrocytes. Lab. Invest. 88 (8), 816–830.

Rezaei, M., Keshtzar, E., Khodayar, M.J., Javadipour, M., 2019. SirT3 regulates diabetogenic effects caused by arsenic: an implication for mitochondrial complex II modification. Toxicol. Lett. 18793169. 301, 24–33. Available from: http://www.elsevier.com/locate/toxlet. doi:10.1016/j.toxlet.2018.10.025.

Santra, A., Bishnu, D., Santra, S., Ghatak, S., Mukherjee, P.S., Dhali, G.K., Chowdhury, A., 2022. Arsenic-induced injury of mouse hepatocytes through lysosome and mitochondria: an in vitro study. Int. J. Hepatol. 2022(1), 1546297.

Sarkar, D., Imam, F., Kumar, A., Mukherjee, A., Purohit, P., Kiesewetter, G., Klimont, Z., Ghosh, S., Balakrishnan, K., Chowdhury, S., 2025a. Pathways for India to reduce ambient air pollution health burden and achieve the sustainable development goal (SDG-3.4). Environ. Sci. Technol. 59 (10), 4765–4777.

Sarkar, O., Islam, S., Mukherjee, S., Chattopadhyay, A., 2025b. Combined effects of lead and chromium at environmentally relevant concentrations in zebrafish (Danio rerio) liver: role of Nrf2-Keap1-ARE pathway. J. Appl. Toxicol. 45 (7), 1331–1347.

Sarkar, S., Malovic, E., Harischandra, D.S., Ngwa, H.A., Ghosh, A., Hogan, C., Rokad, D., Zenitsky, G., Jin, H., Anantharam, V., Kanthasamy, A.G., Kanthasamy, A., 2018. Manganese exposure induces neuroinflammation by impairing mitochondrial dynamics in astrocytes. NeuroToxicology. 18729711. 64, 204–218. Available from: https://www.elsevier.com/inca/publications/store/6/2/1/3/5/5. doi:10.1016/j.neuro.2017.05.009.

Shamsudduha, M., Joseph, G., Haque, S.S., Khan, M.R., Zahid, A., Ahmed, K.M.U., 2020. Multi-hazard groundwater risks to water supply from shallow depths: challenges to achieving the sustainable development goals in Bangladesh. Expo. Health. 24519685. 12(4), 657–670. Available from: http://link.springer.com/journal/volumesAndIssues/12403. doi:10.1007/s12403-019-00325-9.

Shao, J., Lai, C., Zheng, Q., Luo, Y., Li, C., Zhang, B., Sun, Y., Liu, S., Shi, Y., Li, J., Zhao, Z., Guo, L., 2024. Effects of dietary arsenic exposure on liver metabolism in mice. Ecotoxicol. Environ. Saf. 01476513. 274, 116147. doi:10.1016/j.ecoenv.2024.116147.

Shilpa, O., Anupama, K.P., Antony, A., Gurushankara, H.P., 2021a. Lead (Pb)-induced oxidative stress mediates sex-specific autistic-like behaviour in *Drosophila melanogaster*. Mol. Neurobiol. 58 (12), 6378–6393.

Shilpa, O., Anupama, K.P., Antony, A., Gurushankara, H.P., 2021b. Lead (Pb) induced oxidative stress as a mechanism to cause neurotoxicity in *Drosophila melanogaster*. Toxicology 462, 152959.

Singh, S., Chauhan, K., Baby, T., Jagdale, K., Sharma, S., 2025. Prenatal arsenic exposure alters EZH2/H3K27me3 to induce RKIP/NF-kB/ERK1/2-mediated early-onset kidney disease in mouse offspring. Environ. Sci. Pollut. Res. Int. 32 (13), 8498–8517.

Song, X.B., Liu, G., Liu, F., Yan, Z.G., Wang, Z.Y., Liu, Z.P., Wang, L., 2017. Autophagy blockade and lysosomal membrane permeabilization contribute to lead-induced nephrotoxicity in primary rat proximal tubular cells. Cell Death and Disease. 20414889. 8(6). Available from: https://www.nature.com/cddis/. doi:10.1038/cddis.2017.262.

Stößer, S., Lumpp, T., Fischer, F., Gunesch, S., Schumacher, P., Hartwig, A., 2023. Effect of long-term low-dose arsenic exposure on DNA methylation and gene expression in human liver cells. Int. J. Mol. Sci. 1422-0067. 24 (20), 15238. doi:10.3390/ijms242015238.

Subhavana, K., Keerthana, R., Qureshi, A., 2020. Mercury in marine, freshwater and aquaculture species from south India and human exposure risk assessment. Expo. Health 12 (4), 897–903.

Sun, H.J., Ding, S., Guan, D.X., Ma, L.Q., 2022. Nrf2/Keap1 pathway in countering arsenic-induced oxidative stress in mice after chronic exposure at environmentally-relevant concentrations. Chemosphere. 18791298. 303. Available from: https://www.elsevier.com/locate/chemosphere. doi:10.1016/j.chemosphere.2022.135256.

Tan, X., Guan, H., Yang, Y., Luo, S., Hou, L., Chen, H., Li, J., 2020. Cu (II) disrupts autophagy-mediated lysosomal degradation of oligomeric Aβ in microglia via mTOR-TFEB pathway. Toxicol. Appl. Pharmacol. 401, 115090.

Tang, J., Duan, W., Deng, P., Huijuan, L., Liu, C., Duan, Y., Feng, M., Xu, S., 2021. Cadmium disrupts mitochondrial distribution and activates excessive mitochondrial fission by elevating cytosolic calcium independent of MCU-mediated mitochondrial calcium uptake in its neurotoxicity. Toxicology. 0300483X. 453, 152726. doi:10.1016/j.tox.2021.152726.

Tchounwou, P.B., Yedjou, C.G., Patlolla, A.K., Sutton, D.J., 2012. Heavy metal toxicity and the environment. In: Molecular, Clinical and Environmental Toxicology: Volume 3: Environmental Toxicology, Springer Basel, pp. 133–164.

Teixeira, F.B., de Oliveirade Oliveira, A.C.A., Leão, L.K.R., Fagundes, N.C.F., Fernandes, R.M., Fernandes, L.M.P., da Silva, M.C.F., Amado, L.L., Sagica, F.E.S., de Oliveirade Oliveira, E.H.C., Crespo-Lopez, M.E., Maia, C.S.F., Lima, R.R., 2018. Exposure to inorganic mercury causes oxidative stress, cell death, and functional deficits in the motor cortex. Front.

Mol. Neurosci. 16625099. 11. Available from: https://www.frontiersin.org/articles/10.3389/fnmol.2018.00125/pdf. doi:10.3389/fnmol.2018.00125.

Vieira, M.C., Torronteras, R., Córdoba, F., Canalejo, A., 2012. Acute toxicity of manganese in goldfish *Carassius auratus* is associated with oxidative stress and organ specific antioxidant responses. Ecotoxicol. Environ. Saf. 10902414. 78, 212–217. doi:10.1016/j.ecoenv.2011.11.015.

Wang, L., Cao, J., Chen, D., Liu, X., Hao, L., Liu, Z., 2009. Role of oxidative stress, apoptosis, and intracellular homeostasis in primary cultures of rat proximal tubular cells exposed to cadmium. Biol. Trace Elem. Res. 0163-4984. 127 (1), 53–68. doi:10.1007/s12011-008-8223-7.

Wang, L., Wise, J.T.F., Zhang, Z., Shi, X., 2016. Progress and prospects of reactive oxygen species in metal carcinogenesis. Curr. Pharmacol. Rep. 2198-641X. 2 (4), 178–186. doi:10.1007/s40495-016-0061-2.

Woo, S.Y., Lee, M.Y., Jung, Y.J., Yoo, E.S., Seoh, J.Y., Shin, H.Y., Ahn, H.S., Ryu, K.H., 2006. Arsenic trioxide inhibits cell growth in SH-SY5Y and SK-N-AS neuroblastoma cell lines by a different mechanism. Pediatric Hematology and Oncology. 15210669. 23 (3), 231–243. doi:10.1080/08880010500506818.

Xu, J., Lian, L.J., Wu, C., Wang, X.F., Fu, W.Y., Xu, L.H., 2008. Lead induces oxidative stress, DNA damage and alteration of p53, Bax and Bcl-2 expressions in mice. Food Chem. Toxicol. 02786915. 46 (5), 1488–1494. doi:10.1016/j.fct.2007.12.016.

Yang, F., Pei, R., Zhang, Z., Liao, J., Yu, W., Qiao, N., Han, Q., Li, Y., Hu, L., Guo, J., Pan, J., Tang, Z., 2019. Copper induces oxidative stress and apoptosis through mitochondria-mediated pathway in chicken hepatocytes. Toxicol. Vitro. 08872333. 54, 310–316. doi:10.1016/j.tiv.2018.10.017.

Yang, P., Yang, X., Sun, L., Han, X., Xu, L., Gu, W., Zhang, M., 2022. Effects of cadmium on oxidative stress and cell apoptosis in Drosophila melanogaster larvae. Sci. Rep. 2045-2322. 12(1). doi:10.1038/s41598-022-08758-0.

Yang, Z., Yang, S., Qian, S.Y., Hong, J.-S., Kadiiska, M.B., Tennant, R.W., Waalkes, M.P., Liu, J., 2007. Cadmium-induced toxicity in rat primary mid-brain neuroglia cultures: role of oxidative stress from microglia. Toxicol. Sci. 1096-6080. 98 (2), 488–494. doi:10.1093/toxsci/kfm106.

Yao, Y., Zhao, X., Zheng, S., Wang, S., Liu, H., Shiwen, X., 2021. Subacute cadmium exposure promotes M1 macrophage polarization through oxidative stress-evoked inflammatory response and induces porcine adrenal fibrosis. Toxicology. 0300483X. 461, 152899. doi:10.1016/j.tox.2021.152899.

Ye, F., Li, X., Liu, Y., Jiang, A., Li, X., Yang, L., Chang, W., Yuan, J., Chen, J., 2020. CypD deficiency confers neuroprotection against mitochondrial abnormality caused by lead in SH-SY5Y cell. Toxicol. Lett. 03784274. 323, 25–34. doi:10.1016/j.toxlet.2019.12.025.

Yi, L., Shang, X.J., Lv, L., Wang, Y., Zhang, J., Quan, C., Shi, Y., Liu, Y., Zhang, L., 2022. Cadmium-induced apoptosis of Leydig cells is mediated by excessive mitochondrial fission and inhibition of mitophagy. Cell Death and Disease. 20414889. 13(11). Available from: https://www.nature.com/cddis/. doi:10.1038/s41419-022-05364-w.

Zakir, H.M., Sharmin, S., Akter, A., Rahman, M.S., 2020. Assessment of health risk of heavy metals and water quality indices for irrigation and drinking suitability of waters: a case study of Jamalpur Sadar area, Bangladesh. Environ. Adv. 26667657. 2, 100005. doi:10.1016/j.envadv.2020.100005.

Zhang, G., Zhang, Y., Jing, L., Zhao, H., 2023. Lead exposure induced developmental nephrotoxicity in Japanese quail (Coturnix japonica) via oxidative stress-based PI3K/AKT pathway inhibition and NF-κB pathway activation. Comp. Biochem. Physiol. C Toxicol. Pharmacol. 18781659. 268. Available from: https://www.journals.elsevier.

com/comparative-biochemistry-and-physiology-part-c-toxicology-and-pharmacology. doi:10.1016/j.cbpc.2023.109599.

Zhang, J., Su, P., Xue, C., Wang, D., Zhao, F., Shen, X., Luo, W., 2022. Lead disrupts mitochondrial morphology and function through induction of er stress in model of neurotoxicity. Int. J. Mol. Sci. 1422-0067. 23 (19), 11435. doi:10.3390/ijms231911435.

Zhang, L., Bo, J., Chen, W., Li, S., Wang, Y., Yan, L., Wu, L., Zhang, Y., 2021. The role of Nrf2 on the cognitive dysfunction of high-fat diet mice following lead exposure. Biol. Trace Elem. Res. 0163-4984. 199 (6), 2247–2258. doi:10.1007/s12011-020-02346-x.

Zhang, Y., Pei, X., Jing, L., Zhang, Q., Zhao, H., 2024. Lead induced cerebellar toxicology of developmental Japanese quail (*Coturnix japonica*) via oxidative stress-based Nrf2/Keap1 pathway inhibition and glutathione-mediated apoptosis signaling activation. Environ. Pollut. 02697491. 352, 124114. doi:10.1016/j.envpol.2024.124114.

Zhang, Z.W., Zhi-GangTan, N.Q., Kang, Z.L., Chen, Z.L., Hu, L.M., Yang, Z.M., Li, Y., 2016. Copper-induced spermatozoa head malformation is related to oxidative damage to testes in CD-1 mice. Biol. Trace Elem. Res. 15590720. 173(2), 427–432. Available from: http://www.springer.com/humana+press/journal/12011. doi:10.1007/s12011-016-0675-6.

Zhao, L., Liu, X., Xu, G., Guo, Y., Sun, L., Zhang, C., Li, X., Li, B., 2020. Arsenic induces mTOR-dependent autophagy, whereas it impairs the autophagy–lysosome pathway and the potential role of TFEB in cultured dendritic cells. Metallomics. 1756-5901. 12 (8), 1230–1245. doi:10.1039/d0mt00057d.

Zhong, G., He, Y., Wan, F., Wu, S., Jiang, X., Tang, Z., Hu, L., 2021. Effects of long-term exposure to copper on the Keap1/Nrf2 signaling pathway and msr-related redox status in the kidneys of rats. Biol. Trace Elem. Res. 0163-4984. 199 (11), 4205–4217. doi:10.1007/s12011-020-02557-2.

Chapter 18

Intensive cropping systems reduce heavy metals in cotton fields

Sherif Ibrahim Abdel-Wahab[a], Tamer Ibrahim Abdel-Wahab[a], Eman Ibrahim Abdel-Wahab[b], and Mohamed Mourad Lamlom[a]
[a]*Crop Intensification Research Department, Field Crops Research Institute, Agricultural Research Center (ARC), Giza, Egypt*
[b]*Food Legumes Research Department, Field Crops Research Institute, Agricultural Research Center (ARC), Giza, Egypt*

18.1 Introduction

Heavy metals in the soil, including lead (Pb), nickel (Ni), and cadmium (Cd), can harm both human health and the environment. High levels of heavy metals can affect plant growth, food safety, and water quality, posing risks to health and the environment. Osman et al. (2021) and Sarhan et al. (2021) showed that both natural and human activities have contributed to the heavy metal contamination of Middle Egypt's soil. Soil contamination is also caused by vehicle emissions and Pb-based fuels. These metals can build up in plants, potentially causing toxicity when animals or humans consume them. An excess of Pb accumulation can reduce root growth by up to 42% (Collin et al., 2022). In addition, Ni is a crucial micronutrient for plants, influencing water quality, food safety, and plant growth. However, excessive Ni in the soil can be toxic to plants and contaminate groundwater (Said, 2022; Rizwan et al., 2024). High levels of Cd in soil can lead to contamination of crops and water sources, which poses significant health risks to humans and animals (Haider et al., 2021).

In recent years, the government's primary focus has been on increasing the production of Egyptian cotton (*Gossypium barbadense* L.) during the summer season. The main challenge lies in planting the winter crop first. Ensuring a successful planting and harvest of the winter crop remains the key hurdle before transitioning to the summer crop. Egyptian clover, faba bean (*Vicia faba* L.), and wheat (*Triticum aestivum* L.) are crucial winter crops in Egypt, but they often compete for limited agricultural land and water resources (Mohamed and

The Metallome in Motion. https://doi.org/10.1016/B978-0-443-44299-5.00015-8

Bakheit, 2025). Egyptian clover is valued for its high protein content, making it a crucial crop for feeding livestock during the winter season (Salem et al., 2019). Moreover, the faba bean is a crucial winter crop in Egypt due to its high protein content, making it an affordable and nutritious protein source, especially for individuals with limited incomes (Salman et al., 2024). The two legume crops can fix nitrogen (N) in the soil, which can help reduce metal toxicity and improve soil health overall (Pandey et al., 2022). However, the Nile Delta region in Egypt is a prime location for wheat cultivation due to its fertile soil and abundant water supply from the Nile River. Egypt is one of Africa's leading producers of wheat, with the majority of the grain being used domestically (Abdalla et al., 2022). Because wheat plants' roots may take up heavy metals from the soil and then pass them on to cotton plants through root exudates, wheat can bioaccumulate more heavy metals in cotton fields (Vardumyan et al., 2024).

This competition forms a conflict between using land to grow wheat or faba beans to feed the human population and cultivating Egyptian clover to provide nutritious fodder for livestock. Among major crops, cotton exhibits the highest resistance to abiotic stresses, including heavy metals (Li et al., 2020). Cotton is usually planted in higher regions of Middle Egypt in the spring, though the best times to plant vary slightly based on the location and the weather (El-Adly et al., 2018). Farmers often try to plant between March and May; however, the precise dates vary to align with the ideal growing conditions of sunshine and temperature (EL-Refaey et al., 2022). Despite the negative impact of heavy metal stress on cotton growth, the plant possesses advanced stress-resistance mechanisms. Cotton, being a nonedible fiber-producing crop with significant biomass and efficient heavy metal absorption capabilities, is well-suited for restoring heavy metal-contaminated soils. It offers distinct ecological and economic advantages, making it an ideal choice for remediation efforts with promising application potential.

In Egypt, intercropping field crops with cotton has long been a popular strategy to increase agricultural output and land use efficiency (Metwally et al., 2009, 2012; Lamlom et al., 2018). This approach also improves soil health and reduces nematode pressure, leading to higher overall crop yields (Lamlom et al., 2019). These benefits positively impact the unsaturated fatty acids in cottonseed oil by promoting nutrient uptake and plant growth, resulting in a higher quality product (Lamlom et al., 2020). Various remediation strategies have been utilized to eliminate heavy metals from polluted soil, with phytoremediation being the most prominent. Intercropping sesame (*Sesamum indicum* L.) with cotton can help reduce soil metal levels through phytoremediation, as sesame is known for its high tolerance to heavy metals (Liu et al., 2023). Moreover, intercropping onion (*Allium cepa* L.) with cotton can help reduce metal levels in the soil by taking advantage of the different root systems of the two crops. Onions have shallow roots that can absorb surface metals, while cotton's deeper roots can access metals in lower soil layers (Schuh and Tong, 2025). The study aimed to enhance seed cotton yield, improve seed cotton oil quality, and decrease heavy metal content to produce healthier cooking oil and enhance soil health.

18.2 Materials and methods

A two-year study was conducted at Sids Agricultural Research Station in Beni Sweif Governorate, Agricultural Research Center (ARC), Egypt. Soil samples (0–30 cm) were analyzed by the Water, Soil, and Environment Research Institute, ARC, following the methods of Jackson (1958) and Chapman and Pratt (1961) prior to planting winter crops. Soil pH, available nitrogen, phosphorus, and potassium were 8.32, 13.15, 25.50, and 170.5 ppm, respectively. The soil texture was determined to be clay. Furrow irrigation was the predominant irrigation system used in the region. The winter field crop cultivars included Giza 6 for Egyptian clover, Giza 843 for faba bean, Giza 6 Improved for onion, and Misr 1 for wheat. For summer field crops, the cultivars used were Giza 95 "extra-long staple" for cotton, Cream 1 for cowpea, and Shandweel 3 for sesame. Seeds for Egyptian clover and cowpea were provided by the Forage Crops Research Department, Field Crops Research Institute, ARC. Faba bean seeds were supplied by the Food Legumes Research Department, Field Crops Research Institute, ARC. Onion transplants were obtained from the Onion Research Department at Sids Agricultural Research Station, Field Crops Research Institute, ARC. Wheat grains were sourced from the Wheat Research Department, Field Crops Research Institute, ARC. Cotton seeds were provided by the Cotton Research Institute, ARC, and sesame seeds were supplied by the Oil Crops Research Department, Field Crops Research Institute, ARC. *Rhizobium trifolii* and *Rhizobium leguminosarum* were inoculated into Egyptian clover and faba bean seeds, respectively, prior to seeding during the two winter seasons. Arabic gum was used as a sticking agent. Using Arabic gum as a sticking agent, cowpea seeds were infected with *Rhizobium meliloti* before sowing over the two summer seasons. During the two winter seasons, 476 kg of calcium superphosphate (15.5% P_2O_5) was applied per hectare to prepare the soil. Under intercropping and sole plantings, mineral N fertilizer was applied at rates of 35.7 kg nitrogen per hectare for Egyptian clover, 17.8 and 35.7 kg N per hectare for faba beans, 191.3 and 285.6 kg N per hectare for onions, and 119.5 and 178.5 kg N per hectare for wheat. At 45 and 60 days after cotton planting, two equal dosages of mineral N fertilizer were administered to the cotton plants at a rate of 142.8 kg N per hectare. One equal dose of mineral N fertilizer was applied to cowpea plants 25 days after cowpea planting at rates of 17.8 and 35.7 kg N per hectare under intercropping and sole plantings, respectively. At 25 and 40 days after sesame planting, two equal doses of mineral N fertilizer were applied to the plants at rates of 35.7 and 71.4 kg N per hectare under intercropping and sole plantings, respectively. All of the crops that were examined received the required amount of mineral K fertilizer. The planting and

TABLE 18.1 Sowing and harvest dates of all the studied field crops in the two seasons.

	Season			
	First season		Second season	
Crop	Sowing date	Harvest date	Sowing date	Harvest date
Egyptian clover	21st October	11th March	18th October	7th March
Faba bean	21st October	29th April	18th October	26th April
Onion	21st October	14th April	18th October	12th April
Wheat	21st October	8th May	18th October	5th May
Cotton	22nd March	16th September	18th March	13th September
Cowpea	14th May	27th July	11th May	24th July
Sesame	14th May	30th August	11th May	28th August

harvest dates of winter and summer field crops in the two growing seasons are presented in Table 18.1.

The experiment involved twelve cropping systems as described below: Egyptian clover seeds were broadcast at a rate of 47.6 kg per hectare. After the third cutting of Egyptian clover, cotton seeds were planted on two sides of the bed, with two plants spaced 25 cm apart. This system was referred to as Egyptian clover—cotton in the winter season and cotton in the summer season (traditional cropping system) (Fig. 18.1).

Similarly, Egyptian clover seeds were broadcast at the same rate, and after the third cutting, cotton seeds were planted on two sides of the bed, with two plants spaced 25 cm apart. In addition, two rows of cowpea seeds were planted in the middle of the cotton beds, with two plants spaced 20 cm apart. This system was referred to as Egyptian clover—cotton in the winter season and cotton + cowpea in the summer season (Fig. 18.2).

Furthermore, Egyptian clover seeds were broadcast at the same rate, and after the third cutting, cotton seeds were planted on two sides of the bed, with two plants spaced 25 cm apart. One row of sesame seeds was planted in the middle of the cotton beds, with two plants spaced 20 cm apart. This system was referred to as Egyptian clover–cotton in the winter season and cotton + sesame in the summer season (Fig. 18.3).

In another cropping system, faba bean seeds were planted in two rows in the middle of the bed, with two plants spaced 15 cm apart. Cotton seeds were planted on both sides of the faba bean beds, with two plants spaced 25 cm apart. This cropping system was referred to as faba bean/cotton in the winter season. After the faba bean harvest, cotton continued to grow alone in the summer season (Fig. 18.4).

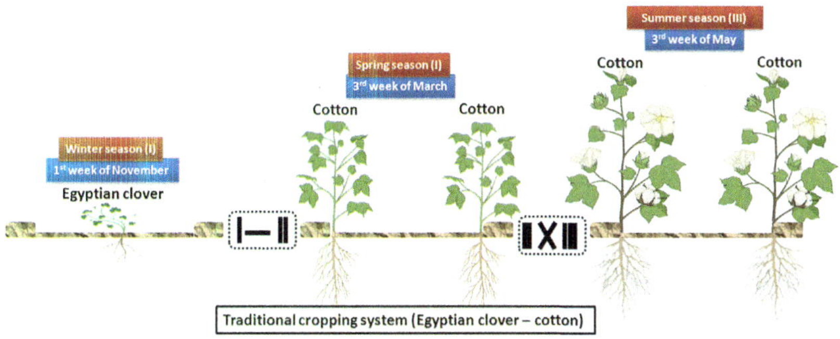

FIG. 18.1 Schematic diagram of traditional cropping system (Egyptian clover—cotton).

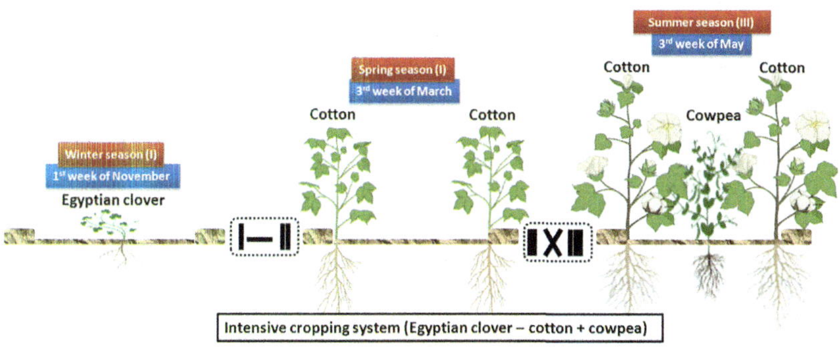

FIG. 18.2 Schematic diagram of an intensive cropping system (Egyptian clover—cotton + cowpea).

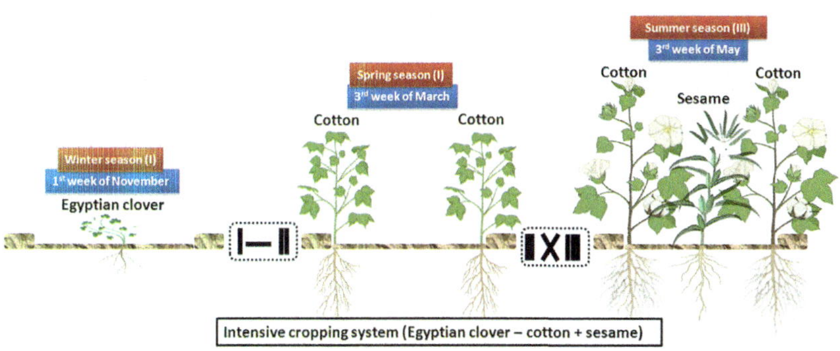

FIG. 18.3 Schematic diagram of an intensive cropping system (Egyptian clover—cotton + sesame).

In another setup, cowpea seeds were planted in two rows in the middle of the cotton beds, with two plants spaced 20 cm apart. This cropping system was known as faba bean/cotton in the winter season and cotton + cowpea in the summer season (Fig. 18.5).

Similarly, sesame seeds were planted in one row in the middle of the cotton beds, with two plants spaced 20 cm apart. This cropping system was referred

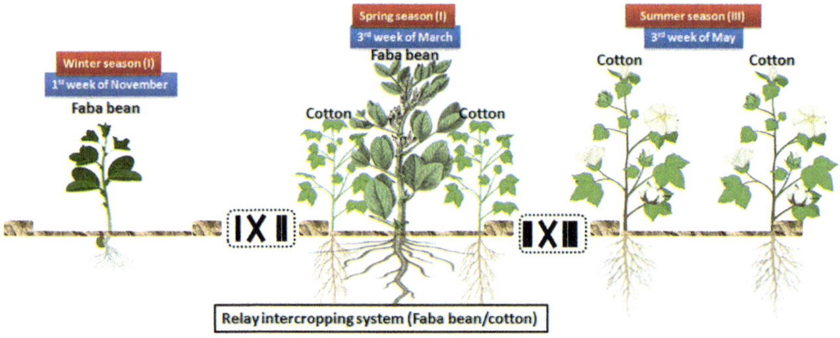

FIG. 18.4 Schematic diagram of relay intercropping system (faba bean/cotton).

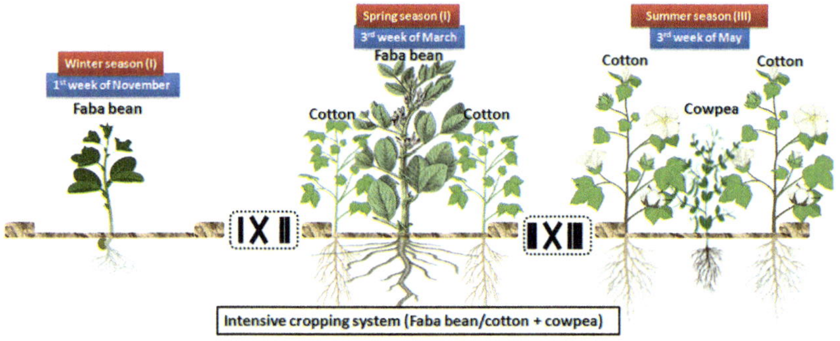

FIG. 18.5 Schematic diagram of an intensive cropping system (faba bean/cotton + cowpea).

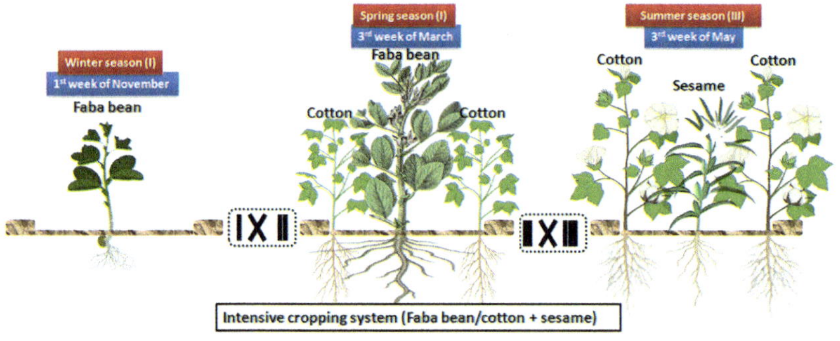

FIG. 18.6 Schematic diagram of intensive cropping system (faba bean/cotton + sesame).

to as faba bean/cotton in the winter season and cotton + sesame in the summer season (Fig. 18.6).

Onion transplants were planted in four rows in the middle of the bed, with each plant spaced 10 cm apart. Cotton seeds were planted on both sides of the onion beds, with two plants spaced 25 cm apart. This cropping system

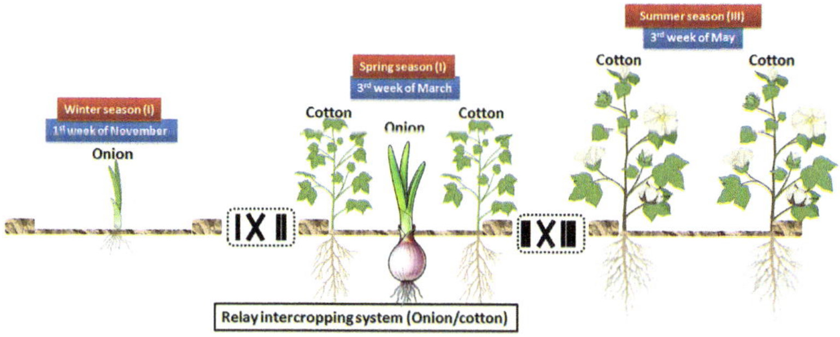

FIG. 18.7 Schematic diagram of relay intercropping system (onion/cotton).

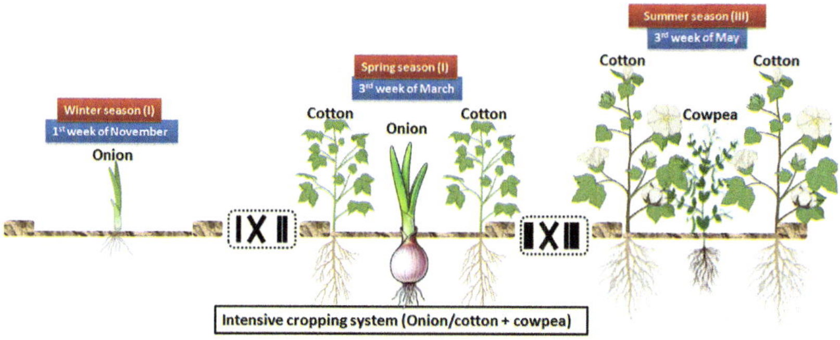

FIG. 18.8 Schematic diagram of an intensive cropping system (onion/cotton + cowpea).

was described as onion/cotton during the winter season. After the onions were uprooted, the cotton continued to grow alone during the summer season (Fig. 18.7).

In another scenario, cowpea seeds were planted in two rows in the middle of the cotton beds, with two plants spaced 20 cm apart. This cropping system was known as onion/cotton in the winter season and cotton + cowpea in the summer season (Fig. 18.8).

In addition, sesame seeds were planted in one row in the middle of the cotton beds, with two plants spaced 20 cm apart. This cropping system was referred to as onion/cotton in the winter season and cotton + sesame in the summer season (Fig. 18.9).

Wheat grains were drilled in four rows in the middle of the bed at a rate of 119.0 kg per hectare. Cotton seeds were planted on both sides of the wheat beds, with two plants spaced 25 cm apart. This cropping system was expressed as wheat/cotton in the winter season. After the wheat harvest, cotton continued to grow alone in the summer season (Fig. 18.10).

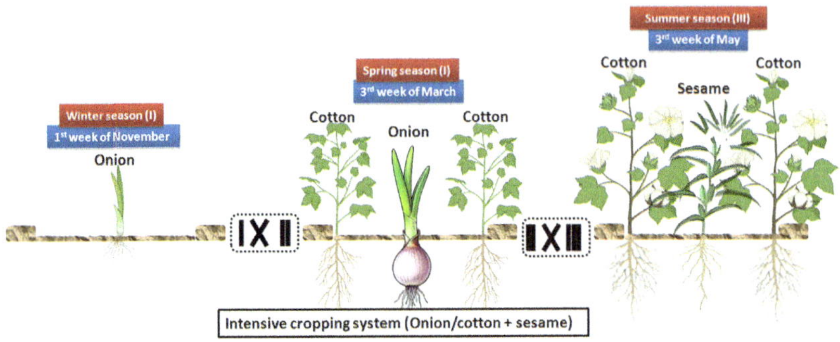

FIG. 18.9 Schematic diagram of an intensive cropping system (onion/cotton + sesame).

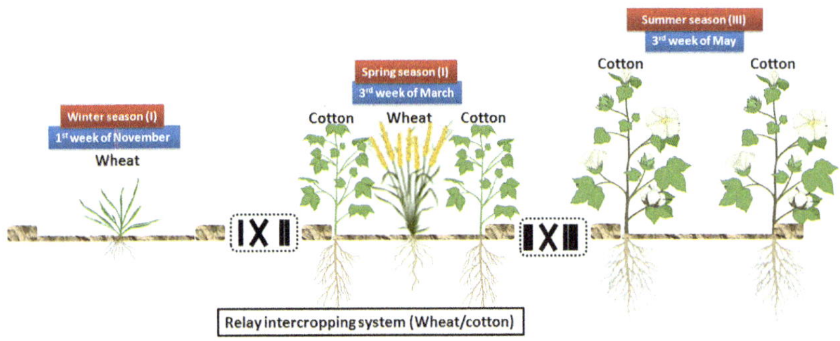

FIG. 18.10 Schematic diagram of relay intercropping system (wheat/cotton).

In another setup, cowpea seeds were planted in two rows in the middle of the cotton beds, with two plants spaced 20 cm apart. This cropping system was known as wheat/cotton in the winter season and cotton + cowpea in the summer season (Fig. 18.11).

Similarly, sesame seeds were planted in one row in the middle of the cotton beds, with two plants spaced 20 cm apart. This cropping system was referred to as wheat/cotton in the winter season and cotton + sesame in the summer season (Fig. 18.12).

In addition, sole Egyptian clover or wheat was grown by broadcasting Egyptian clover seeds or drilling wheat grains at rates of 47.6 or 119.0 kg per hectare, respectively. For Egyptian clover, the fifth cutting was done in the first week of May in both seasons. Sole onion or faba bean was grown by planting three or two rows in ridges, with one or two plants spaced 10 or 25 cm apart, respectively. Sole cowpea or sesame was grown by planting two rows in ridges, with two plants spaced 20 cm apart. The treatments consisted of combinations of four winter cropping systems and two summer cropping systems. The twelve cropping systems were compared using a randomized complete blocks design with three replications. The plot area was 21.6 m^2. For intercropping and sole plantings of wheat and Egyptian clover, each plot contained six raised beds,

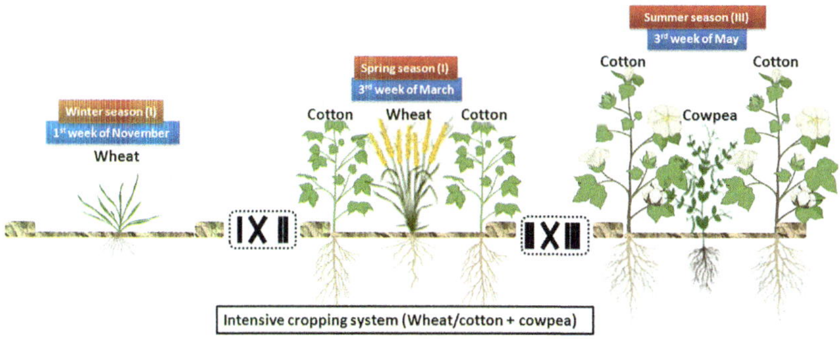

FIG. 18.11 Schematic diagram of intensive cropping system (wheat/cotton + cowpea).

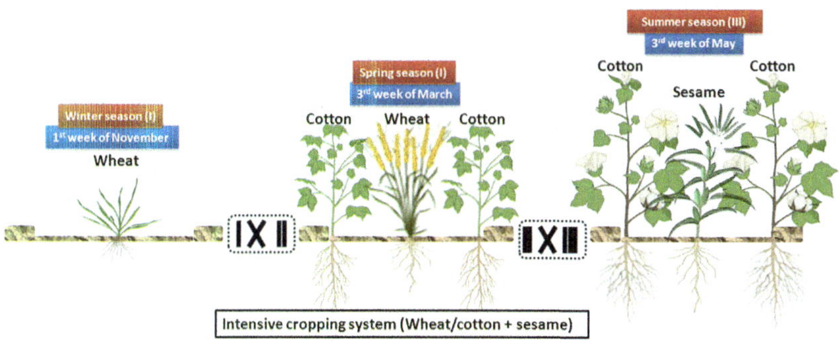

FIG. 18.12 Schematic diagram of an intensive cropping system (wheat/cotton + sesame).

with each bed measuring 3.0 m in length and 1.2 m in width. For sole plantings of faba bean, onion, cowpea, and sesame, each plot contained twelve ridges, with each ridge measuring 3.0 m in length and 0.6 m in width. Seed cotton yield per hectare (t) was recorded based on the subplot area by harvesting all plants in each subplot and converting it to yield per hectare. Fatty acids were separated according to Vogel (1975) and identified using gas liquid chromatography (GLC) on a Trace GC Ultra, Thermo Scientific apparatus. These analyses were conducted by the Regional Center for Food & Feed, ARC, Giza, Egypt. Statistical analysis was performed by conducting an analysis of variance on the obtained results for each season. The measured variables were analyzed using ANOVA with the M-STATC statistical package (Freed, 1991). Mean comparisons were conducted using the least significant differences (LSD) test with a significance level of 5% (Gomez and Gomez, 1984).

18.3 Results

18.3.1 Seed cotton yield per hectare

The traditional cropping system (Egyptian clover—cotton) produced more seed cotton per hectare than the other cropping systems (Fig. 18.13). It should be noted

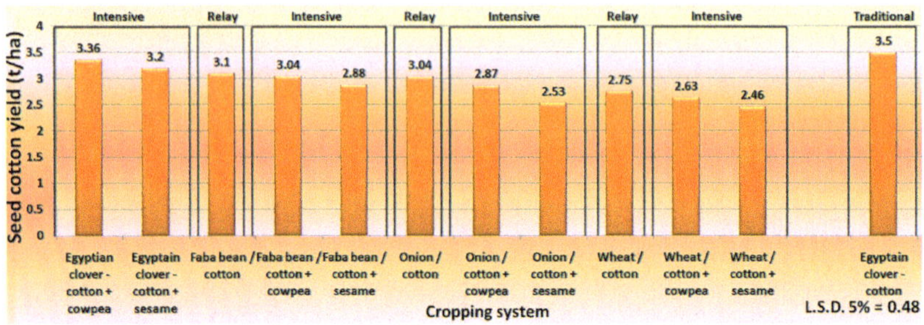

FIG. 18.13 Effect of cropping systems on seed cotton yield per hectare (combined data across the two seasons).

that the traditional cropping system (Egyptian clover—cotton), intensive cropping systems (Egyptian clover—cotton + cowpea, Egyptian clover—cotton + sesame, and Faba bean/cotton + cowpea), and relay intercropping systems (faba bean/cotton and onion/cotton) did not differ significantly. The seed cotton yield of the traditional cropping system (Egyptian clover—cotton), intensive cropping systems (Egyptian clover—cotton + cowpea, Egyptian clover—cotton + sesame, and faba bean/cotton + cowpea), and relay intercropping systems (faba bean/cotton and onion/cotton) were 3.50, 3.36, 3.20, 3.04, 3.10, and 3.04 t per hectare, respectively. The yield of seed cotton per hectare was lower in cropping systems that included wheat. Relay intercropping systems (wheat/cotton) and intensive cropping systems (wheat/cotton + cowpea, wheat/cotton + sesame) had yields of 2.75, 2.63, and 2.46 t per hectare, respectively.

18.3.2 Cotton seed oil's fatty acid content

Cropping systems significantly influenced the saturated fatty acids in seed cotton oil (Table 18.2). Palmitic and stearic fatty acids were found to be lower in the traditional cropping system (Egyptian clover—cotton) and intensive cropping systems (Egyptian clover—cotton + cowpea, Egyptian clover—cotton + sesame, faba bean/cotton + cowpea, and Faba bean/cotton + sesame) compared to other cropping systems. Palmitic fatty acid in cotton seed oil of the traditional cropping system (Egyptian clover—cotton) and intensive cropping systems (Egyptian clover—cotton + cowpea, Egyptian clover—cotton + sesame, faba bean/cotton + cowpea, and faba bean/cotton + sesame) were 20.86%, 20.77%, 20.63%, 20.97%, and 20.84%, respectively.

Meanwhile, stearic fatty acid in cotton seed oil of traditional cropping systems (Egyptian clover—cotton) and intensive cropping systems (Egyptian clover—cotton + cowpea, Egyptian clover—cotton + sesame, faba bean/cotton + cowpea, and faba bean/cotton + sesame) was 2.59%, 2.37%, 2.24%, 2.65%, and 2.51%, respectively. The unsaturated fatty acids in cotton seed oil were found to be lower in intensive cropping systems that included onion or wheat in the winter seasons compared to other cropping systems (Table 18.2). Oleic

TABLE 18.2 Effect of cropping systems on saturated and unsaturated fatty acids in cotton seed oil (combined data across the two seasons).

	Saturated fatty acids (%)		Unsaturated fatty acids (%)	
Cropping system	Plamitic	Stearic	Oleic	Linoleic
Intensive cropping system (Egyptian clover—cotton + cowpea)	20.77	2.37	23.18	55.29
Intensive cropping system (Egyptian clover—cotton + sesame)	20.63	2.24	23.28	55.41
Relay intercropping system (Egyptian clover—cotton)	21.06	2.74	22.88	55.05
Intensive cropping system (Faba bean/ cotton + cowpea)	20.97	2.65	22.99	55.16
Intensive cropping system (Faba bean/ cotton + sesame)	20.84	2.51	23.14	55.26
Relay intercropping system (Onion/cotton)	21.32	3.03	22.65	54.76
Intensive cropping system (onion/cotton + cowpea)	21.22	2.92	22.76	54.88
Intensive cropping system (onion/cotton + sesame)	21.20	2.91	22.68	54.76
Relay intercropping system (Wheat/cotton)	21.46	3.13	22.48	54.54
Intensive cropping system (wheat/cotton + cowpea)	21.34	3.02	22.57	54.64
Intensive cropping system (wheat/cotton + sesame)	21.20	2.91	22.68	54.76
Traditional cropping system (Egyptian clover—cotton)	20.86	2.59	23.03	55.20
L.S.D. 5%	0.44	0.53	0.29	0.22

fatty acid in cotton seed oil of relay intercropping systems (onion/cotton and wheat/cotton) and intensive cropping systems (onion/cotton + cowpea, onion/cotton + sesame, wheat/cotton + cowpea, and wheat/cotton + sesame) was 22.65%, 22.48%, 22.76%, 22.68%, 22.57%, and 22.68%, respectively. Meanwhile, linoleic fatty acid in cotton seed oil of relay intercropping systems (onion/cotton and wheat/cotton) and intensive cropping systems (onion/cotton + cowpea, onion/cotton + sesame, wheat/cotton + cowpea, and wheat/cotton + sesame) was 54.76%, 54.54%, 54.88%, 54.76%, 54.64%, and 54.76%, respectively.

18.4 Discussion

Clover may increase a plant's water usage efficiency, which means it may draw more water from the soil while reducing water loss, according to some research (Barzegar et al., 2016). This is partially because of the plant's large root system, which allows it to obtain water from deeper in the soil profile. As a result, Egyptian clover in traditional cropping systems (Egyptian clover—cotton) plays a role in reducing soil Pb levels through chemical reactions, such as $Pb + 2H_2O + 2e^- \rightarrow Pb(OH)_2 + 2OH^-$ (Tan, 2011), which contribute to soil health and fertility. This emphasizes the potential benefits of incorporating Egyptian clover into crop rotations for sustainable agriculture practices, leading to higher seed cotton yields compared to other cropping systems. Egyptian clover's roots can also absorb chloride (Cl) from the soil, which in turn helps to lower soil Ni levels by binding with Cl (Muhammad et al., 2014). This process is a result of the complex interactions between the soil, plants, and specific forms of Ni. When Cl ions and Ni in the soil combine, they form complexes that decrease the amount of Ni accessible to cotton plants. The plant then absorbs some of these complexes along with Cl. The presence of Egyptian clover in traditional cropping systems (Egyptian clover—cotton) reduces soil Ni levels through chemical reactions, such as $Ni + 2HCl^- \rightarrow NiCl_2 + H_2$ (Iqbal et al., 2025), indicating its positive impact on soil quality and crop productivity. In addition, traditional cropping systems may exhibit better soil nutrient retention compared to other cropping systems. There are no hydroxyl (OH) groups released into the soil by Egyptian clover roots. It is known that Egyptian clover roots fix more atmospheric N into the soil than faba bean roots (Lamlom et al., 2018), even though Egyptian clover grows symbiotically with nitrogen-fixing bacteria in root nodules, releasing OH ions into the soil (Fetyan et al., 2015). The presence of OH ions released by Egyptian clover roots can contribute to soil pH levels and nutrient availability, potentially affecting crop growth and overall soil health. As a result, Egyptian clover in traditional cropping systems (Egyptian clover—cotton) helps reduce soil Cd levels through reactions like $2Cd^{2+} + 2OH^- \rightarrow Cd(OH)_2$ (Wang et al., 2023), potentially contributing to increased seed cotton yields. The lack of significant differences among the cropping systems suggests that farmers have flexibility in choosing winter crops without compromising cotton yield. Traditional cropping systems (Egyptian clover—cotton) can be a sustainable practice for enhancing soil health, fertility, and agricultural productivity. Fig. 18.2 shows that intensive cropping systems (Egyptian clover—cotton + cowpea) can effectively reduce soil Pb levels in cotton fields by increasing the uptake of Pb by cowpea plants and decreasing its availability in the soil for cotton (El-Shamy et al., 2023). This method is a sustainable and environmentally friendly way to remediate contaminated soils. Intensive cropping systems (Egyptian clover—cotton + cowpea) can effectively reduce soil Ni levels in cotton fields by increasing the uptake of Ni by cowpea plants (Lv et al., 2023). This helps to decrease the amount of Ni available in the soil for cotton, leading to improved soil health and increased crop yield in the field. Intensive cropping systems (Egyptian clover—cotton + cowpea) can effectively reduce soil Cd levels in cotton fields by leveraging the N-fixing abilities of cowpea to enhance soil health and decrease Cd uptake by cotton plants (El-Sharawy et al., 2018). This sustainable farming method not only boosts crop yield but also enhances soil fertility in the long run. Meanwhile, Fig. 18.3 shows that intensive cropping systems (Egyptian clover—cotton + sesame) can effectively reduce soil Pb levels in cotton fields by increasing the uptake of Pb by sesame plants and decreasing the amount of Pb available for cotton uptake (Donyavian et al., 2018). This system has shown promising results in reducing soil contamination and improving cotton yield in contaminated areas. Intensive intercropping systems (Egyptian clover—cotton + sesame) can effectively reduce soil Ni levels in cotton fields by increasing the uptake of Ni by sesame plants, which are known to be hyperaccumulators of this metal (Awad et al., 2023). This process can help improve soil quality and reduce the risk of Ni toxicity in cotton plants. Intensive intercropping systems (Egyptian clover—cotton + sesame) can effectively reduce soil Cd levels in cotton fields by increasing the uptake of Cd by sesame plants, preventing it from accumulating in the soil (El-Shamy et al., 2021). This system is a sustainable and environmentally friendly way to improve soil quality in contaminated areas.

Faba bean roots play a crucial role in nutrient cycling by releasing compounds like sulfate (SO_4) into the soil (Manschadi et al., 1998). In a reply intercropping system (faba bean/cotton), the roots of faba beans help reduce soil Pb levels through a chemical reaction: $Pb + 2H_2SO_4 \rightarrow PbSO_4 + 2H_2O + SO_2$ (Blecharczyk et al., 2024) (Fig. 18.4). This reduction in soil Pb levels can benefit soil health and crop productivity in the long run. In addition, in the same relay intercropping system, faba beans can lower soil Ni levels in cotton fields by releasing citric acid from their roots, which binds to in the soil, forming a complex that is less available to cotton plants (Santos et al., 2017). This leads to decreased Ni concentration in the soil, resulting in improved cotton yield and quality. Furthermore, relay intercropping system (faba bean/cotton) can effectively decrease soil Cd levels in cotton fields. Faba bean plants increase the uptake of Cd, which is then removed from the field during harvest, reducing the overall Cd content in the soil (Ghorbi et al., 2023). The deep root system of faba beans also helps alleviate soil compaction, improving water infiltration and nutrient absorption for subsequent cotton crops. By relay intercropping system (faba bean/cotton), soil health can be enhanced, and the risk of Cd contamination minimized, promoting both crop productivity and environmental quality in agricultural systems. Intensive cropping system (faba bean/cotton + cowpea), effectively reduces soil Pb and Ni levels (Fig. 18.5). Cowpea's phytoremediation capabilities absorb Pb, while its N-fixing abilities enhance soil health and reduce Ni and Cd uptake by cotton. This sustainable practice improves soil health, decreases heavy metal contamination in food crops, and can lead to increased crop yield. Intensive cropping system (faba bean/cotton + sesame) effectively reduces soil levels of Pb, Ni, and Cd in cotton fields (Fig. 18.6). This is achieved by enhancing the uptake of these metals by sesame plants, which exhibit hyperaccumulation of Ni, thereby reducing their availability for cotton and preventing soil accumulation. This sustainable practice contributes to improved soil quality and cotton yields in contaminated environments.

Relay intercropping system (onion/cotton) have been shown to effectively reduce soil Pb levels in cotton fields (Fig. 18.7). This is achieved by the increased exudates from onion roots promoting the immobilization of Pb in the soil, thus decreasing its availability for uptake by cotton plants (Cui et al., 2024). In addition, relay intercropping system disrupts pest and disease cycles, improving soil health and reducing the need for chemical inputs. In the case of reducing soil Ni levels in cotton fields, relay intercropping system (onion/cotton) can be beneficial. Onions can help remove Ni from the soil through increased uptake, especially when harvested (Arunachalam et al., 2024). This practice not only enhances soil fertility but also boosts overall crop productivity over time. Similarly, relay intercropping system (onion/cotton) can effectively lower soil Cd levels. By increasing the uptake of Cd by onion plants, the heavy metal is prevented from accumulating in cotton plants (Opriş et al., 2023). This symbiotic relationship between onion and cotton enhances soil health and minimizes environmental contamination. Intensive intercropping system (onion/cotton + cowpea) can also contribute to soil remediation (Fig. 18.8). This practice reduces Pb, Ni, and Cd levels in the soil through phytoremediation, improving soil health and reducing contamination risks in nearby food crops. Furthermore, intensive cropping system (onion/cotton + cowpea) can effectively reduce soil Ni levels by enhancing Ni uptake by cowpea plants, leading to improved soil health and increased crop yield. This sustainable farming approach benefits soil fertility in the long term. Intensive cropping system (onion/cotton + sesame) has also shown promise in reducing soil contamination (Fig. 18.9). Sesame plants can help lower Pb, Ni, and Cd levels in the soil by increasing their uptake of these metals, thereby improving soil quality and crop yield in polluted areas. Overall, intensive cropping systems in cotton fields can play a significant role in reducing soil metal levels, enhancing soil health, and promoting sustainable farming practices.

Fig. 18.10 shows that the relay intercropping system (wheat/cotton) can effectively elevate soil Pb levels in cotton fields by increasing the organic matter content in the soil (Ali et al., 2025). This organic matter helps bind Pb particles, preventing their leaching into groundwater. The relay intercropping system (wheat/cotton) can significantly raise soil Ni levels in cotton fields. This is due to the fact that wheat roots have a greater ability to absorb Ni compared to cotton roots, resulting in the accumulation of Ni in the soil (Naveed et al., 2024). The relay intercropping system (wheat/cotton) can also lead to elevated soil Cd levels in cotton fields. This is because wheat roots release organic acids that mobilize Cd in the soil, increasing its availability for uptake by cotton plants (Rizwan et al., 2016). As a result, cotton tissues may contain higher Cd levels, posing a potential risk to human health if consumed. Conversely, intensive cropping systems (wheat/cotton + cowpea and wheat/cotton + sesame) had lower seed cotton yields than the other cropping systems (Figs. 18.11 and 18.12). While cowpea or sesame can have positive effects on reducing heavy metals in cotton fields, the preceding winter crop, wheat, had a greater impact on increasing heavy metal levels in the soil. This is because wheat has the ability to absorb heavy metals from the soil and release them during decomposition. The root system of wheat may also help move heavy metals closer to the surface, making them more accessible to subsequent crops like cotton. Consequently, the benefits of cowpea or sesame in cotton fields diminish when the soil is contaminated with heavy metals from the wheat crop. This underscores the importance of implementing cropping system strategies to mitigate heavy metal contamination in agricultural fields. Different crops in cropping systems can have diverse effects on soil heavy metal levels.

Oil extracted from seed cotton is less likely to contain soil heavy metals, making it a healthier option for consumption. Oils with low levels of saturated fatty acids are preferred for cooking and baking due to their stability at high temperatures. Cropping systems that involve legumes in winter, even in the presence of high soil heavy metals, provide a safe and viable option for producing healthy cooking oils. These systems help maintain soil health and minimize heavy metal accumulation in the oil. Winter legume cultivation aids in natural soil detoxification and reduces heavy metal levels, promoting a sustainable approach that benefits the environment and ensures a safer and healthier oil product for consumers. The saturated fatty acids in cotton seed oil were found to be higher in intensive cropping systems that included onion or wheat in the winter seasons compared to other cropping systems (Table 18.2). This is due to the elevated levels of soil heavy metals in cotton fields following the harvest of wheat or the uprooting of onion. These findings suggest that winter crops in these cropping systems can directly influence the fatty acid composition of cotton seed oil. The presence of heavy metals in the soil may impact the absorption and distribution of nutrients in cotton plants, thereby affecting the fatty acid profile. In spite of the high levels of heavy metals in the soil, winter cropping systems that use legumes present a chance to boost the amount of healthy unsaturated fatty acids in cotton seed oil. This suggests that crop rotation or intercropping with legumes could be a sustainable practice for improving the nutritional quality of cotton seed oil in areas with heavy metal contamination. Because cotton and wheat or onion crops compete for nutrients and resources, there is less buildup of healthy unsaturated fatty acids in cotton seed oil. Growing wheat or onion in cropping systems with cotton in metal-heavy soil may not be ideal, but it could be a better option in metal-free soil. It is crucial to assess the potential effects of metal contamination on crop yield and quality when designing cropping systems. Conducting soil tests and adopting suitable soil management strategies can help minimize these risks and enhance crop production in metal-heavy soils.

18.5 Conclusion

Legume crops, particularly Egyptian clover and faba bean, significantly improve agricultural systems by enhancing water usage efficiency and soil health through heavy metal reduction (Pb, Ni, Cd). These crops, especially in intercropping and rotation systems with cotton, cowpea, sesame, onion, or wheat, boost seed cotton yields, influence soil pH, and contribute to nutrient availability via N fixation. Legume integration can also lead to healthier cooking oils with reduced heavy metal accumulation and potentially improved fatty acid profiles in cotton seed oil. Managing heavy metal contamination is crucial for sustainable and productive agriculture.

AI disclosure

During the preparation of this work, the author(s) used ChatGPT in order to improve the language. After using this tool/service, the author(s) reviewed and edited the content as needed and take(s) full responsibility for the content of the publication.

References

Abdalla, A., Stellmacher, T., Becker, M., 2022. Trends and prospects of change in wheat self-sufficiency in Egypt. Agriculture. 13 (1), 7.

Ali, A., Jabeen, N., Chachar, Z., Chachar, S., Ahmed, S., Ahmed, N., Laghari, A.A., Sahito, Z.A., Farruhbek, R., Yang, Z., 2025. The role of biochar in enhancing soil health & interactions with rhizosphere properties and enzyme activities in organic fertilizer substitution. Front. Plant Sci. 16, 1595208.

Arunachalam, T., Gade, K., Mahadule, P.A., Soumia, P.S., Govindasamy, V., Gawande, S.J., Mahajan, V., 2024. Optimizing plant growth, nutrient uptake, and yield of onion through the application of phosphorus solubilizing bacteria and endophytic fungi. Front. Microbiol. 15, 1442912.

Awad, M.M., Abdelsatar, M.A., Ibrahim, M.M.A., 2023. Impact of different sesame intercropping dates with cotton on agronomic performance and insect pests infestation. Moroc. J. Agric. Sci. 4 (1). doi:10.5281/ZENODO.8003719.

Barzegar, A., Yousefi, A., Zargoosh, N., 2016. Water stress and soil compaction impacts on clover growth and nutrient concentration. Eurasian J. Soil Sci. 5 (2), 139–145.

Blecharczyk, A., Sawinska, Z., Piechota, T., Idziak, R., 2024. The effect of sustainable tillage systems on faba bean yield in a long-term experiment in Poland. Sustainability. 17 (10), 4293.

Chapman, H.D., Pratt, P.E., 1961. Methods of Analysis for Soil, Plant and Water. Division Agric. Sci, California Univ., U.S.A.

Collin, S., Baskar, A., Geevarghese, D.M., Ali, M.N.V.S., Bahubali, P., Choudhary, R., Lvov, V., Tovar, G.I., Senatov, F., Koppala, S., Swamiappan, S., 2022. Bioaccumulation of lead (Pb) and its effects in plants: a review. J. Hazard. Mater. Lett. 3, 100064.

Cui, F., Li, Q., Shang, S., Hou, X., Miao, H., Chen, X., 2024. Effects of cotton peanut rotation on crop yield soil nutrients and microbial diversity. Sci. Rep. 14, 28072.

Donyavian, H.R., Raii, Y., Jokar, M., 2018. Land equivalent ratio (LER), and competition indices in cotton (*Gossypium hirsutum*)—sesame (*Sesamum indicum*) intercropping system. Egypt. Acad. J. Biol. Sci. 11 (2), 81–88.

El-Adly, H.H., Eissa, A.E.M., Khalif, H.S., Mohamed, A.A., Baker, K.M.A., Said, S.R.N., Soliman, A.M.M., Awad, H.Y., Awaad, M.M., Mohamed, S.A.S., Hussien, F.S., 2018. "Giza 95" a long staple Egyptian cotton variety for Middle and Upper Egypt. Egypt. J. Agric. Res. 96 (2), 717–726.

EL-Refaey, R.A., Emara, M.A.A., Ashri, H.M., El-Sawy, M.A., 2022. Cotton productivity and fiber quality response to nitrogen fertilization levels under different sowing dates. J. Sustain. Agric. Environ. Sci. 1 (1), 27–39.

El-Shamy, M.A., El-Mansoury, M.A.M., El-Bialy, M.A., 2021. Effect of sowing dates, plant density of sesame and intercropping on yield and yield components of cotton and sesame. Alex. Sci. Exch. J. 42 (1), 179–190.

El-Shamy, M.A., El-Tahawe, H.S., Farag, A.A., 2023. Impact of cotton intercropping with cowpea and insecticides on crops characteristics and infestation with *Aphis gossypii* and *Pectinophora gossypiella*. Middle East J. Agric. Res. 12 (01), 163–173.

El-Sharawy, H.H., Mahmoud, M.I., El-Tantawy, E.M., 2018. Organic farming of cowpea (*Vigna unguiculata* L.) under El-Arish region conditions. SINAI J. Appl. Sci. 7 (1), 35–46.

Fetyan, N., Massoud, O.N., Morsy, E.M., Kalil, H.M., 2015. Biological evaluation of soil cultivated with Egyptian clover (*Trifolium alexndrinum* L.) though long term trial at Bahtim region, Egypt. Middle East J. Appl. Sci. 05 (02), 515–525.

Freed, R.D. 1991. MSTATC Microcomputer Statistical Program. Michigan State Univ. East Lansing, Michigan, USA.

Ghorbi, S., Ebadi, A., Parmoon, G., Siller, A., Hashemi, M., 2023. The use of faba bean cover crop to enhance the sustainability and resiliency of no-till corn silage production and soil characteristics. Agronomy. 13 (8), 2082.

Gomez, K.A., Gomez, A.A. 1984. Statistical Procedures for Agricultural Research. John Willey and Sons, New York.

Haider, F.U., Liqun, C., Coulter, J.A., Cheema, S.A., Wu, J., Zhang, R., Wenjun, M., Farooq, M., 2021. Cadmium toxicity in plants: impacts and remediation strategies. Ecotoxicol. Environ. Saf. 211, 111887.

Iqbal, A., Ullah, F., Saleem, M.A., 2025. Yield and quality responses of Egyptian clover (*Trifolium alexandrinum* L.) to changing sowing time and cutting intervals. Discov. Agric. 3, 72.

Jackson, M.L. 1958. Soil Chemical Analysis. Prentice Hall, Englwood Cliffis, New Jersy.

Lamlom, M.M., Abdel-Wahab, S.I., Abdel-Wahab, T.I., Ibrahim, M.A.A., 2018. Crop interference effects of some winter and summer field crops on Egyptian cotton characters. Adv. Crop Sci. Technol. 6 (5), 394.

Lamlom, M.M., Abdel-Wahab, T.I., Abdel-Wahab, S.I., Ibrahim, M.A.A., 2019. Crop diversity in Egyptian cotton for nematodes management. Res. Crops 20 (Issue Suppl), S91–S104.

Lamlom, M.M., Abdel-Wahab, S.I., Abdel-Wahab, T.I., Ibrahim, M.A.A., 2020. Impact of different cropping systems on seed yield and quality of Egyptian cotton. Plant Arch. 20 (1), 1003–1013.

Li, L., Yan, X., Li, J., Tian, Y., Ren, P., 2020. Advances in cotton tolerance to heavy metal stress and applications to remediate heavy metal-contaminated farmland soil. Phyton-Int. J. Exp. Bot. doi:10.32604/phyton.2021.012276.

Liu, Y., Huang, L., Wen, Z., Fu, Y., Liu, Q., Xu, S., Li, Z., Liu, C., Yu, C., Feng, Y., 2023. Effects of intercropping on safe agricultural production and phytoremediation of heavy metal-contaminated soils. Sci. Total Environ. 875 (8), 162700.

Lv, Q., Chi, B., He, N., Zhang, D., Dai, J., Zhang, Y., Dong, H., 2023. Cotton-based rotation, intercropping, and alternate intercropping increase yields by improving root–shoot relations. Agronomy. 13 (2), 413.

Manschadi, A., Sauerborn, J., Stützel, H., Göbel, W., Saxena, M., 1998. Simulation of faba bean (Vicia faba L.) root system development under Mediterranean conditions. Eur. J. Agron. 9 (4), 259–272.

Metwally, A.A., Shafik, M.M., Sherief, M.N., Abdel-Wahab, T.I., 2009. Intercropping maize with Egyptian cotton. Egypt. J. Agron. 31 (2), 179–197.

Metwally, A.A., Shafik, M.M., Sherief, M.N., Abdel-Wahab, T.I., 2012. Effect of intercropping corn on Egyptian cotton characters. J. Cotton Sci. 16 (4), 210–219.

Mohamed, A.A., Bakheit, B.R., 2025. Improving yield and its component traits through mixed intercropping and sowing methods in wheat (*Triticum aestivum* L.) with Egyptian clover (*Trifolium alexandrinum* L.). Egypt. J. Agron. 47 (3), 703–716.

Muhammad, D., Misri, B., EL-nahrawy, M., Khan, S., Serkan, A. 2014. Egyptian Clover (*Trifolium Alexandrinum*), King of Forage Crops. Food and Agriculture Organization of the United Nations, Regional Office of the Near East and North Africa, Cairo.

Naveed, M., Abid, I., Mustafa, F., Ahmad, H.R., Alamri, S., Siddiqui, M.H., Alfagham, A.T., Mustafa, A., 2024. Microbiologically modified bioorganic fertilizer and metal-tolerant *Bacillus sp.* MN54 regulate the nutrient homeostasis and boost phytoextraction efficiency of mustard (*Brassica juncea* L.) in nickel-contaminated soil. Chem. Biol. Technol. Agric. 11 (1), 1–18.

Opriş, O., Lung, I., Gméling, K., Stegarescu, A., Buczkó, N., Culicov, O., Soran, M., 2023. Responses of the *Allium cepa* L. to heavy metals from contaminated soil. Plants. 13 (20), 2913.

Osman, R., Melegy, A., Dawood, Y., Gad, A., 2021. Distribution of some potentially toxic heavy metals in the soil of Shoubra El Kheima, Egypt. Egypt. J. Chem. 64 (4), 1965–1980.

Pandey, A.K., Zorić, L., Sun, T., Karanović, D., Fang, P., Borišev, M., Wu, X., Luković, J., Xu, P., 2022. The anatomical basis of heavy metal responses in legumes and their impact on plant–rhizosphere interactions. Plants. 11 (19), 2554.

Rizwan, M., Ali, S., Abbas, T., Zia-Ur-Rehman, M., Hannan, F., Keller, C., Al-Wabel, M.I., Ok, Y.S., 2016. Cadmium minimization in wheat: a critical review. Ecotoxicol. Environ. Saf. 130, 43–53.

Rizwan, M., Usman, K., Alsafran, M., 2024. Ecological impacts and potential hazards of nickel on soil microbes, plants, and human health. Chemosphere. 357, 142028.

Said, I., 2022. Nickel pollution pathways in small ecosystem, Egypt. Arab. J. Geosci. 15, 988.

Salem, A., Sayed, M.S., Aboelgoud, S.A., Ismail, F.I., 2019. Influence of sowing dates and seeding rates on Egyptian clover forage and seed yields under El-Serw environment. Egypt. J. Appl. Sci. 34 (12), 214–232.

Salman, M.M., Osman, M.A., Mahmoud, G.I., Gaballa, H.S., 2024. Comparative study between chemical and allelochemical treatments on faba bean vegetation growth and broomrape control. Egypt. J. Agron. 46 (2), 281–294.

Santos, S.R., Silva, E.D.-D., Alleoni, L.R.F., Grazziotti, P.H., 2017. Citric acid influence on soil phosphorus availability. J. Plant Nutr. doi:10.1080/01904167.2016.1270312.

Sarhan, M.G.R., Abd Elhafeez, A.M., Bashandy, S.O., 2021. Evaluation of heavy metals concentration as affected by vehicular emission in alluvial soil at Middle Egypt conditions. Egypt. J. Soil Sci. 61 (3), 337–354.

Schuh, M., Tong, C., 2025. Growing onions in home gardens. University of Minnesota Extension, Available from: https://extension.umn.edu/vegetables/growing-onions.

Tan, K.H. 2011. Principles of Soil Chemistry, fourth ed. CRC Press, Taylor & Francis Group.

Vardumyan, H., Singh, A., Rajput, V.D., Minkina, T., El-Ramady, H.R., Ghazaryan, K., 2024. Additive-mediated phytoextraction of copper-contaminated soils using *Medicago lupulina* L. Egypt. J. Soil Sci. 64 (2), 599–618.

Vogel, A.J., 1975. A Text Book of Practical Organic Chemistry, third ed. English Language Book Society And Longman Group Ltd, London, pp. 969–971.

Wang, Z., Teng, Y., Wang, X., Xu, Y., Li, R., Hu, W., Li, X., Zhao, L., Luo, Y., 2023. Removal of cadmium and polychlorinated biphenyls by clover and the associated microbial community in a long-term co-contaminated soil. Sci. Total Environ. 871, 161983.

Chapter 19

Molecular toxicology of metal exposure: Oxidative stress induction and cytotoxic mechanistic pathways

Maneesh Kumar[a], Bibekananda Bhoi[b], and Suman Kumar[a,c]
[a]*State-Virus Research and Diagnostic Laboratory, Department of Microbiology, All India Institute of Medical Sciences, Deoghar, Jharkhand, India*
[b]*Tata Memorial Centre, Homi Bhabha Cancer Hospital and Research Centre, Muzaffarpur, Bihar, India*
[c]*Department of Microbiology, All India Institute of Medical Sciences, Deoghar, Jharkhand, India*

19.1 Introduction

Environmental metal contamination and microbial infections are a complex and increasingly interconnected subject of toxicological and ecological interest. The pressure on living organisms is heightened when they are exposed to both living organisms and heavy metals (HMs) in biological systems, as both can cause harm (Singh et al., 2022). This interaction triggers inflammation and cell death within the host, making it more difficult for the host to cope with the damage and causing the host to produce reactive oxygen species (ROS), which can further damage cells and molecules (Maldonado et al., 2020). Hostile, metal-tolerant *Escherichia coli* and *Candida albicans* can survive in areas with high levels of harmful metals such as iron (Fe), copper (Cu), cadmium (Cd), or mercury (Hg) from industrial waste, mining, and urban pollution, while *Leishmania donovani* and some viruses are negatively affected by these elevated metal levels in polluted areas (Kanekar and Kanekar, 2022; Ahmed et al., 2023; Sánchez-Corona et al., 2025; Rodríguez et al., 2017). Germs exploit the stress caused by metals to evolve, becoming more dangerous and better at surviving, which disrupts the host's cellular functions, leading to deoxyribonucleic acid (DNA) damage and oxidative stress that impair the host's normal functioning. The creation of ROS, which occurs when metals and microbes interact, is the primary effect of this interaction (Sahu et al., 2022; Nair et al., 2025). Pathogens produce specific enzymes, such as oxido-reductases, peroxidases, and laccases, in the

The Metallome in Motion. https://doi.org/10.1016/B978-0-443-44299-5.00019-5

presence of redox-active metals, which assist them in generating harmful substances. These reactions produce H_2O^2, O_2^-, and OH. For instance, sites rich in Fe exacerbate the damage *E. coli* inflicts on gut cells, and when *C. albicans* grows on surfaces contaminated with metals, there is increased production of ROS, which damages tissue and causes stress (Mousavi et al., 2021; Asif et al., 2024). In addition to damaging host macromolecules, these ROS also disrupt microbial metabolism, creating cycles of oxidative amplification. Beyond generating ROS, environmental HMs can effectively induce microorganisms to secrete toxins, which intensify oxidative and genetic stress (Mansoor et al., 2023). It has been reported that toxic metals such as Cd, lead (Pb), and arsenic (As) upregulate the expression of virulence-encoded genes in bacteria, fungi, and viruses (Sánchez-Corona et al., 2025). For example, Ni and Fe stimulate *E. coli* to produce Shiga toxin, which is responsible for a potentially deadly disease called haemolytic-uraemic syndrome, while Cd induces *E. coli* to produce *Aspergillus flavus* aflatoxins, increasing the likelihood of mutations in the plants and animals it inhabits (Bunnell et al., 2017; Joseph et al., 2020; Pickova et al., 2021). Viral infections such as hepatitis B and C also enhance the production of proteases and replication in the presence of excessive metals, which can lead to changes in cancer development and DNA strand breaks (Isaguliants et al., 2021). Proteins that bind to metals and certain elements that detect metals, such as fur in bacteria or metal-responsive regions in fungal genes, often initiate the release of toxins, which can result in issues like chromosomal breaks and DNA damage (Steingard and Helmann, 2023; Nnaji et al., 2024).

Metal pollution reveals itself in the form of higher levels of microbial infection compared to other areas, and those microbial infections stress host cells to maintain a correct balance of chemicals within them. Metals weaken the body's natural defenses by lowering glutathione (GSH) levels and inhibiting the function of important enzymes such as cytosolic superoxide dismutase (SOD) and mitochondrial manganese-dependent SOD (Chandra and Roychoudhury, 2020; Wróblewski et al., 2024). Pathogens exploit these redox networks to enhance their intracellular persistence. Similarly, it has been reported that the most virulent pathogens, *Mycobacterium tuberculosis* and *L. donovani*, utilize host iron (Fe) to generate ROS, which hinder the ability of macrophages to limit the growth and survival of parasites that depend on phagolysosomes. This occurs by preventing the action of the cytoprotective agent GSH and increasing the sensitivity and vulnerability of macrophage proteins (Kumari et al., 2017; Dickson and Zhou, 2020; Mansoor et al., 2023).

Nuclear factor-κB (NF-κB) is a target for toxicants. Several toxic metals, such as arsenic (As) and Hg, overactivate NF-κB and suppress nuclear factor erythroid 2–related factor 2 (Nrf2) signaling, leading to cellular damage and inflammation (Buha et al., 2021). The effects of this interaction are deleterious, damaging the mitochondria and resulting in issues with membrane potential as well as the electron transport chain due to ROS from heavy metals (HMs) and toxins of pathogens (Sun et al., 2022; Mansoor et al., 2023). Red blood cells infected with *Plasmodium falciparum* significantly reduce adenosine triphosphate (ATP) production in mitochondria by creating an unusual type of ATP when there is an excess of Fe. Lipid bilayers containing polyunsaturated fatty acids exhibit high specific susceptibility to lipid peroxidation, which is potentiated by metal ions (Fe, Cu, and Hg) and microbial pathogens (Fraser et al., 2021; Abd Elnabi et al., 2023). Enhanced vascular permeability, inflammation, and immune escape result from cytotoxicity caused by the stiffening of the cell membrane and changes in receptor signaling. These processes are centered on programmed cell death, including apoptosis, pyroptosis, and ferroptosis (Wautier and Wautier, 2022; Bedoui et al., 2020). Cytochrome c, a molecule involved in apoptosis, is triggered by its release due to ROS and metals. The activation of gasdermin D in pxome- and metal-induced pyroptosis is the newest finding in pxome's activities outside the nucleus (Rana, 2008; Kalpage et al., 2018). ROS application potentiates pyroptosis and acute inflammation (Circu and Aw, 2010). Ferroptosis occurs when Fe, along with lipid ROS and Fe^{2+}, gets into cells, causing more tissue damage than apoptosis and suppressing the immune response. The findings reveal metal–bacterial interactions and indicate potential applications in risk assessment and therapeutic interventions (Feng et al., 2023). It is necessary to study these molecular mechanisms to understand the potential risks to the environment and health associated with infections and metals. This information provides valuable insights for targeted therapy and environmental detoxification (Tang et al., 2023). It is one way to prevent the possible destruction of waterways, ecosystems, flora and fauna, and human health by deadly metals.

19.2 Metal–microbe synergy in ROS generation: Catalysis of oxidative stress

The relationship between microbial infections and HM pollution in the environment is one of the major contributors to the generation of ROS and oxidative stress in biological systems. Since the very early history of aerobic metabolism, ROS has posed a significant threat to all forms of life (Mansoor et al., 2023). Recent studies have revealed that ROS actually have two critical functions in cells: they not only cause oxidative damage but are also utilized in many cellular processes (Sies et al., 2022). Novel data, however, now reveal the continuum of complexity and flexibility of ROS signaling particularly in species that have adapted to extreme environments (Checa and Aran, 2020). HMs are present in soils under natural conditions, but the progression of industrialization and human activities, including the excessive use of agrochemicals, has significantly increased their concentration on a global scale (Alengebawy et al., 2021). Because most toxic HMs are nonbiodegradable and persistent, they are catastrophic to the environment and pose serious threats to human health. Utilization of microorganisms for the removal of HMs appears to be an attractive option to mitigate this industrial pollution (Das et al., 2023; Zhou et al., 2023).

Mechanism of microbe-mediated remediation is important for immobilization of HMs, the mobilization of metals (leached into systems), and the ease of extraction (Verma et al., 2023). In this context, current developments in microbe-mediated HM removal have positioned bioremediation as a promising alternative to traditional practices. Hence, to remediate the toxicity of these metallic poisons, a few selected microorganisms have developed complex detoxification strategies that offer a ray of hope for aquatic recovery (Mallick et al., 2019).

The pollution of HMs is a worldwide problem and has serious implications for plants and animals in numerous freshwater ecosystems, as well as for human health. HM pollution in aquatic systems has become a significant environmental issue due to its high persistence, bioaccumulation, and biomagnification. These metals originate from both natural and man-made sources (Madhav et al., 2019; Okereafor et al., 2020). The toxicity of HMs poses a serious environmental sustainability challenge for all species in the fish-breeding industry, affecting fish growth, reproduction, and physiology. There are various forms of exposure to HMs, each with different implications for environmental damage. However, exposure can still be critical for human health, either due to the direct effects of poisoning or for less direct reasons (Bhat et al., 2025). One of the outcomes is the excessive production of ROS, which are essential molecules that mediate the functions of pathogens and contribute to oxidative stress conditions. This can eventually lead to the development and worsening of numerous harmful diseases in the human body (Yadav et al., 2024). HMs are a group of elements with high density, specifically densities greater than 5000 kg/m^3, which are at least five times greater than that of water (Huber et al., 2021). These elements predominantly include transition metals, along with some metalloids, actinides, and lanthanides (Babula et al., 2009; Ali and Khan, 2018; Huber et al., 2021). HMs, often referred to as trace elements, generally exist in the ecosystem in trace amounts (<10 ppm) (Bandara and Manage, 2022; Aslam et al., 2024). Several HMs, such as copper (Cu), iron (Fe), cobalt (Co), zinc (Zn), molybdenum (Mo), nickel (Ni), manganese (Mn), vanadium (V), and selenium (Se), are required by biological systems to maintain health. However, higher levels of these metals can be toxic and cause harm to the cells of living organisms (Ding et al., 2022; Botle et al., 2025). On the other hand, many other HMs, such as cadmium (Cd), arsenic (As), lead (Pb), mercury (Hg), and chromium (Cr), are not essential for life forms and become toxic at ultra-low concentrations due to their nondegradability (Rahman and Singh, 2019). In the presence of microbial communities (including pathogenic or toxin-producing bacteria, fungi, viruses, and parasites), these metals can enhance oxidative injury, where hydrogen peroxide (H_2O_2) and redox-active Fe^{2+} are converted to hydroxyl radicals (OH) (Khezerlou et al., 2018; Olo Ndela, 2025). Most situations involving the interaction of even gas-phase stresses differ by the generation of reactive oxygen metabolites (ROMs: radical and nonradical ROS generation) by bacterial species. common environmental bacteria, such as *Pseudomonas aeruginosa* and

E. coli, in effluent wastewater and metal-contaminated terrestrial environments, produce H_2O_2 during their metabolism (Buonocore et al., 2010; Ranjan et al., 2024). by-products of metal excess directly promote the generation of ROS, causing disturbances to microbial communities, local plants, aquatic organisms, and human cells, which are subsequently transferred through the food or water chain (Mishra et al., 2018; Ding et al., 2022).

Exposure to metals, such as those listed above, can enhance the level of oxidative stress and therefore increase the toxicity of other compounds during fungal infections by toxigenic fungal species such as *A. flavus* and *Fusarium* spp. (Egbuta et al., 2017). For instance, soil-borne cadmium or lead contamination induces the enhancement of aflatoxin biosynthesis, which is accompanied by changes in the antioxidant systems of the host plants or insects (Yaakoub et al., 2022; Iqbal et al., 2024). However, this double hit of fungal toxin and metal-induced ROS generation can be harmful to plant roots and the beneficial microbes around them, and subsequently could affect crop production and favor more disease outbreaks (Mansoor et al., 2023). Moreover, the parasite metabolism, such as *L. donovani* and *P. falciparum*, determines their metal metabolism as well, especially when exposed to higher levels of Fe or Co than anticipated, both of which may be stressful to the host's immune or red cells (Maya-Maldonado et al., 2021). On the contrary, heavy metals exacerbate oxidant stress-induced hepatocyte injury and disrupt oxidative signaling pathways involved in the regulation of viral replication and immune evasion in a metal-contaminated aquatic environment (Navarro et al., 2025) (Fig. 19.1).

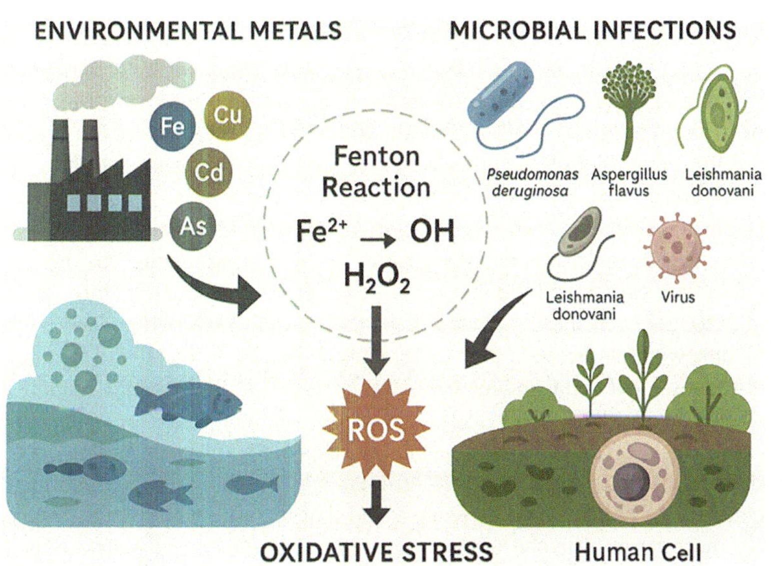

FIG. 19.1 Environmental metals and microbial infections initiate Fenton reactions, generating ROS responsible for oxidative stress and cellular toxicity.

The relationship between metals and microbes is particularly significant in aquatic ecosystems receiving runoff from mines or industries, such that water containing HMs and water containing organic pollutants and pathogenic microbes coexist (Pawłowska et al., 2023). For instance, estuaries situated near tanneries or electroplating plants may serve as vectors of cadmium (Cd), along with microbial activities showing peroxidative stress in mollusks as well as fish. Blue-green algae that form blooms, e.g., *Microcystis aeruginosa* in eutrophic iron (Fe)-rich waters, generate microcystins, which may induce oxidative stress in aquatic animals (Xiao et al., 2021). These metabolic pathways are affected by the responses to being exposed to metals, which increase the toxicity in the metabolism of microorganisms. This, in turn, becomes alien to the environment and amplifies the impact on the food chain. Therefore, it is essential to study further how metals and microorganisms interact to cause oxidative stress, so we can work toward creating a better environment and potentially a safer ecosystem, free from such toxic effects (Mohan et al., 2022; Ganguly et al., 2024).

19.3 Metal-enhanced toxin secretion and oxidative DNA damage

HMs and metal-containing nanoparticles: Metal-based nanoparticles are being increasingly acknowledged for their multiple effects in biological scenarios, mainly including the modulation of oxidative stress-related activities, promotion of microbial secretory toxin release, and hampering of DNA fidelity (Karimi, 2019; Min et al., 2023). In the case of bacteria, metals, including manganese, are not only nutrients required for growth, but they are requisitioned as tools to control survival behavior. An exemplary system is vector-encoded Mn-binding and its secretion in *Burkholderia thailandensis*, which is mediated through T6SS-4, and the deployment of a ferrotoxin (TseM) delivered during Fenton-type killing (Si et al., 2017; Lin et al., 2021). This protein serves to scavenge Mn^{2+} for the promotion of antioxidant defenses and is an example of how metal availability can be exploited for pathogenesis. Conversely, metal excess—Fe and Zn in particular—can interfere with crucial DNA repair pathways, such as the base excision repair (BER) pathway, by compromising enzyme activity, and they can extend the duration of oxidatively generated lesions (Sharma et al., 2025). Such metal-induced damages are not always attenuated by antioxidants, which indicates a direct interaction between the metal and the enzyme and suggests that metal-induced genotoxic stress is still complex (Chandra and Roychoudhury, 2020).

The pace of technological advances, especially in microbiology, seems to be breakneck fast, yet we have little knowledge about the health effects of metal nanoparticles. Previous work found that metallic nanoparticles are possibly more harmful to the lungs compared to micrometer particles (Sánchez-López et al., 2020). Cytotoxic and genotoxic effects of metal nanoparticles, as well as DNA damage after exposure, have been investigated in vitro in human

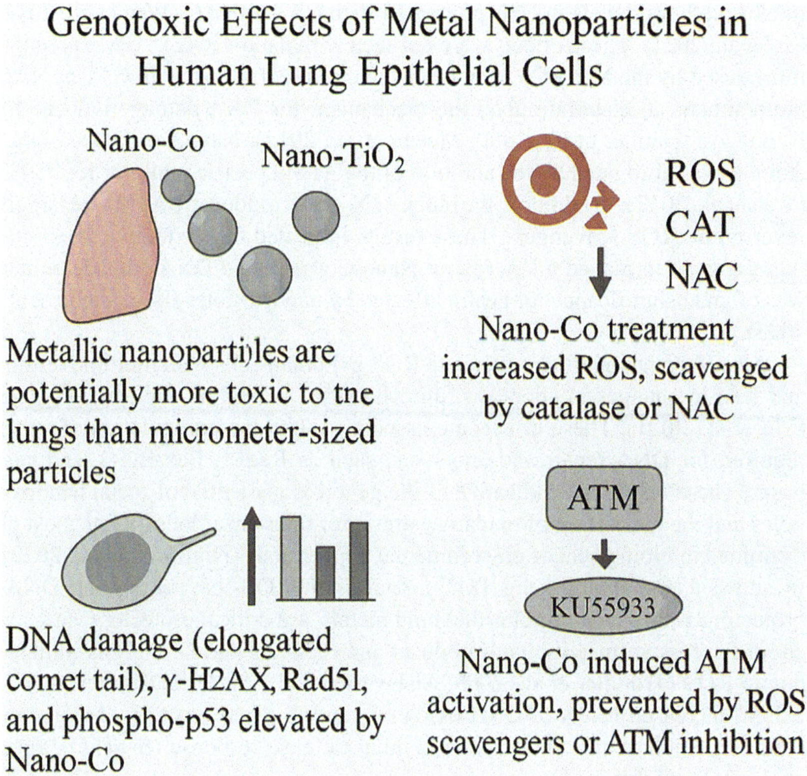

FIG. 19.2 The toxicity of Nano-Co increases ROS, activates ATM, and induces DNA damage in A549 cells; alleviated by catalase, NAC, or KU55933.

lung epithelial cells (A549) (Rosário et al., 2020). Nanotoxicology studies have demonstrated that engineered metal-based nanoparticles, such as cobalt (Co) and zinc oxide (ZnO), pose significant genotoxic risks (Zhang et al., 2022; Li et al., 2022). Cobalt nanoparticles generate high levels of ROS in lung epithelial cells, resulting in DNA strand breaks and the upregulation of damage response proteins, including γ-H2AX and phospho-p53, which are mediated by ataxia-telangiectasia mutated (ATM) kinase (Hassanen et al., 2024) (Fig. 19.2).

The genotoxicity of nanoparticles of cobalt (Nano-Co) and titanium dioxide (Nan-TiO(2)) was investigated in this work (Alaraby et al., 2020). The ROS of ND minerals was significantly higher than that in other groups. The ROS generated after the Nano-Co treatment could be scavenged after the addition of the ROS inhibitor or scavenger, and both catalase (CAT) and N-acetylcysteine (NAC) were able to scavenge ROS. Nano-Co had the DNA of A549 cells damaged (Liu et al., 2017; Aishwarya et al., 2021). Expressions of the phosphorylated form of histone H2AX (γ-H2AX), radiation-sensitive 51 (Rad51), and phospho-p53 were upregulated upon Nano-Co treatment; these levels dropped to close to basal levels in cells pretreated with CAT or NAC (Wan et al., 2012; Mo et al., 2021). These effects were not seen with nano-TiO(2). ATM upregulation caused by the Nano-Co, which was inversely correlated with CAT or NAC pretreatment, to elaborate upon the mechanism for DNA damage induced by Nano-Co (Trouiller et al., 2009; Meena et al., 2012). Nano-Co-induced DNA damage was abrogated by the addition of the ATM-specific inhibitor KU55933 (Wan et al., 2012). In addition, the block of Nano-Co-induced pATM was largely reversed by ROS scavengers. These results indicated that oxidative stress and ATM activation played a key role in Nano-Co-mediated DNA damage, which was of great significance for health affected by nanoparticles (Bastianello et al., 2023).

Also, ZnO nanoparticles generate ROS in human cells with multiple origins and lead to changes in apoptosis, mitochondria, as well as nuclear DNA loss (Mo et al., 2021). These effects are associated with the upregulation of genes required for DNA repair and apoptosis, such as Rad51, Bax/Bcl-2, and caspases. These results are indicative of the genotoxic potential of metal nanoparticles and the generation of oxidative stress, for their hazardous effects must be examined in biomedical or environmental applications (Nikiforov et al., 2022). In addition, metallothioneins (MTs), a class of ROS-scavenging and DNA-protecting antioxidant proteins that bind metals, are critical protectors via scavenging excessive metallic end-products and reducing the DNA lysis initiated due to ROS (Trouiller et al., 2009; Aishwarya et al., 2021). MT-deficient cells exhibit increased levels of DNA oxidation, and this is reversed by MT reconstitution, emphasizing their role in cellular defense response (Sánchez-López et al., 2020) (Table 19.1).

Chronic HM exposure can cause oxidative stress and DNA damage, which may, in turn, induce epigenetic pathways, resulting in cellular remodeling and senescence. Exposure to welding fumes (sources containing metals such as Cr-, Ni, and Mn) is linked with oxidative stress, as well as shortening of telomere length and alterations in DNA methylation in peripheral blood mononuclear cells (PBMNCs) (Shoeb et al., 2017; Adegbola and Adetutu, 2024; Marrugo et al., 2019). In addition, epigenetic and telomeric alterations are predispositions for aging-related diseases and tumorigenesis, with a lifelong impact on health. Furthermore, epigenetic and telomeric changes indicate tendencies toward age-related diseases and tumorigenesis, demonstrating long-term health consequences (Bellizzi et al., 2019). Certain metals, including Cd and Ni, can replace cofactors or interfere with DNA repair enzymes [e.g., X-ray repair cross-complementing protein 1 (XRCC1) and 8-oxoguanine DNA glycosylase 1 (OGG1)] during nucleotide excision repair and BER pathways of DNA repair, whereas the binding of others, such as arsenic, to DNA may lead to compromised recognition and repair of lesions. Arsenic (As) is a cocarcinogen that enhances the mutagenicity of other compounds and contributes to DNA methylation disorders (Alcántara-Mejía et al., 2024). These changes and their resultant effects could lead to genomic instability, thus emphasizing the necessity

TABLE 19.1 Metals' effects on toxin secretion, oxidative damage, and repair.

Metal/ context	Effect on toxin/stress	Oxidative DNA damage	DNA repair impact
Nano-Co (Cobalt)	No direct toxin	↑ ROS, γ-H2AX, ATM/p53 signaling	ROS scavengers mitigate damage
ZnO nanoparticles	No toxin secretion	↑ γ-H2AX, Rad51, apoptosis	Indirect interference via mitochondrial → DNA damage
Metal overload (Fe^{2+}/Zn^{2+})	N/A	Delay in the clearance of oxidized DNA	Direct inhibition of BER enzymes (polymerase β, FEN1)
Welding fumes (Cr, Ni, Mn, Fe)	Inflammation-mediated ROS	Telomere shortening, methylation changes	Long-term genomic instability
MT-mediated protection	Protective	↓ Oxidative DNA lesions	Scavenging and sequestration buffering effect

of monitoring environmental and occupational exposures to metals, as well as protecting against their effects with antioxidant therapy, overexpressing MT, and/or modulating their impact with chelating agents in order to maintain genome integrity.

19.4 Redox imbalance in host cells infected by metal-interacting pathogens

Metal-scavenging microorganisms have evolved efficient strategies to manipulate the redox equilibrium of host cells, using metal ions not only for their role in enzymatic activities but also as agents of immune subversion. These pathogens subvert host metal homeostasis networks, especially for Fe, Cu, and Zn, while infecting, growing more virulent, and evading immune surveillance (Adegbola and Adetutu, 2024). For instance, *M. tuberculosis* assimilates host Fe for its metabolism by producing siderophores (mycobactin) to take up the Fe from host ferritin and transferrin (Sritharan and Margolin, 2016). Pathogen uptake of Fe enhances the Fenton reaction, leading to an increase in hydroxyl radical (OH) production and oxidative stress in infected macrophages (Dickson and Zhou, 2020). Likewise, *Salmonella enterica* triggers macrophages to overaccumulate Cu in the phagolysosome as an antimicrobial defense. However, as a counter-strategy, the pathogen induces copper efflux pumps and detoxification

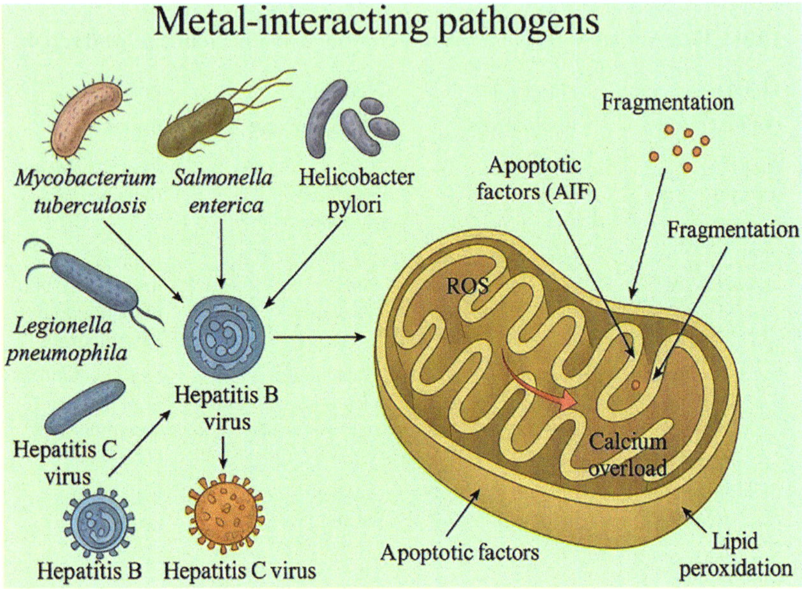

FIG. 19.3 The figure illustrates how pathogen infections interacting with metals induce mitochondrial dysfunctions, leading to redox disorders and imbalance, ROS overproduction, mitochondrial fragmentation, and apoptosis in host cells, mediated by the toxicities of certain enzymes, toxins, and alterations in electron transport.

activities by the host, producing toxic ROS that kill its own host (Mo et al., 2021; Gogoi et al., 2019). *Helicobacter pylori* is another well-described organism that colonizes deep in the gastric mucosa, causing imbalances in metal ion modulation and increased local oxidative stress through its urease-mediated ammonia production and Fe scavenging, where both processes interfere with host antioxidant capacity and induce inflammation (Han et al., 2022). In such infection incidences, overproduction of ROS and reactive nitrogen species (RNS), including nitric oxide (NO) and peroxynitrite ($ONOO^-$) often occurs, causing lipid peroxidation, DNA strand breaks, and protein oxidation (Molteni et al., 2014). Such an imbalance harms organelles such as mitochondria, which act as major centers for redox signaling and energy generation, thereby reinforcing oxidative stress and impeding cell viability (Fig. 19.3).

Other microbes have also adapted ways to modulate the redox state of their host, and not only with the help of redox-active metals, such as Listeria monocytogenes, *E. coli*, *P. aeruginosa,* and *C. albicans* (Dagah et al., 2024). For example, *Listeria* secretes listeriolysin O, a pore-forming toxin that mediates the destruction of the phagosomal membrane as well as affects the release of cytosolic ROS (Nguyen et al., 2019). *E. coli*, particularly uropathogenic and enterotoxigenic strains, induces intracellular ROS generation through the induction of NADPH oxidase- and mitochondria-derived ROS pathways, as well as harboring its own stress response machinery, including SODs or CATs, to survive against oxidative killing (Krawczyk et al., 2025; Bordt and Polster, 2014). *P. aeruginosa* utilizes redox-active phenazine-type pigments such as pyocyanin (PYO) to generate intracellular ROS, which disrupts the host-epithelial barrier function, resulting in chronic inflammation, more intensified in cystic fibrosis patients (Hall et al., 2016; Mudaliar and Bharath Prasad, 2024). The fungal pathogen *C. albicans* is also capable of utilizing various host Fe sources, employing a ferric reductase system and homeostatically controlling its complement of antioxidant defenses to resist the action of neutrophil oxidants (Zheng et al., 2025). Furthermore, the metal-mediated redox balance can also be indirectly modulated by some viral agents, such as the hepatitis C virus (HCV) and memantine human immunodeficiency virus (HIV) (Ruggieri et al., 2013; Sadiq, 2023; Verma et al., 2023). HCV is one such virus because it disturbs Fe homeostasis by upregulating hepatic hepcidin suppression, which enhances free Fe and ROS-mediated liver injury (Chatzikalil et al., 2025). HIV disease is characterized by zinc depletion and thiol imbalance, leading to increased oxidative stress and immunocompetence. These examples demonstrate how pathogens may utilize metal-mediated redox regulation in various reclamation decisions, ultimately resulting in chronic inflammation, immunosuppression, and tissue decay (Oli et al., 2025; Rodrigues et al., 2025). Redox imbalance in host cells infected with metal-interacting pathogens is, therefore, a multipathogen and complex response evoked or introduced through competition for metals, as well as the upregulation or downregulation of ROS/RNS production and antioxidant pathways (Bellanti et al., 2025). Knowledge of this redox-metal-pathogen triad is critical for the development of host-directed therapies (e.g., metal chelators, antioxidant supplements, or agents rebalancing the redox tone) targeting protection from infection-induced cellular damage and for the containment of pathogens. If pathogens survive in infected cells, excessive unnecessary damage, in most circumstances, occurs (Bellanti et al., 2025; Sbodio et al., 2019) (Table 19.2).

19.5 Mitochondrial dysfunction and bioenergetic collapse induced by metals and pathogens

Mitochondria are essential organelles that control energy metabolism by oxidative phosphorylation and apoptosis, redox signalling and innate immunity. But harmful metals and infectious microorganisms have the potential to cause severe damage to mitochondrial structure and function through oxidative stress, ATP decline, and bioenergetic failure (Chen et al., 2018; Lee and Song, 2021). Such a process is known in other contexts of cell damage (by way of infection or metal poisoning) and is at the basis of many diseases, such as neurodegenerative disease, inflammatory conditions or cancers. As, Cd, Hg, Pb and Fe are established HMs for their effects in mitochondria. These metals can accumulate in the mitochondria or, conversely, act by interacting with mitochondrial

TABLE 19.2 Pathogen-mediated redox imbalance via metal interaction.

Pathogen	Targeted metal(s)	Mechanism of redox manipulation	Effects on host cell
M. tuberculosis	Fe	Produces siderophores (mycobactin) to scavenge iron and promotes the Fenton reaction	ROS generation, mitochondrial damage, DNA oxidation, and chronic inflammation
S. enterica	Cu, Zn, Fe	Induces copper influx in phagosomes; activates Cu-efflux pumps and superoxide dismutase	Excess ROS production, macrophage dysfunction, and lipid peroxidation
H. pylori	Fe, Ni	Urease activity increases ammonia and local pH; it scavenges iron from the gastric epithelium	Increased ROS, mucosal damage, chronic gastritis, and gastric cancer risk
L. *monocytogenes*	Fe	Uses listeriolysin O to rupture phagosomes, exposing the cytosol to metal-catalyzed ROS	Cytosolic oxidative burst, cell membrane disruption, apoptosis
E. coli	Fe, Zn	Activates host NADPH oxidase; expresses superoxide dismutase and catalase for ROS detox	Imbalance in redox signaling, mitochondrial ROS, urinary or intestinal inflammation
P. aeruginosa	Fe, Cu	Produces redox-active pigments (e.g., pyocyanin) that shuttle electrons and generate ROS	Disruption of epithelial barriers, neutrophil dysfunction, and chronic lung infections
C. albicans	Fe, Cu, Zn	Employs high-affinity metal uptake systems; resists neutrophil ROS via glutathione and catalase	Escapes oxidative killing, induces ROS in the mucosal tissue, and causes inflammation
HCV	Fe	Inhibits hepcidin expression; increases hepatic Fe storage, leading to oxidative stress	Liver fibrosis, DNA damage, carcinogenesis
HIV	Zn, Se	Causes Zn depletion and thiol imbalance; impairs redox-sensitive immune functions	Oxidative damage to immune cells and increased susceptibility to coinfections

enzymes and, when doing so, inhibit the respiratory complexes (Wu et al., 2025; Huang et al., 2025). For instance, sequestration of cadmium in the complex III (cytochrome bc1 complex) of electron transport chain (ETC) causes electron escape and generation of superoxide radical (O_2^-), a prevailing ROS. As also blocks complexes I and pyruvate dehydrogenase, resulting in the production of NADH and ATP (Branca et al., 2020). When not well-regulated (e.g., in hemochromatosis or a *P. falciparum* infection), essential Fe forms hydroxyl radicals (OH), mitochondrial deoxyribonucleic acid (mtDNA) mutations, and oxidative damage to mitochondrial membranes via Fenton reactions in the mitochondria (Torrentino-Madamet et al., 2011; Fraser et al., 2021; Tang et al., 2021). During degradation, this damage is accumulated with the result of reduction of mitochondrial membrane potential ($\Delta\psi m$), which in turn opens the mPTP and causes leakage of cytochrome *c*, a key event in intrinsic apoptosis (Caroppi et al., 2009). Both Pb and Hg, two widely accepted neurotoxins, have been shown to block mitochondrial antioxidant activities such as glutathione peroxidase (GPx) or SOD that can result in an accumulation of free radicals due to both enhanced oxidative stress effects and a decrease in neuronal energy metabolism or ATP generation, creating neurodevelopmental delays as indicated by the autism haplotype scores employed here (Farina and Aschner, 2019; Manivasagam et al., 2020) (Fig. 19.4).

Many pathogens also subvert the mitochondria during their infection cycle. For example, *Chlamydia trachomatis* and *Legionella pneumophila* release effectors into the host cytoplasm that target mitochondria to manipulate their normal function and inhibit host cell apoptosis. This process is beneficial for the optimal replication of these pathogens in an intracellular compartment with limited environmental monitoring (Mukherjee and Dikic, 2022; Kellermann et al., 2021). This can cause mitochondrial depolarization (MPT) and, therefore, the release of several pro-apoptotic factors from the intermembranous space into the cytoplasm, such as cytochrome *c*, or even into the nucleus, e.g., via AIF (Loterio et al., 2021). *M. tuberculosis* hijacks the fate of host mitochondria by regulating mitofusin and dynamin-related protein 1 (DRP1) to induce fragmentation and energy loss (Mohareer et al., 2020). Viral pathogens such as hepatitis B virus (HBV) and HCV are also responsible for mitochondrial dysfunction: HBV (HBx) transactivates mitochondria by interacting with their membrane, causing calcium overload and ROS production, whereas HCV core proteins inhibit the functioning of the ETC while promoting oxidative lipid peroxidation (Schollmeier et al., 2023).

Bioenergetic failure, characterized by the inability of cells to produce enough ATP, usually occurs after prolonged mitochondrial damage caused by such insults. This disruption results in the general downfall of all energy-dependent cellular functions, such as ion homeostasis, protein synthesis, and repair systems (Choudhuri et al., 2021). In immune cell types, particularly macrophages and dendritic cells, defective mitochondria lead to disrupted clearance of pathogens and imbalanced cytokine responses. In neurons that rely on

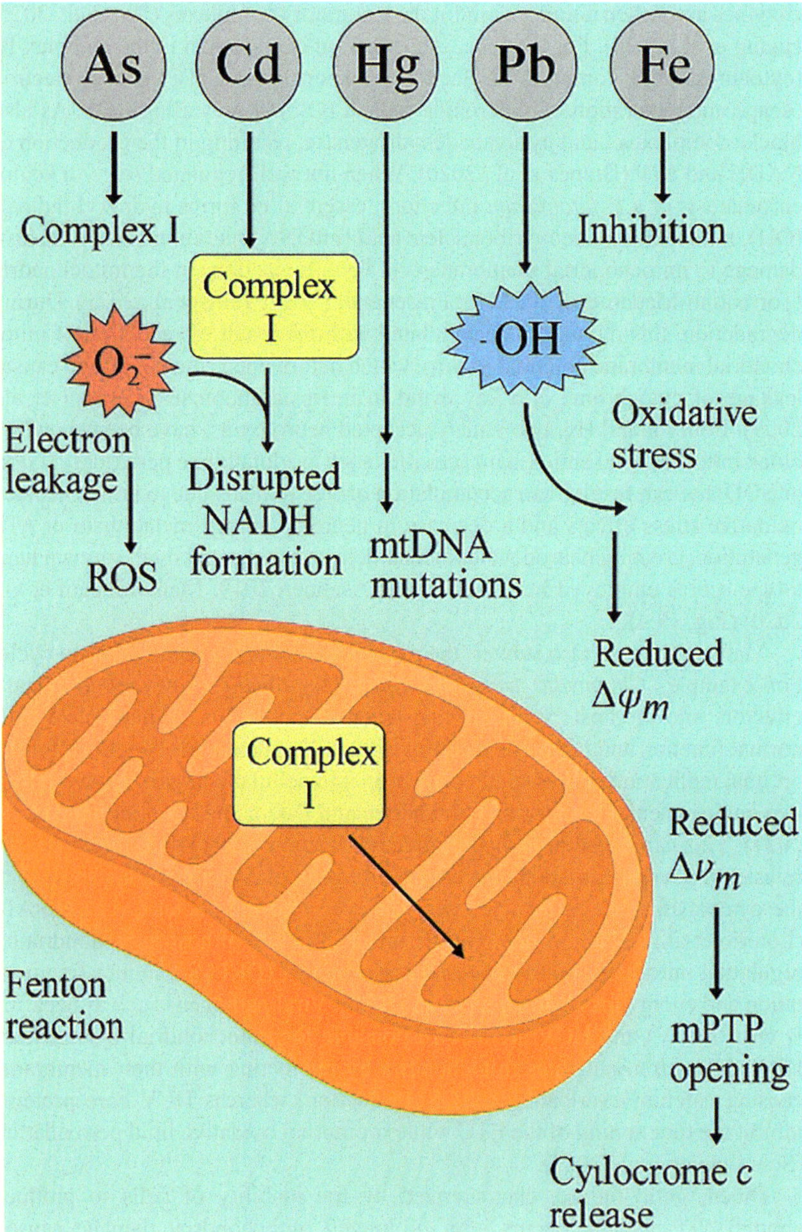

FIG. 19.4 Biological effects of HMs within mitochondria.

oxidative metabolism to a significant extent, bioenergetic failure leads to synaptic failure and ultimately cell death, as observed, for instance, in Alzheimer's or Parkinson's disease. HMs (Co, Cd) cause plant mitochondrial swelling and inhibit ATP synthase activity; excess ROS production in plants affects energy metabolism and growth (Tönnies and Trushina, 2017; Branca et al., 2020; Mishra et al., 2025).

Particularly, the cross-talk between metal toxicity and pathogen infection also induces more impaired mitochondria. For example, in the case of *P. aeruginosa* infections, PYO acts together with Fe to enhance ROS. Understanding these complex relationships has far-reaching implications (Buonocore et al., 2010). There may also be an increase in mitochondrial stress, promoting viral replication. Understanding these complex relationships helps in treating illnesses. Dietary supplements of antioxidants, such as MitoQ, SkQ1 and metal chelators like deferoxamine for Fe, or bioenergetic-stabilizing drugs like nicotinamide riboside or CoQ10, can help lower mitochondrial dysregulation associated with viral illness and exposure to HMs. Cells must regulate mitochondrial homeostasis to evade immune surveillance (Pham et al., 2020; Lin et al., 2023).

19.6 Lipid peroxidation and membrane damage mediated by metal-toxin interactions

Free radical-induced oxidation of polyunsaturated lipids in cellular membranes, known as lipid peroxidation, is a characteristic feature of metal-toxic interactions and a primary agent mediating the harmful effects of mitochondrial damage within cells. In cell biology, this effect is often studied in the context of oxidative stress, where transition metals such as Fe, Co, and others are frequently examined. Transition metals like Fe, Cu, and Cd serve as catalysts in the generation of hydroxyl radicals (OH), one of the most powerful oxidizing agents (Manivasagam et al., 2020; Adegbola and Adetutu, 2024; Jomova et al., 2012). The initiating radicals abstract hydrogen atoms from the fatty acyl chains of membrane phospholipids, generating further lipid radicals that perpetuate the process. This cascade leads to the formation of lipid peroxides and reactive aldehydes, such as malondialdehyde (MDA) and 4-hydroxynonenal (4-HNE), which not only damage membrane structure but also form adducts with DNA and proteins, further contributing to cellular dysfunction (Li et al., 2022). Such enhanced peroxidation causes alterations in the fluidity and permeability of the plasma membrane of hepatocytes, leading to anomalous modulation of ion transport and cell signaling. Fe deposition and the effects of lipid peroxidation in nerve tissues are also suspected to play a significant role in neurodegenerative diseases. These toxic effects highlight the substantial impact that metal-induced oxidative lipid damage can have on cellular homeostasis and underscore the importance of lipid peroxidation as a critical step in pathogenesis (Mansoor et al., 2023; Gallo et al., 2020).

Complexes of metals with microbial or toxic environmental agents also contribute to the enhancement of lipid peroxidation and membrane injury. Some pathogens and their toxins use metal homeostasis within the host cells to cause oxidative stress. For instance, the pathogens *S. enterica* and *M. tuberculosis* alter the Fe status of their hosts to ensure their own survival; however, these conditions upregulate the production of ROS, which leads to the destruction of host cell membranes (Murdoch and Skaar, 2022; Mansoor et al., 2023). Moreover, environmental pollutants such as paraquat or methylmercury also interactively enhance oxidative damage and exposure to metals (Fe or Cu) were reported. Mitochondria, being especially enriched in unsaturated lipids and redox-active metal centres, can potentially lead to membrane potential collapse and loss of ATP synthesis due to lipid peroxidation (Sahoo and Sharma, 2023). It is demonstrated in hepatic cells exposed to a combination of cadmium and organophosphate that mitochondrial membrane peroxidation leads to the release of cytochrome *c* from mitochondria and apoptosis. Moreover, ferroptosis—a form of programmed cell death that is characterised by the Fe-dependent accumulation of lipid-based ROS production—underscores the cytotoxic dimensionality this crosstalk conveys (Sahoo and Sharma, 2023; Lokesh and Raichur, 2024). Ferroptosis has become an anti-cancer therapy target in cancer cell biology, as the build-up of pro-oxidant metals drives death of malignant cells through oxidative damage to membrane lipids. Peroxidative damage depends on cell type, subcellular metal location and the particular toxin(s) involved. Importantly, these cells have antioxidant defence mechanisms like GPx, CAT and SOD, although excessive exposure to a combination of metal-toxins could overwhelm them, resulting in permanent membrane damage (Bedoui et al., 2020) (Fig. 19.5).

Considering the broader cellular picture, lipid peroxidation is more than just damage—it is a crucial signaling process. Peroxidation aldehydes have the capacity to activate proinflammatory pathways, alter transcription factors, and change gene expression (Yadav and Ramana, 2013). Disruption of the lipid bilayer, in turn, affects membrane-bound receptors, ion channels, and signal transduction cascades, where it can influence everything from cell proliferation to immune responses (Gęgotek and Skrzydlewska, 2019). In cell systems in vitro, the epiradical generated by metal ions and lipophilic toxins often causes blebbing of the plasma membrane, membrane rupture, and loss of cytoplasm, which are also characteristic of necrosis/apoptosis. For instance, human lung epithelial cells treated with Cr and benzo[a]pyrene experience membrane oxidation, influx of calcium, and cell death—evidence that inhalants cause cellular damage (Saxena et al., 2019). Pesticide and metal cooperation induces lipid peroxidation in the gill and liver, thus disturbing respiration and detoxification in aquatic organisms. Hence, the combined metal and toxicity effects model, in relation to membrane lipid peroxidation, is important for understanding this cellular susceptibility and adaptation network. The understanding of molecular patho-mechanisms of cell injury and cell death has not only expanded but is also providing valuable information for future developments in therapeutic

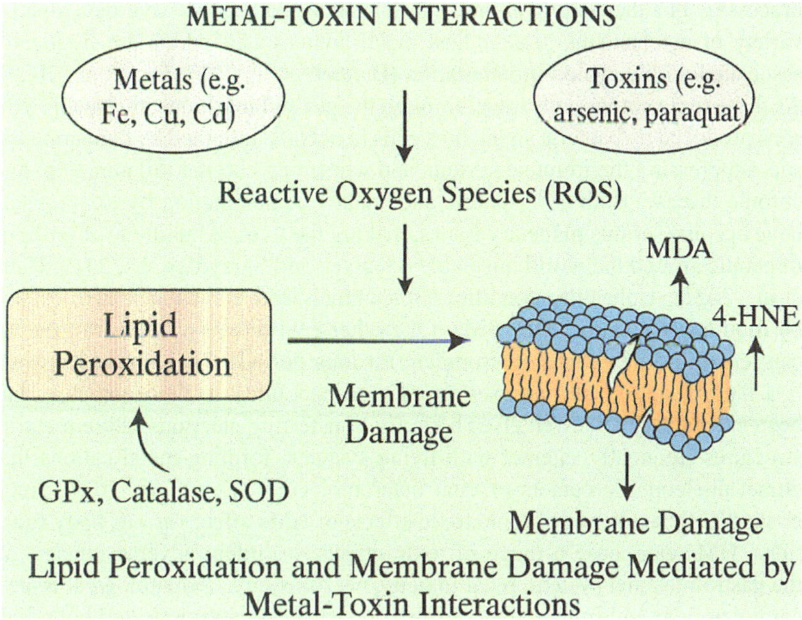

FIG. 19.5 Metal-toxin interaction during membrane damage.

interventions and biomarker discoveries in toxicology, as well as in disease processes (Martini et al., 2023; Sahoo and Sharma, 2023).

19.7 Inflammatory cascade amplification by metal-activated microbial pathways

Metal-mediated microbial pathways and the rise of inflammation are increasingly being considered a source of information for understanding how cells respond to disease. The body's immune system reacts to infections and injuries, removing whatever is causing cell damage and initiating the healing process as a result of inflammation (Jomova et al., 2022). In this way, inflammation serves to protect us but needs to be very carefully modulated. Laboratory tests and computer simulations additionally enhance the body's defenses and suppress harmful infections during rapid inflammation, preserving tissue health and promptly mitigating the inflammatory response (Buha et al., 2021). Metal-based nanomaterials already show tremendous potential to overcome these problems, as they are capable of killing a broad spectrum of bacteria, assisting the immune system, and triggering tissue regeneration (Kaur et al., 2023). Moreover, another aspect worth noting is their multifaceted mechanism of action for antibacterial, anti-inflammatory, and tissue regeneration of metal nanomaterials. HMs present significant environmental risks to human health, with exposure levels rising due to industrialization, human activities, and other modern technological processes. For their survival and multiplication, pathogens have developed a variety of mechanisms to alter host metal homeostasis, which are frequently associated with elevated inflammation (Bunnell et al., 2017; Das et al., 2023). As these toxic compounds travel through the gut and intestines, the deadly poisons produced by bacteria signal host cells to become inflamed by damaging tissue, suppressing the immune system, and worsening chronic inflammation and chronic disease. Both atmospheric and aquatic contamination by toxic metals have become serious planetary issues, making the lives of hundreds of millions of people around the world miserable (Gęgotek and Skrzydlewska, 2019; Buha et al., 2021). Unhealthy conditions for animals and humans are also caused by food contamination with HMs. Like other environmental toxicants, metals can remain in the natural environment for long periods. Thus, metal exposure is a fact of human life, and sex-specific susceptibility to these toxicants has been extensively reviewed elsewhere. By transferring electrons, these metallic structures frequently interact with living systems, forming metal cations that attract nucleophilic centers of vital macromolecules (Zhu et al., 2018; Singh et al., 2022). Acute and chronic toxic effects of HMs affect various body functions. HMs can cause a range of toxic effects, including adverse impacts on the gastrointestinal system, renal toxicity, neurotoxicity, dermatological issues, cardiovascular and immunotoxic problems, as well as abortions and both malformations and carcinogenic effects (Cheng et al., 2025). Synergistic effects are possible when several metals are exposed simultaneously. Long-term exposure to HMs, especially with severe intoxication, may lead to severe or fatal outcomes, such as colic, bloody diarrhea, and acute renal failure. Conversely, low-dose chronic exposure is often referred to as the silent killer unless it manifests through noticeable syndromes or symptoms, such as neuropsychiatric disorders that significantly impact intelligence quotient (IQ) and cognitive functions in children. One of the reasons for these chronic exposures is that some metals are classified as human carcinogens. The precise mechanisms are unknown, but cytogenetic changes and modifications in the genome and gene expression appear to be of paramount importance (Kellermann et al., 2021). Toxic metal exposure (e.g., As, Cd, and Cr) contrasts with the suppression of DNA synthesis and its repair processes. HM toxicity and carcinogenicity are known to be dose-related. At high exposure levels, animals and humans experience a variety of responses, including rapid progression of DNA damage, severe mental disorders, and chronic wounds, all of which may constitute serious threats (Buha et al., 2021; Kumar et al., 2024). Thus, infection with bacteria and the reduction of ROS are also necessary for wound healing. As enzyme-like nanomaterials, nanozymes can transform natural molecules into highly harmful substances, such as ROS, to eliminate bacteria and biofilms without leading to drug resistance. However, the current nanozyme models that function as only one type of enzyme are insufficient to meet the complex needs of anthroposophic medicine (AM) therapy (Sies et al., 2022; Gallo et al., 2020).

This amplification is, in part, mediated by the activation of toll-like receptors (TLRs) and inflammation in immune cells. For example, *S. enterica* and *M. tuberculosis* may affect iron and copper levels in macrophages to induce intracellular ROS production, which can then activate the NLRP3 inflammasome (Weiss and Schaible, 2015). This activation leads to high levels of interleukin-1β (IL-1β) and IL-18 release, cytokines required in the inflammatory response. In addition, transition metals induce Fenton chemistry to further potentiate ROS generation, which enhances oxidative injury and prolongs the activation of NF-κB and MAPK pathways. This, in concert, induces the expression of pro-inflammatory factors such as TNF-α, IL-6, and iNOS (Song et al., 2023). Enteric pathogens—like *E. coli*—hitchhike on gut inflammation. Fe-laden conditions, favoring the expression of pathogenic factors and biofilm production by enteric bacteria, further heighten mucosal inflammation in conditions like inflammatory bowel disease (IBD) (Asif et al., 2024). In addition, the crosstalk between environmental metals and microbial elements could be a strong inducer of overresponses. For example, exposure to As in human subjects (individuals from endemic areas) is capable of sensitizing innate immune cells for hyperresponsiveness to bacterial lipopolysaccharide. This priming condition results in higher tumor necrosis factor alpha (TNF-α) and IL-1β production, leading to systemic inflammation and even septic-like conditions. In the case of an airborne infection, inhaled metal particles (as with a contaminated industrial environment) coupled with bacterial infections may overstimulate alveolar macrophages, leading to sensitivity to acute respiratory distress syndrome (ARDS) (Gęgotek, and Skrzydlewska, 2019). Similarly, excessive use of Zn and Fe in gingival tissues under the status of periodontal disease disturbs local immunity against *Porphyromonas gingivalis*, leading to higher matrix metalloproteinase activity and tissue destruction. At the molecular level, metals and pathogen-induced signaling crosstalk to affect redox-sensitive transcription factors and inflammatory gene programs. Pathogens themselves often hijack host cell systems for the transport of metals (e.g., NRAMP1, DMT1) to avoid immune responses; this transgression is known to result in excess metal content and oxidant stress as well. At the same time, pathogens utilize microbial secretion systems (e.g., Type III secretion system components in *P. aeruginosa*) to secrete effector proteins into host cells and subvert metal-sensing pathways and inflammation (Wessling-Resnick, 2015). Moreover, cumulative mitochondrial damage via combined HM poisoning and microbial insult triggers the loss of mtDNA and secondary proinflammatory signals. Collectively, metal-activated microbial pathways are an important nexus in inflammation biology (Kumar et al., 2024). Inflammation amplification by these mechanisms is not limited to infection but also involves chronic noninfectious diseases—neurodegeneration, autoimmunity, and cancer. Understanding how this dance of inflammation takes place puts us in a position to potentially develop targeted therapeutics that break these vicious cycles of increased inflammation, which include treatments such as metal chelators, antioxidant therapies, or drugs that block inflammasome signaling, restore immune homeostasis, and minimize tissue damage.

19.8 Future prospective

Potential future avenues of investigation may be directed toward elucidating the interplay between HMs and microbial toxins with respect to the regulation of cellular signaling pathways, including NF-κB and Nrf2. As the crosstalk between these two regulatory networks determines inflammation-antioxidant homeostasis, further research should focus on molecular checkpoints that can be targeted by drugs to restore this balance. Identification of novel pharmacological or nanotherapeutic agents that can specifically control NF-κB activation and upregulate Nrf2-mediated ROS scavenging functions may become an attractive future therapeutic approach. For example, plant polyphenols such as curcumin, resveratrol, and quercetin have been shown to be effective in preventing perturbations in NF-κB/Nrf2 pathways along with oxidative stress in preclinical models of metal toxicity. Furthermore, the most recent data from molecular imaging (omics), including proteomics, transcriptomics, and metabolomics approaches, should be utilized to unravel detailed pathways of HM-induced mitochondrial dysfunctions as well as oxidative damage in DNA. Computational modeling that integrates AI-guided analyses could also be employed to infer how toxicants interact with cellular defense networks and guide the design of personalized interventions. In environmental and occupational health settings, the discovery of biomarkers for NF-κB/Nrf2 dysregulation and mitochondrial impairment would support surveillance programs aimed at early warning and risk profiling in metal exposure. Moreover, it would be desirable for further studies to investigate the combinatorial effects of metal nanoparticles and microbial toxins under realistic conditions in which coexposure occurs. On the whole, this research area holds the potential not only to contribute to a better mechanistic understanding of toxicant-induced pathophysiology but also to build a foundation for intervention strategies that may promote mitochondrial health and augment antioxidant defenses in combating chronic inflammation associated with environmental toxicants.

19.9 Conclusion

The study highlights the intricate engagement of toxic metals and microbial toxins in cross-talk with host cell signaling cascades. In contrast, HMs (As and Hg) also lead to NF-κB hyperactivation, but they inhibit Nrf2 antioxidant defense these agents induce persistent oxidative stress and inflammation. The asymmetric distribution of these protein complexes is not only toxic to cellular macromolecules but also fatal for mitochondrial structure, including membrane potential and the ETC. Excessive ROS generation also exacerbates mitochondrial dysfunction and cellular power outages, leading to the progression of chronic inflammatory and degenerative diseases. Additionally, combined effects between microbial toxins and metal-induced oxidative stress could enhance cell injury patterns while impairing endogenous protective systems. These results indicate that there is potential for developing a therapy that can focus on the balance of NF-κB/Nrf2, reduce oxidative stress, and maintain mitophagy. Further study using a combination of molecular, biochemical, and computational approaches may lead to the development of targeted therapies against HM-related toxicity and inflammation. Taken together, the study offers important knowledge about the molecular mechanisms responsible for metal-induced cellular toxicity and brings new opportunities for developing successful antioxidant and anti-inflammatory drugs.

Acknowledgement

We extend our gratitude to the Department of Health, Government of India, for their support in this study.

References

Abd Elnabi, M.K., Elkaliny, N.E., Elyazied, M.M., Azab, S.H., Elkhalifa, S.A., Elmasry, S., Mouhamed, M.S., Shalamesh, E.M., Alhorieny, N.A., Elaty, A.E.A., Elgendy, I.M., Etman, A.E., Saad, K.E., Tsigkou, K., Ali, S.S., Kornaros, M., Mahmoud, Y.A.G., 2023. Toxicity of heavy metals and recent advances in their removal: a review. Toxics. 2305-6304. 11 (7). Available from: http://www.mdpi.com/journal/toxics. doi:10.3390/toxics11070580.

Adegbola, P.I., Adetutu, A., 2024. Genetic and epigenetic modulations in toxicity: the two-sided roles of heavy metals and polycyclic aromatic hydrocarbons from the environment. Toxicol. Rep. 2214-7500. 12, 502–519. Available from: https://www.sciencedirect.com/science/journal/22147500. doi:10.1016/j.toxrep.2024.04.010.

Ahmed, G., Jamal, F., Tiwari, R.K., Singh, V., Rai, S.N., Chaturvedi, S.K., Pandey, K., Singh, S.K., Kumar, A., Narayan, S., Vamanu, E., 2023. Arsenic exposure to mouse visceral leishmaniasis model through their drinking water linked to the disease exacerbation via modulation in host protective immunity: a preclinical study. Sci. Rep. 2045-2322. 13 (1). Available from: https://www.nature.com/srep/. doi:10.1038/s41598-023-48642-z.

Aishwarya, V., Solaipriya, S., Sivaramakrishnan, V., 2021. Role of ellagic acid for the prevention and treatment of liver diseases. Phytother. Res. 35 (6), 2925–2944.

Alaraby, M., Demir, E., Domenech, J., Velázquez, A., Hernández, A., Marcos, R., 2020. In vivo evaluation of the toxic and genotoxic effects of exposure to cobalt nanoparticles using Drosophila melanogaster. Environ. Sci. Nano. 2051-8161. 7 (2), 610–622. Available from: http://pubs.rsc.org/en/journals/journal/en. doi:10.1039/c9en00690g.

Alcántara-Mejía, V.A., Álvarez-Barrera, L., Mateos-Nava, R.A., Rodríguez-Mercado, J.J., 2024. Metal-induced DNA damage, its impact on health, and activation of repair mechanisms: an overview. Toxicology. 20, 1–18.

Alengebawy, A., Abdelkhalek, S.T., Qureshi, S.R., Wang, M.Q., 2021. Heavy metals and pesticides toxicity in agricultural soil and plants: ecological risks and human health implications. Toxics. 2305-6304. 9 (3), 1–34. Available from: https://www.mdpi.com/2305-6304/9/3/42/pdf. doi:10.3390/toxics9030042.

Ali, H., Khan, E., 2018. What are heavy metals? Long-standing controversy over the scientific use of the term 'heavy metals'–proposal of a comprehensive definition. Toxicol. Environ. Chem. 1029-0486. 100 (1), 6–19. Available from: http://www.tandfonline.com/loi/gtec20. doi:10.1080/02772248.2017.1413652.

Asif, M., Arshad, I., Javed, M., Tauqeer, M., 2024. Iron redox chemistry and its environmental impacts. Int. Res. J. Manag. Soc. Sci. 5 (2), 524–536.

Aslam, H., Umar, A., Khan, M.U., Honey, S., Ullah, A., Ashraf, M.A., Ayesha, G., Nusrat, N., Jamil, M., Khan, S., Abid, A., 2024. A review on heavy metals in ecosystems, their sources, roles, and impact on plant life. J. Genet. Med. 2994, 256X.

Babula, P., Adam, V., Opatrilova, R., Zehnalek, J., Havel, L., Kizek, R., 2009. Uncommon heavy metals, metalloids and their plant toxicity: a review. In: Organic farming, pest control and remediation of soil pollutants. pp. 275–317. doi:10.1007/s10311-008-0159-9.

Bandara, K.R., Manage, P.M., 2022. Heavy metal contamination in the coastal environment and trace level identification. In: Mancuso, M., Bottari, T., Abdelhafez, A.A. (Eds.), Marine Pollution: Recent Developments. IntechOpen, pp. 1–16.

Bastianello, G., Porcella, G., Beznoussenko, G.V., Kidiyoor, G., Ascione, F., Li, Q., Cattaneo, A., Matafora, V., Disanza, A., Quarto, M., Mironov, A.A., Oldani, A., Barozzi, S., Bachi, A., Costanzo, V., Scita, G., Foiani, M., 2023. Cell stretching activates an ATM mechano-transduction pathway that remodels cytoskeleton and chromatin. Cell Rep. 2211-1247. 42 (12). Available from: https://www.sciencedirect.com/science/journal/22111247. doi:10.1016/j.celrep.2023.113555.

Bedoui, S., Herold, M.J., Strasser, A., 2020. Emerging connectivity of programmed cell death pathways and its physiological implications. Nat. Rev. Mol. Cell Biol. 21 (11), 678–695.

Bellanti, F., Coda, A.R.D., Trecca, M.I., Buglio, A.L., Serviddio, G., Vendemiale, G., 2025. Redox imbalance in inflammation: the interplay of oxidative and reductive stress. Antioxidants. 2076-3921. 14 (6). Available from: www.mdpi.com/journal/antioxidants. doi:10.3390/antiox14060656.

Bellizzi, D., Guarasci, F., Iannone, F., Passarino, G., Rose, G., 2019. Epigenetics and ageing. In: Caruso, C. (Ed.), Centenarians: An Example of Positive Biology. Springer International Publishing, Italy, pp. 99–133. Available from: https://link.springer.com/book/10.1007/978-3-030-20762-5. doi:10.1007/978-3-030-20762-5_7.

Bhat, I.A., Rather, M.A., Ahmad, I., Ahmad, I., Mir, I.N., Hussna, 2025. Impact of shifting abiotic factors in aquaculture on fish breeding and reproduction: a review. Blue Biotechnol. 2948-2364. 2 (1). doi:10.1186/s44315-025-00027-9.

Bordt, E.A., Polster, B.M., 2014. NADPH oxidase-and mitochondria-derived reactive oxygen species in proinflammatory microglial activation: a bipartisan affair? Free Radic. Biol. Med. 76, 34–46.

Botle, A., Salgaonkar, S., Tiwari, R., Barabde, G., 2025. Health concerns and issues associated with toxic heavy metals. In: Mehmood, M.A., Bhat, R.A, Dar, G.H. (Eds.), Global Perspectives of Toxic Metals in Bio Environs: Volume 1: Environmental Impact, Ecotoxicology, Health Concerns, and Modelling. Springer, Cham, p. 161.

Branca, J.J.V., Pacini, A., Gulisano, M., Taddei, N., Fiorillo, C., Becatti, M., 2020. Cadmium-induced cytotoxicity: effects on mitochondrial electron transport chain. Front. Cell Dev. Biol. 2296-634X. 8. Available from: https://www.frontiersin.org/journals/cell-and-developmental-biology#. doi:10.3389/fcell.2020.604377.

Buha, A., Baralić, K., Djukic-Cosic, D., Bulat, Z., Tinkov, A., Panieri, E., Saso, L., 2021. The role of toxic metals and metalloids in Nrf2 signaling. Antioxidants. 2076-3921. 10 (5), 630. doi:10.3390/antiox10050630.

Bunnell, B.E., Escobar, J.F., Bair, K.L., Sutton, M.D., Crane, J.K., 2017. Zinc blocks SOS-induced antibiotic resistance via inhibition of RecA in *Escherichia coli*. PLoS ONE 1932-6203. 12 (5). Available from: http://journals.plos.org/plosone/article/file?id=10.1371/journal.pone.0178303&type=printable. doi:10.1371/journal.pone.0178303.

Buonocore, G., Perrone, S., Tataranno, M.L., 2010. Oxygen toxicity: chemistry and biology of reactive oxygen species. Semin. Fetal Neonatal Med. 1744-165X. 15 (4), 186–190. doi:10.1016/j.siny.2010.04.003.

Caroppi, P., Sinibaldi, F., Fiorucci, L., Santucci, R., 2009. Apoptosis and human diseases: mitochondrion damage and lethal role of released cytochrome c as proapoptotic protein. Curr. Med. Chem. 0929-8673. 16 (31), 4058–4065. doi:10.2174/092986709789378206.

Chandra, S., Roychoudhury, A., 2020. Role of selenium and manganese in mitigating oxidative damages. In: Roychoudhury, A., Tripathi, D.K. (Eds.), Protective Chemical Agents in the Amelioration of Plant Abiotic Stress: Biochemical and Molecular Perspectives. Wiley, India, pp. 597–621. Available from: https://onlinelibrary.wiley.com/doi/book/10.1002/9781119552154. doi:10.1002/9781119552154.ch30.

Chatzikalil, E., Arvanitakis, K., Kalopitas, G., Florentin, M., Germanidis, G., Koufakis, T., Solomou, E.E., 2025. Hepatic iron overload and hepatocellular carcinoma: new insights into pathophysiological mechanisms and therapeutic approaches. Cancers. 2072-6694. 17 (3), 392. doi:10.3390/cancers17030392.

Checa, J., Aran, J.M., 2020. Reactive oxygen species: drivers of physiological and pathological processes. J. Inflamm. Res. 1178-7031. 13, 1057–1073. Available from: https://www.dovepress.com/getfile.php?fileID=64356. doi:10.2147/JIR.S275595.

Chen, Y., Zhou, Z., Min, W., 2018. Mitochondria, oxidative stress and innate immunity. Front. Physiol. 1664-042X. 9. Available from: http://www.frontiersin.org/Physiology/archive/. doi:10.3389/fphys.2018.01487.

Cheng, Y.F., Zhao, Y.J., Chen, C., Zhang, F., 2025. Heavy metals toxicity: mechanism, health effects, and therapeutic interventions. MedComm. 2688-2663. 6 (9). Available from: http://onlinelibrary.wiley.com/journal/26882663. doi:10.1002/mco2.70241.

Choudhuri, S., Chowdhury, I.H., Garg, N.J., 2021. Mitochondrial regulation of macrophage response against pathogens. Front. Immunol. 1664-3224. 11. Available from: https://www.frontiersin.org/journals/immunology#. doi:10.3389/fimmu.2020.622602.

Circu, M.L., Aw, T.Y., 2010. Reactive oxygen species, cellular redox systems, and apoptosis. Free Radic. Biol. Med. 0891-5849. 48 (6), 749–762. doi:10.1016/j.freeradbiomed.2009.12.022.

Dagah, O.M.A., Silaa, B.B., Zhu, M., Pan, Q., Qi, L., Liu, X., Liu, Y., Peng, W., Ullah, Z., Yudas, A.F., Muhammad, A., Zhang, X., Lu, J., 2024. Exploring immune redox modulation in bacterial infections: insights into thioredoxin-mediated interactions and implications for understanding host–pathogen dynamics. Antioxidants. 2076-3921. 13 (5). Available from: www.mdpi.com/journal/antioxidants. doi:10.3390/antiox13050545.

Das, S., Sultana, K.W., Ndhlala, A.R., Mondal, M., Chandra, I., 2023. Heavy metal pollution in the environment and its impact on health: exploring green technology for remediation. Environ. Health Insights. 1178-6302. 17. Available from: https://journals.sagepub.com/home/EHI. doi:10.1177/11786302231201259.

Dickson, K.B., Zhou, J., 2020. Role of reactive oxygen species and iron in host defense against infection. Front. Biosci. (Landmark Ed.) 2768-6698. 25 (8), 1600–1616. Available from: https://www.bioscience.org/fbs/getfile.php?FileName=/2020/v25/af/4869/4869.pdf. doi:10.2741/4869.

Ding, C., Chen, J., Zhu, F., Chai, L., Lin, Z., Zhang, K., Shi, Y., 2022. Biological toxicity of heavy metal(loid)s in natural environments: from microbes to humans. Front. Environ. Sci.

2296-665X. 10. Available from: http://journal.frontiersin.org/journal/environmental-science. doi:10.3389/fenvs.2022.920957.

Egbuta, M.A., Mwanza, M., Babalola, O.O., 2017. Health risks associated with exposure to filamentous fungi. Int. J. Environ. Res. Public Health 14 (7), 719.

Farina, M., Aschner, M., 2019. Glutathione antioxidant system and methylmercury-induced neurotoxicity: an intriguing interplay. Biochim. Biophys. Acta Gen. Subj. 0304-4165. 1863 (12), 129285. doi:10.1016/j.bbagen.2019.01.007.

Feng, S., Tang, D., Wang, Y., Li, X., Bao, H., Tang, C., Dong, X., Li, X., Yang, Q., Yan, Y., Yin, Z., Shang, T., Zheng, K., Huang, X., Wei, Z., Wang, K., Qi, S., 2023. The mechanism of ferroptosis and its related diseases. Mol. Biomed. 2662-8651. 4 (1). Available from: https://www.springer.com/journal/43556. doi:10.1186/s43556-023-00142-2.

Fraser, M., Matuschewski, K., Maier, A.G., 2021. Of membranes and malaria: phospholipid asymmetry in Plasmodium falciparum-infected red blood cells. Cell. Mol. Life Sci. 1420-9071. 78 (10), 4545–4561. Available from: http://link.springer.de/link/service/journals/00018/index.htm. doi:10.1007/s00018-021-03799-6.

Gallo, G., Sprovieri, P., Martino, G., 2020. 4-hydroxynonenal and oxidative stress in several organelles and its damaging effects on cell functions. J. Physiol. Pharmacol. 71 (1), 15–33.

Ganguly, D., Kumar, P., Kumari, A., Kumar, M., 2024. Importance of microbial consortia and green chemistry in the removal of xenobiotics from the environment. In: Srivastav, A.L., Grewal, A.S., Tiwari, M., Pham, T.D. (Eds.), Role of Green Chemistry in Ecosystem Restoration to Achieve Environmental Sustainability. Elsevier, pp. 11–21.

Gęgotek, A., Skrzydlewska, E., 2019. Biological effect of protein modifications by lipid peroxidation products. Chem. Phys. Lipids 1873-2941. 221, 46–52. Available from: www.elsevier.com/locate/chemphyslip. doi:10.1016/j.chemphyslip.2019.03.011.

Gogoi, M., Shreenivas, M.M., Chakravortty, D., 2019. Hoodwinking the big-eater to prosper: the Salmonella-macrophage paradigm. J. Innate Immun. 11 (3), 289–299.

Hall, S., McDermott, C., Anoopkumar-Dukie, S., McFarland, A.J., Forbes, A., Perkins, A.V., Davey, A.K., Chess-Williams, R., Kiefel, M.J., Arora, D., Grant, G.D., 2016. Cellular effects of pyocyanin, a secreted virulence factor of Pseudomonas aeruginosa. Toxins. 2072-6651. 8 (8). Available from: http://www.mdpi.com/2072-6651/8/8/236/pdf. doi:10.3390/toxins8080236.

Han, L., Shu, X., Wang, J., 2022. Helicobacter pylori-mediated oxidative stress and gastric diseases: a review. Front. Microbiol. 13, 811258.

Hassanen, E.I., Abdelrahman, R.E., Aboul-Ella, H., Ibrahim, M.A., El-Dek, S., Shaalan, M., 2024. Mechanistic approach on the pulmonary oxido-inflammatory stress induced by cobalt ferrite nanoparticles in rats. Biol. Trace Elem. Res. 1559-0720. 202 (2), 765–777. Available from: https://www.springer.com/journal/12011. doi:10.1007/s12011-023-03700-5.

Huang, Y., Zhang, P., Wang, H., Chen, Y., Liu, T., Luo, X., 2025. Genetic code expansion: recent developments and emerging applications. Chem. Rev. 1520-6890. 125 (2), 523–598. Available from: http://pubs.acs.org/journal/chreay. doi:10.1021/acs.chemrev.4c00216.

Huber, F., Korotenko, E., Šyc, M., Fellner, J., 2021. Material and chemical composition of municipal solid waste incineration bottom ash fractions with different densities. J. Mater. Cycles Waste Manag. 1611-8227. 23 (1), 394–401. Available from: http://link.springer.de/link/service/journals/10163/index.htm. doi:10.1007/s10163-020-01109-z.

Iqbal, N., Czékus, Z., Ördög, A., Poór, P., 2024. Fusaric acid-evoked oxidative stress affects plant defence system by inducing biochemical changes at subcellular level. Plant Cell Rep. 1432-203X. 43 (1). Available from: https://www.springer.com/journal/299. doi:10.1007/s00299-023-03084-9.

Isaguliants, M., Bayurova, E., Avdoshina, D., Kondrashova, A., Chiodi, F., Palefsky, J.M., 2021. Oncogenic effects of HIV-1 proteins, mechanisms behind. Cancers. 2072-6694. 13 (2), 1–24. Available from: https://www.mdpi.com/2072-6694/13/2/305/pdf. doi:10.3390/cancers13020305.

Jomova, K., Baros, S., Valko, M., 2012. Redox active metal-induced oxidative stress in biological systems. Transit. Met. Chem. 37 (2), 127–134.

Jomova, K., Makova, M., Alomar, S.Y., Alwasel, S.H., Nepovimova, E., Kuca, K., Rhodes, C.J., Valko, M., 2022. Essential metals in health and disease. Chem. Biol. Interact. 1872-7786. 367. Available from: www.elsevier.com/locate/chembioint. doi:10.1016/j.cbi.2022.110173.

Joseph, A., Cointe, A., Kurkdjian, P.M., Rafat, C., Hertig, A., 2020. Shiga toxin-associated hemolytic uremic syndrome: a narrative review. Toxins. 2072-6651. 12 (2), 67. doi:10.3390/toxins12020067.

Kalpage, H.A., Bazylianska, V., Recanati, M.A., Fite, A., Liu, J., Wan, J., Mantena, N., Malek, M.H., Podgorski, I., Heath, E.I., Vaishnav, A., 2018. Tissue-specific regulation of cytochrome c by post-translational modifications: respiration, the mitochondrial membrane potential, ROS, and apoptosis. FASEB J. 33 (2), 1540.

Kanekar, P.P., Kanekar, S.P., 2022. Metallophilic, metal-resistant, and metal-tolerant microorganisms. In: Kanekar, P.P., Kanekar, S.P. (Eds.), Diversity and Biotechnology of Extremophilic Microorganisms from India. Springer Nature Singapore, Singapore, pp. 187–213.

Karimi, E., 2019. Antimicrobial activities of nanoparticles. In: Panpatte, D.G., Jhala, Y.K. (Eds.), Nanotechnology for Agriculture: Crop Production & Protection. Springer Singapore, Iran, pp. 171–206. doi:10.1007/978-981-32-9374-8_10.

Kaur, R., Kaur, K., Alyami, M.H., Lang, D.K., Saini, B., Bayan, M.F., Chandrasekaran, B., 2023. Combating microbial infections using metal-based nanoparticles as potential therapeutic alternatives. Antibiotics. 2079-6382. 12 (5). Available from: http://www.mdpi.com/journal/antibiotics. doi:10.3390/antibiotics12050909.

Kellermann, M., Scharte, F., Hensel, M., 2021. Manipulation of host cell organelles by intracellular pathogens. Int. J. Mol. Sci. 22 (12), 6484.

Khezerlou, A., Alizadeh-Sani, M., Azizi-Lalabadi, M., Ehsani, A., 2018. Nanoparticles and their antimicrobial properties against pathogens including bacteria, fungi, parasites and viruses. Microb. Pathog. 1096-1208. 123, 505–526. Available from: http://www.elsevier.com/inca/publications/store/6/2/2/9/1/5/index.htt. doi:10.1016/j.micpath.2018.08.008.

Krawczyk, B., Wityk, P., Burzyńska, M., Majchrzak, T., Markuszewski, M.J., 2025. Uropathogenic *Escherichia coli* associated with risk of urosepsis—genetic, proteomic, and metabolomic studies. Int. J. Mol. Sci. 1422-0067. 26 (12), 5681. doi:10.3390/ijms26125681.

Kumar, M., Bhoi, B., Kumar, H., Bhardwaj, H., 2024. Fungi's involvement in metal NPS synthesis and environmentally sustainable practices. In: Bhardwaj, A.K., Srivastav, A.L., Rai, S. (Eds.), Biogenic Wastes-Enabled Nanomaterial Synthesis: Applications in Environmental Sustainability. Springer Nature, India, pp. 149–170. Available from: https://link.springer.com/book/10.1007/978-3-031-59083-2. doi:10.1007/978-3-031-59083-2_6.

Kumari, A., Singh, K.P., Mandal, A., Paswan, R.K., Sinha, P., Das, P., Ali, V., Bimal, S., Lal, C.S., 2017. Intracellular zinc flux causes reactive oxygen species mediated mitochondrial dysfunction leading to cell death in Leishmania donovani. PLoS ONE. 1932-6203. 12 (6). Available from: http://journals.plos.org/plosone/article/file?id=10.1371/journal.pone.0178800&type=printable. doi:10.1371/journal.pone.0178800.

Lee, J., Song, C.-H., 2021. Effect of reactive oxygen species on the endoplasmic reticulum and mitochondria during intracellular pathogen infection of mammalian cells. Antioxidants. 2076-3921. 10 (6), 872. doi:10.3390/antiox10060872.

Li, Y., Zhao, T., Li, J., Xia, M., Li, Y., Wang, X., Liu, C., Zheng, T., Chen, R., Kan, D., Xie, Y., 2022. Oxidative stress and 4-hydroxy-2-nonenal (4-HNE): implications in the pathogenesis and treatment of aging-related diseases. J. Immunol. Res. 2022 (1), 2233906.

Lin, J., Guo, Z., Zheng, Z., Hou, L., Xu, J., Liu, Q., Du, T., Guo, F., Jing, X., 2023. Desferoxamine protects against hemophilic arthropathy through the upregulation of HIF-1α-BNIP3 mediated mitophagy. Life Sci. 0024-3205. 312, 121172. doi:10.1016/j.lfs.2022.121172.

Lin, J., Xu, L., Yang, J., Wang, Z., Shen, X., 2021. Beyond dueling: roles of the type VI secretion system in microbiome modulation, pathogenesis and stress resistance. Stress Biol. 1 (1), 11.

Liu, Y., Yang, X., Wang, W., Wu, X., Zhu, H., Liu, F., 2017. Melatonin counteracts cobalt nanoparticle-induced cytotoxicity and genotoxicity by deactivating reactive oxygen species-dependent mechanisms in the NRK cell line. Mol. Med. Rep. 1791-3004. 16 (4), 4413–4420. Available from: https://www.spandidos-publications.com/mmr/16/4/4413/download. doi:10.3892/mmr.2017.7309.

Lokesh, K.N., Raichur, A.M., 2024. Bioactive nutraceutical ligands and their efficiency to chelate elemental iron of varying dynamic oxidation states to mitigate associated clinical conditions. Crit. Rev. Food Sci. Nutr. 1549-7852. 64 (2), 517–543. Available from: https://www.tandfonline.com/loi/bfsn20. doi:10.1080/10408398.2022.2106936.

Loterio, R.K., Zamboni, D.S., Newton, H.J., 2021. Keeping the host alive–lessons from obligate intracellular bacterial pathogens. Pathog. Dis. 79 (9), ftab052.

Madhav, S., Ahamad, A., Singh, A.K., Kushawaha, J., Chauhan, J.S., Sharma, S., Singh, P., 2019. Water pollutants: sources and impact on the environment and human health. Sensors Water Pollut. Monit. Role Mater. 1, 43–62.

Maldonado, E., Rojas, D.A., Morales, S., Miralles, V., Solari, A., 2020. Dual and opposite roles of reactive oxygen species (ROS) in chagas disease: beneficial on the pathogen and harmful on the host. Oxid. Med. Cell. Longev. 1942-0994. 2020. Available from: http://www.hindawi.com/journals/oximed/. doi:10.1155/2020/8867701.

Mallick, I., Ghosh, A., Ghosh, A., 2019. Microbe-mediated removal of heavy metals for sustainable agricultural practices. In: Giri, B., Prasad, R., Wu, Q.-S., Varma, A. (Eds.), Biofertilizers for Sustainable Agriculture and Environment. Springer International Publishing, Cham, pp. 521–544.

Manivasagam, T., Arunadevi, S., Essa, M.M., SaravanaBabu, C., Borah, A., Thenmozhi, A.J., Qoronfleh, M.W., 2020. Role of oxidative stress and antioxidants in autism. In: Personalized Food Intervention and Therapy for Autism Spectrum Disorder Management. pp. 193–206. doi:10.1007/978-3-030-30402-7_7.

Mansoor, S., Ali, A., Kour, N., Bornhorst, J., AlHarbi, K., Rinklebe, J., Moneim, D.A.E., Ahmad, P., Chung, Y.S., 2023. Heavy metal induced oxidative stress mitigation and ROS scavenging in plants. Plants. 2223-7747. 12 (16). Available from: www.mdpi.com/journal/plants. doi:10.3390/plants12163003.

Marrugo, D.G., León-Méndez, D., Silva, J.P., Granados-Conde, C., León-Méndez, G., 2019. Metal fumes: exposure to heavy metals, their relationship with oxidative stress and their effect on health. Producción+ Limpia. 14 (2), 8–20.

Martini, S., Aceti, A., Della Gatta, A.N., Beghetti, I., Marsico, C., Pilu, G., Corvaglia, L., 2023. Antenatal and postnatal sequelae of oxidative stress in preterm infants: a narrative review targeting pathophysiological mechanisms. Antioxidants. 2076-3921. 12 (2), 422. doi:10.3390/antiox12020422.

Maya-Maldonado, K., Cardoso-Jaime, V., González-Olvera, G., Osorio, B., Recio-Tótoro, B., Manrique-Saide, P., Rodríguez-Sánchez, I.P., Lanz-Mendoza, H., Missirlis, F., Hernández-Hernández, F.D.L.C., 2021. Mosquito metallomics reveal copper and iron as critical factors for Plasmodium infection. PLoS Negl. Trop. Dis. 15 (6), e0009509.

Meena, R., Rani, M., Pal, R., Rajamani, P., 2012. Nano-TiO_2-induced apoptosis by oxidative stress-mediated DNA damage and activation of p53 in human embryonic kidney cells. Appl. Biochem. Biotechnol. 1559-0291. 167 (4), 791–808. doi:10.1007/s12010-012-9699-3.

Min, Y., Suminda, G.G.D., Heo, Y., Kim, M., Ghosh, M., Son, Y.O., 2023. Metal-based nanoparticles and their relevant consequences on cytotoxicity cascade and induced oxidative stress. Antioxidants. 2076-3921. 12 (3). Available from: www.mdpi.com/journal/antioxidants. doi:10.3390/antiox12030703.

Mishra, S., Bharagava, R.N., More, N., Yadav, A., Zainith, S., Mani, S., Chowdhary, P., 2018. Heavy metal contamination: an alarming threat to environment and human health. In: Sobti, R.C., Arora, N.K., Kothari, R. (Eds.), Environmental Biotechnology: For Sustainable Future. Springer Singapore, Singapore, pp. 103–125.

Mishra, Y., Kumar, A., Kaundal, R.K., 2025. Mitochondrial dysfunction is a crucial immune checkpoint for neuroinflammation and neurodegeneration: mtDAMPs in focus. Mol. Neurobiol. 1559-1182. 62 (6), 6715–6747. Available from: https://www.springer.com/journal/12035. doi:10.1007/s12035-024-04412-0.

Mo, Y., Zhang, Y., Zhang, Y., Yuan, J., Mo, L., Zhang, Q., 2021. Nickel nanoparticle-induced cell transformation: involvement of DNA damage and DNA repair defect through HIF-1α/miR-210/Rad52 pathway. J. Nanobiotechnol. 1477-3155. 19 (1). Available from: http://www.jnanobiotechnology.com/start.asp. doi:10.1186/s12951-021-01117-7.

Mohan, H., Vadivel, S., Rajendran, S., 2022. Removal of harmful algae in natural water by semiconductor photocatalysis—a critical review. Chemosphere. 0045-6535. 302, 134827. doi:10.1016/j.chemosphere.2022.134827.

Mohareer, K., Medikonda, J., Vadankula, G.R., Banerjee, S., 2020. Mycobacterial control of host mitochondria: bioenergetic and metabolic changes shaping cell fate and infection outcome. Front. Cell. Infect. Microbiol. 2235-2988. 10. Available from: http://www.frontiersin.org/Cellular_and_Infection_Microbiology/archive. doi:10.3389/fcimb.2020.00457.

Molteni, C.G., Principi, N., Esposito, S., 2014. Reactive oxygen and nitrogen species during viral infections. Free Radic. Res. 48 (10), 1163–1169.

Mousavi, S.M., Hashemi, S.A., Moezzi, S.M.I., Ravan, N., Gholami, A., Lai, C.W., Chiang, W.H., Omidifar, N., Yousefi, K., Behbudi, G., 2021. Recent advances in enzymes for the bioremediation of pollutants. Biochem. Res. Int. 2090-2255. 2021. Available from: http://www.hindawi.com/journals/bcri/. doi:10.1155/2021/5599204.

Mudaliar, S.B., Prasad, A.S.B., 2024. A biomedical perspective of pyocyanin from Pseudomonas aeruginosa: its applications and challenges. World J. Microbiol. Biotechnol. 1573-0972. 40 (3). Available from: https://www.springer.com/journal/11274. doi:10.1007/s11274-024-03889-0.

Mukherjee, R., Dikic, I., 2022. Regulation of host-pathogen interactions via the ubiquitin system. Annu. Rev. Microbiol. 1545-3251. 76, 211–233. Available from: http://www.annualreviews.org/journal/micro. doi:10.1146/annurev-micro-041020-025803.

Murdoch, C.C., Skaar, E.P., 2022. Nutritional immunity: the battle for nutrient metals at the host–pathogen interface. Nat. Rev. Microbiol. 1740-1534. 20 (11), 657–670. Available from: https://www.nature.com/nrmicro/. doi:10.1038/s41579-022-00745-6.

Nair, A.V., Singh, A., Chakravortty, D., 2025. Defence warriors: exploring the crosstalk between polyamines and oxidative stress during microbial pathogenesis. Redox Biol. 83, 103648.

Navarro, M., Daniel, L.V., Colina-Vegas, L., Visbal, G., 2025. Zinc from an essential element to an antiparasitic therapeutic agent. ACS Omega. 2470-1343. 10 (3), 2393–2414. Available from: http://pubs.acs.org/journal/acsodf. doi:10.1021/acsomega.4c07331.

Nguyen, B.N., Peterson, B.N., Portnoy, D.A., 2019. Listeriolysin O: a phagosome-specific cytolysin revisited. Cell. Microbiol. 21 (3), e12988.

Nikiforov, V.S., Blinova, E.A., Kotikova, A.I., Akleyev, A.V., 2022. Transcriptional activity of repair, apoptosis and cell cycle genes (TP53, MDM2, ATM, BAX, BCL-2, CDKN1A, OGG1, XPC, PADI4, MAPK8, NF-KB1, STAT3, GATA3) in chronically exposed persons with different intensity of apoptosis of peripheral blood lymphocytes. Vavilov J. Genet. Breed. 2500-3259. 26 (1), 50–58. doi:10.18699/vjgb-22-08.

Nnaji, N.D., Anyanwu, C.U., Miri, T., Onyeaka, H., 2024. Mechanisms of heavy metal tolerance in bacteria: a review. Sustainability. 2071-1050. 16 (24), 11124. doi:10.3390/su162411124.

Okereafor, U., Makhatha, M., Mekuto, L., Uche-Okereafor, N., Sebola, T., Mavumengwana, V., 2020. Toxic metal implications on agricultural soils, plants, animals, aquatic life and human health. Int. J. Environ. Res. Public Health. 1660-4601. 17 (7), 2204. doi:10.3390/ijerph17072204.

Oli, A.H., Maduka, H.C.C., Maduka, I.C., Obaji, M.U., Otakagu, E.C., Oli, A.N., 2025. The role of antioxidant enzymes and micronutrients in mitigating HIV-associated oxidative stress in Sub-Saharan African populations. J. Curr. Biomed. Res. 2659-0352. 5 (3, May-June), 2110–2135. doi:10.54117/dc1k0k80.

Olo Ndela, E., 2025. Microorganisms thriving together as communities. Nat. Rev. Microbiol. 1740-1526. 23 (9), 550. doi:10.1038/s41579-025-01199-2.

Pawłowska, M., Mila-Kierzenkowska, C., Szczegielniak, J., Woźniak, A., 2023. Oxidative stress in parasitic diseases—reactive oxygen species as mediators of interactions between the host and the parasites. Antioxidants. 13 (1), 38.

Pham, T., MacRae, C.L., Broome, S.C., D'souza, R.F., Narang, R., Wang, H.W., Mori, T.A., Hickey, A.J.R., Mitchell, C.J., Merry, T.L., 2020. MitoQ and CoQ10 supplementation mildly suppresses skeletal muscle mitochondrial hydrogen peroxide levels without impacting mitochondrial function in middle-aged men. Eur. J. Appl. Physiol. 1439-6327. 120 (7), 1657–1669. Available from: http://link.springer.de/link/service/journals/00421/index.htm. doi:10.1007/s00421-020-04396-4.

Pickova, D., Ostry, V., Toman, J., Malir, F., 2021. Aflatoxins: history, significant milestones, recent data on their toxicity and ways to mitigation. Toxins. 2072-6651. 13 (6), 399. doi:10.3390/toxins13060399.

Rahman, Z., Singh, V.P., 2019. The relative impact of toxic heavy metals (THMs) (arsenic (As), cadmium (Cd), chromium (Cr) (VI), mercury (Hg), and lead (Pb)) on the total environment: an overview. Environ. Monit. Assess. 1573-2959. 191 (7). Available from: https://link.springer.com/journal/10661. doi:10.1007/s10661-019-7528-7.

Rana, S.V.S., 2008. Metals and apoptosis: recent developments. J. Trace Elem. Med. Biol. 0946-672X. 22 (4), 262–284. doi:10.1016/j.jtemb.2008.08.002.

Ranjan, P., Kumar, M., Bhardwaj, H., Kumari, P., Kumari, A., 2024. Application of enzymes in biomass waste management. In: Srivastav, A.L., Bhardwaj, A.K., Kumar, M. (Eds.), Valorization of Biomass Wastes for Environmental Sustainability: Green Practices for the Rural Circular Economy. Springer, India, pp. 189–205. Available from: https://link.springer.com/book/10.1007/978-3-031-52485-1. doi:10.1007/978-3-031-52485-1_10.

Rodrigues, S.S., Bocchi, M., de Oliveira, D.M., Fernandes, E.V., 2025. Importance of trace elements in the immunometabolic health of people living with HIV/AIDS: a literature review. Mol. Biol. Rep. 1573-4978. 52 (1). Available from: https://www.springer.com/journal/11033. doi:10.1007/s11033-024-10186-4.

Rodríguez, I.A., Cárdenas-González, J.F., Juárez, V.M.M., Pérez, A.R., Zarate, M.D.G.M., Castillo, N.C.P., 2017. Biosorption of heavy metals by Candida albicans. Adv. Bioremed. Phytoremed. 3, 43–63.

Rosário, F., Bessa, M.J., Brandão, F., Costa, C., Lopes, C.B., Estrada, A.C., Tavares, D.S., Teixeira, J.P., Reis, A.T., 2020. Unravelling the potential cytotoxic effects of metal oxide nanoparticles and metal(Loid) mixtures on a549 human cell line. Nanomaterials. 2079-4991. 10 (3). Available from: https://www.mdpi.com/2079-4991/10/3/447/pdf. doi:10.3390/nano10030447.

Ruggieri, A., Anticoli, S., Nencioni, L., Sgarbanti, R., Garaci, E., Palamara, A.T., 2013. Interplay between hepatitis C virus and redox cell signaling. Int. J. Mol. Sci. 1422-0067. 14 (3), 4705–4721. Available from: http://www.mdpi.com/1422-0067/14/3/4705/pdf. doi:10.3390/ijms14034705Italy.

Sadiq, I.Z., 2023. Free radicals and oxidative stress: signaling mechanisms, redox basis for human diseases, and cell cycle regulation. Curr. Mol. Med. 23 (1), 13–35.

Sahoo, K., Sharma, A., 2023. Understanding the mechanistic roles of environmental heavy metal stressors in regulating ferroptosis: adding new paradigms to the links with diseases. Apoptosis. 1573-675X. 28 (3-4), 277–292. Available from: https://www.springer.com/journal/10495. doi:10.1007/s10495-022-01806-0.

Sahu, P.K., Jayalakshmi, K., Tilgam, J., Gupta, A., Nagaraju, Y., Kumar, A., Hamid, S., Singh, H.V., Minkina, T., Rajput, V.D., Rajawat, M.V.S., 2022. ROS generated from biotic stress: effects on plants and alleviation by endophytic microbes. Front. Plant Sci. 1664-462X. 13. Available from: https://www.frontiersin.org/journals/plant-science. doi:10.3389/fpls.2022.1042936.

Sánchez-Corona, C.G., Gonzalez-Avila, L.U., Hernández-Cortez, C., Rojas-Vargas, J., Castro-Escarpulli, G., Castelán-Sánchez, H.G., 2025. Impact of heavy metal and resistance genes on antimicrobial resistance: ecological and public health implications. Genes. 2073-4425. 16 (6). Available from: http://www.mdpi.com/journal/genes/. doi:10.3390/genes16060625.

Sánchez-López, E., Gomes, D., Esteruelas, G., Bonilla, L., Lopez-Machado, A.L., Galindo, R., Cano, A., Espina, M., Ettcheto, M., Camins, A., Silva, A.M., Durazzo, A., Santini, A., Garcia, M.L., Souto, E.B., 2020. Metal-based nanoparticles as antimicrobial agents: an overview. Nanomaterials. 2079-4991. 10 (2). Available from: https://www.mdpi.com/2079-4991/10/2/292/pdf. doi:10.3390/nano10020292.

Saxena, A., Sonowal, H., Ramana, K.V., 2019. Transcriptional factor modulation by lipid peroxidation-derived aldehydes. In: Patel, V.B. (Ed.), The Molecular Nutrition of Fats. Academic Press, pp. 419–431.

Sbodio, J.I., Snyder, S.H., Paul, B.D., 2019. Redox mechanisms in neurodegeneration: from disease outcomes to therapeutic opportunities. Antioxid. Redox Signal. 30 (11), 1450–1499.

Schollmeier, A., Glitscher, M., Hildt, E., 2023. Relevance of HBx for hepatitis B virus-associated pathogenesis. Int. J. Mol. Sci. 1422-0067. 24 (5), 4964. doi:10.3390/ijms24054964.

Sharma, P., Jha, A.B., Dubey, R.S., 2025. Utilizing manganese-based nanoparticles for enhancing environmental stress resilience and productivity of plants. Environ. Sci. Nano 2051-8161. 12 (5), 2580–2602. Available from: http://pubs.rsc.org/en/journals/journal/en. doi:10.1039/d5en00292c.

Shoeb, M., Kodali, V.K., Farris, B.Y., Bishop, L.M., Meighan, T.G., Salmen, R., Eye, T., Friend, S., Schwegler-Berry, D., Roberts, J.R., Zeidler-Erdely, P.C., Erdely, A., Antonini, J.M., 2017. Oxidative stress, DNA methylation, and telomere length changes in peripheral blood mononuclear cells after pulmonary exposure to metal-rich welding nanoparticles. NanoImpact. 2452-0748. 5, 61–69. Available from: http://www.journals.elsevier.com/nanoimpact/. doi:10.1016/j.impact.2017.01.001.

Si, M., Zhao, C., Burkinshaw, B., Zhang, B., Wei, D., Wang, Y., Dong, T.G., Shen, X., 2017. Manganese scavenging and oxidative stress response mediated by type VI secretion system in Burkholderia thailandensis. Proc. Natl. Acad. Sci. U. S. A. 0027-8424. 114 (11). doi:10.1073/pnas.1614902114.

Sies, H., Belousov, V.V., Chandel, N.S., Davies, M.J., Jones, D.P., Mann, G.E., Murphy, M.P., Yamamoto, M., Winterbourn, C., 2022. Defining roles of specific reactive oxygen species (ROS) in cell biology and physiology. Nat. Rev. Mol. Cell Biol. 1471-0080. 23 (7), 499–515. Available from: https://www.nature.com/molcellbio. doi:10.1038/s41580-022-00456-z.

Singh, A., Sharma, A., Verma, R.K., Chopade, R.L., Pandit, P.P., Nagar, V., Aseri, V., Choudhary, S.K., Awasthi, G., Awasthi, K.K., Sankhla, M.S., 2022. Heavy metal contamination of water and their toxic effect on living organisms. In: Dorta, D.J. (Ed.), The Toxicity of Environmental Pollutants. IntechOpen, pp. 1–19.

Song, Y., You, Q., Chen, X., 2023. Transition metal-based therapies for inflammatory diseases. Adv. Mater. 0935-9648. 35 (39). doi:10.1002/adma.202212102.

Sritharan, M., Margolin, W., 2016. Iron homeostasis in mycobacterium tuberculosis: mechanistic insights into siderophore-mediated iron uptake. J. Bacteriol. 0021-9193. 198 (18), 2399–2409. doi:10.1128/jb.00359-16.

Steingard, C.H., Helmann, J.D., 2023. Meddling with metal sensors: fur-family proteins as signaling hubs. J. Bacteriol. 1098-5530. 205 (4). Available from: https://journals.asm.org/doi/10.1128/jb.00022-23. doi:10.1128/jb.00022-23.

Sun, Q., Li, Y., Shi, L., Hussain, R., Mehmood, K., Tang, Z., Zhang, H., 2022. Heavy metals induced mitochondrial dysfunction in animals: molecular mechanism of toxicity. Toxicology. 0300-483X. 469, 153136. doi:10.1016/j.tox.2022.153136.

Tang, D., Chen, X., Kang, R., Kroemer, G., 2021. Ferroptosis: molecular mechanisms and health implications. Cell Res. 1748-7838. 31 (2), 107–125. Available from: http://www.nature.com/cr/index.html. doi:10.1038/s41422-020-00441-1.

Tang, Z., Wang, H.Q., Chen, J., Chang, J.D., Zhao, F.J., 2023. Molecular mechanisms underlying the toxicity and detoxification of trace metals and metalloids in plants. J. Integr. Plant Biol. 1744-7909. 65 (2), 570–593. Available from: http://onlinelibrary.wiley.com/journal/10.1111/(ISSN)1744-7909. doi:10.1111/jipb.13440.

Tönnies, E., Trushina, E., 2017. Oxidative stress, synaptic dysfunction, and Alzheimer's disease. J. Alzheimers Dis. 1875-8908. 57 (4), 1105–1121. Available from: www.iospress.nl/journal/journal-of-alzheimers-disease/. doi:10.3233/JAD-161088.

Torrentino-Madamet, M., Alméras, L., Desplans, J., Priol, Y.L., Belghazi, M., Pophillat, M., Fourquet, P., Jammes, Y., Parzy, D., 2011. Global response of Plasmodium falciparum to hyperoxia: a combined transcriptomic and proteomic approach. Malar. J. 1475-2875. 10. doi:10.1186/1475-2875-10-4.

Trouiller, B., Reliene, R., Westbrook, A., Solaimani, P., Schiestl, R.H., 2009. Titanium dioxide nanoparticles induce DNA damage and genetic instability in vivo in mice. Cancer Res. 0008-5472. 69 (22), 8784–8789. doi:10.1158/0008-5472.CAN-09-2496.

Verma, S., Bhatt, P., Verma, A., Mudila, H., Prasher, P., Rene, E.R., 2023. Microbial technologies for heavy metal remediation: effect of process conditions and current practices. Clean Technol. Environ. Policy. 1618-9558. 25 (5), 1485–1507. Available from: https://www.springer.com/journal/10098. doi:10.1007/s10098-021-02029-8.

Wan, R., Mo, Y., Feng, L., Chien, S., Tollerud, D.J., Zhang, Q., 2012. DNA damage caused by metal nanoparticles: involvement of oxidative stress and activation of ATM. Chem. Res. Toxicol. 1520-5010. 25, 1402–1411. doi:10.1021/tx200513t.

Wautier, J.L., Wautier, M.P., 2022. Vascular permeability in diseases. Int. J. Mol. Sci. 1422-0067. 23 (7). Available from: https://www.mdpi.com/1422-0067/23/7/3645/pdf. doi:10.3390/ijms23073645.

Weiss, G., Schaible, U.E., 2015. Macrophage defense mechanisms against intracellular bacteria. Immunol. Rev. 1600-065X. 264 (1), 182–203. Available from: http://onlinelibrary.wiley.com/journal/10.1111/(ISSN)1600-065X. doi:10.1111/imr.12266Austria.

Wessling-Resnick, M., 2015. Nramp1 and other transporters involved in metal withholding during infection. J. Biol. Chem. 0021-9258. 290 (31), 18984–18990. doi:10.1074/jbc.r115.643973.

Wróblewski, M., Wróblewska, W., Sobiesiak, M., 2024. The role of selected elements in oxidative stress protection: key to healthy fertility and reproduction. Int. J. Mol. Sci. 1422-0067. 25 (17), 9409. doi:10.3390/ijms25179409.

Wu, K., Chen, Y., Huang, W., 2025. Combined molecular toxicity mechanism of heavy metals mixtures. Toxicol. Assess. Comb. Chem. Environ. 1, 125–172.

Xiao, L.J., Lei, L.M., Peng, L., Lin, Q.Q., Naselli-Flores, L., 2021. Iron operates as an important factor promoting year-round diazotrophic cyanobacteria blooms in eutrophic reservoirs in the tropics. Ecol. Indic. 1470-160X. 125. Available from: http://www.elsevier.com/locate/ecolind. doi:10.1016/j.ecolind.2021.107446.

Yaakoub, H., Mina, S., Calenda, A., Bouchara, J.P., Papon, N., 2022. Oxidative stress response pathways in fungi. Cell. Mol. Life Sci. 1420-9071. 79 (6). Available from: http://link.springer.de/link/service/journals/00018/index.htm. doi:10.1007/s00018-022-04353-8.

Yadav, N.K., Patel, A.B., Singh, S.K., Mehta, N.K., Anand, V., Lal, J., Dekari, D., Devi, N.C., 2024. Climate change effects on aquaculture production and its sustainable management through climate-resilient adaptation strategies: a review. Environ. Sci. Pollut. Res. 1614-7499. 31 (22), 31731–31751. Available from: https://www.springer.com/journal/11356. doi:10.1007/s11356-024-33397-5.

Yadav, U.C., Ramana, K.V., 2013. Regulation of NF-κB-induced inflammatory signaling by lipid peroxidation-derived aldehydes. Oxid. Med. Cell. Longev. 2013 (1), 690545.

Zhang, N., Xiong, G., Liu, Z., 2022. Toxicity of metal-based nanoparticles: challenges in the nano era. Front. Bioeng. Biotechnol. 10, 1001572.

Zheng, D., Zhang, X., Ding, J., Yue, D., Yang, F., Li, Y., 2025. Mechanisms and regulation of iron uptake and the role of iron in pathogenesis of Candida albicans. Crit. Rev. Microbiol. 1549-7828. 51 (6), 1384–1401. Available from: https://www.tandfonline.com/loi/imby20. doi:10.1080/1040841X.2025.2510256.

Zhou, B., Zhang, T., Wang, F., 2023. Microbial-based heavy metal bioremediation: toxicity and eco-friendly approaches to heavy metal decontamination. Appl. Sci. 13 (14), 8439.

Zhu, T., Sha, Y., Yan, J., Pageni, P., Rahman, M.A., Yan, Y., Tang, C., 2018. Metallo-polyelectrolytes as a class of ionic macromolecules for functional materials. Nat. Commun. 2041-1723. 9 (1). Available from: http://www.nature.com/ncomms/index.html. doi:10.1038/s41467-018-06475-9.

Chapter 20

Molecular mechanism of metal-induced oxidative stress and cytotoxicity

Auroshree Sadhu[a], Surajit Ghosh[a], Kishore Dhara[b], Nimai Chandra Saha[c], Surjyo Jyoti Biswas[d], and Shubhajit Saha[a]

[a]*Ecotoxicology Research Laboratory, Department of Zoology, The University of Burdwan, Burdwan, West Bengal, India*

[b]*Department of Fisheries, Government of West Bengal, Kolkata, West Bengal, India*

[c]*Harichand Guruchand University, Thakurnagar, West Bengal, India*

[d]*Genetics and Cell Biology Laboratory, Department of Zoology, Sidho-Kanho-Birsha University, Purulia, West Bengal, India*

20.1 Introduction

Metal ions are required to keep biological creatures functioning properly. For ages, people have utilized metals for everyday purposes without contemplating their disadvantages and repercussions. Consequently, along with harming the entire biome, metal ions poison water supplies, besides having had a considerable impact on plant as well as animal life. Nowadays, metal pollution is mostly generated by acid rain, mining, fossil fuel residues, industrial effluent, urban waste, fertilizers, and pesticides (Nurchi et al., 2020; Samajdar et al., 2023; Saha et al., 2025; Sharma et al., 2025).

Heavy metals (HMs) are elements whose density exceeds 5 g/mL (Jarup, 2003; Kim et al., 2019). They have been employed in a variety of applications for years (Sadhu et al., 2025). The most frequent metals are Cr, Hg, Pb, Cu, Cd, and Zn. Furthermore, because its physical and chemical characteristics are comparable to those of HMs, it can be placed in this category (Festa and Thiele, 2011; Kucuk and Gulcin, 2016; Kocyigit et al., 2018; Caglayan et al., 2019). Mn, Fe, and Co are less prevalent HMs. HMs can be divided into two categories founded on their toxicity (essential and non-essential). Essential HMs like Zn, Fe, Cu, and Co are less effective or relatively hazardous in little quantities. Non-essential HMs, such as Cd, As, Hg, and Cr, are very hazardous also at low levels (Dhara et al., 2022a, 2022b, 2022c; Saha et al., 2023). HMs, such as Cu,

The Metallome in Motion. https://doi.org/10.1016/B978-0-443-44299-5.00018-3

Zn, and Fe, are required for the biological activities of many proteins as well as enzymes as cofactors in specific biological as well as physiological processes. Cu, Zn, Fe, and Co play important roles in oxygen transport, cell development, enzymatic processes, biomolecule production, and immune system maintenance (Kishore et al., 2022). An overabundance of HMs in the cytoplasm can disturb the intracellular redox balance, affect the cytoplasm's pH, modify protein structure, and impair enzyme performance. This condition can certainly result in cell malfunction, necrosis, or apoptosis. Furthermore, HMs can react with proteins' thiol, carboxyl, as well as imidazole groups (Jomova and Valko, 2011; Caglayan et al., 2020).

The rising abundance of HMs in our environment, owing mostly to industrialization, agriculture, and inappropriate waste management, poses a substantial and ongoing threat to all forms of life (Kaur et al., 2019; Sadhu et al., 2024; Ghosh et al., 2025a; Mandal et al., 2025a; Mukherjee et al., 2025; Sharma et al., 2025). HMs, unlike many organic contaminants, are not biodegradable, causing them to accumulate in biological systems and then biomagnify via food chains. This extensive exposure necessitates a thorough understanding of how these elements harm cells and molecules. Oxidative stress induction is a key and ubiquitous mechanism underpinning HM toxicity. This crucial imbalance arises when the creation of highly reactive oxygen species (ROS)—like superoxide anions, hydroxyl radicals, and hydrogen peroxide—outnumbers the cell's inherent antioxidant defense systems (Bhattacharya, 2014). The resulting sequence of events causes considerable damage to critical cellular components, impairing cellular function and integrity, a condition known as cytotoxicity (Mandal et al., 2026; Sadhu et al., 2026). This cellular damage can be observed as decreased metabolic activities, structural abnormalities, and, in severe situations, programmed cell death (apoptosis) or necrosis (Angelé-Martínez et al., 2014; Mandal et al., 2025b).

This article will investigate the underlying molecular processes by which different HMs cause and perpetuate oxidative stress, resulting in cytotoxicity. We'll look at how metals produce ROS through mechanisms like Fenton and Haber-Weiss reactions, direct electron transfer, and by affecting mitochondrial function. Furthermore, we will examine how these metals undermine the cell's antioxidant defenses and cause broad oxidative damage to essential macromolecules, including proteins, lipids, and nucleic acids. Understanding these complex molecular processes is critical for creating effective techniques for diagnosing, mitigating, and treating the negative health effects of metal exposure in many species.

20.2 Metal exposure pathways

To determine the risk assessment of metals, it is critical to understand the way metals interact with and travel through the environment. HMs penetrate the environment through a variety of natural geological processes and, more importantly, human-caused activities. Generally, HMs comprise naturally occurring elements derived from the Earth's crust, typically found in igneous and sedimentary rocks. For example, basaltic igneous rocks can have copper (Cu) concentrations that range from 48 to 240 parts per million (ppm), whereas granite igneous rocks generally contain 5 to 140 ppm of Cu. Sedimentary rocks such as clays and shales can contain 18 to 180 ppm of Cu, with black shales having greater quantities ranging from 34 to 1500 ppm of Cu (Angon et al., 2024). Natural events add to the release of these metals into the environment. Weathering, erosion, and leaching from rocks are all natural causes of metal presence in soil as well as water bodies (Angon et al., 2024). Volcanic eruptions are projected to release 820 tonnes of cadmium (Cd) per year, whereas forest fires contribute around 70 tonnes of Cd each year (Dashtey, 2021). Biological processes, terrestrial activities, and surface winds all promote the natural dispersion of HMs across landscapes (Piwowarska et al., 2024). Despite the natural existence of HMs, anthropogenic (human-caused) activities are the most common source of environmental pollution (Saha et al., 2020, 2021; Chakraborty et al., 2024a; Saha et al., 2024b; Chakraborty et al., 2025; Ghosh et al., 2025a) and subsequent human exposure (Table 20.1).

Beyond direct discharges, environmental contamination occurs through processes that are frequently exacerbated by human activity, such as metal corrosion, atmospheric accumulation, HM leaching, metal ion soil erosion, sediment re-suspension, and the evaporation of metals from water bodies to soil and groundwater (Kaur et al., 2019). Human and ecological exposure principally occurs through inhalation, assimilation of food and water, and dermal contact. This might lead to biodiversity loss, habitat degradation, and impaired ecosystem functionality, with profound impacts on foundational components like soil microbial communities and aquatic organisms (Chu, 2018; Musah, 2025). For humans, exposure can result in a wide array of severe health issues, such as neurological damage, organ dysfunction, and increased cancer risk (Mahurpawar, 2015).

20.3 Metal-induced toxicity in organisms

HMs, like lead, mercury, cadmium, copper, silver, and zinc, are examples of environmental contaminants that may cause chronic and occasionally acute toxic poisoning when humans are exposed to them via water and food (Ghosh et al., 2025; Mandal et al., 2024). The expression and severity of metal poisoning are greatly dependent on the absorbed dosage, the precise route of exposure, and the period of exposure (acute or chronic) (Jaishankar et al., 2014). Regardless of the metal, bioaccumulation, or buildup within individual organisms, frequently results in an extensive range of toxic effects on numerous body tissues as well as organs (Balali-Mood et al., 2021). It interferes with biological functioning, resulting in potentially fatal symptoms if not treated promptly. The effects are systemic and may affect several organ systems (Table 20.2).

TABLE 20.1 Anthropogenic sources that release heavy metals.

Source	Activities	Associated heavy metals	References
Mining & Smelting Operations	Ore extraction, metal refining	Lead (Pb), Chromium (Cr), Nickel (Ni), Mercury (Hg), Copper (Cu), Cadmium (Cd), Arsenic (As), Zinc (Zn)	Kaur et al. (2019)
Industrial Production & Use	Fossil fuel combustion (coal, petroleum), electroplating, iron and steel production, chemical industries, textile industry, paints and pigments, battery manufacturing, plastics, microelectronics.	Lead (Pb), Chromium (Cr), Nickel (Ni), Mercury (Hg), Copper (Cu), Cadmium (Cd), Arsenic (As), Zinc (Zn)	Kaur et al. (2019)
Agricultural Activities	Phosphate fertilizers, pesticides (insecticides, herbicides, fungicides), biosolids, farm manures, wastewater irrigation	Lead (Pb), Chromium (Cr), Nickel (Ni), Mercury (Hg), Cadmium (Cd), Copper (Cu), Arsenic (As), Zinc (Zn)	Kaur et al. (2019)
Waste Disposal	Incineration of industrial/municipal waste, unauthorized dumping, landfills	Lead (Pb), Chromium (Cr), Nickel (Ni), Mercury (Hg), Copper (Cu), Cadmium (Cd), Arsenic (As), Zinc (Zn)	Jaishankar et al. (2014)
Other Diffuse Sources	Metal corrosion, urban runoff, vehicle emissions	Chromium (Cr), Copper (Cu), Lead (Pb), Cadmium (Cd), Zinc (Zn)	Balali-Mood et al. (2021)

The abundance and quantity of HMs in the environment, predominantly in aquatic ecosystems and in aquatic species, i.e., in aquatic flora and fauna used as human food, are determined by human nature and actions. Fish and other seafood always contain HMs as a result of their aquatic habitat. The ratio of expected HM concentrations to HM concentrations due to anthropogenic activities in fish fluctuates by element. In contaminated areas, where water does not exchange sufficiently with the world's seas, the concentration of HMs is significantly greater than usual in estuaries, rivers, and especially in sites adjacent

TABLE 20.2 Health hazards due to some of the metals and their sources.

Metal	Principal sources	Key health hazards/Impacts	References
Lead (Pb)	Contaminated water (pipes), old paint, batteries, gasoline, construction materials, firing ranges, cosmetics.	Neurological damage (brain damage, memory loss, neurodevelopmental deficits in children), anemia, kidney damage, liver damage, cardiovascular dysfunction (hypertension, arrhythmia), gastrointestinal pain, reproductive issues (miscarriage)	Chandra et al. (1984) and Saha et al. (2024a).
Mercury (Hg)	Fluid in thermometers, lightbulbs, dental amalgam, seafood (methylmercury from pollution), topical antiseptics, and coal combustion	Central nervous system injuries (focal degeneration of neurons, neurodevelopmental delays, ataxia, memory loss), renal dysfunction, gastrointestinal ulceration, hepatotoxicity, immune system damage, cardiovascular issues, and teratogenic effects	Chandra et al. (1984) and Saha et al. (2023)
Arsenic (As)	Contaminated water, seafood, topical creams, algae, herbicides, pesticides, insecticides, fungicides, enamels, glass, paints, smelting processes, wood preservatives, volcanic eruptions	Cancer (skin, lungs, bladder, kidneys, liver), vascular diseases, diabetes, neurobehavioral disorders, developmental abnormalities, reproductive toxicity, blood diseases, and nervous system diseases	Parida and Patel (2023)
Cadmium (Cd)	Cigarette smoke, metal plating, batteries, spray painting, vegetables, seeds, shellfish, plastics production	Renal cancer, bronchiolitis, chronic obstructive pulmonary disease (COPD), emphysema, fibrotic bone damage (Itai-itai disease), cardiovascular effects (hypertension, peripheral arterial disease), reproductive toxicity, lung/prostate/kidney cancer	Parida and Patel (2023)
Thallium (Tl)	Rodenticides, pesticides, fireworks, coal combustion, semiconductor manufacturing, exhaust emissions	Highly toxic; clinical presentation varies by dose, age, and exposure	Fatima et al. (2025)
Chromium (Cr)	Stainless steel manufacturing, chrome plating, leather tanning, dyes, cleaning solutions, anticorrosive, industrial exposure	Kidney dysfunction, DNA damage, respiratory tract cancer (hexavalent form), allergies, asthma	Fatima et al. (2025)
Copper (Cu)	Industrial effluents, contaminated water	Increased blood pressure, breathing difficulties, kidney or liver damage, spasms, convulsions, vomiting (at high concentrations); essential at low concentrations	Fatima et al. (2025)
Zinc (Zn)	Industrial effluents, contaminated water	Gastric nausea, skin irritation, spasms, vomiting, anemia (at high concentrations); essential at low concentrations	Fatima et al. (2025)

to industrial operations (Forouhar Vajargah et al., 2018; Vajargah, 2021). Table 20.3 provides an organized outline of the many biomarkers available, emphasizing their use in a variety of biological systems as well as their value in detecting toxicity phases.

20.4 Fundamental molecular mechanisms of metal-induced oxidative stress

HMs cause oxidative stress in animals via a complex network of molecular processes, fundamentally upsetting cellular homeostasis. This process is distinguished by a disparity between the production of ROS and the cell's capability to neutralize them using antioxidants (Jaishankar et al., 2014). Metals with significant toxicity and carcinogenicity, like arsenic, lead, mercury, cadmium, and chromium, are typically associated with oxidative stress resulting from ROS production (Ondrasek et al., 2025).

20. 4.1 Reactive oxygen species generation

HMs like lead, cadmium, arsenic, mercury, and chromium are strong inducers of ROS and other free radicals (Wang et al., 2024). This excessive ROS generation, which comprises superoxide anions, hydrogen peroxide, and hydroxyl radicals, can be caused by a variety of intracellular sources (Oros et al., 2025).

20.4.1.1 Fenton and haber-weiss reactions (e.g., Fe, Cu)

Fenton and Haber-Weiss reactions, which create highly reactive species like hydroxyl radicals (OH) and hydrogen peroxide (H_2O_2), are a major source of ROS (Ondrasek et al., 2025). These reactions are frequently catalyzed by transition metals like copper and iron, which may cycle between different oxidation states, resulting in the constant creation of free radicals (Ondrasek et al., 2025). For example, arsenic may create superoxide, hydrogen peroxide, and peroxyl radicals, all of which contribute to oxidative stress. In the presence of HM ions (Cu or Fe) and O_2, H_2O_2 forms $OH\cdot$ by the distinguished Fenton reaction (Fenton, 1894; Ghosh et al., 2024). On the contrary, the Haber–Weiss reaction generates $OH\cdot$ from O_2^- and H_2O_2, catalyzed by ferrous ions. This reaction was initially proposed by Fritz Haber along with his student (Haber and Weiss, 1934).

$$Fe^{2+} + H_2O_2 \rightarrow Fe^{3+} + OH^- + OH \text{ (Fenton reaction)}$$

$$O_2^- + H_2O_2 \rightarrow O_2 + H_2O + OH \text{ (Haber–Weiss reaction)}$$

In subsequent research, it was established that both of the reactions are key sources of radicals as well as being accountable for cellular impairment.

TABLE 20.3 Structured overview of biomarkers for metal exposure and effects in different organisms.

Organism type	Biomarker category	Specific biomarker	Significance	References
Mammals/ Humans	Exposure	Methylmercury (MeHg) levels	Direct measurement of mercury exposure, especially neurotoxic forms	Chandra et al. (1984)
		Blood lead (Pb) levels	Direct measurement of lead exposure correlates with neurological effects.	
	Effect	Elevated liver enzymes (ALT, AST)	Liver damage (hepatotoxicity)	Balali-Mood et al. (2021)
		Renal dysfunction markers (proteinuria)	Kidney damage (nephrotoxicity)	
		Anemia	Impaired heme biosynthesis (e.g., by lead)	
		Cognitive impairment tests	Neurotoxicity, brain damage	
Aquatic Life	Exposure	Metallothioneins (MTs)	Induction by metals (Cd, Zn, Hg, Cu, Pb, As) indicates metal sequestration and detoxification response.	Oros et al. (2025)
		Acetylcholinesterase (AChE) activity	Inhibition by neurotoxic metals (Pb, Hg) indicates neurotoxicity and behavioral disruption.	
	Effect	Lipid Peroxidation (LPO)/Malondialdehyde (MDA)	Oxidative membrane injury	Sabullah et al. (2015)
		Micronuclei formation	Chromosomal damage, genomic instability	
		Histopathological alterations (gills, liver, kidney)	Structural damage, tissue necrosis, inflammation	
	Susceptibility/ Condition	Hepatosomatic Index (HSI)/ Gonadosomatic Index (GSI)	Energy status, reproductive investment, overall physiological health.	Wang et al. (2024)
		Vitellogenin (VTG) induction	Endocrine disruption, particularly by estrogenic metals (Cd, As).	

Continued

Table 20.3 Structured overview of biomarkers for metal exposure and effects in different organisms—cont'd

Organism type	Biomarker category	Specific biomarker	Significance	References
Plants	Effect	Chlorophyll content reduction	Photosynthesis impairment	Jaishankar et al. (2014) and (Nawab et al., 2022)
		Reduced growth/yield	Overall plant health and productivity	
		Reactive Oxygen Species (ROS) levels	Oxidative stress	
		Nutrient uptake efficiency	Interference with nutrient assimilation	
		Enzyme activity (e.g., antioxidant enzymes)	Disruption of metabolic processes, oxidative stress response.	

20.4.1.2 Direct electron transfer and redox cycling (e.g., Cr, As)

HMs cause oxidative stress by direct electron transfer and redox cycling, in which they gain or lose electrons, resulting in free radicals. This mechanism involves metals interacting with biomolecules containing sulfur, nitrogen, and oxygen, impairing proteins, enzymes, and numerous other cellular components (Balali-Mood et al., 2021). Metals like chromium, arsenic, etc., are known to engage in redox cycling, which results in the ongoing formation of ROS as well as oxidative damage to cellular macromolecules (Hameed et al., 2020).

20.4.1.3 Mitochondrial dysfunction and ROS production

Mitochondrial failure contributes significantly to intracellular ROS production caused by HMs (Wang et al., 2024). Metals can affect mitochondrial processes by binding to the electron transport chain and reducing oxygen, resulting in the production of superoxide (O_2-) as well as other ROS (Balali-Mood et al., 2021). This reduction in ATP generation (Fig. 20.1) and altered mitochondrial membrane potential exacerbates oxidative stress (Oros et al., 2025). Furthermore, HMs can activate enzymes such as NADPH oxidase as well as protein kinase C, increasing the production of intracellular ROS (Ondrasek et al., 2025).

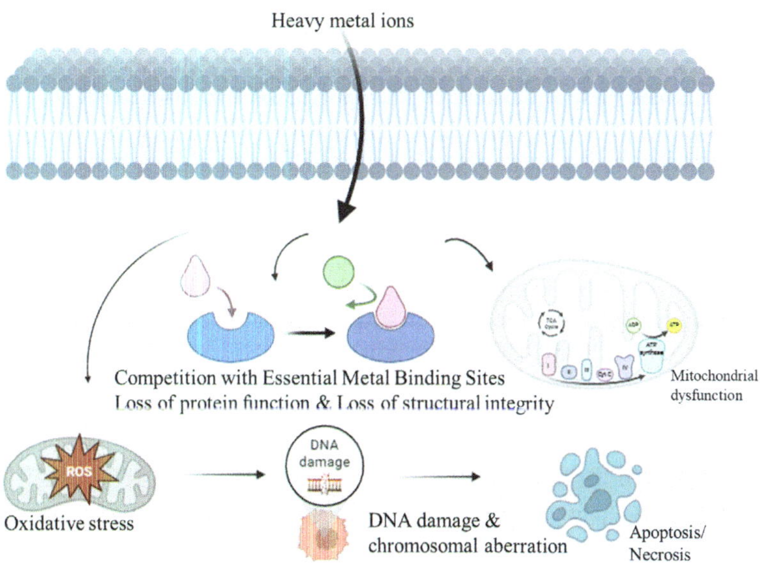

FIG. 20.1 Schematic representation of the molecular changes caused by metal toxicity inside a cell.

20.4.2 Interaction with sulfhydryl groups in proteins and enzymes

HMs directly disrupt important biological components, including enzymes and proteins, which are required for proper organ function. These metals regularly react with biological systems by losing electrons, thereby producing metal cations, which have a high affinity for nucleophilic sites on essential macromolecules (Balali-Mood et al., 2021). Proteins are major focuses; HMs interfere with their physiological functioning by creating stable complexes with functional side chain groups (e.g., sulfhydryl groups on cysteine residues) or by shifting essential metal ions from metalloproteins (Tamás et al., 2014). HMs bind to sulfhydryl (-SH) groups in proteins and alter cysteine residues. For example, metals such as mercury and methylmercury attach to the sulphur in cysteinyl residues in proteins (Tamás et al., 2014). This interaction with biomolecules containing sulphur, nitrogen, and oxygen can change the structure and function of enzymes, proteins, and hormones. Lead binds selectively to sulfhydryl groups in proteins, interfering with enzyme function and cellular signalling pathways (Tamás et al., 2014).

20.4.2.1 Enzyme inactivation and functional disruption

HM binding to proteins and enzymes causes inactivation and functional disruption, preventing critical organs from functioning properly (Fig. 20.1). HMs impair biological functions, including growth, proliferation, differentiation, damage repair, and apoptosis (Balali-Mood et al., 2021). Specific examples demonstrate this interference: Lead interacts with aminolevulinic acid dehydratase and ferrochelatase, two essential enzymes in heme production, inhibiting them and leading to anemia (Balali-Mood et al., 2021). Mercury can deactivate enzymes by strongly adhering to the sulfur atoms in cysteine-containing proteins (Jaishankar et al., 2014). Arsenic inhibits pyruvate dehydrogenase, which disrupts the Krebs cycle and oxidative phosphorylation (Balali-Mood et al., 2021).

In addition to direct inactivation, metals can hinder the in vitro refolding of chemically damaged proteins and meddle with protein folding in vivo. They increase nascent protein aggregation, which severely disturbs cellular protein homeostasis, eventually jeopardizing cell survival. HMs can reduce enzyme activity via lipid peroxidation (Wang et al., 2024). They can operate as enzyme cofactors, but in high concentrations, they tend to limit enzyme activity by binding to particular amino acids at proteins' active and allosteric regions (Sabullah et al., 2015). HMs, if internalized, interfere with macromolecular functions and enzyme activity (Oros et al., 2025).

20.4.2.2 Impairment of antioxidant defense systems (e.g., Glutathione depletion)

HMs impair the cell's natural defense systems by depleting endogenous cellular antioxidants like glutathione (GSH) and decreasing the function of crucial antioxidant enzymes, including catalase (CAT), superoxide dismutase (SOD), and glutathione peroxidase (GPx) (Wang et al., 2024). Lead exposure, for example, lowers GSH, SOD, CAT, and GPx levels (Balali-Mood et al., 2021). HMs like arsenic, cadmium, and mercury may reduce thiol groups in GSH, a key antioxidant that neutralizes ROS. This leads to reduced availability for ROS scavenging (Oros et al., 2025). The GSH system is an important part of cellular defense; GSH, a tripeptide, binds non-enzymatically to metals like lead, cadmium, and mercury, generating less reactive and more excretable conjugates. This system also supports enzymatic pathways, including GPx, and GST, which reduce ROS-induced damage and help remove electrophilic metal species. While acute exposure may initially activate these enzymes as a compensatory response, chronic metal pollution can overload or block these systems, resulting in long-term oxidative damage (Chakraborty et al., 2024b; Wang et al., 2024; Oros et al., 2025).

20.4.3 Competition with essential metal-binding sites

HMs can disrupt biological functions by competing with necessary metal ions for binding sites on proteins and enzymes. This rivalry upsets the delicate balance of mineral homeostasis inside the cell, resulting in functional deficits.

20.4.3.1 Displacement of essential ions (e.g., Zn, Ca, Fe, Cu)

Toxic HMs frequently imitate necessary metal ions due to their resemblance in ionic radii and electronic configurations, enabling them to attach to protein sites that were not designed for them. This results in the displacement of critical metals like zinc, calcium, iron, and copper from their normal binding sites (Jaishankar et al., 2014). For example, beryllium (Be^{2+}) can substitute magnesium (Mg^{2+}) in some enzymes, resulting in toxicity. Cadmium (Cd) can mimic critical elements such as zinc, disrupting calcium, zinc, and iron homeostasis (Tchounwou et al., 2012). HMs can also enter cells via ion channels and transporters, imitating important elements like sodium, calcium, and potassium, exacerbating their disruptive effects (Oros et al., 2025).

20.4.3.2 Disruption of metalloprotein function

The displacement of vital metal ions or the binding of hazardous metals to crucial protein sites has a direct impact on the physiological functioning of metalloproteins, which require a metal ion to function (Witkowska et al., 2021). This interference has the potential to cause cell dysfunction and, eventually, toxicity (Fig. 20.1). HMs, for example, can interfere with macromolecular processes and impair enzyme activity once they enter the body. The disruption of metalloprotein activity is a primary method by which HMs harm human health, causing structural and functional changes inside cells (Fu and Xi, 2020).

20.5 Molecular mechanisms leading to cytotoxicity

20.5.1 Overview of cytotoxicity mechanisms

HMs impair biological functions, including growth, proliferation, differentiation, damage repair, and apoptosis (Waalkes et al., 2000; Parida and Patel, 2023). They cause cytotoxicity through a variety of molecular pathways, including oxidative stress linked to mitochondrial malfunction, apoptosis, necrosis, and endoplasmic reticulum (ER) stress, all of which are interrelated (Madkour, 2020; Rana, 2020). These metals may penetrate cells and tissues and attach to biomolecules like proteins and DNA, resulting in cellular damage, inflammation, and programmed cell death (Madkour, 2020). High metal concentrations in biological systems impact enzymatic activities as well as cell organelles and their components, such as the mitochondria, nucleus, cell membrane, and enzymes, leading to DNA damage, cell cycle alterations, carcinogenesis, and cell death (Parida and Patel, 2023). Molecular and biochemical indicators frequently appear before visual symptoms of disease, providing a sensitive foundation for early diagnosis and biomonitoring. These reactions disrupt cellular homeostasis, resulting in tissue damage, immunological suppression, and reduced physiological performance (Balabekova et al., 2024).

20.5.1.1 DNA damage and genomic instability

HMs can cause considerable genotoxicity, either directly or indirectly, by overproducing ROS (Tabassum et al., 2021). These impacts include numerous types of DNA damage, including strand breakage, base alterations, and chromosomal abnormalities (Kocadal et al., 2020). The single-cell gel electrophoresis (Comet) along with micronucleus assays are frequently employed to assess these damages (D'Costa et al., 2019). HMs have been shown to interact with nuclear proteins and DNA, resulting in site-specific damage. This can happen through "direct" damage, in which the metal stimulates structural changes in biomolecules, or "indirect" damage, which arises from the generation of reactive oxygen as well as nitrogen species (Kocadal et al., 2020; Tabassum et al., 2021). HM binding to DNA as well as nuclear proteins is the primary lead to oxidative degradation in biological macromolecules (Fig. 20.1). Chromium, cadmium, and arsenic are well recognised to cause genomic instability (Filipič, 2012; Wise and Wise, 2012). Accumulated HMs, particularly at high concentrations or after prolonged exposure, can harm tissues and cause the production of ROS and electrophilic metabolites, which then merge with DNA molecules, resulting in oxidative attack, lipid peroxidation, genetic material changes, and ribose oxidation, eventually leading to cell death or carcinogenesis (Sytar et al., 2013; Ghosh et al., 2025b).

20.5.1.2 Oxidative DNA damage

HMs trigger oxidative DNA damage predominantly through the production of ROS. These reactive species may directly target DNA molecules, causing strand breakage and base alterations like 8-hydroxy-2'-deoxyguanosine (8-oxodG) (White, 2005). The oxidative degradation of biological macromolecules is instigated by HMs binding to DNA and nuclear proteins (Dutta et al., 2018). HMs have also been shown to activate signaling pathways, which contribute to this harm (Nickcrk ct al., 2024).

20.5.1.3 Interference with DNA repair mechanisms

Metal-induced genotoxicity is characterized by its capacity to interfere with DNA repair pathways (Hartwig, 1994). Faults in DNA repair, which are frequently the result of induced oxidative stress and direct DNA damage, are thought to be the major cause of some metals' carcinogenicity (Filipič, 2012; Wise and Wise, 2012). Carcinogenic metals like cadmium, arsenic, and chromium have been shown to impair both DNA synthesis and repair mechanisms within cells (Sytar et al., 2013).

20.5.1.4 Chromosomal aberrations and carcinogenesis

HMs, specifically cadmium, chromium, and arsenic, are known to initiate genomic instability, which can result in chromosomal abnormalities (Filipič, 2012; Wise and Wise, 2012; Parida and Patel, 2023). The specific mechanism is frequently unknown; however, abnormal alterations in the genome as well as gene expression are proposed as underlying mechanisms. These metals can cause DNA damage, such as single and double-strand breaks, DNA-protein crosslinks, interstrand crosslinks, and p53 point mutations (Andrés et al., 2023). Furthermore, HMs are recognized to cause epigenetic changes, like changes in DNA methylation as well as histone modification, which affect gene expression without changing the DNA sequence (Chervona and Costa, 2012). In aquatic creatures, accumulated HMs can cause genetic modification and changes in species diversity, as well as DNA damage, resulting in gene mutations, chromosomal abnormalities, and even cancer (Jha, 2004; Mishra et al., 2010). For example, iron ions may promote high methylation of DNA, whereas lead, copper, and zinc ions can limit methyltransferase activity, and lead can result in low methylation of DNA (Vidal et al., 2015). Certain toxic metals, like arsenic and cadmium, are considered human carcinogens and have been linked to a variety of malignancies, including bladder, lung, and liver cancer (Parida and Patel, 2023).

20.5.2 Lipid peroxidation and membrane damage

HMs cause oxidative stress, which results in extensive oxidative damage to essential biological macromolecules like lipids (Ercal et al., 2001). Lipid peroxidation increases the destruction of cell membranes.

20.5.2.1 Disruption of membrane integrity and permeability

Lipid peroxidation directly impairs cellular membrane integrity, resulting in structural damage and functional problems (Catalá and Díaz, 2016). HMs can disrupt general membrane function and nutrient uptake, aggravating cellular stress (Ercal et al., 2001). They can also modify cell membrane fluidity and the permeability of ion pumps, lower cell membrane stability, and interfere with important cellular processes such as phagocytic function.

20.5.2.2 Formation of toxic aldehydes

Toxic aldehydes are produced as a substantial byproduct of lipid peroxidation. Malondialdehyde (MDA) is a regularly detected indicator of lipid peroxidation, and it often accumulates during HM-induced oxidative stress (Okieke, 2017). These aldehydes are highly reactive and can further harm cellular components, contributing to overall cytotoxicity.

20.5.3 Protein oxidation and aggregation

Proteins are considered the main targets of HM toxicity, with the general opinion being that metals interfere with their physiological activities. HMs affect protein function and activity in a variety of ways, including direct binding and oxidative destruction (Hasan et al., 2017).

20.5.3.1 Loss of protein function and structural integrity

HMs directly disrupt important biological components, including enzymes and proteins, which are required for proper organ function (Wu et al., 2016). These metals commonly interact with biological systems, generating metal cations with a high affinity for nucleophilic sites on essential macromolecules, such as sulfhydryl groups on cysteine residues (Henkel and Krebs, 2004). This binding causes proteins and enzymes to become inactivated and functionally disrupted, preventing critical organs from functioning normally (Blundell and Jenkins, 1977). HMs can also reduce enzyme activity via lipid peroxidation. While certain metals can function as enzyme cofactors, at high concentrations, they frequently impede enzyme activity by binding to particular amino acids at proteins' active and allosteric regions. HMs, if internalized, interfere with macromolecular functions and enzyme activity. Beyond direct binding, metal-induced oxidative stress can cause protein misfolding, aggregation, and damage, affecting their structure and function (Tamás et al., 2014).

20.5.3.2 Activation of unfolded protein response

HMs as well as metalloids have been shown to hinder the in vitro refolding of chemically damaged proteins, hamper protein folding in vivo, and increase the aggregation of newly formed proteins (Tamás et al., 2014). Unfolded proteins with motile backbones as well as side chains are far more likely to form stable, pluridented metal complexes than native proteins with well-defined 3D structures. HM ions and metalloids have a significant impact on protein homeostasis and cell survival because they disrupt the folding process (Tamás et al., 2014). This imbalance can instigate cellular stress responses, like ER stress, which is linked to oxidative stress, mitochondrial malfunction, and apoptosis (Madkour, 2020; Rana, 2020). Cells activate molecular chaperones, like heat shock proteins, to help them survive and regulate unfolded proteins, indicating a biological response to keep protein quality under control (Papsdorf and Richter, 2014).

20.5.4 Disruption of cellular homeostasis

The overall mechanism of HM toxicity is the breakdown of metabolic equilibrium at the cellular level. HMs disrupt significant cellular processes like DNA synthesis and repair, protein synthesis, and signal transduction pathways, resulting in cellular malfunction and pathology (Kocadal et al., 2020). These metals interfere with essential biological processes like growth, proliferation, differentiation, and damage repair, which frequently result in programmed cell death (apoptosis) (Hartwig et al., 2002). Metal exposure causes reactions that disturb general cellular homeostasis, resulting in tissue damage, immunological suppression, and reduced physiological performance (Balabekova et al., 2024). HMs impair critical biochemical as well as structural processes, resulting in organelle destruction, energy imbalance, and physiological malfunction. Mitochondria are particularly sensitive, with reduced adenosine triphosphate (ATP) generation and altered membrane potential (Balali-Mood et al., 2021; Wang et al., 2024). Autophagy, a lysosome-dependent mechanism, is initiated to destroy damaged organelles, but long-term exposure can decrease lysosomal functionality (Trivedi et al., 2020). HMs can also inhibit important enzymes such as carbonic anhydrase and proteasomal enzymes (Lionetto et al., 2012). They can also block ion-regulatory enzymes like Na+/K+-ATPase and Ca2+-ATPase, which disrupts nerve impulse transmission and ion homeostasis (Chandra et al., 1984). Cadmium, for example, may imitate important elements like as zinc and bind to albumin, disrupting calcium, zinc, and iron homeostasis (Moulis, 2010).

20.6 Conclusion

The extensive presence of HMs in our environment, arising from both natural processes and, more importantly, human activity, poses a complicated and growing hazard to all living creatures. Unlike organic contaminants, these elements are not biodegradable, resulting in long-term accumulation, bioaccumulation within individual species, and biomagnification up the food chain. This fundamental trait ensures extensive exposure and cascading ecological impacts, posing significant threats to ecosystem health and human well-being (Sadhu et al., 2025). HM toxicity is caused by a complex network of molecular and cellular pathways. These include direct competition with important metal-binding sites, which causes the displacement of crucial ions such as zinc, calcium, iron, and copper, affecting the function of critical metalloproteins. Furthermore, HMs have a strong affinity for sulfhydryl groups in proteins and enzymes, inactivating them and compromising important physiological activities such as antioxidant defense mechanisms. Oxidative stress is a key and unifying mechanism that is characterized by the excessive formation of ROS via mechanisms such as Fenton and Haber-Weiss reactions, direct electron transfer, and mitochondrial malfunction. This massive creation of ROS, along with the depletion of cellular antioxidants, causes extensive oxidative damage to critical macromolecules, including DNA, lipids, and proteins, resulting in cytotoxicity. This cellular damage manifests as lipid peroxidation, DNA strand breakage, protein aggregation, and a general disturbance in cellular homeostasis, which frequently results in programmed cell death.

This molecular disruption influences a wide range of biological systems. HM exposure in animals can cause significant neurological impairments, renal and hepatic damage, cardiovascular problems, and an increased risk of numerous malignancies, with youngsters and pregnant women being especially susceptible. Aquatic creatures experience reduced development and reproduction, physiological and metabolic abnormalities, immunotoxicity, and genetic changes, with biomagnification having the potential to exacerbate these impacts further up the food chain. Plants, too, suffer considerable growth decreases, reduced photosynthesis, and altered nutrient absorption when grown in polluted soil. Despite tremendous advances in understanding metal toxicity, obstacles remain, particularly in determining the long-term effects of chronic, low-level exposure. Future efforts must prioritize further research into novel biomarkers and innovative remediation technologies, as well as the development and harmonization of international and national regulatory regimes. Finally, a proactive and comprehensive plan combining scientific knowledge, strong policy, and technical innovation is required to mitigate the ubiquitous danger of metal-induced toxicity and protect both environmental integrity and public health for future generations.

References

Andrés, C.M.C., Lastra, J.M.P.D.L., Juan, C.A., Plou, F.J., Pérez-Lebeña, E., 2023. Chemical insights into oxidative and nitrative modifications of DNA. Int. J. Mol. Sci. 1422-0067. 24 (20). Available from: http://www.mdpi.com/journal/ijms. doi:10.3390/ijms242015240.

Angelé-Martínez, C., Goodman, C., Brumaghim, J., 2014. Metal-mediated DNA damage and cell death: mechanisms, detection methods, and cellular consequences. Metallomics. 1756-591X. 6 (8), 1358–1381. Available from: http://www.rsc.org/Publishing/Journals/MT/index.asp. doi:10.1039/c4mt00057a.

Angon, P.B., Islam, M.S., KC, S., Das, A., Anjum, N., Poudel, A., Suchi, S.A., 2024. Sources, effects and present perspectives of heavy metals contamination: soil, plants and human food chain. Heliyon. 2405-8440. 10 (7). Available from: https://www.sciencedirect.com/science/journal/24058440. doi:10.1016/j.heliyon.2024.e28357.

Balabekova, M.K., Kairanbayeva, G.K., Stankevicius, E., Koks, S., Tokusheva, A.N., Sycheva, Y.S., Myrzagulova, S.E., Yu, V.K., 2024. Toxic effects of heavy metals on the immune system and new approaches to restoring homeostasis. J. Med. Chem. Sci. 7 (11), 1411–1421.

Balali-Mood, M., Naseri, K., Tahergorabi, Z., Khazdair, M.R., Sadeghi, M., 2021. Toxic mechanisms of five heavy metals: mercury, lead, chromium, cadmium, and arsenic. Front. Pharmacol. 1663-9812. 12. Available from: http://www.frontiersin.org/Pharmacology. doi:10.3389/fphar.2021.643972.

Bhattacharya, S., 2014. Reactive oxygen species and cellular defense system. In: Rani, V., Yadav, U. (Eds.), Free Radicals in Human Health and Disease. Springer, New Delhi, pp. 17–29. doi:10.1007/978-81-322-2035-0_2.

Blundell, T.L., Jenkins, J.A., 1977. The binding of heavy metals to proteins. Chem. Soc. Rev. 0306-0012. 6 (2), 139–171. doi:10.1039/CS9770600139.

Caglayan, C., Taslimi, P., Türk, C., Gulcin, İ., Kandemir, F.M., Demir, Y., Beydemir, Ş., 2020. Inhibition effects of some pesticides and heavy metals on carbonic anhydrase enzyme activity purified from horse mackerel (Trachurus trachurus) gill tissues. Environ. Sci. Pollut. Res. 1614-7499. 27 (10), 10607–10616. Available from: https://link.springer.com/journal/11356. doi:10.1007/s11356-020-07611-z.

Caglayan, C., Taslimi, P., Türk, C., Kandemir, F.M., Demir, Y., Gulcin, İ., 2019. Purification and characterization of the carbonic anhydrase enzyme from horse mackerel (Trachurus trachurus) muscle and the impact of some metal ions and pesticides on enzyme activity. Comp. Biochem. Physiol. C Toxicol. Pharmacol. 1878-1659. 226. Available from: https://www.journals.elsevier.com/comparative-biochemistry-and-physiology-part-c-toxicology-and-pharmacology. doi:10.1016/j.cbpc.2019.108605.

Catalá, A., Díaz, M., 2016. Impact of lipid peroxidation on the physiology and pathophysiology of cell membranes. Front. Physiol. 7, 423.

Chakraborty, D., Ghosh, S., Mandal, A.H., Roy, T., Sadhu, A., Paria, D.S., Saha, N.C., Sopjani, M., Saha, S., Faggio, C., 2025. Sodium Dodecylbenzenesulfonate-induced oxidative stress and tissue damage in Tubifex tubifex: a comprehensive toxicological study. Environ. Toxicol. Pharmacol. 1872-7077. 118. Available from: https://www.sciencedirect.com/science/journal/13826689. doi:10.1016/j.etap.2025.104778.

Chakraborty, D., Mandal, A.H., Ghosh, S., Sadhu, A., Das, D., Saha, N.C., Saha, S., 2024b. The physiological effects of acute and sub-lethal exposure to phenol on antioxidant enzyme activity in the freshwater sludge worm Tubifex tubifex. Toxicol. Rep. 2214-7500. 13. Available from: https://www.sciencedirect.com/science/journal/22147500. doi:10.1016/j.toxrep.2024.101717.

Chakraborty, D., Saha, S., Podder, S., Saha, N.C., Faggio, C., 2024a. Generation of oxidative stress in freshwater oligochaete Tubifex tubifex due to exposure to aniline: time and concentration dependent toxicity assessment. Chem. Ecol. 1029-0370. 40 (3), 260–275. Available from: www.tandf.co.uk/journals/titles/02757540.asp. doi:10.1080/02757540.2024.2304806.

Chandra, S.V., Murthy, R.C., Husain, T., Bansal, S.K., 1984. Effect of interaction of heavy metals on (Na+-K+) ATPase and the uptake of 3H-DA and 3H-NA in rat brain synaptosomes. Acta Pharmacol. Toxicol. 1600-0773. 54 (3), 210–213. doi:10.1111/j.1600-0773.1984.tb01919.x.

Chervona, Y., Costa, M., 2012. The control of histone methylation and gene expression by oxidative stress, hypoxia, and metals. Free Radic. Biol. Med. 1873-4596. 53 (5), 1041–1047. doi:10.1016/j.freeradbiomed.2012.07.020.

Chu, D., 2018. Effects of heavy metals on soil microbial community. IOP Conf. Ser. Earth Environ. Sci. 1755-1307. 113 (1), 012009. doi:10.1088/1755-1315/113/1/012009.

D'Costa, A., Kumar, M.K.P., Shyama, S.K., 2019. Genotoxicity assays: the micronucleus test and the single-cell gel electrophoresis assay. In: Surya, N.M., Milind, M.N. (Eds.), Advances in Biological Science Research: A Practical Approach. Elsevier, India, pp. 291–301. doi:10.1016/B978-0-12-817497-5.00018-5.

Dashtey, A., 2024. Fate and transport of heavy metals in soil, surface water, and groundwater: implications for environmental management. Int. J. Sci. Res. Manag. 2321-3418. 12 (12), 202–215. doi:10.18535/ijsrm/v12i12.c01.

Dhara, K., Chukwuka, A.V., Saha, S., Saha, N.C., Faggio, C., 2022b. Effects of short-term selenium exposure on respiratory activity and proximate body composition of early-life stages of Catla catla, Labeo rohita and Cirrhinus mrigala. Environ. Toxicol. Pharmacol. 1872-7077. 90. Available from: www.elsevier.com/locate/etap. doi:10.1016/j.etap.2021.103805.

Dhara, K., Saha, S., Chukwuka, A.V., Pal, P., Saha, N.C., Faggio, C., 2022c. Fluoride sensitivity in freshwater snail, Bellamya bengalensis (Lamarck, 1882): an integrative biomarker response assessment of behavioral indices, oxygen consumption, haemocyte and tissue protein levels under environmentally relevant exposure concentrations. Environ. Toxicol. Pharmacol. 1872-7077. 89. Available from: www.elsevier.com/locate/etap. doi:10.1016/j.etap.2021.103789.

Dhara, K., Saha, S., Pal, P., Chukwuka, A.V., Panigrahi, A.K., Saha, N.C., Faggio, C., 2022a. Biochemical, physiological (haematological, oxygen-consumption rate) and behavioural effects of mercury exposures on the freshwater snail, Bellamya bengalensis. Comp. Biochem. Physiol. C Toxicol. Pharmacol. 1878-1659. 251. Available from: https://www.journals.elsevier.com/comparative-biochemistry-and-physiology-part-c-toxicology-and-pharmacology. doi:10.1016/j.cbpc.2021.109195.

Dutta, S., Mitra, M., Agarwal, P., Mahapatra, K., De, S., Sett, U., Roy, S., 2018. Oxidative and genotoxic damages in plants in response to heavy metal stress and maintenance of genome stability. Plant Signal. Behav. 1559-2324. 13 (8), 1–49. doi:10.1080/15592324.2018.1460048.

Ercal, N., Gurer-Orhan, H., Aykin-Burns, N., 2001. Toxic metals and oxidative stress part I: mechanisms involved in metal-induced oxidative damage. Curr. Top. Med. Chem. 1568-0266. 1 (6), 529–539. doi:10.2174/1568026013394831.

Fatima, G., Raza, A.M., Dhole, P., 2025. Heavy metal exposure and its health implications: a comprehensive review. Indian J. Clin. Biochem. 0974-0422. 41 (2), 152–180. Available from: https://www.springer.com/journal/12291. doi:10.1007/s12291-025-01322-3.

Fenton, H.J.H., 1894. LXXIII.—oxidation of tartaric acid in presence of iron. J. Chem. Soc. Trans. 0368-1645. 65, 899–910. doi:10.1039/CT8946500899.

Festa, R.A., Thiele, D.J., 2011. Copper: an essential metal in biology. Curr. Biol. 0960-9822. 21 (21), R877. Available from: http://www.elsevier.com/journals/current-biology/0960-9822. doi:10.1016/j.cub.2011.09.040.

Filipič, M., 2012. Mechanisms of cadmium induced genomic instability. Mutat. Res. Fundam. Mol. Mech. Mutagen. 1386-1964. 733 (1–2), 69–77. doi:10.1016/j.mrfmmm.2011.09.002.

Forouhar Vajargah, M., Mohamadi Yalsuyi, A., Sattari, M., Hedayati, A., 2018. Acute toxicity effect of glyphosate on survival rate of common carp, Cyprinus carpio. Environ. Health Eng. Manag. 2423-3765. 5 (2), 61–66. doi:10.15171/ehem.2018.09.

Fu, Z., Xi, S., 2020. The effects of heavy metals on human metabolism. Toxicol. Mech. Methods 1537-6524. 30 (3), 167–176. Available from: http://www.tandfonline.com/loi/itxm20. doi:10.1080/15376516.2019.1701594.

Ghosh, S., Dey, S., Mandal, A.H., Sadhu, A., Saha, N.C., Barceló, D., Pastorino, P., Saha, S., 2025b. Exploring the ecotoxicological impacts of microplastics on freshwater fish: a critical review. J. Contam. Hydrol. 1873-6009. 269. Available from: https://www.sciencedirect.com/science/journal/01697722. doi:10.1016/j.jconhyd.2025.104514.

Ghosh, S., Sadhu, A., Mandal, A.H., Biswas, J.K., Sarkar, D., Saha, S., 2025a. Copper oxide nanoparticles as an emergent threat to aquatic invertebrates and photosynthetic organisms: a synthesis of the known and exploration of the unknown. Curr. Pollut. Rep. 2198-6592. 11 (1). Available from: https://www.springer.com/journal/40726. doi:10.1007/s40726-024-00334-6.

Ghosh, S., Sadhu, A., Mandal, A.H., Dey, S., Saha, N.C. and Saha, S., 2025. Metabolomics profiling and hazard prediction of spinosyn-based agricultural products: A computational approach. Sci. Total Environ. 959, 178279. doi:10.1016/j.scitotenv.2024.178279.

Haber, F., Weiss, J., 1934. The catalytic decomposition of hydrogen peroxide by iron salts. Proc. R. Soc. Lond. A Math. Phys. Sci. 147 (861), 332–351. doi:10.1098/rspa.1934.0221.

Hameed, M., Dijoo, Z.K., Bhat, R.A., Qayoom, I., 2020. Concerns and threats of heavy metals' contamination on aquatic ecosystem. In: Bhat, R.A., Hakeem, K.R. (Eds.), Bioremediation and Biotechnology: Techniques for Noxious Substances Remediation, vol. 4. Springer International Publishing, India, pp. 1–19. doi:10.1007/978-3-030-48690-7_1.

Hartwig, A., 1994. Role of DNA repair inhibition in lead- and cadmium-induced genotoxicity: a review. Environ. Health Perspect. 0091-6765. 102 (suppl 3), 45–50. doi:10.1289/ehp.94102s345.

Hartwig, A., Asmuss, M., Ehleben, I., Herzer, U., Kostelac, D., Pelzer, A., Schwerdtle, T., Bürkle, A., 2002. Interference by toxic metal ions with DNA repair processes and cell cycle control: molecular mechanisms. Environ. Health Perspect. 0091-6765. 110 (suppl 5), 797–799. doi:10.1289/ehp.02110s5797.

Hasan, M.K., Cheng, Y., Kanwar, M.K., Chu, X.Y., Ahammed, G.J., Qi, Z.Y., 2017. Responses of plant proteins to heavy metal stress—a review. Front. Plant Sci. 1664-462X. 8. Available from: http://journal.frontiersin.org/article/10.3389/fpls.2017.01492/full. doi:10.3389/fpls.2017.01492.

Henkel, G., Krebs, B., 2004. Metallothioneins: zinc, cadmium, mercury, and copper thiolates and selenolates mimicking protein active site features—structural aspects and biological implications. Chem. Rev. 104 (2), 801–824. doi:10.1021/cr020620d.

Jaishankar, M., Tseten, T., Anbalagan, N., Mathew, B.B., Beeregowda, K.N., 2014. Toxicity, mechanism and health effects of some heavy metals. Interdiscip. Toxicol. 1337-9569. 7 (2), 60–72. Available from: http://versita.com/science/medicine/it/. doi:10.2478/intox-2014-0009.

Jarup, L., 2003. Hazards of heavy metal contamination. Br. Med. Bull. 68, 167–182. Find this article online.

Jha, A.N., 2004. Genotoxicological studies in aquatic organisms: an overview. Mutat. Res. Fundam. Mol. Mech. Mutagen. 0027-5107. 552 (1-2), 1–17. doi:10.1016/j.mrfmmm.2004.06.034.

Jomova, K., Valko, M., 2011. Advances in metal-induced oxidative stress and human disease. Toxicology. 0300-483X. 283 (2–3), 65–87. doi:10.1016/j.tox.2011.03.001.

Kaur, R., Sharma, S., Kaur, H., 2019. Heavy metals toxicity and the environment. J. Pharmacogn. Phytochem. 1, 247–249.

Kim, J.J., Kim, Y.S., Kumar, V., 2019. Heavy metal toxicity: an update of chelating therapeutic strategies. J. Trace Elem. Med. Biol. 1878-3252. 54, 226–231. Available from: www.urban-fischer.de/journals/jtraceelm/trace.htm. doi:10.1016/j.jtemb.2019.05.003.

Kishore, D., Shubhajit, S., Chukwuka, A.V., Chandra, S.N., 2022. Behavioural toxicity and respiratory distress in early life and adult stage of walking catfish Clarias batrachus (Linnaeus) under acute fluoride exposures. Toxicol. Environ. Health Sci. 2233-7784. 14 (1), 33–46. Available from: www.springer.com/journal/13530. doi:10.1007/s13530-021-00115-4.

Kocadal, K., Alkas, F.B., Battal, D., Saygi, S., 2020. Cellular pathologies and genotoxic effects arising secondary to heavy metal exposure: a review. Hum. Exp. Toxicol. 0960-3271. 39 (1), 3–13. doi:10.1177/0960327119874439.

Kocyigit, U.M., Taslimi, P., Gulçin, İ., 2018. Characterization and inhibition effects of some metal ions on carbonic anhydrase enzyme from Kangal Akkaraman sheep. J. Biochem. Mol. Toxicol. 1099-0461. 32 (8). Available from: http://onlinelibrary.wiley.com/journal/10.1002/(ISSN)1099-0461. doi:10.1002/jbt.22172.

Kucuk, M., Gulcin, I., 2016. Purification and characterization of the carbonic anhydrase enzyme from Black Sea trout (Salmo trutta Labrax Coruhensis) kidney and inhibition effects of some metal ions on enzyme activity. Environ. Toxicol. Pharmacol. 1872-7077. 44, 134–139. Available from: www.elsevier.com/locate/etap. doi:10.1016/j.etap.2016.04.011.

Lionetto, M.G., Caricato, R., Giordano, M.E., Erroi, E., Schettino, T., 2012. Carbonic anhydrase and heavy metals. In: Biochemistry, first ed. Intech, Rijeka, pp. 205–224.

Madkour, L.H., 2020. Reactive Oxygen Species (ROS), Nanoparticles, and Endoplasmic Reticulum (ER) Stress-Induced Cell Death Mechanisms. Elsevier, Egypt, pp. 1–753. Available from: https://www.elsevier.com/books/reactive-oxygen-species-ros-nanoparticles-and-endoplasmic-reticulum-er-stress-induced-cell-death-mechanisms/madkour/978-0-12-822481-6. doi:10.1016/C2019-0-04102-7.

Mahurpawar, M., 2015. Effects of heavy metals on human health. Int J Res Granthaalayah. 530 (516), 1–7.

Mandal, A.H., Ghosh, S., Adhurjya, D., Chatterjee, P., Samajdar, I., Mukherjee, D., Dhara, K., Saha, N.C., Piccione, G., Multisanti, C.R., Saha, S., Faggio, C., 2024. Exploring the impact of zinc oxide nanoparticles on fish and fish-food organisms: a review. Aquac. Rep. 2352-5134. 36. Available from: https://www.sciencedirect.com/science/journal/23525134. doi:10.1016/j.aqrep.2024.102038.

Mandal, A.H., Sadhu, A., Ghosh, S., Acharya, D., Ghosh, K., Saha, N.C. and Saha, S., 2026. Evaluation of acetamiprid toxicity on tubifex tubifex: cytotoxic, physiological, histopathological, and ultrastructural approach. Sci. Total Environ. 1014, 181293. doi:10.1016/j.scitotenv.2025.181293.

Mandal, A.H., Sadhu, A., Ghosh, S., Saha, N.C., Mossotto, C., Pastorino, P., Saha, S., Faggio, C., 2025b. Evaluating the impact of neonicotinoids on aquatic non-target species: a comprehensive review. Environ. Toxicol. Pharmacol. 1872-7077. 113. Available from: https://www.sciencedirect.com/science/journal/13826689. doi:10.1016/j.etap.2024.104606.

Mandal, A.H., Sadhu, A., Ghosh, S., Saha, N.C., Saha, S., 2025a. Carbonsulfan-induced physiological, histopathological, and ultrastructural alterations in tubifex tubifex (müller, 1774). Sci. Rep. 2045-2322. 15 (1). Available from: https://www.nature.com/srep/. doi:10.1038/s41598-025-11463-3.

Mishra, S., Dwivedi, S.P., Singh, R.B., 2010. A review on epigenetic effect of heavy metal carcinogens on human health. Open Nutraceuticals J. 1876-3960. 3 (1), 188–193. doi:10.2174/18763960010030100188.

Moulis, J.M., 2010. Cellular mechanisms of cadmium toxicity related to the homeostasis of essential metals. BioMetals. 0966-0844. 23 (5), 877–896. Available from: www.wkap.nl/journalhome.htm/0966-0844. doi:10.1007/s10534-010-9336-y.

Mukherjee, D., Ghosh, S., Mandal, A.H., Saha, N.C., Faggio, C., Pastorino, P., Saha, S., 2025. Silent threats beneath the surface: unraveling the impact of organophosphate toxicity on fish. Sci. Total Environ. 1879-1026. 985. Available from: https://www.sciencedirect.com/science/journal/00489697. doi:10.1016/j.scitotenv.2025.179725.

Musah, B.I., 2025. Effects of heavy metals and metalloids on plant-animal interaction and biodiversity of terrestrial ecosystems—an overview. Environ. Monit. Assess. 1573-2959. 197 (1). Available from: https://www.springer.com/journal/10661. doi:10.1007/s10661-024-13490-5.

Nawab, J., Ghani, J., Khan, S., Khan, M.A., Ali, A., Rahman, Z., Alam, M., Hesham, A.E.L., Lei, M., 2022. Nutrient uptake and plant growth under the influence of toxic elements. In: Mahmood, Q. (Ed.), Sustainable Plant Nutrition under Contaminated Environments. Springer, pp. 75–101. doi:10.1007/978-3-030-91499-8_5.

Niekerk, L.A., Gokul, A., Basson, G., Badiwe, M., Nkomo, M., Klein, A., Keyster, M., 2024. Heavy metal stress and mitogen activated kinase transcription factors in plants: exploring heavy metal-ROS influences on plant signalling pathways. Plant Cell Environ. 1365-3040. 47 (8), 2793–2810. Available from: http://onlinelibrary.wiley.com/journal/10.1111/(ISSN)1365-3040. doi:10.1111/pce.14926.

Nurchi, V.M., Cappai, R., Crisponi, G., Sanna, G., Alberti, G., Biesuz, R., Gama, S., 2020. Chelating agents in soil remediation: a new method for a pragmatic choice of the right chelator. Front. Chem. 2296-2646. 8. Available from: http://journal.frontiersin.org/journal/chemistry. doi:10.3389/fchem.2020.597400.

Okieke, O., 2017. Effect of Food Chain Mediated Exposure to Cadmium and Arsenic on Some Oxidative Stress Markers in Rat Models. Delta State University, Abraka.

Ondrasek, G., Shepherd, J., Rathod, S., Dharavath, R., Rashid, M.I., Brtnicky, M., Shahid, M.S., Horvatinec, J., Rengel, Z., 2025. Metal contamination—a global environmental issue: sources, implications & advances in mitigation. RSC Adv. 2046-2069. 15 (5), 3904–3927. Available from: http://pubs.rsc.org/en/journals/journal/ra. doi:10.1039/d4ra04639k.

Oros, A., Coatu, V., Damir, N., Danilov, D., Ristea, E., Lazar, L., 2025. Molecular mechanisms and biomarker-based early-warning indicators of heavy metal toxicity in marine fish. Fishes. 2410-3888. 10 (7). Available from: www.mdpi.com/journal/fishes/. doi:10.3390/fishes10070339.

Papsdorf, K., Richter, K., 2014. Protein folding, misfolding and quality control: the role of molecular chaperones. Essays Biochem. 0071-1365. 56 (1), 53–68. Available from: http://essays.biochemistry.org/bsessays/056/0053/0560053.pdf. doi:10.1042/BSE0560053.

Parida, L., Patel, T.N., 2023. Systemic impact of heavy metals and their role in cancer development: a review. Environ. Monit. Assess. 1573-2959. 195 (6). Available from: https://www.springer.com/journal/10661. doi:10.1007/s10661-023-11399-z.

Piwowarska, D., Kiedrzyńska, E., Jaszczyszyn, K., 2024. A global perspective on the nature and fate of heavy metals polluting water ecosystems, and their impact and remediation. Crit. Rev. Environ. Sci. Technol. 1547-6537. 54 (19), 1436–1458. Available from: www.tandf.co.uk/journals/titles/10643389.asp. doi:10.1080/10643389.2024.2317112.

Rana, S.V.S., 2020. Endoplasmic reticulum stress induced by toxic elements—a review of recent developments. Biol. Trace Elem. Res. 0163-4984. 196 (1), 10–19. doi:10.1007/s12011-019-01903-3.

Sabullah, M.K., Ahmad, S.A., Shukor, M.Y., Gansau, A.J., Syed, M.A., Sulaiman, M.R., Shamaan, N.A., 2015. Heavy metal biomarker: fish behavior, cellular alteration, enzymatic reaction and proteomics approaches. Int. Food Res. J. 2231-7546. 22 (2), 435–454. Available from: http://www.ifrj.upm.edu.my/22%20(02)%202015/(2).pdf.

Sadhu, A., Ghosh, S., Mandal, A.H., Chatterjee, S., Saha, N.C., Biswas, J.K. and Saha, S., 2026. Toxicological profile of titanium dioxide nanoparticles: properties, production and potential toxic effects on non-target aquatic organisms. Water Air Soil Pollut. 237 (9). doi:10.1007/s11270-026-09165-1.

Sadhu, A., Ghosh, S., Mandal, A.H., Nayak, S., Saha, N.C., Mitra, A., Saha, S., 2025. Effects of covid-19 pandemic on blue economy in India: impacts, opportunities and challenges. Proc. Zool. Soc. 0974-6919. 78 (3), 251–266. Available from: https://www.springer.com/journal/12595. doi:10.1007/s12595-025-00580-6.

Sadhu, A., Mandal, A.H., Ghosh, S., Lakdawala, P., Saha, S., 2024. Dimethoate-induced toxicity: a comprehensive review of its aquatic environmental hazards. Toxicol. Environ. Health Sci. 2233-7784. 16 (3), 243–258. Available from: https://www.springer.com/journal/13530. doi:10.1007/s13530-024-00228-6.

Saha, N.C., Chatterjee, A., Banerjee, P., Bhattacharya, R., Sadhu, A., Pastorino, P., Saha, S., 2024a. Toxic effects of lead exposure on freshwater climbing perch, anabas testudineus, and bioremediation using ocimum sanctum leaf powder. Toxics. 2305-6304. 12 (12). Available from: http://www.mdpi.com/journal/toxics. doi:10.3390/toxics12120927.

Saha, S., Chukwuka, A.V., Mukherjee, D., Patnaik, L., Nayak, S., Dhara, K., Saha, N.C., Faggio, C., 2021. Chronic effects of diazinon exposures using integrated biomarker responses in freshwater walking catfish, Clarias batrachus. Appl. Sci. 2076-3417. 11 (22), 10902. doi:10.3390/app112210902.

Saha, S., Dhara, K., Chukwuka, A.V., Pal, P., Saha, N.C., Faggio, C., 2023. Sub-lethal acute effects of environmental concentrations of inorganic mercury on hematological and biochemical parameters in walking catfish, Clarias batrachus. Comp. Biochem. Physiol. C Toxicol. Pharmacol. 1878-1659. 264. Available from: https://www.journals.elsevier.com/comparative-biochemistry-and-physiology-part-c-toxicology-and-pharmacology. doi:10.1016/j.cbpc.2022.109511.

Saha, S., Dhara, K., Pal, P., Saha, N.C., Faggio, C. and Chukwuka, A.V., 2023. Longer-term adverse effects of selenate exposures on hematological and serum biochemical variables in air-breathing fish channa punctata (Bloch, 1973) and non-air breathing fish ctenopharyngodon idella (Cuvier, 1844): an integrated Biomarker Response Approach. Biol. Trace. Elem. Res. 201 (7), 3497–3512. doi:10.1007/s12011-022-03449-3.

Saha, S., Mukherjee, D., Dhara, K., Saha, N.C., 2020. Captan-induced toxicity and behavioural alterations on oligochaete worm, Branchiura sowerbyi. J. Aquat. Biol. Fish. 8, 37–40.

Saha, S., Saha, S., Mistri, A., Saha, N.C., 2024b. Antioxidant enzyme activity and pathophysiological consequences in the sludge worm Tubifex tubifex under acute and sub-lethal exposures to the fungicide Tilt. Pestic. Biochem. Physiol. 1095-9939. 198. Available from: https://www.sciencedirect.com/science/journal/00483575. doi:10.1016/j.pestbp.2023.105738.

Saha, S., Saha, S., Pastorino, P., Saha, N.C., 2025. Effects of difenoconazole on tubifex tubifex: antioxidant activity, insights from GUTS predictions, and multi-biomarker analysis. Biology. 2079-7737. 14 (3). Available from: www.mdpi.com/journal/biology. doi:10.3390/biology14030302.

Samajdar, I., Saha, S., Mandal, D.K., 2023. Chlorpyrifos induced oxidative stress responses and alteration of acetylcholinesterase activity in the olfactory organ of freshwater minor carp, Labeo bata. Iranian J. Ichthyol. 2383-0964. 10 (4), 248–263. Available from: https://www.ijichthyol.org/index.php/iji/article/view/998/677. doi:10.22034/iji.v10i4.998.

Sharma, P., Saha, S., Chatterjee, S., Mandal, A.H., Ghosh, S., Saha, N.C., Piccione, G., Impellitteri, F., Faggio, C., 2025. Toxicological and physiological impact and bioremediation strategies for polycyclic aromatic hydrocarbons (PAHs). Chem. Ecol. 1029-0370. 41 (6), 843–866. Available from: www.tandf.co.uk/journals/titles/02757540.asp. doi:10.1080/02757540.2025.2490035.

Sytar, O., Kumar, A., Latowski, D., Kuczynska, P., Strzałka, K., Prasad, M.N.V., 2013. Heavy metal-induced oxidative damage, defense reactions, and detoxification mechanisms in plants. Acta Physiol. Plant. 0137-5881. 35 (4), 985–999. Available from: https://rd.springer.com/journal/11738. doi:10.1007/s11738-012-1169-6.

Tabassum, Jeena, A.S., Pandey, D., 2021. Metal induced genotoxicity and oxidative stress in plants, assessment methods, and role of various factors in genotoxicity regulation. In: Khan, Z., Ansari, M.Y.K, Shahwar, D. (Eds.), Induced Genotoxicity and Oxidative Stress in Plants. Singapore, Springer Nature, pp. 133–149. doi:10.1007/978-981-16-2074-4_5.

Tamás, M.J., Sharma, S.K., Ibstedt, S., Jacobson, T., Christen, P., 2014. Heavy metals and metalloids as a cause for protein misfolding and aggregation. Biomolecules. 2218-273X. 4 (1), 252–267. doi:10.3390/biom4010252.

Tchounwou, P.B., Yedjou, C.G., Patlolla, A.K., Sutton, D.J., 2012. Heavy metal toxicity and the environment. In: Molecular, Clinical and Environmental Toxicology: Volume 3: Environmental Toxicology. Experientia Supplementum, vol. 101. Springer, Basel, pp. 133–164. doi:10.1007/978-3-7643-8340-4_6.

Trivedi, P.C., Bartlett, J.J., Pulinilkunnil, T., 2020. Lysosomal biology and function: modern view of cellular debris bin. Cells. 2073-4409. 9 (5). doi:10.3390/cells9051131.

Vajargah, M.F., 2021. A review on the effects of heavy metals on aquatic animals. J. Biomed. Res. Environ. Sci. 2766-2276. 2 (9), 865–869. doi:10.37871/jbres1324.

Vidal, A.C., Semenova, V., Darrah, T., Vengosh, A., Huang, Z., King, K., Nye, M.D., Fry, R., Skaar, D., Maguire, R., Murtha, A., Schildkraut, J., Murphy, S., Hoyo, C., 2015. Maternal cadmium, iron and zinc levels, DNA methylation and birth weight. BMC Pharmacol. Toxicol. 2050-6511. 16 (1). Available from: http://www.biomedcentral.com/bmcpharmacoltoxicol/. doi:10.1186/s40360-015-0020-2.

Waalkes, M.P., Fox, D.A., States, J.C., Patierno, S.R., McCabe, M.J., 2000. Metals and disorders of cell accumulation: modulation of apoptosis and cell proliferation. Toxicol. Sci. 1096-6080. 56 (2), 255–261. Available from: http://toxsci.oxfordjournals.org/. doi:10.1093/toxsci/56.2.255.

Wang, Y., Noman, A., Zhang, C., AL-Bukhaiti, W.Q., Abed, S.M., 2024. Effect of fish-heavy metals contamination on the generation of reactive oxygen species and its implications on human health: a review. Front. Mar. Sci. 2296-7745. 11. Available from: https://www.frontiersin.org/journals/marine-science#. doi:10.3389/fmars.2024.1500870.

White, B., 2005. Analysis of 8 oxo 7, 8-dihydroGuanine formation and oxidation mediated by Fenton reaction induced DNA oxidative stress. Dublin, Dublin City University. Available from: https://doras.dcu.ie/18276/1/Bl%C3%A0naid_White.pdf.

Wise, S.S., Wise, J.P., 2012. Chromium and genomic stability. Mutat. Res. Fundam. Mol. Mech. Mutagen. 0921-8262. 733 (1–2), 78–82. doi:10.1016/j.mrfmmm.2011.12.002.

Witkowska, D., Słowik, J., Chilicka, K., 2021. Heavy metals and human health: possible exposure pathways and the competition for protein binding sites. Molecules. 1420-3049. 26 (19), 6060. doi:10.3390/molecules26196060.

Wu, X., Cobbina, S.J., Mao, G., Xu, H., Zhang, Z., Yang, L., 2016. A review of toxicity and mechanisms of individual and mixtures of heavy metals in the environment. Environ. Sci. Pollut. Res. 1614-7499. 23 (9), 8244–8259. Available from: http://www.springerlink.com/content/0944-1344. doi:10.1007/s11356-016-6333-x.

Chapter 21

Metal-binding proteins in toxicodynamics: Functional roles of metalloproteins and metallochaperones

S. Sharma and A. Bobbili
Amity Institute of Food Technology, Amity University, Noida, Uttar Pradesh, India

21.1 Introduction

21.1.1 Metalloprotein: Structure, function and application

Metalloproteins constitute nearly one-third to one-half of all known proteins, highlighting their essential contributions to biological systems and accounting for an estimated **30%–50% of all known proteins.** Their ubiquity across all domains of life reflects the indispensable roles played by metal ions in supporting biochemical reactions, structural rigidity, electron transport, signal transduction, and gene regulation (Waldron et al., 2009b). Metalloproteins, along with many of the most intricate and vital biological functions—including photosynthesis, respiration, water splitting, oxygen reduction, and nitrogen fixation—are carried out by their metal-binding centres. Applying this knowledge to develop new metalloproteins that can mimic the structures and functions of their natural counterparts is currently the main challenge (Barker, 2003; Lu et al., 2001; Lu, 2006). Many proteins rely on metal ions to maintain and stabilise their structural framework (Miller et al., 1985; Tan et al., 2014). To directly participate in the metabolic activities they catalyse, others require metal ions (Bellomo et al., 2014; Rowlett, 2014). The biological functions of metalloproteins can be signalled or mediated by participating in bimetallic (two metal ions involved) or multimetallic (more than two metal ions involved) interactions. In recent years, some biomedical applications have been developed, but they are restricted to Fe or Co bimetallic complexes or ortho- and para-complexes of metalloporphyrins or metallosapphyrins (Jeong et al., 2023). Metalloprotein research began in the 19th century when haemoglobin, one of the first structurally and functionally defined examples of a metal-dependent biological macromolecule, was

The Metallome in Motion. https://doi.org/10.1016/B978-0-443-44299-5.00020-1

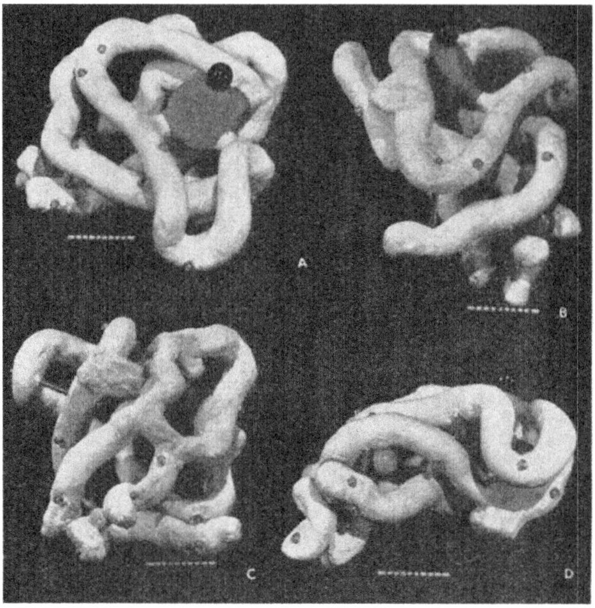

FIG. 21.1 Three-dimensional model of the myoglobin molecule obtained by X-ray analysis (Kendrew et al., 1958).

identified as an iron-coordinating protein responsible for reversible oxygen binding and transport in vertebrate blood (Sheftel et al., 2013). The development of X-ray crystallography (Fig. 21.1) 1950s marked a fundamental advancement in modern structural understanding. The conceptual framework of metal–protein interactions was drastically altered when the first atomic-resolution structures of myoglobin (1958) and haemoglobin (1960) revealed the exact coordination geometry of heme-bound iron. These seminal findings shifted the field's focus from primarily biochemical description to meticulous molecular and electronic mechanistic investigation (Shi, 2014).

Interest in metalloproteins has increased dramatically over the last thirty years, coinciding with rapid developments in contemporary analytical methods that enable thorough investigation of the connections between their structures and functions. Many new areas within the bioinorganic chemistry of metalloproteins are anticipated to grow even more as the need for metalloprotein-focused research rises, especially in the creation of new medicinal agents and remedies for environmental problems (Kunkle and Skaar, 2023). Because of the complex interactions resulting from their coordinating surroundings and ligand field effects, biomolecules' dynamic trajectories frequently differ significantly from those deduced from bulk data. In this regard, the quest for a thorough understanding of metalloproteins may approach a theoretical complexity comparable to the traditional "three-body problem" in celestial mechanics, where the interdependent forces make accurate prediction extremely difficult (Andreini et al., 2022).

In its broadest definition, bioinorganic chemistry is the study of the interactions between biological molecules and inorganic substances. The function of metals in biochemical systems is a major area of study. Bioinorganic chemistry has historically been separated into two primary areas. The first examines the metabolic processing of harmful inorganic species, as well as the role, uptake, transport, and final destiny of vital biological components, such as transition metal ions and metalloids. The creation and use of metal-based medicines, diagnostic tools, metal tracers for tissue imaging, and contrast agents for magnetic resonance imaging comprise the second domain (Zhang et al., 2022).

21.1.1.1 Structure and functions of metalloproteins

Proteins that include one or more metal ions as cofactors necessary for their structural integrity or biological activity are known as metalloproteins. This class includes a sizable fraction of all proteins. Zinc-binding domains are present in at least 1000 of the roughly 20,000 proteins in the human proteome; however, the total number of zinc-dependent metalloproteins is thought to be as high as 3000 (Banci, 2013). With a primary focus on metalloproteins, the molecular structures and related functional activities of biological macromolecules that bind metals have been extensively studied (Rosato et al., 2016). In metalloproteins, donor atoms like nitrogen, oxygen, or sulfur that come from amino acid residues inside the protein usually coordinate metal ions. The side chains of particular amino acids are most frequently responsible for these coordinating groups. Among these, the carboxylate group of aspartate residues, the thiolate group of cysteine residues, and the imidazole group of histidine residues are especially crucial for metal binding (Cangelosi et al., 2017). One or more metal ions are thought to be present in about half of all proteins. According to other estimates, between 25% and 33% of all proteins need metal ions in order to function biologically. As a result, metalloproteins are involved in many different physiological functions, such as signal transduction, enzymatic catalysis, host-pathogen interactions linked to infectious illnesses, and metal storage and transport (Carver, 2013). Due to the pivotal activities they undertake, interest in examining the structural features of metal-binding biological macromolecules and their complexes with substrates, inhibitors, and metal ions has expanded considerably (Anandhan et al., 2025). Metals have unique spectroscopic properties that are fundamentally different from those of organic groups. This has been widely utilized at many different spatial scales, from the macroscopic level to the atomic size. Clarifying the structures of biomolecules has advanced significantly, especially in relation to their cooperative, dynamic, and multiscale behaviors; further developments in this area are expected in the future (Doroudian and Gailer, 2022).

Metalloproteins that have one or more metal ions as essential parts of their structure or function are known as metalloproteins. These metal ions may stabilize protein structure, promote electron transport, control biological activity, or directly engage in enzymatic catalysis (Bertini et al., 1994; Lippard and Berg , 1984). Metalloproteins are categorized based on a variety of factors, such as the kind of metal ion, nature of the prosthetic group or metal cluster, biological function, manner of metal binding, and coordination environment, due to the great diversity of metal ions and biological roles (Messerschmidt et al., 2001). Because of their various oxidation states and coordination flexibility, which allow for redox chemistry and catalytic activity, transition metals like iron, copper, zinc, manganese, cobalt, nickel, and molybdenum are often involved (Bertini et al., 1994; Crichton, 2019). While copper proteins are mostly linked to oxidative catalysis and electron transfer, iron-containing proteins are crucial for oxygen transport, electron transfer, and metabolism (Solomon et al., 2014). While manganese, cobalt, nickel, and molybdenum are essential elements of specialized metabolic enzymes, zinc proteins frequently aid in structural stabilization and hydrolytic catalysis (Ragsdale, 2009; Hille, 1996). Table 21.1 illustrates the classification of metalloproteins based on metal ion, biological function, mode of metal binding, and coordination environment.

21.1.1.2 Application of metalloproteins

Considering their unique ability to utilize the chemical characteristics of metal ions, metalloproteins are essential components of biological, medicinal, industrial, and environmental systems. Functions, which include redox chemistry, substrate activation, electron transfer, and structural stabilization are made possible by the presence of metal cofactors and cannot be effectively carried out by purely organic proteins (Bertini et al., 1994; Lippard and Berg, 1994). As a result, metalloproteins have found extensive use in industrial catalysis, biotechnology, medicine, and environmental cleanup (Table 21.2).

21.2 Metallochaperones: Structure, classification and applications

A unique class of metal-binding proteins called metallochaperones helps move metal ions safely and selectively inside cells. In contrast to metalloproteins, which directly use metal ions for structural or catalytic functions, metallochaperones are mostly involved in metal transport and trafficking, making sure that necessary metals get to their proper cellular locations while avoiding toxicity (O'Halloran and Culotta, 2000a; Robinson and Winge, 2010). Although transition metals like copper, zinc, iron, manganese, and nickel are essential for biological metabolism, their presence as free ions can be extremely hazardous. As a result, free metal pools are essentially nonexistent, and intracellular metal concentrations are strictly controlled. By binding metals as soon as they are absorbed and delivering them straight to particular target proteins through regulated protein–protein interactions, metallochaperones are essential to this regulation (Waldron and Robinson, 2009a). By exerting kinetic control over

TABLE 21.1 Classification of metalloproteins with examples.

Basis of classification	Class/category	Key characteristics	Representative examples	References
Type of metal ion	**Iron (Fe) metalloproteins**	Redox activity, oxygen binding, electron transfer	Hemoglobin, myoglobin, cytochromes, ferritin, catalase	(Bertini et al., 1994; Nelson and Cox, 2021)
	Copper (Cu) metalloproteins	Electron transfer, oxygen activation	Plastocyanin, azurin, ceruloplasmin, hemocyanin	(Solomon et al., 2014)
	Zinc (Zn) metalloproteins	Structural stabilization and catalysis	Carbonic anhydrase, carboxypeptidase, zinc-finger proteins	(Vallee and Auld, 1990; Klug, 2010)
	Manganese (Mn) metalloproteins	Redox reactions, photosynthetic oxygen evolution	Mn-superoxide dismutase, oxygen-evolving complex (PSII)	(Yano and Yachandra, 2014)
	Cobalt (Co) metalloproteins	Cobalamin-dependent catalysis	Vitamin B_{12} enzymes, methionine synthase	(Marsh, 1999)
	Nickel (Ni) metalloproteins	Hydrolysis and redox metabolism (mostly microbial)	Urease, Ni–Fe hydrogenase	(Ragsdale, 2009)
	Molybdenum (Mo) metalloproteins	Redox metabolism	Xanthine oxidase, nitrate reductase	(Hille, 1996)
	Calcium (Ca) metalloproteins	Signaling, conformational regulation	Calmodulin, troponin C, cadherins	(Kretsinger, 1976)
	Magnesium (Mg) metalloproteins	ATP binding, enzyme activation	Kinases, DNA/RNA polymerases	(Cowan, 2002)

Continued

Table 21.1 Classification of metalloproteins with examples—cont'd

Basis of classification	Class/category	Key characteristics	Representative examples	References
Prosthetic group/cluster	**Heme proteins**	Iron–porphyrin prosthetic group	Hemoglobin, cytochrome P450, peroxidases	(Ortiz de Montellano, 2015)
	Iron–sulphur proteins	[2Fe–2S], [4Fe–4S] clusters for ET	Ferredoxin, aconitase, nitrogenase	(Beinert et al., 1997; Johnson et al., 2005)
	Blue copper proteins	Unique Cu coordination, high ET efficiency	Plastocyanin, azurin	(Solomon et al., 2014)
	Zinc finger proteins	Zn stabilizes DNA/RNA-binding motifs	TFIIIA, nuclear receptors	(Klug, 2010)
Biological function	**Metalloenzymes**	Metal directly involved in catalysis	Carbonic anhydrase (Zn), urease (Ni), nitrogenase (Fe/Mo)	(Lippard and Berg, 1994)
	Electron transfer proteins	Shuttle electrons in metabolism	Cytochromes, ferredoxins	(Gray and Winkler, 1996)
	Oxygen transport/ storage proteins	Bind and transport oxygen	Hemoglobin, myoglobin, hemerythrin	(Nelson and Cox, 2021)
	Metal transport proteins	Transport metal ions	Transferrin, ceruloplasmin	(Andreini et al., 2009)
	Regulatory/signaling proteins	Metal-dependent activity regulation	Calmodulin (Ca^{2+}), Zn-finger TFs	(Kretsinger et al., 1976; Klug, 2010)

Mode of metal binding	**Tightly bound metals**	Integral, permanent metal binding	Carbonic anhydrase, nitrogenase	(Bertini et al., 1994)
	Loosely bound metals	Reversible, regulatory binding	Ca^{2+} in signaling proteins	(Nelson and Cox, 2021)
	Apo vs. holo forms	Metal-free vs. metal-bound forms	Apo-/holo-carbonic anhydrase	(Lippard and Berg, 1994)
Coordination environment	**Ligand type**	Cys, His, Asp, Glu coordination	Zn-fingers (Cys-rich), Cu enzymes (His-rich)	(Vallee and Auld, 1990)
	Coordination geometry	Determines metal reactivity	Tetrahedral (Zn), octahedral (Fe), square planar (Ni)	(Bertini et al., 1994)
	Polynuclear metal centres	Multiple metal ions act cooperatively	Mn_4Ca cluster (PSII), Ni–Fe hydrogenase	(Yano and Yachandra, 2014)

TABLE 21.2 Applications of metalloproteins with representative examples.

Application area	Role of metalloproteins	Representative metalloproteins/ examples	References
Physiological & biological functions	Oxygen transport and storage	Hemoglobin, myoglobin, hemocyanin	(Nelson and Cox, 2021)
	Electron transfer in metabolism	Cytochromes, ferredoxins, iron–sulphur proteins	(Beinert et al., 1997; Gray and Winkler, 1996)
	Detoxification of reactive oxygen species	Superoxide dismutase (Cu/Zn, Mn), catalase (Fe)	(McCord and Fridovich, 1988)
	Carbon dioxide metabolism	Carbonic anhydrase (Zn)	(Vallee and Auld, 1990)
Medical & pharmaceutical applications	Drug metabolism and detoxification	Cytochrome P450 enzymes	(Ortiz de Montellano, 2015)
	Therapeutic enzymes	Superoxide dismutase, catalase	(McCord and Fridovich, 1988)
	Disease biomarkers and drug targets	Matrix metalloproteinases (MMPs)	(Nagase et al., 2006)
	Blood substitutes	Hemoglobin-based oxygen carriers	(Winslow, 2000)
Biotechnology & industrial applications	Biocatalysis in chemical synthesis	Alcohol dehydrogenase, monooxygenases	(Sheldon and Woodley, 2018)
	Biofuel production	Hydrogenases, dehydrogenases	(Ragsdale, 2009)
	Food and detergent industries	Metalloproteases	(Rao et al., 1998)
Environmental applications	Bioremediation of pollutants	Laccases, peroxidases	(Claus, 2004)
	Phytoremediation	Phytochelatin synthase, metal-binding proteins	(Cobbett and Goldsbrough, 2002)
Agricultural applications	Biological nitrogen fixation	Nitrogenase (Fe/Mo)	(Howard and Rees, 2006)
	Soil nutrient cycling	Metalloenzymes in microbial metabolism	(Bertini et al., 1994)
Biosensing & diagnostics	Clinical and environmental biosensors	Glucose oxidase, horseradish peroxidase, cytochrome c	(Turner et al., 1987; Willner and Katz, 2000)
Nanotechnology & materials science	Nanoparticle synthesis and delivery	Ferritin nanocages	(Uchida et al., 2007)
	Bio-templated nanomaterials	Metalloprotein scaffolds	(Messerschmidt et al., 2001)

metalation and ensuring that metals reach their proper biological destinations before being sequestered or ejected, metallochaperones play a crucial role in this intracellular metal economy. Metallochaperones participate in hierarchical metal allocation networks instead of serving as passive carriers, giving priority to critical pathways under metal limitation and limiting access during metal excess (Waldron and Robinson, 2009a). Specialized intracellular proteins called metallochaperones bind metal ions and transport them to particular target proteins in a safe and targeted manner. Their main function is metal trafficking, which ensures that necessary metals get to the right metalloproteins without creating hazardous free metal pools, rather than metal storage or catalysis (O'Halloran and Culotta, 2000b). Table 21.3 illustrates the classification of metallochaperones.

21.2.1 Application of metallochaperones

Specialized intracellular proteins called metallochaperones bind and transfer metal ions to certain target proteins, guaranteeing precise metallation while averting metal-induced toxicity. They are used in biotechnology, toxicology, human health, and basic biological processes. Table 21.4 exhibits the main uses of metallochaperones.

21.3 Metalloprotein and metallochaperones: Functional role in toxicodynamic

Toxicodynamic refers to the biochemical, molecular, and cellular mechanisms by which toxic substances exert various adverse effects in the system. In pharmacology, it is sometimes confined to beneficial or therapeutic effects and diagnostics; they are also considered essential components in life processes. Likewise, in toxicology, it refers to adverse or injurious effects. In terms of metals and metalloids, toxicity is not governed solely by exposure but primarily by how they interact with bio-macromolecules. Metalloproteins and metallochaperones play a central role in regulating metal availability, distribution, reactivity, and cellular targets, thereby determining the nature and severity of metal-induced toxicity.

Metalloproteins play a major role by becoming direct targets for toxic metals or by serving as a crucial part of the body's defense and detoxification mechanisms. The toxicity mechanism involves the displacement of essential metals, the disruption of normal metalloproteins, interference with their synthesis, or the generation of oxidative stress.

- **Metal Ion Sequestration and Buffering (Detoxification** vs. **Retention)**: Metalloproteins, such as metallothioneins (MTs) bind metals like Cd, Hg, Zn, and Cu, etc., lowering free metal ion concentrations and reducing acute cellular damage. However, MT–metal complexes can alter metal distribution and lead to long biological half-lives (e.g., Cd-MT accumulation in the

TABLE 21.3 Classification of metallochaperones.

Class of metallochaperone	Metal ion handled	Representative metallochaperones	Major target proteins/pathways	Physiological role	Key references (within table)
Copper metallochaperones (cytosolic antioxidant pathway)	Cu^{+}	CCS	Cu/Zn Superoxide dismutase (SOD1)	Copper insertion and activation of antioxidant defense enzymes	(Culotta et al., 1997; Rae et al., 1999a)
Copper metallochaperones (secretory pathway)	Cu^{+}	Atox1	ATP7A, ATP7B (Golgi Cu-transporting ATPases)	Copper delivery to secreted and membrane-bound cuproenzymes	(Hamza et al., 2001a; Lutsenko, 2010)
Copper metallochaperones (mitochondrial respiration)	Cu^{+}	Cox17, Sco1, Sco2, Cox11	Cytochrome c oxidase (Complex IV)	Assembly of copper centers in the mitochondrial respiratory chain	(Horng et al., 2004; Cobine et al., 2006)
Iron–sulfur (Fe–S) cluster chaperones	Fe^{2+}/Fe–S clusters	IscU, Nfu1, Grx5	Aconitase, respiratory enzymes, and DNA repair proteins	Biogenesis and delivery of Fe–S clusters	(Lill and Freibert, 2020; Rouault and Maio, 2017)
Heme metallochaperones	Heme (Fe-protoporphyrin IX)	CcmE, HRG1, Hbp1	Cytochromes, hemoproteins	Heme trafficking and insertion into target proteins	(Kranz et al., 2009a)

Nickel metallochaperones	Ni^{2+}	HypA, HypB, UreE	[NiFe]-hydrogenase, Urease	Nickel delivery for metalloenzyme maturation	(Maier et al., 2007; Zambelli et al., 2011)
Zinc metallochaperones	Zn^{2+}	HypA, ZNG1	Zinc-dependent enzymes and transcription factors	Targeted zinc delivery and buffering	(Eide, 2011; Capdevila et al., 2017)
Manganese metallochaperones	Mn^{2+}	MtmA, PhpP-associated proteins	Mn-dependent SOD, kinases	Manganese homeostasis and enzyme activation	(Kehres and Maguire, 2003; Aswathy et al., 2009)
Cobalt metallochaperones	Co^{2+}	CobW, CobN	Vitamin B_{12} biosynthetic enzymes	Cobalt insertion during cobalamin synthesis	(Moore et al., 2013)
Molybdenum metallochaperones	Mo	MogA, MoeA	Molybdoenzymes (xanthine oxidase, nitrate reductase)	Molybdenum cofactor biosynthesis and delivery	(Schwarz et al., 2009; Hille et al., 2014)

TABLE 21.4 Application of metallochaperones.

Application area	Metal/ metallochaperone	Representative example	Application/role	References
Antioxidant defense	Cu—CCS	CCS-mediated copper delivery to Cu/Zn SOD1	Activates superoxide dismutase, reducing oxidative stress	(Culotta et al., 1997; Rae et al., 1999b)
Mitochondrial respiration	Cu—Cox17, Sco1, Sco2	Copper insertion into cytochrome *c* oxidase	Ensures proper assembly of respiratory Complex IV and ATP production	(Horng et al., 2004; Cobine et al., 2006)
Secretory pathway and copper homeostasis	Cu—Atox1	Copper delivery to ATP7A/ATP7B	Metallation of secreted cu-proenzymes and prevention of copper toxicity	(Hamza et al., 2001b; Lutsenko, 2010)
Iron–sulfur cluster biogenesis	Fe–S—IscU, Nfu1, Grx5	Assembly of Fe–S proteins	Maturation of enzymes involved in respiration and DNA repair	(Lill and Freibert, 2020; Rouault and Maio, 2017)
Heme trafficking and erythropoiesis	Heme—CcmE, HRG1	Heme delivery to hemoproteins	Supports hemoglobin synthesis and cytochrome function	(Kranz et al., 2009b; Hamza and Dailey, 2012)
Metalloenzyme activation in microbes	Ni—HypA, HypB	Nickel insertion into hydrogenase and urease	Enables functionality of key microbial enzymes	(Maier et al., 2007; Zambelli et al., 2011)
Zinc homeostasis and buffering	Zn—ZNG1, zinc chaperones	Zinc delivery to Zn-dependent enzymes	Maintains zinc balance and prevents metal toxicity	(Eide, 2011; Capdevila et al., 2017)
Neurodegenerative disease research	Cu—CCS, Atox1	Copper trafficking in neurons	Understanding mis-metallation in ALS and Alzheimer's disease	(Lutsenko, 2010; Tokuda et al., 2015)
Antimicrobial target development	Fe, Cu, Ni chaperones	Bacterial IscU, HypA	Disruption impairs pathogen survival and virulence	(Zambelli et al., 2011; Freibert and Lill, 2020)
Biotechnology and synthetic biology	Engineered metallochaperones	Controlled metal delivery systems	Improves folding and activity of recombinant metalloproteins	(Waldron and Robinson, 2009a)

gastrointestinal tract), which subsequently influence chronic toxicity. These proteins are rich in cysteine residues, which have a high affinity for heavy metals. They sequester these toxic metals in vital tissues such as the kidneys and liver; positively, they neutralize them and prevent their accumulation in the brain, which is the most sensitive organ.

- **Metal-induced oxidative stress**: The imbalance between the formation of free radicals and their elimination by defense systems is termed oxidative stress. Transition metal ions are key elements of various bio-processes that range from oxygen formation to sensing hypoxia, and hence, their homeostasis is maintained within limits through regulated mechanisms like uptake, storage, and secretion. Breakdown of metal homeostasis leads to the formation of reactive oxygen species (ROS) via the Fenton reaction, which produces hydroxyl radicals, and RNS (reactive nitrogen species), which can cause damage to bio-macromolecules such as DNA, proteins, and lipids.
- **Biomarkers:** Metalloproteins/Matrix metalloproteinases (MMPs) are a class of extracellular zinc peptidases involved in various processes, both physiological and pathological. These enzymes serve as excellent biomarkers for the identification of various diseases, including cancers and periodontitis. They also serve as prognostic markers, which help determine how much a disease has progressed. In addition, they are potential candidate biomarkers for conditions like type 2 diabetes mellitus (T2DM), such as ceruloplasmin.

Metallochaperones are small periplasmic proteins that act as metal carriers. They not only isolate toxic free metal ions but also ensure the correct delivery to their targets. However, some provide protection against multiple metals. Metallochaperones mitigate the toxicodynamics of essential and non-essential heavy metals by acting as highly specific intracellular carriers. They are involved in several key functions, such as maintaining homeostasis, preventing misallocations, minimizing oxidative stress, and facilitating transport for efflux. **Maintaining homeostasis and prevention of misevaluation: Chaperones ensure that metals like copper and zinc (essential metals) are delivered to their correct target proteins and to their proper cellular compartments. This mechanism is vital for many biological functions, such as antioxidant defense, respiration**, etc. **Proper allocation prevents metal dysregulation. Chaperones also prevent highly reactive metals, especially toxic ones like cadmium or lead, from binding to and inactivating incorrect proteins. This is a key aspect of preventing toxicity.**

- **Role in neuro-protection:** Chaperones primarily include target delivery, detoxification, and prevention of aggregation by controlling free metal concentrations, helping to prevent them from binding to and promoting the aggregation of pathological proteins. Metals like arsenic, copper, and zinc, which are toxic, are bound and buffered by metallothionein, hence acting as a defense mechanism. They ensure the precise delivery of metalloenzymes and allow them to function correctly.

- **Iron homeostasis: Excess iron accumulation and disturbance in balance lead to iron homeostasis, which can cause the formation of Fenton reactions, generate harmful free radicals, and promote the aggregation of proteins.** An imbalance in metal ions, whether excessive or insufficient, contributes to neuronal death through ferroptosis (an iron-dependent form of programmed cell death driven by iron-catalyzed accumulation), leading to oxidative damage and the collapse of cell membranes.

21.4 Challenges and future perspective of the functional role of metalloproteins and metallochaperones

As they control metal ion absorption, intracellular trafficking, utilization, and detoxification, metalloproteins and metallochaperones are essential to toxicodynamics. Toxic metals like cadmium, lead, mercury, and arsenic interfere with these well-controlled processes and have negative biological effects, whereas essential metals like iron, copper, zinc, and manganese are necessary for regular cellular function. Metal mimicry is one of the main obstacles to comprehending the function of metalloproteins and metallochaperones in toxicodynamics. Toxic metals can attach to metalloproteins inappropriately because they frequently have ionic radius and charge similarities to necessary metals. Cadmium, for instance, can take the place of zinc in zinc-finger transcription factors, changing gene expression and causing a decrease in DNA-binding capacity. Lead can also affect neuronal signaling by interfering with calcium-binding proteins. The mis-metallation of proteins is another significant problem. In situations of metal overload or toxic exposure, metallochaperones may unintentionally aid in the distribution of hazardous metals to delicate cellular compartments. Normally, metallochaperones guarantee targeted and secure metal transport. Enzyme inactivation, protein misfolding, and compromised cellular metabolism are the outcomes of this. Another issue is the redox activity of metals. ROS can be produced via Fenton and Haber-Weiss reactions involving iron and copper-containing metalloproteins. This process is made worse by toxic metals, which result in DNA damage, oxidative stress, lipid peroxidation, and mitochondrial dysfunction. It is still very difficult to distinguish between secondary oxidative damage and direct metal poisoning. Moreover, the mechanisms involved in metal homeostasis are intricately linked. Toxicodynamic reactions are complicated and systemic because disruption of one metal frequently impacts others. Developmental variations and tissue-specific metalloprotein expression further restrict the use of experimental results for risk assessment in human health.

According to recent research, metallochaperones serve as protective regulators of metal toxicity in addition to being metal carriers. Knowing their specific functions may enable targeted control to stop the buildup of hazardous metals and restore proper protein metallation. By providing real-time tracking of metal–protein interactions and metal fluxes within cells, emerging fields, including metallomics, metalloproteomics, and systems toxicology, are predicted to transform toxicodynamic research. These methods will replace conventional concentration-based evaluations in toxicology with mechanism-driven models based on metalloprotein functional disruption. Targeting metallochaperones presents interesting therapeutic approaches, such as enhanced cellular metal-buffering capacity, regulated chelation, and selective metal reprogramming. In addition to influencing metalloprotein stability, nutritional modification of necessary metals may lessen vulnerability to exposure to hazardous metals.

21.5 Conclusion

A vital link between metal exposure and biological reaction is represented by metalloproteins and metallochaperones. Emerging technologies in metallomics, systems biology, and molecular toxicology present an unprecedented opportunity to redefine toxicodynamics, despite the fact that their complexity presents significant experimental and interpretive obstacles. In order to establish metalloproteins and metallochaperones as both targets and instruments in toxicological science, future research should move away from metal-centric toxicity models and toward protein- and pathway-centric frameworks. Identifying metal-induced toxicity, as well as developing effective intervention techniques, necessitates an understanding of metalloproteins and metallochaperones. In general, comprehending metal-induced toxicity and creating effective preventive and therapeutic measures depend on clarifying the functions of metalloproteins and metallochaperones in toxicodynamics.

References

Anandhan, A., Jali, B.R., Durairaj, P., 2025. Advanced Inorganic Chemistry: Structure, Reactivity and Applications, Addition Publishing House.

Andreini, C., Arnesano, F., Rosato, A., 2022. The zinc proteome of SARS-CoV-2. Metallomics 14 (7).

Andreini, C., Bertini I., Rosato A., 2009. Metalloproteins: a bioinformatic approach. Acc. Chem. Res. 42 (10), 1471–1479.

Aswathy, A., Varghese S., Imlay J.A., 2009. Manganese import is a key element of the OxyR response to hydrogen peroxide in Escherichia coli. Molecular Microbiology 72, 844–858.

Banci, L., 2013. Metallomics and the cell: some definitions and general comments. In: Sigel, A., Sigel, H., Sigel, R.K. (Eds.), Metallomics and the Cell. Metal Ions in Life Sciences, vol. 12. Springer, pp. 1–13.

Barker, P.D., 2003. Designing redox metalloproteins from bottom-up and top-down perspectives. Curr. Opin. Struct. Biol. 0959440X. 13 (4), 490–499. Available from: http://www.elsevier.com/locate/sbi. doi:10.1016/S0959-440X(03)00108-8.

Beinert, H., Holm, R.H., Münck, E., 1997. Iron-sulfur clusters: nature's modular, multipurpose structures. Science 277 (5326), 653–656.

Bellomo, E., Massarotti, A., Hogstrand, C., Maret, W., 2014. Zinc ions modulate protein tyrosine phosphatase 1B activity. Metallomics. 1756-5901. 6 (7), 1229–1239. doi:10.1039/c4mt00086b.

Bertini, I., Gray, H.B., Stiefel, E.I., Valentine, J.S., 1994. Biological Inorganic Chemistry: Structure and Reactivity, University Science Books.

Cangelosi, V., Ruckthong, L., Pecoraro, V.L., 2017. Lead (II) binding in natural and artificial proteins. In: Metal Ions in Life Sciences, Vol. 17, pp. 271–318.

Capdevila, D.A., Edmonds, K.A., Giedroc, D.P., 2017. Metallochaperones and metalloregulation in bacteria. Trends Biochem. Sci. 42 (3), 215–233.

Carver, P.L., 2013. Metal ions and infectious diseases. An overview from the clinic. In: Sigel, A., Sigel, H., Sigel, R. (Eds.), Interrelations Between Essential Metal Ions and Human Diseases. Metal Ions in Life Sciences, vol. 13. Springer.

Claus, H., 2004. Laccases: structure, reactions, distribution. Micron 35 (1–2), 93–96.

Cobbett, C., Goldsbrough, P., 2002. Phytochelatins and metallothionein: roles in heavy metal detoxification and homeostasis. Annu. Rev. Plant Biol. 53, 159–182.

Cobine, P.A., Ojeda, L.D., Rigby, K.M., Winge, D.R., 2006. Yeast contain a non-proteinaceous pool of copper in the mitochondrial matrix. J. Biol. Chem. 281 (20), 14447–14455.

Cowan, J.A., 2002. Magnesium chemistry and biochemistry. Bimetals 15, 203–210.

Crichton, R., 2019. Biological Inorganic Chemistry: A New Introduction to Molecular Structure and Function, third ed. Academic Press.

Culotta, V.C., Klomp, L.W.J., Strain, J., Casareno, R.L.B., Krems, B., Gitlin, J.D., 1997. The copper chaperone for superoxide dismutase. J. Biol. Chem. 272 (38), 23469–23472.

Doroudian, M., Gailer, J., 2022. Integrative metallomics studies of toxic metal (loid) substances at the blood plasma-red blood cell-organ/tumour nexus. Inorganics 10 (11).

Eide, D.J., 2011. The oxidative stress of zinc deficiency. Metallomics 3 (11), 1124–1129.

Freibert, S.A., Lill, R., 2020. Biogenesis of iron–sulfur proteins in eukaryotes. Annu. Rev. Biochem. 89, 471–499.

Gray, H.B., Winkler, J.R., 1996. Electron transfer in proteins. Annu. Rev. Biochem. 65, 537–561.

Hamza, I., Dailey, H.A., 2012. One ring to rule them all: trafficking of heme and heme synthesis intermediates in the metazoans. Biochim. Biophys. Acta Mol. Cell Res. 1823 (9), 1617–1632.

Hamza, I., Prohaska, J., Gitlin, J.D., 2001a. The metallochaperone Atox1 plays a critical role in perinatal copper homeostasis. Proc. Natl. Acad. Sci. USA 98 (12), 6848–6852.

Hamza, I., Schaefer, M., Klomp, L.W.J., Gitlin, J.D., 2001b. Interaction of the copper chaperone HAH1 with the Wilson disease protein is essential for copper homeostasis. Proc. Natl. Acad. Sci. USA 98 (12), 6848–6852.

Hille, R., 1996. The mononuclear molybdenum enzymes. Chem. Rev. 96 (7), 2757–2816.

Hille, R., Hall, J., Basu, P., 2014. The mononuclear molybdenum enzymes. Chem. Rev. 114 (7), 3963–4038.

Horng, Y.C., Cobine, P.A., Maxfield, A.B., Carr, H.S., Winge, D.R., 2004. Specific copper transfer from the Cox17 metallochaperone to Sco1 and Cox11. J. Biol. Chem. 279 (34), 35334–35340.

Howard, J.B., Rees, D.C., 2006. How many metals does it take to fox N2? A mechanistic overview of biological nitrogen fixation. PNAS 103 (46), 17088–17093.

Jeong, W.J., Lee, J., Eom, H., Song, W.J., 2023. A specific guide for metalloenzyme designers: introduction and evolution of metal-coordination spheres embedded in protein environments. Acc. Chem. Res. 56 (18), 2416–2425.

Johnson, D.C., Dean, D.R., Smith, A.D., Johnson, M.K., 2005. Structure, function, and formation of biological iron-sulfur clusters. Annu. Rev. Biochem. 74, 247–281.

Kehres, D.G., Maguire, M.E., 2003. Emerging themes in manganese transport, biochemistry and pathogenesis in bacteria. FEMS Microbiol. Rev. 27 (2–3), 263–290.

Kendrew, J.C., Bodo, G., Dintzis, H.M., Parrish, R.G., Wyckoff, H., Phillips, D.C., 1958. A three-dimensional model of the myoglobin molecule obtained by X-ray analysis. Nature 181, 662–666.

Klug, A., 2010. The discovery of zinc fingers and their applications in gene regulation and genome manipulation. Annu. Rev. Biochem. 79, 213–231.

Kranz, R.G., Fogal, C.R., Taylor, J.S., Rawley, E.R., 2009a. Cytochrome c biogenesis: mechanisms for covalent modifications and trafficking of heme and for heme-iron redox control. Microbiol. Mol. Biol. Rev. 73 (3), 510–528.

Kranz, R.G., Richard-Fogal, C., Taylor, J.S., Frawley, E.R., 2009b. Cytochrome c biogenesis: mechanisms for covalent modifications and trafficking of heme and for heme–iron redox control. Microbiol. Mol. Biol. Rev. 73 (3), 510–528.

Kretsinger, R.H., 1976. Calcium-binding protein. Annu. Rev. Biochem. 45, 239–266.

Kunkle, D.E., Skaar, E.P., 2023. Moving metals: how microbes deliver metal cofactors to metalloproteins. Mol. Microbiol. 120 (4), 547–554.

Lill, R., Freibert, S.A., 2020. Mechanisms of mitochondrial iron–sulfur protein biogenesis. Annu. Rev. Biochem. 89, 471–499.

Lippard, S.J., Berg, J.M., 1984. Principles of Bioinorganic Chemistry. University Science Books.

Lippard, S.J., Berg, J.M., 1994. Principles of Bioinorganic Chemistry, University Science Books.

Lu, Y., 2006. Metalloprotein and metallo-DNA/RNAzyme design: current approaches, success measures and future challenges. Inorg. Chem. 45, 9930–9940. doi:10.1021/ic052007t.

Lu, Y., Berry, S.M., Pfister, T.D., 2001. Engineering novel metalloproteins: design of metal-binding sites into native protein scaffolds. Chem. Rev. 101, 3047–3080. doi:10.1021/cr0000574.

Lutsenko, S., 2010. Human copper homeostasis: a network of interconnected pathways. Curr. Opin. Chem. Biol. 14 (2), 211–217.

Maier, T., Jacobi, A., Sauter, M., Böck, A., 2007. The product of the hypB gene, required for nickel insertion into hydrogenases, is a novel guanine nucleotide-binding protein. J. Biol. Chem. 282 (2), 13297–13306.

Marsh, E.N.G., 1999. Coenzyme B12 (cobalamin)-dependent enzymes. Essays Biochem. 34, 139–54.

McCord, J.M., Fridovich, I., 1988. Superoxide dismutase: the first twenty years (1968-1988). Free Radic. Biol. Med. 5 (506), 363–369.

Messerschmidt, A., et al., 2001. Handbook of Metalloproteins. Wiley.

Miller, J., McLachlan, A.D., Klug, A., 1985. Repetitive zinc-binding domains in the protein transcription factor IIIA from Xenopus oocytes. EMBO J. 4 (6), 1609–1614.

Moore, S.J., Lawrence, A.D., Biedendieck, R., Deery, E., Frank, S., Howard, M.J., Rigby, S.E., Warren, M.J., 2013. Elucidation of the anaerobic pathway for the corrin component of cobalamin (vitamin B_{12}). Proc. Natl. Acad. Sci. 110 (37), 14906–14911.

Nagase, H., Visse, R., Murphy, G., 2006. Structure and function of matrix metalloproteinases and TIMPs. Cardiovasc. Res. 69 (3), 562–573.

Nelson, D.L., Cox, M.M., 2021. Lehninger Principles of Biochemistry, W. H. Freeman.

O'Halloran, T.V., Culotta, V.C., 2000a. Metallochaperones, an intracellular shuttle service for metal ions. J. Biol. Chem. 75 (33), 25057–25060.

O'Halloran, T.V., Culotta, V.C., 2000b. Metallochaperones: an intracellular shuttle service for metal ions. J. Biol. Chem. 275 (33), 25057–25060.

Ortiz de Montellano, P.R., 2015. Cytochrome P450: Structure, Mechanism, and Biochemistry, Springer.

Rae, T.D., Schmidt, P.J., Pufahl, R.A., Culotta, V.C., O'Halloran, T.V., 1999a. Undetectable intracellular free copper: the requirement of a copper chaperone for superoxide dismutase. Science 284 (5415), 805–808.

Rae, T.D., Schmidt, P.J., Pufahl, R.A., Culotta, V.C., O'Halloran, T.V., 1999b. Undetectable intracellular free copper: the requirement of a copper chaperone for superoxide dismutase. Science 284 (5415), 805–808.

Ragsdale, S.W., 2009. Nickle-based enzyme systems. J. Biol. Chem. 284 (10), 18571–18575.

Rao, M.B., Tansale, A.M., Ghatge, M.S., Deshpande, V.V., 1998. Molecular and biotechnological aspect of microbial proteases. Microbiol. Mol. Biol. Rev. 62 (3), 597–635.

Robinson, N.J., Winge, D.R., 2010. Copper metallochaperones. Annu. Rev. Biochem. 79, 537–562.

Rosato, A., Valasatava, Y., Andreini, C., 2016. Minimal functional sites in metalloproteins and their usage in structural bioinformatics. Int. J. Mol. Sci. 17 (5), 67.

Rouault, T.A., Maio, N., 2017. Biogenesis and functions of mammalian iron-sulfur proteins in the regulation of iron homeostasis and pivotal metabolic pathways. J. Biol. Chem. 292 (31), 12744–12753.

Rowlett, R.S., 2014. Structure and catalytic mechanism of beta-carbonic anhydrases. Subcell. Biochem. 75, 53–76.

Schwarz, G., Mendel, R.R., Ribbe, M.W., 2009. Molybdenum cofactors, enzymes and pathways. Nature 460, 839–847.

Sheftel, A.D., Mason, A.B., Ponka, P., 2013. The long history of Iron in the Universe and in health and disease. Biochim. Biophys. Acta 1820 (3), 161–187.

Sheldon, R.A., Woodley, J.M., 2018. Role of biocatalysis in sustainable chemistry. Chem. Rev. 118 (2), 801–838.

Shi, Y., 2014. A glimpse of structural biology through X-ray crystallography. Cell 159 (5), 995–1014.

Solomon, E.I., Heppner, D.E., Johnston, E.M., Ginsach, J.W., Cirera, J., Qayyum, M., Emmons, M.T.K., Kjaregaard, C.H., Hadt, R.G., Li, T., 2014. Copper active sites in biology. Chem. Rev. 114 (7), 3659–3853.

Tan, D., Zhou, M., Kiledjian, M., Tong, L., 2014. The ROQ domain of Roquin recognizes mRNA constitutive-decay element and double-stranded RNA. Nat. Struct. Mol. Biol.

Tokuda, E., Ono, S., Ishige, K., Mizuno, Y., 2015. Copper chaperone for superoxide dismutase and neurodegeneration. J. Neurosci. Res. 93 (4), 503–509.

Turner, A.P.F., et al., 1987. Biosensors: fundamentals and applications. Anal. Chim. Acta 201, 363–364.

Uchida, M., et al., 2007. Biological containers: protein cages as multifunctional nanoplatforms. Adv. Mater. 19 (8), 1025–1042.

Vallee, B.L., Auld, D.S., 1990. Zinc coordination, function, and structure of zinc enzymes and other protein. Biochemistry 29 (24), 5647–5659.

Waldron, K.J., Robinson, N.J., 2009a. How do bacterial cells ensure that metalloproteins get the correct metal? Nat. Rev. Microbiol. 7 (1), 25–35.

Waldron, K.J., Rutherford, J.C., Ford, D., Robinson, N.J., 2009b. Metalloproteins and metal sensing. Nature 460 (7257), 823–830.

Willner, I., Katz, E., 2000. Integration of layered redox protein and conductive supports for bioelectronic applications. Angew. Chem. Int. Ed. 39 (7), 1180–1218.

Winslow, R.M., 2000. Blood Substitutes. Adv. Drug Deliv. Rev. 40 (3), 131–142.

Yano, J., Yachandra, V.K., 2014. Mn4Ca cluster in photosynthesis: where and how water is oxidized to dioxygen. Chem. Rev. 114 (8), 4175–4205.

Zambelli, Musiani, F., Ciurli, S., Maier, T., 2011. Nickel trafficking and incorporation into metalloenzymes. Chem. Rev. 111 (6), 3472–3514.

Zhang, H., Zhang, W., Huang, S., Xu, P., Cao, Z., Chen, M., Lin, X., 2022. The potential role of plasma membrane proteins in response to Zn stress in rice roots based iTRAQ and PRM under low Cd condition. J. Hazard. Mater. 5, 429–128324.

Index

Note: Page numbers followed by "*f*" indicate figures, "*t*" indicate tables.

F

G

H

N

S

T

U

V

W

X

Printed and bound by CPI Group (UK) Ltd, Croydon, CR0 4YY
14/09/2026
02216409-0007